Introduction to
SPORTS MEDICINE
and
ATHLETIC TRAINING
Third Edition

Robert C. France

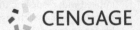

CENGAGE

Australia • Brazil • Japan • Korea • Mexico • Singapore • Spain • United Kingdom • United States

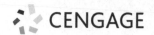

Introduction to Sports Medicine and Athletic Training, **Third Edition**
Robert C. France

SVP, GM Skills & Global Product Management: Jonathan Lau

Product Director: Matthew Seeley

Product Manager: Laura Stewart

Product Assistant: Nicholas Scaglione

Executive Director, Content Design: Mara Bellegarde

Learning Design Manager: Juliet Steiner

Senior Learning Designer: Deb Myette-Flis

Vice President, Strategic Marketing Services: Jennifer Ann Baker

Marketing Manager: Jonathan Sheehan

Senior Director, Content Delivery: Wendy Troeger

Senior Content Manager: Kenneth McGrath

Digital Delivery Lead: Lisa Christopher

Senior Designer: Angela Sheehan

Cover image credits: iStockPhoto.com/ PALMIHELP; iStockPhoto.com/Wavebreakmedia; iStockPhoto.com/teekid; iStockPhoto.com/ Mehmet Hilmi Barcin; Maya2008/ShutterStock .com; ER_09/ShutterStock.com; sunlight19/ ShutterStock.com

For product information and technology assistance, contact us at **Cengage Customer & Sales Support, 1-800-354-9706 or support.cengage.com.**

For permission to use material from this text or product, submit all requests online at **www.cengage.com/permissions.**

Library of Congress Control Number: 2018959063

ISBN: 978-0-357-37916-5

Cengage
20 Channel Center Street
Boston, MA 02210
USA

Cengage is a leading provider of customized learning solutions with employees residing in nearly 40 different countries and sales in more than 125 countries around the world. Find your local representative at **www.cengage.com.**

Cengage products are represented in Canada by Nelson Education, Ltd.

To learn more about Cengage platforms and services, register or access your online learning solution, or purchase materials for your course, visit **www.cengage.com.**

Notice to the Reader

Publisher does not warrant or guarantee any of the products described herein or perform any independent analysis in connection with any of the product information contained herein. Publisher does not assume, and expressly disclaims, any obligation to obtain and include information other than that provided to it by the manufacturer. The reader is expressly warned to consider and adopt all safety precautions that might be indicated by the activities described herein and to avoid all potential hazards. By following the instructions contained herein, the reader willingly assumes all risks in connection with such instructions. The publisher makes no representations or warranties of any kind, including but not limited to, the warranties of fitness for particular purpose or merchantability, nor are any such representations implied with respect to the material set forth herein, and the publisher takes no responsibility with respect to such material. The publisher shall not be liable for any special, consequential, or exemplary damages resulting, in whole or part, from the readers' use of, or reliance upon, this material.

Printed at CLDPC, USA, 03-23

CONTENTS

UNIT TWO

Roles and Responsibilities in Athletic Training 54

CHAPTER 5

CHAPTER 6

CHAPTER 7

UNIT THREE

Injury Assessment and Management 201

CHAPTER 17

The Foot, Ankle, and Lower Leg . . 267

CHAPTER 18

The Knee 288

PREFACE

Introduction to Sports Medicine and Athletic Training, Third Edition, is written for individuals interested in athletics and the medical needs of athletes. This book is unique in that it covers four distinct disciplines in an easy-to-understand format: sports medicine, athletic training, anatomy, and physiology. This all-in-one resource allows the individual to grasp the concepts of anatomy and physiology, and then apply them to sports medicine and athletic training. Each discipline is fully presented and uniquely sequenced to give the user a full understanding of this exciting field. There are comprehensive chapters on nutrition and sports psychology, as well as kinesiology and therapeutic modalities. Instructors will find the textbook organized in a systematic and logical manner that makes it comprehensive, easily understood, presented, and taught. As a full-concept book, an entire course can be created using this sole resource.

Instructors will find that Introduction to Sports Medicine and Athletic Training is fully compliant with the National Athletic Trainers Association secondary curriculum guidelines.

Introduction to Sports Medicine and Athletic Training, Third Edition, was born out of necessity. Today's students are exposed to a field that is still expanding in both relevance and purpose. The discipline of sports medicine and athletic training is growing at a pace far exceeding other disciplines. Finding quality teaching materials written for high school and undergraduate students has been elusive so far in the marketplace. This textbook is designed and written specifically for beginning and mid-level students.

Forty-six years of experience and teaching have gone into the development of this text. Numerous experts from the fields of sports medicine and athletic training have assisted in the organization and content of the manuscript. Experience, coupled with the latest research in these fields, has shaped and molded *Introduction to Sports Medicine and Athletic Training*, Third Edition, into a book that continues to be the standard in classrooms across the United States.

Organization of the Text

Introduction to Sports Medicine and Athletic Training, Third Edition, is organized into four units. Each unit contains several chapters organized around the unit theme. Unit 1 introduces students to the rapidly growing fields of sports medicine and athletic training. Unit 2 examines the roles and responsibilities in athletic training. Unit 3 covers injury assessment and management. The chapters in Unit 3 also present a strong anatomy and physiology component to assist the student in understanding and identifying various structures and functions of the body. Finally, Unit 4 looks at special considerations in athletics. The content and organization allow for a logical flow of material that will interest students and allow them to grasp important concepts.

Changes to the Third Edition

The third edition has been completely updated with the newest, cutting-edge facts and advances in sports medicine and athletic training. Below are major chapter-specific changes to the this edition.

- Chapter 1: Updated sections on professions associated with sports medicine and sport science.
- Chapter 2: Includes the newest salary and employment studies for sports medicine professionals and the newest trends in this exciting field of study.
- Chapter 5: Includes the newest emergency preparedness plans and protocols across the United States.
- Chapter 8: Revised and updated nutrition information using the most up-to-date information available, including the newest MyPlate guidelines.
- Chapter 9: Updated and enhanced dietary supplements and performance enhancers; includes the newest information on local, college, and professional responses to performance enhancement. A revised Athletic Code of Ethics.
- Chapters 11 and 12: Revised assessment and evaluation, as well as therapeutic modalities; including the newest CPR guidelines.
- Chapters 15–22: Updated and revised content based on current standards and practices; including the newest guidelines by the American Red Cross and the National Safety Council.
- Chapter 23: Updated and revised. The section on concussions has been totally re-written to include the latest best practices on recognition and management.
- Chapter 25: Special updates on diabetes and eating disorders, including a new section detailing manorexia. A new section titled, Athlete's with Disabilities; this material will shed light on a long-dismissed notion that athletes with disabilities cannot participate in athletics.

Alignment to Precision Exams Standards for Exercise Science and Sports Medicine

This edition of *Introduction to Sports Medicine and Athletic Training* is aligned to Precision Exams' Exercise Science and Sports Medicine exam, part of the Health Science Career Cluster. The Health Science pathway connects industry with skills taught in the classroom to help students successfully transition from high school to college and/or career. Working together, Precision Exams and National Geographic Learning, a part of Cengage, focus on preparing students for the workforce, with exams and content that is kept up to date and relevant to today's jobs. To access a corresponding correlation guide, visit the accompanying Instructor Companion Website for this title. For more information on how to administer the Exercise Science and Sports Medicine exam or any of the 170+ exams available to your students, contact your local NGL/Cengage Sales Consultant.

PRECISION
EXAMS

The National Athletic Trainers' Association (NATA)

This edition of *Introduction to Sports Medicine and Athletic Training* complies universally with the stated goals of the National Athletic Trainers' Association (NATA) Secondary School Sports Medicine Course Outline.

Learning Supplements

Student Companion Website

Online resources are available to enhance the learning experience. Additional resources include:

- Slides created in Power Point®
- Anatomy, physiology, and pathophysiology animations that enhance student's understanding of difficult concepts
- Additional content to help students prepare for the *Exercise Science and Sports Medicine exam* administered by Precision Exams

To access the online companion, go to: http://www.delmarhealthcare.com/companions

Instructor Resources

Instructor Companion Website

A comprehensive package of instructor tools was designed to assist you in teaching the content, assessing your students' mastery of the material, and elevating students' learning.

- *The Instructor's Manual* provides an annotated chapter lecture outline with key concepts and key terms presented as they are encountered in the text. Suggested teaching strategies provide alternate methods for approaching the subjects of sports medicine beyond those already presented in the text. A complete set of textbook answers also accompany each chapter, as well as lists of equipment and supplies.
- The Cognero® Testbank contains 1,000 questions. You can use these questions to create your own tests.
- Instructor slides created in PowerPoint® are designed to help you plan your class presentations.

MindTap

MindTap is a fully online, interactive learning experience built upon authoritative Cengage Learning content. By combining readings, multimedia and assessments into a singular learning path, MindTap elevates learning by providing real-world application to better engage students. Instructors customize the learning path by selecting Cengage Learning resources and adding their own content via apps that integrate into the MindTap framework seamlessly with many learning management systems.

The guided learning path demonstrates the relevance of sports medicine and athletic training principles through engagement activities, interactive exercises, anatomy, physiology and pathophysiology animations, and taping and wrapping videos with relevant scenarios and assessments. Learners apply an understanding of sports medicine and athletic training through. *Think It Through* scenarios. The scenarios and assessments elevate the study of sports medicine and athletic training by challenging students to apply concepts to practice.

To learn more, visit www.cengage.com/mindtap.

About the Author

Robert C. France is a retired certified and registered athletic trainer in Washington state. His vast knowledge of sports medicine and athletic training has been derived from extensive training from some of the finest colleges in the United States and Europe. His training as an emergency medical technician has helped him to design disaster preparedness programs and assist in their implementation. Registered and certified as an advanced instructor with the National Safety Council, Robert has instructed hundreds of high schools, colleges, and professionals in first aid, CPR, and advanced instructor training.

Robert's unique three-year high school sports medicine program has been recognized nationally for its excellence and preparation of students in the fields of sports medicine and athletic training. Students graduating from his program are now physicians, physical therapists, and certified athletic trainers throughout the United States. He has helped dozens of high schools across the country design and implement similar sports medicine programs.

Robert has lectured throughout the United States and in Europe. In 1996, he was selected as a member of the medical staff for the Olympic Games in Atlanta, Georgia. Athletic Trainer of the Year and Teacher of the Year are just two of the many awards he has received during his career. Since the first edition of *Introduction to Sports Medicine and Athletic Training*, he has written *Introduction to Physical Education and Sport Science* (2009). Robert currently serves as a national consultant on high school sports medicine programs.

Acknowledgments

Revising this textbook has been an enjoyable and challenging task. As this discipline continues to evolve, it is important that students have a resource that is readable and that students can learn from and enjoy reading. Needless to say, it would not have been possible without the unique skills and assistance of many people. I would like to sincerely thank the following individuals for their time and expertise in assisting me.

I would like to thank my family for their patience and support during the lengthy process of revising this book.

I would also like to thank everyone at Cengage Learning for their hard work and incredible expertise on the project.

Special thanks to all the people that spent a great deal of time modeling for this book. Program director/athletic trainer Steven Bunt from Irving High School, Irving, Texas, thank you and your students for allowing me to highlight a very special program, and one of the finest I've found in the United States.

There were four people whose support and relentless prodding helped me understand that writing a textbook would be a good thing. Thank you, Carla Boone, Doug Patrick, John Schroeder, Jim Stapp, and Dr. Cindy Waltman, Ph.D., for all the sleepless nights of worrying about deadlines.

Lastly, I would like to thank my parents, Richard and Carole, for instilling in me the desire to always do my best. Mom and Dad, I think I did.

Robert C. France

Reviewers

Abigail Hansberger, ATC, VATL
Head Athletic Trainer
Teacher

Angela Dahl, MPA, LAT, ATC
Assistant Athletic Trainer
Adjunct Professor

Kathleen M. Laquale, PhD, ATC, LAT, LDN
Professor
Nutrition Minor Coordinator

Wendi Leas, BS
Science Teacher

Rick Leitner, MS
Program Director and University Department Chair
Sports Medicine and Fitness Technology

Julie A. Snyder, MS, ACE CPT, ACE MES, NASM CES
University Department Chair
Sports Medicine & Fitness Technology

How to Use This Book

There are many features of *Introduction to Sports Medicine and Athletic Training*, Third Edition, designed specifically to enhance comprehension and add some elements of fun into the learning process.

Objectives: Objectives begin each chapter and set the stage for the content you are expected to learn in the chapter.

Key Terms: Key Terms are listed and defined at the beginning of each chapter.

Key Concepts: Key Concepts, presented in boxes, correspond directly to the objectives presented in the beginning of each chapter. Key Concepts highlight important material you need to understand at the completion of the chapter.

Anatomy and Physiology: Unit 3 places a strong emphasis on anatomy and physiology. You must become familiar with these concepts to be better prepared to work with athletes and athletic needs related to training, injury prevention, and injury rehabilitation.

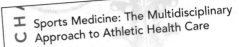

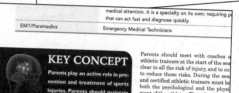

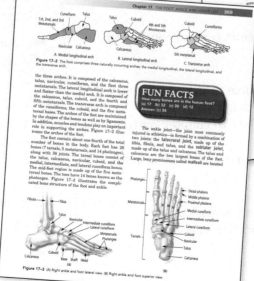

Techniques: Procedures are explained in a step-by-step manner. Each step is illustrated with a photo to enhance understanding.

Fun Facts and Did You Know: Fun Facts and Did You Know? boxes are scattered throughout the chapters to highlight tidbits and interesting facts about the fields of sports medicine, athletic training, and anatomy and physiology. These are designed to add some humor and fun to the learning process.

Chapter 13 TAPING AND WRAPPING **185**

Figure 13–29 Measure another piece of tape the width of the forefoot. This piece of tape is placed in the middle of the last piece measured. The two pieces of tape must be placed adhesive side to adhesive side.

Figure 13–30 Place the tape along the line of the metatarsal phalangeal joints on the top of the forefoot.

Figure 13–31 Place the tape underneath the forefoot on the lateral side.

Figure 13–32 Bring the tape across the top of the forefoot. With the heel of your hand pushing the foot upward, place the other end of the tape under the medial side of the foot.

Figure 13–33 When the athlete puts the foot in plantar flexion, a gap should be created on top of the forefoot. This acts as a "break," keeping the athlete from excessively dorsiflexing the foot.

Figure 13–34 When low-dye taping is finished, there should be a gap between the first and second digits.

for the athletes" safety. Proper care will the best possible outcome as they resume or competition.

DID YOU KNOW? According to the U.S. Department of Labor, careers in the health care industry are among the fastest-growing fields for employment and are expected to expand by 19% through the year 2024.

massage to treat disease and maintain health. Massage spread from the East to Europe and flourished in Greece before 300 B.C.E. Hippocrates, known as the "father of Western medicine," discussed and taught massage, and believed that all physicians

FUN FACTS In ancient Babylonia, every man considered himself a physician. According to Herodotus, anyone who wished could give advice freely to a sick or injured man who was willing to exhibit himself to passersby in the public square.

End-of-Chapter Features:

- The **Conclusion** is a succinct textual conclusion of basic chapter concepts.

- **Review Questions** reinforce material learned by testing comprehension through structured questions that directly relate to chapter content.

- **Projects and Activities** provide ideas for additional examination of the content.

- **Learning Links** suggests websites or web searches for further exploration of chapter content.

Chapter 1 SPORTS MEDICINE: THE MULTIDISCIPLINARY APPROACH TO ATHLETIC HEALTH CARE **11**

CONCLUSION

Sports and exercise have been a part of culture since long before the first Olympic Games in ancient Greece. Today's athletes range in age from early adolescence through the later stages of life. Athletes require specialized care that addresses a variety of concerns. This care is best rendered by an array of specialists whose primary goal is helping athletes return safely and quickly to activity and competition.

REVIEW QUESTIONS

1. Explain the role sports medicine plays in athletics today.
2. You are asked to design a sports medicine program for a large high school. Assuming you have the luxury to include anyone you would like, what would your sports medicine team look like? What would be their responsibilities?
3. Of the medical specialties associated with sports medicine, which interests you the most? Why?
4. What role should coaches play in caring for injured athletes?
5. What role should parents play in the athletic health care of their children?
6. Compare the four certification programs for the personal trainer.

PROJECTS AND ACTIVITIES

1. Interview a local sports medicine physician. Ask why he or she chose this field, and how the care he or she renders to the athlete differs from that of a regular family physician.
2. Select one of the sports medicine professions highlighted in this chapter. Research the role this profession plays in athletics today.
3. Research each of the four certifying organizations for personal trainers. What organization most interests you? Why?

LEARNING LINKS

Use the Internet to find additional information on the field of sports medicine and careers associated with sports medicine.
- Investigate more on the mission of the American College of Sports Medicine at http://www.acsm.org.
- Get an overview of the careers discussed in this chapter by visiting the Occupational Outlook Handbook at http://www.bls.gov/oco/.
- Learn more about the field of physical therapy and requirements for the study of physical therapy at http://www.apta.org.
- Learn more about the field of massage therapy and the requirements for study of massage therapy at http://www.amtamassage.org.
- Learn more about certification as a strength and conditioning trainer at http://www.nsca-lift.org.
- Learn more about the American Council on Exercise at http://www.acefitness.org/.
- Learn more about the National Academy of Sports Medicine at http://www.nasm.org/.

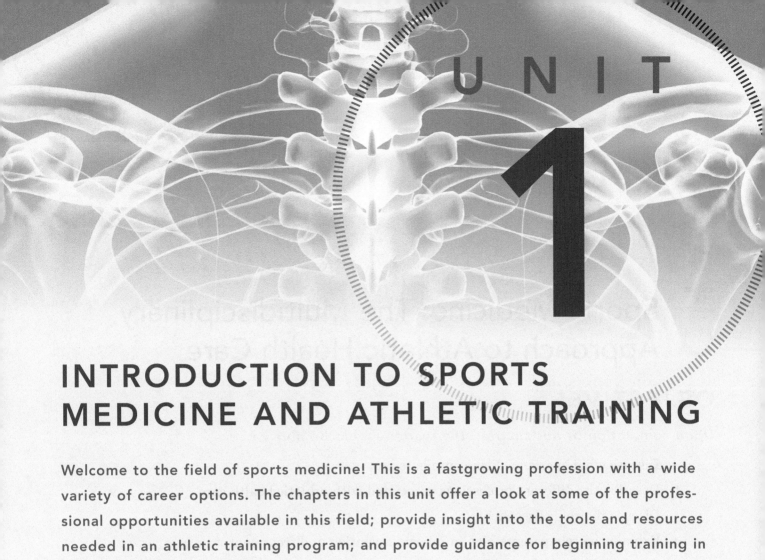

UNIT 1

INTRODUCTION TO SPORTS MEDICINE AND ATHLETIC TRAINING

Welcome to the field of sports medicine! This is a fastgrowing profession with a wide variety of career options. The chapters in this unit offer a look at some of the professional opportunities available in this field; provide insight into the tools and resources needed in an athletic training program; and provide guidance for beginning training in the field of sports medicine and athletic training.

Your journey begins here!

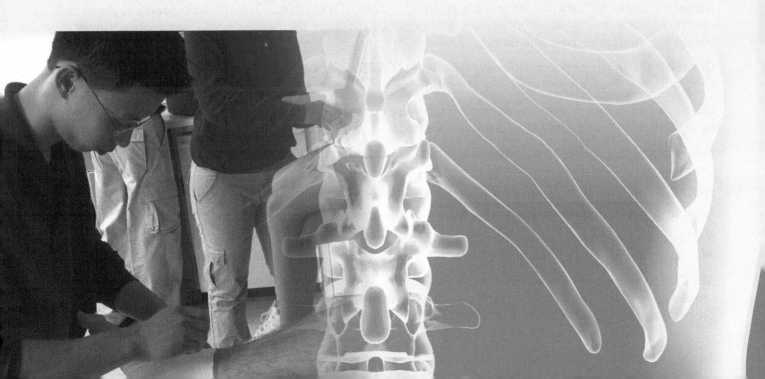

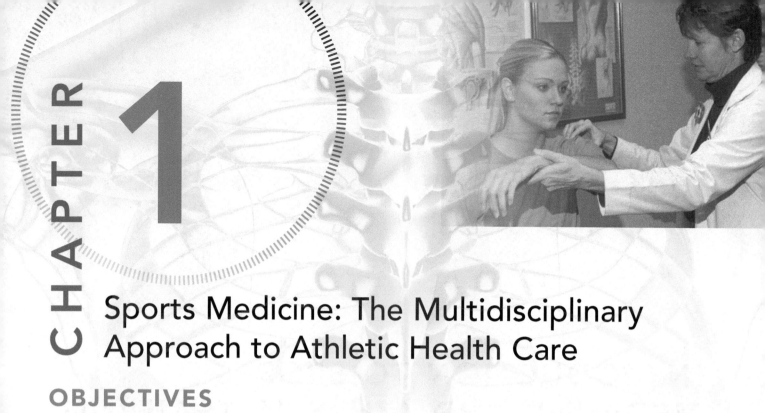

CHAPTER 1

Sports Medicine: The Multidisciplinary Approach to Athletic Health Care

OBJECTIVES

Upon completion of this chapter, the reader should be able to:

- Discuss what sports medicine entails today
- Describe the different professions associated with athletic health care
- Discuss the role of coaches
- Explain the role parents play in injury prevention and treatment

KEY TERMS

American Council on Exercise (ACE) *Fitness certifying organization founded in 1985. Provides certification for Personal Trainer, Group Fitness Instructor, and Lifestyle and Weight Management Consultant.*

Athlete's Circle of Care *All individuals involved in care of the athlete; may include coaches, parents, certified athletic trainer, family physician, school nurse, massage therapist, sports psychologist, physical therapist, nutritionist, personal trainers, and chiropractor.*

Certified Strength and Conditioning Specialist (CSCS) *A specialist who designs and implements safe, effective strength and conditioning programs.*

chiropractor *A health care specialist who provides conservative management of neuromusculoskeletal disorders and functional clinical conditions.*

family physician *The primary physician in the care of the athlete; works in cooperation with the team physician.*

National Academy of Sports Medicine (NASM) *Founded in 1987, it provides education and credentials for fitness, sports performance, and sports medicine professionals.*

National Strength and Conditioning Association Certified Personal Trainer (NSCA-CPT) *A specialist who designs and implements safe, effective strength and conditioning programs with individual clients.*

physical therapist (PT) *A health care specialist who is responsible for performing treatments that require special training in therapeutic exercises, hydrotherapy, and electrotherapy; and for performing procedures dealing with individual muscles and muscular movement.*

KEY TERMS CONTINUED

physical therapy assistant (PTA) *A health care specialist who works with physical therapists to assist in developing treatment plans for the rehabilitation of injury.*

physician assistant (PA) *A midlevel health care practitioner who works interdependently with physicians to provide diagnostic and therapeutic care.*

sports medicine *The study and application of scientific and medical knowledge to aspects of exercise and injury prevention.*

sports nutritionist *A health care specialist who designs special diets with the goal of enhancing athletic performance.*

sports psychologist *A specialist who works with athletes to recover from serious injury through emotional support, and also assists in goal setting and motivation.*

team physician *A physician who specializes in sports medicine and helps the athlete maximize function and minimize time away from sports, work, or school; works in cooperation with the family physician.*

SPORTS MEDICINE

Sports medicine, simply put, is the multidisciplinary approach to health care for those seriously involved in exercise and sport. Today's sports medicine specialists elicit the help of many different disciplines in the care of their patients. These disciplines include family and team physicians, physician assistants, certified athletic trainers, physical therapists and physical therapy assistants, chiropractors, massage therapists, certified strength and conditioning specialists, sports nutritionists, and sport psychologists. In broad terms, sports medicine is the study and application of scientific and medical knowledge to aspects of exercise and athletics. Sports medicine aims to promote health and fitness while preventing, treating, and rehabilitating injury.

The History of Sports Medicine

Sports medicine began developing into a recognized field in the early twentieth century, as physical training and rehabilitation of military veterans became a major concern. The desire to understand and extend the limits of human performance increased during the late nineteenth and early twentieth centuries; one of the first known meetings aimed at pursuing this endeavor was the Sports Physician's Congress, held in Germany in 1912.

In 1954, the American College of Sports Medicine (ACSM) was officially founded. It was intended to guide the convergence of different fields with a common focus directed toward the goal of national health and fitness. Since then, the ACSM has grown to include professionals from many fields in medicine and science. The ACSM promotes the idea that athletes require a broadly trained physician as their first point of contact when dealing with injury.

As athletic competition and participation mushroomed in the last few decades, the need for specialized care became apparent. The term *sports medicine* began to take on many different connotations and gain in popularity. Many health professionals began to advertise themselves as "sports medicine specialists" as a marketing tool to gain new business. However, these specialists

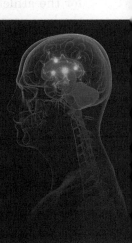

KEY CONCEPT

Sports medicine is a multidisciplinary approach to health care for those seriously involved in exercise and sport. Health care professionals from many disciplines are involved in the care of the athlete.

lacked the training needed to ensure proper care for their patients. Even today, many individuals ask how sports medicine differs from the medical treatment nonathletes receive. Professional sports medicine specialists have training that allows them to specifically address the needs of the athlete.

Sports Medicine Today

Society today is largely focused on physical performance and the condition of one's body. More than at any other time in history, athletics and exercise have been placed at the forefront of the American lifestyle, as well as that of countries worldwide. A person who aims to get and stay in shape will almost always include strenuous exercise and athletic participation in the weekly regimen. Furthermore, today's physically active members of society compromise all ages, both male and female. Although extreme physical activity and athletic competition have become a large component of a healthy lifestyle, they inherently carry with them a high level of risk.

Modern competitive sports have indisputably gone above and beyond the athletic activities of the past in terms of business value, strength of athletes, and the level of importance placed on success. Many athletes in major professional sports are multimillion-dollar commodities, and any hindrance to their performance is a hindrance to the business organization to which they are bound. At the high school, college, and amateur levels, athletes often place enormous emphasis on their ability to compete and perform. Injury is often devastating to these individuals and must be treated quickly, with the ultimate concern being for the athletes" safety. Proper care will allow for the best possible outcome as they resume exercise or competition.

PROFESSIONS ASSOCIATED WITH SPORTS MEDICINE

Sports medicine and athletic training combine for a team approach. Because athletes use many different approaches to their personal care, certified athletic trainers rely on a host of health professionals to aid in their treatment. These professionals are vitally important in the holistic approach to athletic health care. Health professionals range from the school nurse, family physician, and chiropractor to specialists who provide advanced care. Because athletes use many different approaches to their personal care, certified athletic trainers use a team approach for treatment.

The **Athlete's Circle of Care** illustrates the team approach (Figure 1–1). The athlete reports to the coaching staff with a medical complaint. The coaching staff then refers the athlete to the athletic training staff for treatment. The athletic training staff assesses the injury and, if needed, refers the athlete to the family physician. The training staff communicates with the athlete's parents. The athlete may then be referred to a specialist by the family physician (often with input from the training staff). Specialists give care and refer the athlete back to the athletic training staff to monitor progress or give treatment. The athletic training staff communicates with the coaching staff as to the athlete's status.

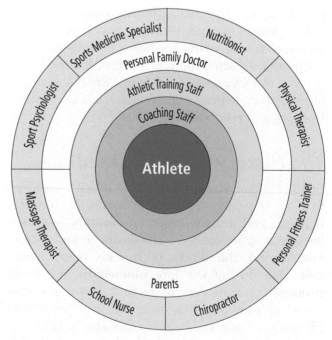

Figure 1–1 The Athlete's Circle of Care. Courtesy of PhotoDisc.

Family and Team Physician

Medical care for all athletes must be directed by the **team** or **family physician** (Figure 1–2). Team physicians are among the greatest assets of an athletic program. Their primary role is to promote lifelong fitness and wellness, and to encourage prevention of illness and injury. Physicians help patients maximize function and minimize disability and time away from sports, work, or school.

Physicians involved in sports medicine may have a primary specialty in family practice, internal medicine, emergency medicine, pediatrics, or physical medicine and rehabilitation, and most have one to two years of additional training in sports medicine through accredited fellowship (subspecialty) programs in sports medicine. Physicians who are board-certified in family practice, internal medicine, emergency medicine, or pediatrics are then eligible to take a subspecialty qualification examination in sports medicine. Additional education, which adds to the expertise of a sports medicine physician, includes continuing education in sports medicine, as well as membership and participation in sports medicine societies.

Physicians have two pathways toward their certification and licensure; MD (medical doctor), and DO (doctor of osteopathic medicine). Both are legally recognized and carry the same privileges.

Team physicians refer athletes back to their family physicians for primary care. They also monitor progress and consult with the family physician on an ongoing basis. Family physicians have a complete medical history of their patients and can better supervise long-term care. The balance between the two is very important and ensures the best possible care. The family physician often sends the patient back to the team physician, as the team physician may have a better understanding of the unique needs of athletic competition.

Physician Assistant

The **physician assistant (PA)** profession originated at Duke University in the mid-1960s. Dr. Eugene A. Stead, Jr., then chairman of the Department of Medicine, believed that midlevel practitioners could increase consumer access to health services by extending the time and skills of the physician. Today, physician assistants are well-recognized and highly sought after members of the health care team. Working interdependently with physicians, PAs provide diagnostic and therapeutic patient care in virtually all medical specialties and settings. They take patient histories, perform physical examinations, order laboratory and diagnostic studies, and develop patient treatment plans. In most states, PAs have the authority to write prescriptions. Their job descriptions are as diverse as those of their supervising physicians and may include patient education, medical education, health administration, and research. Many team physicians use physician assistants to help with patient care. Today, many PAs work in the sports medicine environment. Their services can be a valuable asset to the sports medicine team.

Physical Therapist

Physical therapy is a health care profession that helps people with many different types of medical afflictions. The **physical therapist (PT)** has become an increasingly important member of the health

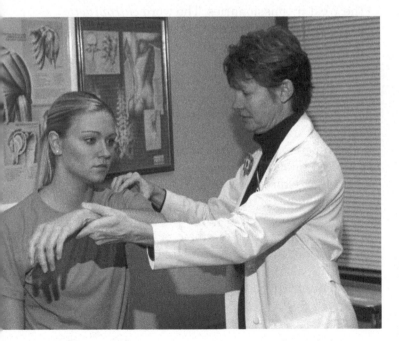

Figure 1–2 The family doctor or team doctor helps treat athletic injury and encourages injury prevention. Courtesy of PhotoDisc.

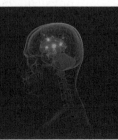

KEY CONCEPT

Physician assistants work interdependently with a physician to aid in patient care.

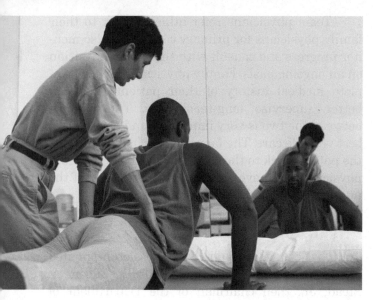

Figure 1–3 The physical therapist works with athletes to rehabilitate injuries through mechanical manipulation of the muscles.

care team (Figure 1–3). The first physical therapists, known as restorative aides, were active in providing care during World War I. However, it was during the polio epidemic of the 1950s that the demand for physical therapists increased. According to the U.S. Department of Labor's Bureau of Labor Statistics (2014), there are more than 210,900 physical therapists in America. Physical therapy programs number approximately 200 throughout the United States. Physical therapists can now specialize in pediatrics, sports medicine, neurology, home health, geriatrics, orthopedics, aquatic therapy, wound care, women's health, acute care, education, administration, research, or cardiopulmonary rehabilitation.

Physical therapists work in a variety of settings, including hospitals, nursing homes, schools, outpatient clinics, fitness facilities, home environments, and even industrial companies.

Physical Therapy Assistant

The **physical therapy assistant (PTA)** works with physical therapists to provide patient care under the direct supervision of a licensed physical therapist. A PTA's responsibilities include assisting in the development of treatment plans and documenting the progress of treatment. PTAs also make modifications in accordance with patient status and within the scope of treatment plans established by a physical therapist. Physical therapy assistants work under the supervision of a physical therapist. They are not responsible for the initial evaluation of a patient, progress notes to the physician, or discharge summaries. Instead, the PTA notes the patient's responses to treatment and reports the outcome to the physical therapist.

Physical therapists and physical therapy assistants use many specialized techniques to aid their patients in recovering from injuries and in improving overall function. These techniques include manual therapy, myofascial release, proprioceptive neuromuscular facilitation, and neurodevelopmental techniques. Working in conjunction with physicians, nurses, athletic trainers, nutritionists, and other members of the health care team, PTs and PTAs are trained to improve movement and function, relieve pain, and expand mobility potential. Through evaluation and treatment programs, physical therapists and physical therapy assistants help with existing problems and provide preventive health care for a variety of needs.

Chiropractor

Chiropractic is a natural form of health care. Spinal manipulation, chiropractic's primary treatment, is used instead of drugs or surgery to promote the body's natural healing process. One of the earliest mentions of soft-tissue manipulation appears in the ancient Chinese *Kong Fou* document written circa 2700 B.C.E., which was brought to the West by missionaries. The word *chiropractic* is derived from the Greek words *cheir* and *praktos*, meaning "done by hand." Chiropractic became more sophisticated as formal educational programs evolved, schools developed requirements, and states established governing laws.

The **chiropractor** provides conservative management of neuromusculoskeletal disorders and related functional clinical conditions, including but not limited to back pain, neck pain, and headaches (Figure 1–4). Chiropractors provide adjustment and manipulation of the articulations and adjacent tissues of the human body, particularly of the spinal column. Included is the treatment of intersegmental aberrations for alleviation of related functional disorders. They also utilize a variety of manual, mechanical, and electrical therapeutic modalities.

Certified Athletic Trainer

The role of the certified athletic trainer as a member of the sports medicine team is discussed in detail in Chapter 2.

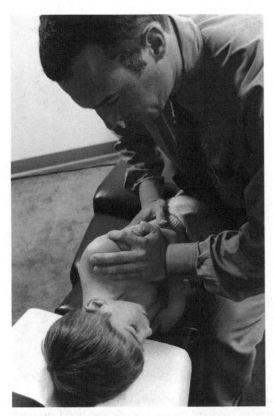

Figure 1–4 Chiropractors aid athletes of all ages in treatment of neuromusculoskeletal disorders and functional clinical conditions.

Massage Therapist

Massage is one of the oldest known methods for providing relief of pain and discomfort. Massage therapy was practiced by the Chinese as early as 3000 B.C.E. The ancient book *The Kong Fou of Tao-Tse* contained information about medicinal plants, exercises, and massage to treat disease and maintain health. Massage spread from the East to Europe and flourished in Greece before 300 B.C.E. Hippocrates, known as the "father of Western medicine," discussed and taught massage, and believed that all physicians should be trained in massage as a healing method. Massage arts were incorporated into Roman healing arts to relieve headaches, strengthen muscles, and combat paralysis. The prominent medical theorist Galen wrote books on hygienic health, exercise, and massage to maintain a healthy body and mind. His books were in use for more than 1,000 years.

The popularity of massage in the late nineteenth century also spawned unscrupulous uses and practices that caused a temporary decline in its reputation during the early twentieth century. There was a revival in the use of massage during World Wars I and II in Armed Forces hospitals, as it was found helpful during rehabilitation. Today, massage is continuing a renaissance that began in the 1960s with an increasing awareness of the need for physical and mental fitness and preventative health care.

Massage is now considered an important aspect in promoting wellness and reducing stress (Figure 1–5). Massage began to emerge as a profession in the 1970s and 1980s, as private schools developed. Many states require professional licensing for massage therapists and schools. Today's massage therapist works with physicians, nurses, and physical therapists to promote health and healing, and to help manage stress. According to the Bureau of Labor Statistics, the number of massage therapists in the

FUN FACTS

In ancient Babylonia, every man considered himself a physician. According to Herodotus, anyone who wished could give advice freely to a sick or injured man who was willing to exhibit himself to passersby in the public square.

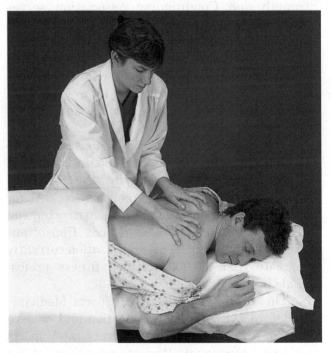

Figure 1–5 Massage therapists promote health and relaxation through therapeutic touch and manipulation of muscles.

United States in 2016 is approximately 168,800. The employment outlook is for an increase of 36,500 jobs through 2024.

Certified Strength and Conditioning Specialist/ Personal Trainer

Many athletes today turn to specialized fitness instructors to monitor and modify their conditioning and strength training. Several organizations offer certification for personal training. Anyone interested in pursuing this career should research which path is best suited to them. Four of the top accredited certifications for the Personal Trainer credential are the **Certified Strength and Conditioning Specialist (CSCS)**; the **National Strength and Conditioning Association Certified Personal Trainer (NSCA-CPT)**; the **American Council on Exercise (ACE)**; and the **National Academy of Sports Medicine (NASM)**. These credentials signify that the recipient has advanced training and meets the national standard for the field.

The Certified Strength and Conditioning Specialist program was created in 1985 to identify individuals who possess the knowledge and skills to design and implement safe, effective strength and conditioning programs. The National Strength and Conditioning Association serves more than 45,000 members in 72 countries. The National Strength and Conditioning Association Certified Personal Trainer credential is designed for individuals who work one-on-one with clients (Figure 1–6). This may occur in a variety of settings including schools, health and fitness clubs, and the client's home.

The American Council on Exercise is a nonprofit organization founded in 1985. In 2003, ACE was granted accreditation by the National Commission for Certifying Agencies (NCCA) for its Personal Trainer, Group Fitness Instructor, and Lifestyle and Weight Management Consultant certification programs. This organization currently has more than 70,000 certified fitness professionals in over 83 countries.

The National Academy of Sports Medicine, founded in 1987, provides education and credentials for fitness, sports performance, and sports medicine professionals. It boasts more than 52,698 members in 53 countries. In addition to its accredited Certified Personal Trainer certification,

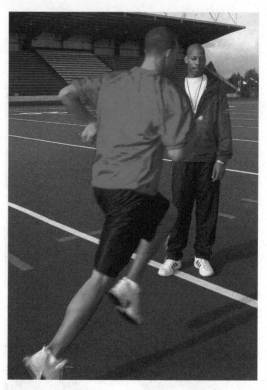

Figure 1–6 Personal trainers work one-on-one with athletes to pinpoint training needs and build strength and endurance.

NASM also offers a progressive career track with access to advanced specializations in sports performance and injury prevention, continuing education courses, and accredited Bachelor and Master's degree programs.

The certified athletic trainer, who may be certified with one or more of these credentials, can work with skilled strength and conditioning specialists to design specific workouts and allocate time to areas to that best meet an athlete's or program's needs.

Sports Nutritionist

The nutrition field has seen an explosion of interest recently. Proper nutrition and dieting have become a national obssssion in recent years. As Americans become more sedentary, they often look for a quick fix to alleviate growing waistlines and lack of exercise.

Television, radio, and newsprint ads all promote the latest quick-fix remedy. Billions of dollars are spent each year on a variety of products, each of which claims to be the newest breakthrough to lose weight, gain weight, gain muscle, or improve other areas of the body. A licensed **sports nutritionist** plays a vital role in ensuring a correct diet and properly instructing athletes on supplements and dietary aids. The nutritionist can help enhance athletic performance by designing special diets that allow the athlete to achieve his or her best results in events. Whether the sport is running the marathon or throwing the discus, proper diet can result in better performance.

Sports Psychologist

The professional **sports psychologist** can be instrumental in helping athletes return to their sport after a serious injury. These experts in the psychology of sport are well-versed in athletics, motivation, and performance (Figure 1–7). Goal setting and imagery are two of the tools sports psychologists use to help their athletes gain a competitive edge.

Sports psychologists are employed in clinical settings, educational institutions, and private practice. Most professional sports teams have sports psychologists on staff. Many work with Olympic athletes, in sports where a slight edge can be the difference between a gold medal and no medal. *The Occupational Outlook Handbook*

estimates that there are approximately 173,900 psychologists in the United States today. This number is expected to grow by 19% through the year 2024.

The Role of Coaches in the Athlete's Circle of Care

Coaches teach and direct activities in which the athlete participates. Whether participation is with a professional athletic team or at the youngest league level, it is the coach who teaches the athlete how to compete without injury. In the younger age group, the coach is frequently the trainer as well as the person responsible for first aid, protective devices, and equipment. Coaches should refer athletes to the certified athletic trainer or family physician as soon as an injury occurs. Good communication among the athlete, coach, parent, and certified athletic trainer ensures the best care for the athlete.

The Role of Parents in the Athlete's Circle of Care

Parents should assume an active role in the prevention and treatment of their children's injuries. Good communication among parents, coaches, and medical staff will be helpful if an injury occurs.

Figure 1–7 The sports psychologist can help the athlete work through the emotional trauma associated with severe injury, or help to keep the athlete motivated within a chosen sport.

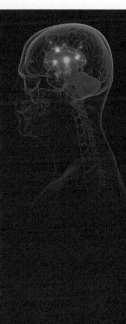

KEY CONCEPT

The primary role of the health care providers involved in the care of athletes is to promote lifelong fitness and wellness, and to encourage prevention of illness and injury. The professionals involved come from a variety of specialty areas, such as physician sassisting, physical therapy, nutrition, chiropractic, and sports psychology.

Table 1–1 Other Occupations Associated with Sports Medicine and Athletic Training

Physical Therapy Aide	Physical Therapy Aids or assistants work under the supervision of a licensed physical therapist and perform many of the same duties.
Occupational Therapist	These therapists treat patients that are recovering from injuries, illnesses or disabilites. This is done through utilizing everyday activities to allow the patient to return to their job or regular life.
Occupational Therapy Assistant	Occupational Therapy Aides or Assistants work under the supervision of a licensed Occupational Therapist.
Exercise Physiologist	Exercise Physiologists design specific exercise programs for athletes in their particular sport. This also includes athletes that have sustained an injury or chronic illness.
Nurse Practitioner	Nurse Practitioners are also referred to as advanced practice registered nurses (APRN). They coordinate patient care and perform duties persuant to specific state regulations.
Biomechanist	Biomechanics is considered a sub-field within the broader discipline of kinesiology, or the study of how people move. Biomechanics is largely a research discipline, but practical applications exist as well.
Orthotist/Prosthetist	These professionals design and manufacture supportive devices including orthotics, braces, protective equipment, artificial limbs; as well as surgical and medical devices.
Emergency Medicine	Emergency Medicine involves treating a patient requiring immediate medical attention. It is a specialty on its own; requiring practitioners that can act fast and diagnose quickly.
EMT/Paramedics	Emergency Medical Technicians

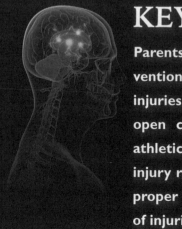

KEY CONCEPT

Parents play an active role in prevention and treatment of sports injuries. Parents should maintain open communication with the athletic training staff regarding injury risk, athletic development, proper nutrition, and treatment of injuries.

Parents should meet with coaches and certified athletic trainers at the start of the season to make clear to all the risk of injury, and to outline actions to reduce those risks. During the season, coaches and certified athletic trainers must be involved in both the psychological and the physical development of the athletes. They should teach athletes to distinguish between discomfort and the pain of injury.

Proper nutrition and conditioning should be discussed within the family before the first day of practice. Parents and coaches should not pressure the athlete to "work through pain" because untreated injuries can lead to permanent damage.

CONCLUSION

Sports and exercise have been a part of culture since long before the first Olympic Games in ancient Greece. Today's athletes range in age from early adolescence through the later stages of life. Athletes require specialized care that addresses a variety of concerns. This care is best rendered by an array of specialists whose primary goal is helping athletes return safely and quickly to activity and competition.

REVIEW QUESTIONS

1. Explain the role sports medicine plays in athletics today.
2. You are asked to design a sports medicine program for a large high school. Assuming you have the luxury to include anyone you would like, what would your sports medicine team look like? What would be their responsibilities?
3. Of the medical specialties associated with sports medicine, which interests you the most? Why?
4. What role should coaches play in caring for injured athletes?
5. What role should parents play in the athletic health care of their children?
6. Compare the four certification programs for the personal trainer.

PROJECTS AND ACTIVITIES

1. Interview a local sports medicine physician. Ask why he or she chose this field, and how the care he or she renders to the athlete differs from that of a regular family physician.
2. Select one of the sports medicine professions highlighted in this chapter. Research the role this profession plays in athletics today.
3. Research each of the four certifying organizations for personal trainers. What organization most interests you? Why?

LEARNING LINKS

Use the Internet to find additional information on the field of sports medicine and careers associated with sports medicine.

- Investigate more on the mission of the American College of Sports Medicine at http://www.ascm.org.
- Get an overview of the careers discussed in this chapter by visiting the Occupational Outlook Handbook at http://www.bls.gov/oco/.
- Learn more about the field of physical therapy and requirements for the study of physical therapy at http://www.apta.org.
- Learn more about the field of massage therapy and the requirements for study of massage therapy at http://www.amtamassage.org.
- Learn more about certification as a strength and conditioning trainer at http://www.nsca-lift.org.
- Learn more about the American Council on Exercise at http://www.acefitness.org/.
- Learn more about the National Academy of Sports Medicine at http://www.nasm.org/.

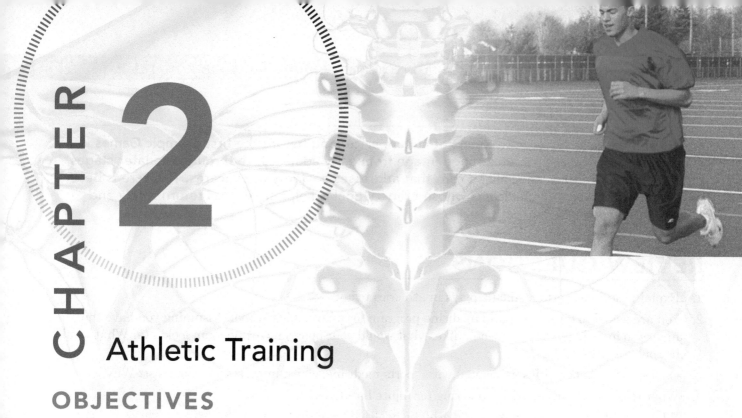

CHAPTER 2

Athletic Training

OBJECTIVES

Upon completion of this chapter, the reader should be able to:

- Describe the history and development of athletic training
- Describe the role certified athletic trainers play in the athletic health care system
- Explain the different qualifications and skills required to be a certified athletic trainer
- Describe the job market and opportunities that exist for certified athletic trainers
- List various professional organizations available to certified athletic trainers
- Discuss the Athlete's Bill of Rights
- Discuss liability and risk management and how they pertain to athletic training
- Explain the importance of HIPAA and FERPA legislation

KEY TERMS

allied health profession *Any area of health care that contributes to or assists the professions of physical medicine, dentistry, optometry pharmacy, and podiatry.*

Athlete's Bill of Rights *Policies and standards for fair treatment of athletes.*

athletic training *The rendering of specialized care (prevention, recognition, evaluation, and care of injuries) to individuals involved in exercise and athletics.*

certified athletic trainer (ATC) *A professional who has attained a standard level of competence in the field of athletic training. The ATC is involved in the prevention, recognition, and evaluation of injuries, and works closely with others in rehabilitation from injuries.*

Hippocratic Oath *Declaration made to Hippocrates, the "father of Western Medicine," by his students; it has become a fundamental part of the practice of medicine.*

Title IX *Federal legislation that prohibits discrimination on the basis of sex as to participation in athletics in schools receiving federal funds.*

WHAT IS ATHLETIC TRAINING?

Athletic training is the rendering of specialized care to individuals involved in exercise and athletics. This specialized care includes the prevention, recognition, evaluation, and care of injuries associated with exercise and sport. Many certified athletic trainers are also involved closely in rehabilitation of the athlete's injuries and preparation for return to activity. A professional who has worked to attain certification in the field of athletic training is designated **Athletic Trainer Certified (ATC)**. This certification indicates to the public that the individual with this level of training is competent at, engaged in, and recognized by the profession. In 1991, the American Medical Association recognized athletic training as an allied health profession. With this designation came the advent of athletic training as a legitimate career.

THE NEED FOR ATHLETIC TRAINERS

Never has there been a greater need for athletic trainers than today. In 1972, federal legislation was enacted that prohibited discrimination on the basis of sex as to participation in athletics in schools. **Title IX**, as it was called, also governed overall equity of treatment and opportunity to participate. This legislation accorded female athletes equal treatment under the law. Since the enactment of Title IX, the number of females participating in athletics has grown substantially. Youth sports have also seen a large increase in participation. With the number of individuals participating in athletics at an all-time high, the need for qualified people to support their overall well-being is considerable.

The National Federation of High School Associations (2017) estimates that nearly 8 million students play high school sports. The National Alliance for Youth Sports estimates that over 30 million youngsters participate in nonschool athletics. Add to this the number of college and professional athletes, and you will see why athletic training professionals are in high demand and will continue to be so well into this century.

THE HISTORY AND DEVELOPMENT OF ATHLETIC TRAINING

Athletic trainers have been working with athletes for centuries in one capacity or another. The physician and philosopher Galen, born in 129 C.E., is considered one of the greatest physicians of the classical period. He and Hippocrates, born 589 years earlier, both contributed volumes to the science of medicine. Galen was a trainer and physician to gladiators in ancient Rome. After the fall of the Roman Empire in approximately 500 C.E., Europe entered the Middle Ages. During this medieval era, which lasted almost 1,000 years, records were few and advancements in medicine scarce. Not until the Renaissance was the human body actively studied again. The preeminent scientist of the Renaissance was Leonardo da Vinci, whose contributions to the science of the human body outshone all who preceded him.

The athletic training profession is evolving. As educational requirements continue to increase, and the public continues to insist on highly skilled professionals specializing in sport and medicine, the athletic training profession continues to assert itself in mainstream health care.

The American Medical Association recognized athletic training as an **allied health profession** in 1991. An allied health profession is one that contributes to or assists the professions of physical medicine, dentistry, optometry, pharmacy, and podiatry. Allied health professions provide health care access and delivery throughout the health care system.

The certified athletic trainer is a highly educated, skilled professional who specializes in the prevention, treatment, and rehabilitation of injuries. In cooperation with physicians and other allied health personnel, the certified athletic

FUN FACTS

Galen was encouraged to pursue the study of medicine after his father dreamed that the god Asclepius told him his son should go into the field of medicine.

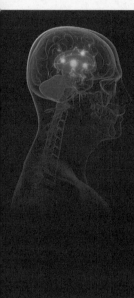

KEY CONCEPT

Athletic training has a long history that dates back to the care Galen provided to gladiators in ancient Rome. However, athletic training was not recognized as an allied health profession until 1991. Because more and more people are becoming involved in athletics, the field of athletic training is still developing. The future of athletic training promises growth.

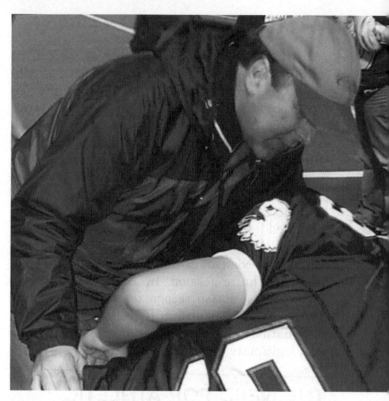

Figure 2–1 Certified athletic trainers must remain calm and be able to communicate with an injured athlete. Reprinted with permission of the National Athletic Trainers' Association.

trainer functions as an integral member of the athletic health care team in secondary schools, colleges and universities, sports medicine clinics, professional sport programs, industrial settings, and other health care environments.

Athletic training will continue to evolve as long as athletes compete and injuries occur. Advancements in medical science and the creation of new products will help everyone involved in sports and exercise stay healthier and active longer in life. The profession of athletic training will continue to outpace many others as interest and participation in sports and activities continue to grow.

QUALIFICATIONS OF A SUCCESSFUL CERTIFIED ATHLETIC TRAINER

Certified athletic trainers are individuals who enjoy exercise, sport, and recreation. They possess skills that allow them to work with people, solve problems, work under stress, analyze injuries, and communicate in a clear, precise manner (Figure 2–1). Athletic training is a highly rewarding profession. A major benefit is knowing that you make a difference in the life of an athlete.

Certified athletic trainers must be willing to work "beyond the clock"; that is, work outside the

traditional workday. Apart from the clinical setting, trainers typically work varying schedules that often exceed 40 hours per week.

Code of Ethics

As allied health professionals, certified athletic trainers adhere to a strict code of ethics and professionalism. ATCs must abide by the rules and procedures of their certifying organization. If licensure

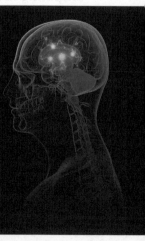

KEY CONCEPT

The certified athletic trainer is a highly educated, skilled professional specializing in the prevention, treatment, and rehabilitation of injuries. The ATC works in cooperation with physicians and other allied health personnel.

KEY CONCEPT

Skills required for athletic training include:

- **Problem-solving ability**
- **Deductive reasoning skills**
- **Good judgment**
- **Good decision-making skills**
- **Proficient knowledge of anatomy, physiology, biology, and advanced first aid**
- **Motor skills**
- **Communication skills**
- **Ability to work well with people**
- **Ability to work well under stressful conditions**
- **Ability to maintain poise in emergencies**

Tasks undertaken during athletic training include:

- **Analyzing injuries**
- **Taping and bandaging**
- **Implementing exercise and rehabilitation programs**
- **Monitoring rehabilitation programs**
- **Demonstrating physical and rehabilitative movements**
- **Using various modalities (methods of treatment) and training equipment**
- **Recording, organizing, and storing information on injuries and rehabilitation**

or certification is required by the state in which they work, they must also abide by the requirements established by legislative action. Failure to act in accordance with these rules can result in disciplinary action or termination. The accompanying box contains the Code of Ethics from the National Athletic Trainers' Association.

Education

Certified athletic trainers have, at a minimum, a bachelor's degree from an accredited, professional, athletic training program. In addition, athletic trainers study human anatomy, human physiology, biomechanics, exercise physiology, athletic training, nutrition, and psychology/counseling. They also participate in extensive clinical experiences with athletic teams, under appropriate supervision.

Certification

Certified athletic trainers have fulfilled the requirements for certification established by the

DID YOU KNOW? March is National Athletic Training Month! Visit the NATA website for information on events taking place during National Athletic Training Month. What can you do to promote the field of athletic training?

National Athletic Trainers' Association Board of Certification, Inc. (NATABOC). The certification examination administered by NATABOC consists of a written portion with multiple-choice questions; a practical section that evaluates the skill components of the domains within athletic training; and a written simulation test, consisting of athletic training-related situations designed to approximate real-life decision making. This last portion of the test evaluates athletic trainers' ability to resolve cases similar to those they might encounter in actual practice.

NATIONAL ATHLETIC TRAINERS' ASSOCIATION CODE OF ETHICS

September 28, 2005, Revised 2016

Preamble

The National Athletic Trainers' Association Code of Ethics states the principles of ethical behavior that should be followed in the practice of athletic training. It is intended to establish and maintain high standards and professionalism for the athletic training profession. The principles do not cover every situation encountered by the practicing athletic trainer, but are representative of the spirit with which athletic trainers should make decisions. The principles are written generally; the circumstances of a situation will determine the interpretation and application of a given principle and of the Code as a whole. When a conflict arises between the Code and the law, the law prevails.

1. MEMBERS SHALL PRACTICE WITH COMPASSION, RESPECTING THE RIGHTS, WELFARE, AND DIGNITY OF OTHERS

    1.1. Members shall render quality patient care regardless of the patient's race, religion, age, sex, ethnic or national origin, disability, health status, socioeconomic status, sexual orientation, or gender identity.

    1.2. Member's duty to the patient is the first concern, and therefore members are obligated to place the welfare and long-term well-being of their patient above other groups and their own self-interest, to provide competent care in all decisions, and to advocate for the best medical interest and safety of their patient at all times as delineated by professional statements and best practices.

    1.3. Members shall preserve the confidentiality of privileged information and shall not release or otherwise publish in any form, including social media, such information to a third party not involved in the patient's care without a release unless required by law.

2. MEMBERS SHALL COMPLY WITH THE LAWS AND REGULATIONS GOVERNING THE PRACTICE OF ATHLETIC TRAINING, NATIONAL ATHLETIC TRAINERS' ASSOCIATION (NATA) MEMBERSHIP STANDARDS, AND THE NATA CODE OF ETHICS

    2.1. Members shall comply with applicable local, state, federal laws, and any state athletic training practice acts.

    2.2. Members shall understand and uphold all NATA Standards and the Code of Ethics.

    2.3. Members shall refrain from, and report illegal or unethical practices related to athletic training.

    2.4. Members shall cooperate in ethics investigations by the NATA, state professional licensing/regulatory boards, or other professional agencies governing the athletic training profession. Failure to fully cooperate in an ethics investigation is an ethical violation.

    2.5. Members must not file, or encourage others to file, a frivolous ethics complaint with any organization or entity governing the athletic training profession such that the complaint is unfounded or willfully ignore facts that would disprove the allegation(s) in the complaint.

(continues)

(continued)

    2.6. Members shall refrain from substance and alcohol abuse. For any member involved in an ethics proceeding with NATA and who, as part of that proceeding is seeking rehabilitation for substance or alcohol dependency, documentation of the completion of rehabilitation must be provided to the NATA Committee on Professional Ethics as a requisite to complete a NATA membership reinstatement or suspension process.

3. MEMBERS SHALL MAINTAIN AND PROMOTE HIGH STANDARDS IN THEIR PROVISION OF SERVICES

    3.1. Members shall not misrepresent, either directly or indirectly, their skills, training, professional credentials, identity, or services.

    3.2. Members shall provide only those services for which they are qualified through education or experience and which are allowed by the applicable state athletic training practice acts and other applicable regulations for athletic trainers.

    3.3. Members shall provide services, make referrals, and seek compensation only for those services that are necessary and are in the best interest of the patient as delineated by professional statements and best practices.

    3.4. Members shall recognize the need for continuing education and participate in educational activities that enhance their skills and knowledge and shall complete such educational requirements necessary to continue to qualify as athletic trainers under the applicable state athletic training practice acts.

    3.5. Members shall educate those whom they supervise in the practice of athletic training about the Code of Ethics and stress the importance of adherence.

    3.6. Members who are researchers or educators must maintain and promote ethical conduct in research and educational activities.

4. MEMBERS SHALL NOT ENGAGE IN CONDUCT THAT COULD BE CONSTRUED AS A CONFLICT OF INTEREST, REFLECTS NEGATIVELY ON THE ATHLETIC TRAINING PROFESSION, OR JEOPARDIZES A PATIENT'S HEALTH AND WELL-BEING.

    4.1. Members should conduct themselves personally and professionally in a manner that does not compromise their professional responsibilities or the practice of athletic training.

    4.2. All NATA members, whether current or past, shall not use the NATA logo in the endorsement of products or services, or exploit their affiliation with the NATA in a manner that reflects badly upon the profession.

    4.3. Members shall not place financial gain above the patient's welfare and shall not participate in any arrangement that exploits the patient.

    4.4. Members shall not, through direct or indirect means, use information obtained in the course of the practice of athletic training to try and influence the score or outcome of an athletic event, or attempt to induce financial gain through gambling.

    4.5. Members shall not provide or publish false or misleading information, photography, or any other communications in any media format, including on any social media platform, related to athletic training that negatively reflects the profession, other members of the NATA, NATA officers, and the NATA office.

Reprinted with permission of the National Athletic Trainers' Association.

The examination covers a variety of topics within the six practice domains of athletic training:

- Prevention
- Recognition, evaluation, and assessment
- Immediate care
- Treatment, rehabilitation, and reconditioning
- Organization and administration
- Professional development and responsibility

Once athletic trainers pass the certification examination proving skills and knowledge within each domain, they use the ATC (Athletic Trainer Certified) designation.

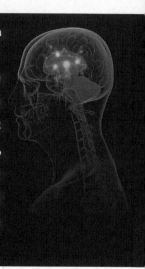

KEY CONCEPT

Certified athletic trainers work in a wide variety of settings, which encompass assisting athletes at various levels of competition, from high school to college, as well as in amateur to professional programs. ATCs can also work in clinic and industrial settings.

WORK SETTINGS FOR THE CERTIFIED ATHLETIC TRAINER

Certified athletic trainers work in a variety of settings, including sports medicine clinics, public and private high schools, colleges and universities, amateur and professional sports teams, health and fitness centers, businesses, Olympic teams and training centers, and hospitals and medical clinics. Each setting has its own rewards and time commitments. For example, when working in a clinical setting, the athletic trainer can expect to work 40 hours each week and see between 15 and 25 patients per day. In a high school setting, the work week may be from 40 to 60 hours, and the athletic trainer may have contact with dozens of athletes. The clinical setting typically does not involve evenings, but the high school position could require work on as many as three to five nights each week.

The many jobs comprising athletic training allow great flexibility in the search for work. Having the option to work in a variety of settings enables the athletic trainer to find a job that fits his or her particular circumstances.

According to the National Athletic Trainers' Association (NATA), salaries for athletic trainers averaged $54,832 in 2016 for work in the high school setting and more than $80,000 for work in certain professional sports (Table 2–1). Individuals with more than 20 years in the profession average more than $68,000 per year. Salaries differ greatly among different regions in the United States. Most jobs offer full benefits.

Table 2–1	Primary Job Market for Athletic Trainers			
	HIGH SCHOOL	COLLEGE	PROFESSIONAL	CLINICAL
Salary*	$52,935	$66,252	$50,000–128,438	$53,881
Days/week	5	5+	6+	5
Hours/week	40–60	40–60	50+	40
Evenings	yes	yes	yes	no
Athletes/day	>30	>30	>45	>20

*Estimated average for the United States. Salary information based on NATA 2011 salary data survey results. Salaries include benefits and bonuses.

PROFESSIONAL ORGANIZATIONS FOR CERTIFIED ATHLETIC TRAINERS

Many organizations provide important resources for health care professionals. These organizations offer a wealth of information and educational opportunities to interested parties.

National Athletic Trainers' Association

The National Athletic Trainers' Association was founded in 1950 by a group of approximately 200 athletic trainers. The NATA, headquartered in Dallas, Texas, has a membership of more than 44,000 worldwide. It is the largest certifying organization for athletic trainers in the United States.

Regional, State, and Local Trainers' Associations

Most states have regional or local associations devoted to the athletic training profession. Such associations promote athletic training, wellness, and the safety of athletes at the local level. This enhances awareness and visibility of athletic trainers throughout the health care system and the sports arena.

KEY CONCEPT

Many professional organizations support the field of sports medicine and athletic training. The most widely known organization, NATA, certifies most athletic trainers in the United States. Many states have their own professional organizations that promote the professional development of athletic trainers.

As an example of one state's association, athletic trainers in Ohio founded the Ohio Athletic Trainers Association (OATA) in 1984. This organization, like many others, provides educational opportunities for athletic trainers, physicians, school administrators, athletic directors, coaches, parents, and athletes. The OATA also encourages professional development of its members and provides a means for the exchange of ideas. The OATA's mission statement (2003) sums up the aims of athletic training associations across the United States: "To advance, encourage and improve the athletic training profession by developing the common interests of its members for the purpose of enhancing the quality of health care for the physically active." The Athletic Training And Sports Medicine Organizations box later in this chapter provides contact information for some national organizations devoted to sports medicine.

ATHLETE'S BILL OF RIGHTS

It is vitally important to recognize athletes' rights regarding participation in athletics. Though the **Athlete's Bill of Rights** has existed for some time, there is no single standard to what these "rights" are and how they may be enforced. The Secondary School Student Athletes' Bill of Rights was introduced as House Resolution 72 (H. Res. 72) into the U.S. House of Representatives on February 15, 2013 by Rep. Jim Gerlach (PA-6) and supported by the Youth Sports Safety Alliance. It was originally co-sponsored by Rep. Devin Nunes (CA-22). This bill creates a national action plan for athlete's rights that assures safe practice and competition environments. The primary reason athletes participate in athletics is for enjoyment and personal satisfaction. A Bill of Rights takes something that is assumed and defines it into something tangible. Common components of an Athlete's Bill of Rights include:

- Right to have fun through sports
- Right to participate at a level commensurate with their maturity level
- Right to qualified adult leadership
- Right to participate in a safe and healthy environment
- Right to competent care and treatment of injuries

ATHLETIC TRAINING AND SPORTS MEDICINE ORGANIZATIONS

American College of Sports Medicine
P.O. Box 1440
Indianapolis, IN 46206
Phone: 317-637-9200
Fax: 317-634-7817
http://www.acsm.org

American Orthopaedic Society for Sports Medicine
6300 N. River Road, Suite 200
Rosemont, IL 60018
Phone: 847-292-4900
Fax: 847-292-4905
http://www.sportsmed.org

American Physical Therapy Association
1111 North Fairfax Street
Alexandria, VA 22314-1488
Phone: 703-684-2782
Fax: 703-684-7343
http://www.apta.org

American Red Cross
431 18th Street NW
Washington, DC 20006
Phone: 202-639-3520
http://www.redcross.org

The Institute for the Study of Youth Sports
213 IM Sports Circle Building
Department of Kinesiology
Michigan State University
East Lansing, MI 48824-1049
Phone: 517-353-6689
Fax: 517-353-5363
http://edwp.educ.msu.edu/isys

International Federation of Sports Medicine
FIMS Business Office
c/o Human Kinetics
P.O. Box 5076
Champaign, IL 61 825-5076
Phone: 1-800-747-4457
Fax:217-351-1549
http://www.fims.org

National Association for Intercollegiate Athletics
23500 West 105th Street
P.O. Box 1 325
Olathe, KS 66051
Phone: 913-791-0044
http://www.naia.org

National Athletic Trainers Association
2952 Stemmons Freeway
Dallas, TX 75247-691 6
Phone: 800-879-6282
Fax:214-637-2206
http://www.nata.org

National Coalition for Promoting Physical Activity
1010 Massachusetts Avenue,
Suite 350
Washington, DC 20001
Phone: 202-454-7521
Fax: 202-454-7598
http://www.ncppa.org

National Collegiate Athletic Association
700 West Washington Street
Indianapolis, IN 46206
Phone: 317-917-6222
Fax: 317-917-6888
http://www.ncaa.org

National Federation of State High School Associations
P.O. Box 690
Indianapolis, IN 46206
Phone: 317-972-6900
Fax: 317-822-5700
http://www.nfhs.org

National Safety Council
P.O. Box 690
1121 Spring Lake Drive
Itasca, IL 60143-3201
Phone: 630-285-1121
Fax: 630-285-1315
http://www.nsc.org

National Strength and Conditioning Association
1955 N. Union Blvd.
Colorado Springs, CO 80909
Phone: 71 9-632-6722
Fax: 719-632-6367
http://www.nsca-lift.org

United States Olympic Committee
Colorado Springs Olympic Training Center
National Headquarters

One Olympic Plaza
Colorado Springs, CO 80909
Phone: 719-866-4500
http://www.olympic-usa.org

Women's Sports Foundation
Eisenhower Park
East Meadow, NY 11554
Phone: 800-227-3988
Fax: 516-542-4716
http://www.womenssportsfoundation.org

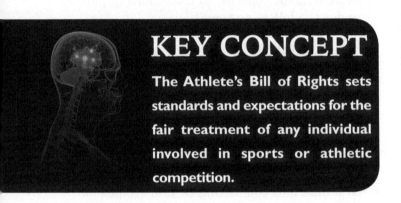

KEY CONCEPT

The Athlete's Bill of Rights sets standards and expectations for the fair treatment of any individual involved in sports or athletic competition.

- Right to share in the leadership and decision making of their sport
- Right to participate in a sport regardless of ability or income level
- Right to proper preparation for participation
- Right to equal opportunity to strive for success
- Right to be treated with dignity
- Right to say "no"

Athletes consider these "rights" to be more standards than written decrees. Coaches and parents must recognize that the needs of the athlete are paramount and take precedence over other needs, desires, and agendas.

LIABILITY AND RISK MANAGEMENT

Hippocratic Oath: "I will follow that system of regimen [use treatment to help the sick] which, according to my ability and judgment, I consider

for the benefit of my patients, and abstain from whatever is deleterious and mischievous [I will never use it to wrong them]" (*Taber's*, 2001). This portion of the famous oath that Hippocrates demanded from his students was written in 400 B.C.E. Medical professionals today regard it as fundamental to the practice of medicine.

Liable means "obligated according to law or equity; responsible" (*Webster's*, 1993). Anyone who works outside the scope of practice and expertise can be found negligent and therefore liable for his or her actions.

Statistics published by the United States Department of Labor (2016) show that more than 778,700 people are employed in legal professions today. With the population of the United States estimated at 324 million, this translates to 1 lawyer for every 416 people. The United States has more lawyers than any other country in the world. With this in mind, it is important that athletic trainers take proper precautions to minimize their exposure to lawsuits. Some of these precautions are to:

- Work within the scope of knowledge and expertise
- Closely follow HIPAA and FERPA procedures
- Keep proper documentation and maintain accurate records
- Follow proper training-room rules and procedures
- Always have adequate training-room supervision
- Keep in close contact with coaches, administration, and parents of athletes

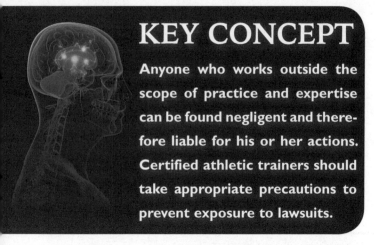

KEY CONCEPT

Anyone who works outside the scope of practice and expertise can be found negligent and therefore liable for his or her actions. Certified athletic trainers should take appropriate precautions to prevent exposure to lawsuits.

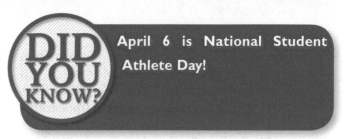

April 6 is National Student Athlete Day!

- Inspect practice and game facilities daily
- Establish a return-to-play protocol
- Involve the team physician in all aspects of the program
- Establish an advisory committee with members of all involved parties (e.g., head trainer, student athletic trainer, team doctor, administrator, coach, and parent)
- Establish and practice an emergency action plan

HIPAA and FERPA Legislation

The Health Insurance Portability and Accountability Act (HIPAA) of 1996 was enacted to protect patients' privacy, and to provide privacy standards to protect patients' medical records and other health information provided to health plans, doctors, hospitals, and other health care providers. Generally, secondary schools, K-12, are not HIPAA-covered entities. The HIPAA Privacy Rule only applies to health plans, health care clearinghouses, and health care providers that transmit health information electronically in connection with certain administrative and financial transactions. Covered transactions are those for which the U.S. Department of Health and Human Services has adopted a standard, such as health care

claims submitted to a health plan. Thus, even though a school employs school nurses, physicians, psychologists, or other health care providers (i.e., certified athletic trainers), a school is not generally a HIPAA-covered entity because the providers do not engage in any of the covered transactions, such as billing a health plan electronically for their services.

The Federal Education Rights and Privacy Act (FERPA) was enacted to protect the privacy rights of student records. Generally, schools must have written permission from the parent or eligible student (age 18 or older) in order to release any information from a student's education record. However, FERPA allows schools to disclose those records, without consent, to the following parties or under the following conditions:

- School officials with legitimate educational interest
- Other schools to which a student is transferring
- Specified officials for audit or evaluation purposes
- Appropriate parties in connection with financial aid to a student
- Organizations conducting certain studies for or on behalf of the school
- Accrediting organizations
- To comply with a judicial order or lawfully issued subpoena
- Appropriate officials in cases of health and safety emergencies
- State and local authorities, within a juvenile justice system, pursuant to specific State law

It is very important that the Certified Athletic Trainer closely adheres to all state and federal laws pertaining to athlete care, record keeping, and dissemination of personal information. The Certified Athletic Trainer must also carefully instruct anyone assisting them in their duties; such as Athletic Training Student Aides (chapter 4).

As careful and prudent as the certified athletic trainer may be, at some point in time he or she may become involved in a lawsuit. Thus, it is advisable to obtain liability insurance. Several companies carry coverage for certified athletic trainers. This coverage could help the ATC avoid financial disaster.

A DAY IN THE LIFE OF A CERTIFIED ATHLETIC TRAINER

Morning's here a little earlier than expected. 5:50 a.m., after the second alarm goes off. I'm on the road by 6:45 and at school by 7:00 for first-period planning. Checking the school district e-mail and grading yesterday's homework comes first, followed by getting equipment organized for two health and fitness classes and the two classroom sections of sports medicine.

Students for my first class arrive at the fitness center at 8:00 a.m. Most begin warming up and stretching on their own, though I need to assist a few in getting started. Some of the newer students need to be reminded to warm up first, and many are too busy socializing to remember to do more than just a few simple stretches. It takes time to educate them enough that they prevent their own injuries. Within 10 or 15 minutes, most move on to their main workout for the day. Again I spend most of my time assisting the newer or younger students in proper techniques. I also work with two students on setting personal workout plans and goals. Each has to identify how they would measure their progress toward their goals and what sort of workout they need to perform to accomplish these goals. My second period, the school's third, is also managing the fitness center. This group of students is organized much the same way, though I have fewer new students. I did not need to create new personal workout plans for them today; instead, one student completes his minimum credit requirements. We spend several minutes reviewing his progress toward the goals he had identified at the beginning of his program. His next step is to complete his evaluative essay for inclusion in his senior portfolio.

Fourth period is officially my planning period, but I come in early to plan and take advantage of our pool to swim laps before lunch. After closing the fitness center, I have approximately 40 minutes to swim before my lunch period. That will be my only time to exercise today. After swimming, showering, and getting dressed in khakis and polo shirt for tonight's game, I have lunch with other department members. This counts as our department meeting and keeps each of us informed as to what is going on.

Fifth period is the first section of sports medicine for today. We have been working on emergency procedures, and today students will be practicing primary and secondary surveys. Since we had already introduced the materials, most students will be able to practice in two- or three-person groups. One student will be the patient and another the rescuer. A little gentle reminder that the first time they do this for real may be at a packed basketball or football game is enough to get most to work a little harder. The students of the second section of Sports Medicine are working on the same skills.

The bell signals the end of school at 2:00. Seventh period, the "after-school" period, officially begins at 2:05. A line of athletes is already waiting before I can walk the 200 feet from the Sports Medicine classroom to the Training Room. C-Team basketball players are anxious to get taped and out to their game, so they get first priority, even over the varsity wrestlers. There are also a few injured athletes, including a gymnast from this morning's practice. Our gymnasts work out at 5:30 in the morning, with only their coach to prepare them for practice. Possible emergencies always get a 911 call, while other problems get ice and directions to see me after school. At 2:35, I am able to move on to evaluating injured athletes. Student athletic trainers finish taping the last of the athletes preparing for practice.

Game equipment preparation begins without much direction on my part while I continue evaluations. Some of the more experienced student athletic trainers also monitor rehabilitation

(continues)

(*continued*)

workouts and occasionally catch me between evaluations to modify an athlete's rehabilitation plan. Practices conclude with warm-ups by 2:50, and the C-Team basketball game is scheduled to begin at 3:30.

Unfortunately, a head injury in the wrestling room interrupts the triaged athletes. Fortunately, only one athlete, a swimmer, is left to evaluate, and he understands that emergencies come first. After phoning the injured swimmer's mother, I return to the training room to find several junior varsity basketball players getting taped, and the swimmer still needing to be evaluated.

With the pregame taping under control and the last evaluation completed, I finally get out to the basketball court to watch some of the C-Team game and finish paperwork. At halftime, I duck back into the training room and find today's injury report completed by the student athletic trainers. I also take the opportunity to have dinner—a sack lunch I made while eating breakfast this morning. The varsity basketball players are taped just after halftime of the JV game, and I recheck the wrestler with the concussion. I rejoin my remaining student athletic trainer on the bench before the end of the third quarter, followed by an exciting, but fortunately uneventful, conclusion to the junior varsity game. Before the varsity game, the student athletic trainer rechecks ice and water while I introduce myself to the visiting coach.

The varsity game begins at 7:00 p.m., before which I duck over to the pool to drop off towels in the laundry. The first quarter also turns out to be uneventful, but the second ends with an opponent twisting an ankle at the buzzer. At halftime, my student athletic trainer accompanies our team while I escort the visiting injured player to the locker room. The athlete had injured his ankle before but was not wearing any form of ankle protection. A quick evaluation shows no ligament laxity or other signs that would prevent him from returning to the game. I have him perform functional tests, tape him, and advise his coach that he can return to play. The second half proves to be entirely uneventful. We return to the training room around 8:45.

The training room and the game equipment are quickly cleaned while a few of the basketball players are icing. My student athletic trainers leave at 9:10 p.m. After finishing paperwork from this afternoon, I lock up at 9:30 and head home to relax. I have no games scheduled for tomorrow, so I should be able to leave school by 6:00 p.m. I finally turn in by 10:30. Seven hours later, my alarm goes off.

Tom Walker, ATC

CONCLUSION

Certified athletic trainers today possess the skills, knowledge, and professionalism that allow them to be respected members of the sports medicine community. As athletic venues open up to persons of all abilities, athletic trainers will find their market expanding. Working with athletes, parents, coaches, and other medical professionals is a highly rewarding aspect of the profession. Each day is a new experience and adventure that calls for diverse talents and the ability to solve problems in a variety of ways.

Many different career paths are open to certified athletic trainers. Traditional markets include public and private school settings, colleges and universities, and professional sports. Therapy clinics, hospitals, and medical centers are other popular avenues for employment. Beyond the traditional market, athletic trainers may find employment as consultants or personal trainers, with amateur sports teams, United States Olympic teams, international athletic organizations, or health and fitness centers, as well as in corporate settings.

In addition to the National Athletic Trainers' Association, most states have elected to certify or license athletic trainers. Many regional and state associations may be available to athletic trainers, depending on the area in which the trainer is located. These organizations provide regional support and information in areas such as employment, continuing education, and advancement and promotion of the occupation.

REVIEW QUESTIONS

1. Briefly describe the history and development of athletic training.
2. Explain the role certified athletic trainers play in the athletic health care system.
3. What education is needed to be an athletic trainer? What other experiences would be helpful?
4. What are the primary skills required for athletic training? What five do you feel are most important?
5. Certified athletic trainers work in a variety of different settings; describe three.
6. Describe the benefits local associations provide to athletic trainers.
7. Athletic trainers must adhere to a strict code of ethics. Why is this so important?
8. What dictates an athletic trainer's "normal" workday?
9. How is the athletic trainer certified or licensed?
10. What is the Athlete's Bill of Rights?
11. Explain liability issues pertaining to athletic trainers.
12. Explain HIPAA and its importance.
13. How does FERPA protect athletes' information?

PROJECTS AND ACTIVITIES

1. Write a three-page paper on Galen. Cover his contributions to medicine and his method of training gladiators in Rome.
2. Research job opportunities in your area for athletic trainers. Which interests you the most? Why?
3. Call or visit some local athletic trainers. How does the average salary for athletic trainers in your city compare with the national average?
4. Review Table 2–1. What career path most interests you? Why?

LEARNING LINKS

- Increase your understanding of Title IX by reviewing its history and reading about outcomes of lawsuits that have been brought as a result of the legislation. A good overview is presented at the following legal firm website: http://www.schillerlawfirm.com.
- Visit the National Athletic Trainers' Association website at http://www.nata.org for information regarding the educational and certification requirements for becoming a certified athletic trainer. Look for professional organizations in your state that support athletic training.

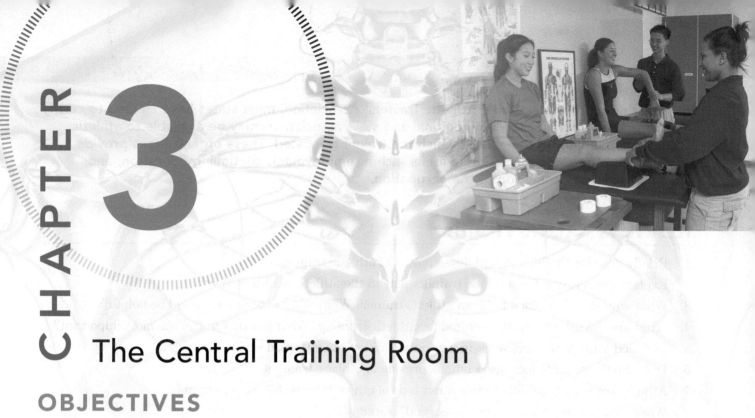

CHAPTER 3

The Central Training Room

OBJECTIVES

Upon completion of this chapter, the reader should be able to:

- Describe the modern central training room and list its specifications
- Understand HIPAA and how it relates to athletic training
- List the various equipment and supply needs of the central training room
- Identify the different modalities used in the central training room
- Describe Occupational Safety and Health Administration (OSHA) standards that apply to the athletic training facility

KEY TERMS

central training room *A multipurpose facility designed to accommodate a variety of athletic training needs.*

electrical modality *A therapeutic treatment technique that involves the use of electrical stimulation; for example, ultrasound, TENS, and e-stim.*

ground fault interrupter (GFI) *A mini circuit breaker that will stop the flow of electricity in the event of a short or contact with water.*

medical kit *A portable storage container for medical supplies such as bandages, gauze, antiseptics, ice packs, gloves, and so on. There are many different varieties: soft-sided bags, fanny packs, and hard-shell boxes.*

mechanical modality *A therapeutic treatment technique that involves manipulation of the muscles in the body; for example, massage, vibration, and mobilization.*

Occupational Safety and Health Administration (OSHA) *A federal agency that develops regulations for employees whose jobs may put them at risk of bloodborne pathogens.*

Sharps equipment *Instruments such as scalpels, blades, razors, and uncapped needles that can penetrate the skin and cause exposure to bloodborne pathogens.*

KEY TERMS CONTINUED

The Health Insurance Portability and Accountability Act (HIPAA) *It was enacted to protect patients' privacy and provide privacy standards to protect patients' medical records and other health information provided to health plans, doctors, hospitals, and other health care providers.*

thermal modality *A therapeutic treatment technique that involves the use of heat or cold; for example, use of the hydrocollator or ice packs.*

THE CENTRAL TRAINING ROOM

The athletic training facility, commonly referred to as the **central training room**, is a multipurpose facility designed to accommodate a variety of needs (Figure 3–1). Training rooms vary greatly from one school to another. Many universities have elaborate training facilities that are both ample in size and stocked with all the latest equipment. Smaller universities and colleges often provide more modest accommodations.

High schools generally operate with little or no formal training-room spaces. Many have facilities that have been converted from closets, storage rooms, and locker-room space.

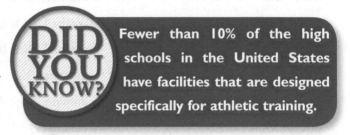

Fewer than 10% of the high schools in the United States have facilities that are designed specifically for athletic training.

Design of the Central Training Room

The central training room must be easily accessible to both male and female athletes. Depending on the size of the school or facility being served, there may also be a need for a smaller satellite facility. When designing a training room or converting space for a training room, careful planning is crucial. Among the many factors to consider in the planning stage are size, lighting, plumbing, electricity, ventilation and heating, telephone access, storage, office space, wet area, taping area, treatment area, and exercise and rehabilitation areas.

Size

The optimum size for any facility will be based on the size of the school and the number of athletes served. High schools with a population of 1,500 to 2,000 students will have approximately 375 athletes, or roughly 25% of the school population. Table 3–1 gives a typical breakdown of sports offered each season and the number of participants that may be on each team for a school of this size.

The size of the central training room for such a school should be approximately 1,200 square feet. Few high school training rooms meet this criterion; most are in the 400- to 800-square-foot range.

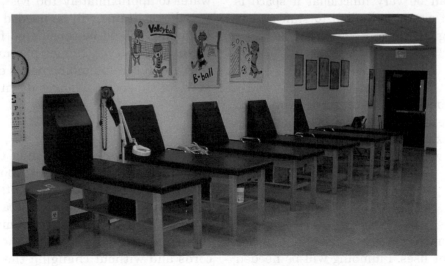

Figure 3–1 The central training room, Irvine High School, Irving, Texas.

Table 3–1 Sports by Season with Anticipated Number of Athletes Competing

FALL	WINTER	SPRING
Football (V) 45	Basketball, Boys (V) 12	Baseball (V) 20
Football (JV) 35	Basketball, Boys (JV) 12	Baseball (JV) 20
Football (C) 50	Basketball, Boys (C) 20	Baseball (C) 20
Cross Country, Boys 35	Basketball, Girls (V) 12	Fastpitch/Softball (V) 25
Cross Country, Girls 35	Basketball, Girls (JV) 12	Fastpitch/Softball (JV) 25
Volleyball (V) 12	Basketball, Girls (C) 20	Fastpitch/Softball (C) 25
Volleyball (JV) 12	Gymnastics 35	Soccer, Boys (V) 20
Volleyball (C) 18	Swimming, Boys 40	Soccer, Boys (JV) 20
Soccer, Girls (V) 20	Wrestling (V) 14	Soccer, Boys (C) 20
Soccer, Girls (JV) 20	Wrestling (JV) 40	Track and Field, Boys 45
Soccer, Girls (C) 20	Wrestling (C) 40	Track and Field, Girls 45
Swimming, Girls 40		Golf, Boys 10
Tennis, Boys 16		Golf, Girls 10
		Tennis, Girls, 16

Cheer team 24 -

Drill/Dance team 45 -

Sports: 14 Athletes: 427	Sports: 11 Athletes: 326	Sports: 11 Athletes: 390

This table is based on a high school of 1,500–2,200 students grades 9–12. (V) varsity; (JV) junior varsity; (C) sophomore or freshman and sophomore.

The most important aspect of a training room is use of space, not square footage (Figure 3–2). A small training room can be very functional if space is used well, and if access is limited to staff and to athletes receiving treatment.

Lighting

The training room must have good lighting to allow for proper examinations and treatment. It is important that examiners not struggle with inadequate lighting, which could result in inaccurate assessments.

Plumbing

The training room requires special plumbing for its many different uses. Plumbing will be needed for the sink (hot and cold water), ice machine, whirlpool, and hydrocollator (a device that heats water to approximately 160°F).

Floor drains will be needed in the wet area. Plumbing should be considered for a dishwasher, washer, and dryer. Proper planning for both current and future plumbing needs can eliminate the need for expensive changes down the line.

Electricity

There will be extensive use of electricity in the training room. An electrician should be consulted as to the specific requirements of the facility. Electrical outlets should be strategically located so that special equipment and modalities used in the training room can operate without extension cords and without changing the configuration of

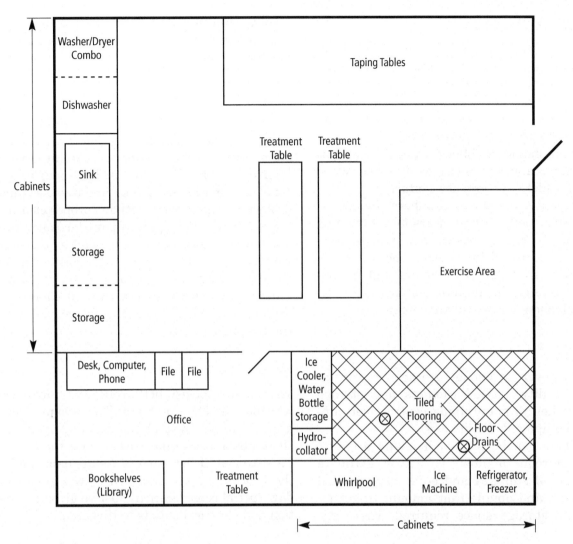

Figure 3–2 Floorplan for the central training room.

the facility to accommodate a particular piece of equipment. **Ground fault interrupters (GFI)** must be used in all areas that are near water (Figure 3–3). GFI circuits are mini circuit breakers that will trip and stop the flow of electricity in the event of a short or contact with water.

Ventilation and Heating

Training rooms are busy areas that place great demands on ventilation and heating systems. Add the use of whirlpools, hydrocollators, and other equipment requiring water, and it is obvious that problems with humidity and heat will quickly arise. Proper ventilation specifically designed for these areas will solve these problems.

The training room should be heated to a comfortable level, taking into account that athletes will be in shorts most of the time.

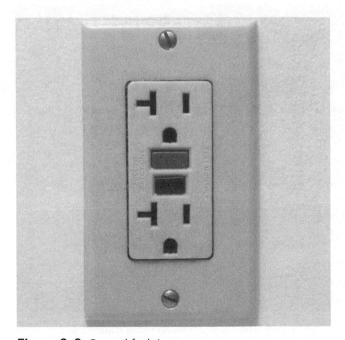

Figure 3–3 Ground fault interrupter.

Telephone Access

A telephone in the training room is important for safety and emergencies. It is best that the phone be installed in the certified athletic trainer's office, with both internal and long-distance lines. A call to the parents of an injured athlete is not always a local call. A specific telephone protocol should be in place and should be followed. Legal as well as professional standards must be followed when calling an athlete's emergency contact.

Emergency telephone numbers should be clearly posted. Cellphone numbers for all training staff should be clearly posted, too, with instructions on whom to call in an emergency. If this is not possible, all trainers (students and adults) must understand the protocol for access to the nearest telephone in case of an emergency.

Storage

There can never be enough storage in a training-room facility. Locked cabinets and storage closets are key to maintaining control over supplies and equipment (Figure 3–4).

Cabinets can be located in many areas of the training room to allow easy access. Estimate the amount of supplies and equipment needed for one year, and double that amount to get an idea of the storage space required. There are always unanticipated needs, and with carryover of items from the previous year, space is always at a premium.

Office Space

An office located within the training room is important for many reasons. There will be a constant need to enter injury and training-room log information into a computer. The security of personal information contained in databases must be protected from anyone without proper clearance.

Private office space allows for consultations and private examinations, as well as conferences with other sports medicine specialists. The office should be large enough for a desk, examination table, file cabinets, bookcases, and some storage (Figure 3–5). This is also the optimal location for the telephone.

Wet Area

The wet area consists of the refrigerator, ice machine, whirlpool, and hydrocollator. This area must be separate from the rest of the training room. There should be a special floor drain, with the floor itself consisting of tile or concrete. As the name indicates, the floor of the wet area will be wet almost every day. Special consideration must be given to ventilation and electrical outlets in this area.

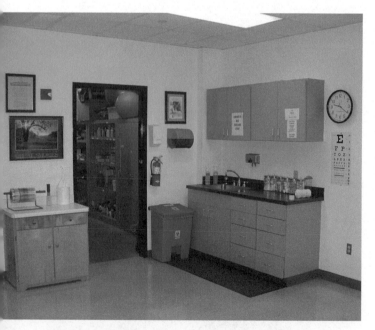

Figure 3–4 The central training room should have adequate storage space.

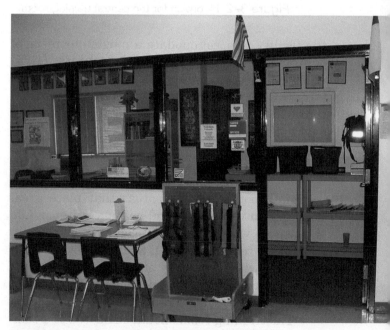

Figure 3–5 Office space within the central training room allows for privacy and security of personal data.

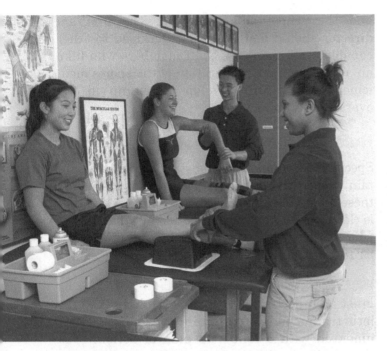

Figure 3–6 The taping/treatment area is the most frequently used space in the central training room.

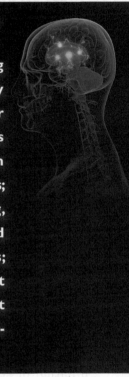

KEY CONCEPT

The modern central training room should be adequately designed to enable the proper care of male and female athletes alike. Specifications for this room include adequate size for needs; adequate lighting, plumbing, electricity, and ventilation and heating; telephone access; storage; office space; and a wet area; a taping area, a treatment area, and an exercise and rehabilitation area.

Taping/Treatment Area

The taping/treatment area will be the most-used area of the training room (Figure 3–6). It is common to have athletes waiting in line to be taped. The training room should have at least six taping tables and provide adequate staffing to handle several athletes at once.

Taping tables are approximately 42 inches long, 24 inches wide, and 38 inches high. Many have storage and drawers underneath to provide easy, quick access to supplies. Tables can be padded and covered in vinyl, or be covered with countertop-type laminate. Cloth should not be used, as it cannot be cleaned and sterilized properly. To allow athletic trainers room to work, there should be approximately 18 to 24 inches between each table.

Treatment Area

The treatment area should consist of at least two treatment tables spaced far enough apart to allow movement of training staff. Treatment tables are approximately 84 inches long, 24 inches wide, and 32 inches high, and are padded with vinyl covering. All taping and treatment tables must be sturdy and able to withstand the heaviest athletes. They will be used on a daily basis and must be durable. All treatment and taping tables must be cleaned and disinfected daily after use.

Exercise and Rehabilitation Areas

If space permits, a separate area in the training room for exercise and rehabilitation equipment is most useful (Figure 3–7). This area should accommodate an exercise bike, elliptical trainer, and special weights and equipment to be used for rehabilitating various areas of the body.

Athletes can exercise under supervision while taping and examinations are in process. Exercise equipment will be used on a continual basis and, if located in the central training room, will allow the athletic training staff to multitask, thus saving time and accomplishing more tasks.

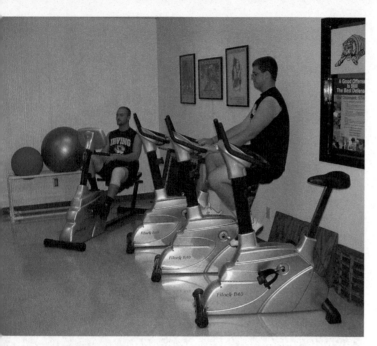

Figure 3–7 Ready access to an exercise area in the central training room allows athletes to work out under supervision, and the athletic training staff to carry out other tasks while supervising the athletes who are rehabilitating.

OPERATION OF THE CENTRAL TRAINING ROOM

The central training room complex requires coordination of staff, athletes, coaches, and custodial workers. It is important to post a schedule to inform everyone involved in the operation of this facility. A well-organized, well-coordinated central training room is a valuable asset to any school or university.

Staffing

The training-room staff consists of a program director, certified athletic trainers, athletic training student aides, and support staff. Support staff consists of team doctors, therapists, and other allied health professionals who visit the training room on an ongoing basis.

PROGRAM DIRECTOR The program director is responsible for the overall operation of the sports medicine program and facility. This includes staffing, central training room, equipment, inventory, budgets, ordering, and recordkeeping, as well as working with athletes, coaches, parents, and the school administration. The program director should distribute the workload to other capable staff members. Staff members who take an active part in the operation of the sports medicine program will develop ownership in the overall program.

Rules and Procedures

Special rules or guidelines must be followed to maintain proper training-room operation. Adhering to these rules will ensure a well-run training room that is clean, operational, and respected by athletes. The following box outlines typical rules and procedures for the central training room.

INJURY MANAGEMENT POLICY All injuries must be reported as soon as possible to the athletic trainer in charge. All injuries must be documented with a follow-up plan of action. It is the certified athletic trainer's responsibility to schedule further medical assistance if necessary. It is important to note that the Certified Athletic Trainer must follow the physician's orders and recommendations as to the care of the athlete.

All athletic training staff shall preserve the confidentiality of privileged information and shall not release such information to any third party not involved in the patient's care.

HEALTH CARE PORTABILITY AND ACCOUNTABILITY ACT The **Health Insurance Portability and Accountability Act** of 1996 (HIPAA) was enacted by Congress on August 21, 1996. This act required the Secretary of Health and Human Services (HHS) to publicize standards for electronic exchange, privacy and security of health information. This provided a national standard for the protection of certain health information.

Most of us believe that our medical and other health information is private and should be protected, and we want to know who has this information. The Privacy Rule, a Federal law, gives you rights over your health information and sets rules and limits on who can look at and receive your health information. The Privacy Rule applies to all forms of individuals' protected health information, whether electronic, written, or oral. The Security Rule is a Federal law that requires security for health information in electronic form.

Most schools and districts are exempt from these laws and are not required to follow them.

It is the sole responsibility of the program director to make decisions about releasing any medical information to a third party. This should be done in conjunction with the school district's legal policy on distribution of medical/injury information.

Athletic training student aides shall not be responsible for making final decisions on the playing status of an athlete. They may pass on information after the certified athletic trainer has

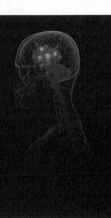

KEY CONCEPT

All athletic training staff shall preserve the confidentiality of privileged information and shall not release such information to a third party not involved in the patient's care.

TRAINING-ROOM RULES AND PROCEDURES

These are examples of rules and expectations you would typically see posted at training-room facilities:

- All injuries are to be reported to the training staff, regardless of severity.
- Treatments are given only after approval by the training staff.
- Treatments are to continue until cleared by medical staff.
- Athletes are not to treat themselves.
- No horseplay or improper language allowed.
- Appropriate dress required: shirt, shorts, and shoes.
- No cleats allowed.
- Do not remove any supplies without the trainer's permission.
- All athletes must sign in before receiving treatment.
- Return all loaned items to the training room.
- No food or drink allowed.
- No use of training equipment without prior approval.
- The telephone is not for personal use.
- Only athletes being treated and their coaches are allowed in the training room.
- Attend and work at the athletic contests and practices assigned.
- Complete daily jobs as assigned.
- Athletes are not to bring their bags or other nonessential personal items into the training room.
- Do not leave the training room or office open when vacant.
- Supervise all treatments.
- Wear gloves whenever your work might involve contact with bodily fluids.
- Wash your hands after working with each athlete.
- Document every injury.

evaluated the athlete and determined his or her status. For example, an athletic training student aide may be asked to provide a player's status update to coaches after the certified athletic trainer has determined it. The certified athletic trainer is solely responsible for decisions on a player's return to play status.

HOUSEKEEPING Daily housekeeping procedures include cleaning all surfaces that come into direct contact with individuals. These surfaces should be cleaned with a suitable disinfectant. All surfaces should be wiped clean with a nonreusable towel. Tables and equipment with high use should be cleaned after each use.

Whirlpools should be cleaned before and after each use. Sinks and countertops should be cleaned each day. All instruments must be cleaned on a daily basis as well.

Handwashing is the best way to prevent the transfer of germs from one person to another. Personnel are to wash their hands thoroughly after each treatment, using warm water and plenty of soap.

Towels and hydrocollator covers should be washed each day, depending on use.

DRESS CODE AND PERSONAL HYGIENE To exhibit professionalism in the central training room, a dress code may be enforced. The following rules are typical of many training programs across the United States:

- Men—a collared shirt; women—a professional shirt that is in good taste
- Pants or shorts, khaki
- Shirts must be tucked into pants
- Socks must be worn with functional shoes
- No open-toed shoes or sandals
- Neat jeans or jean shorts.

Gameday attire will be determined by the head athletic trainer.

Good personal hygiene must be practiced by all sports medicine staff. Taking pride in one's appearance demonstrates professionalism. Facial hair must be kept clean and trimmed. Jewelry must be kept to a minimum at all times, for both practical and hygienic reasons.

Documentation

Proper documentation of injuries and treatments is essential for every central training room. Chapter 11, "Assessment and Evaluation of Sports Injuries," outlines various types of documentation used in the central training room and in the field.

Inventory and Budgeting

One important element of training-room operation is the ordering and inventory of supplies. Most sports medicine budgets are tight and require the use of creative measures to make ends meet. There must be enough inventory to adequately stock the training room with supplies that can be used within a reasonable time period. Many supplies used in the training room have a limited shelf life. Supply and ordering considerations include tracking product expiration dates, identifying purchasing patterns, and establishing relationships with vendors for special pricing. Controlling these matters, and avoiding the purchase of trendy items, will ensure that the facility is always adequately stocked and ready for athletes.

These tips will help in the budgeting, ordering, and use of supplies:

- Create two lists, one for consumable supplies and one for reusable supplies.
- Track all supplies carefully. All training staff are to have ownership in the program and be involved in the inventory and ordering process. This assists in reducing waste and gives each staff member a working knowledge of what is used and when.
- Develop a working relationship with a vendor that understands the needs of the facility. Often the largest companies are those least likely to offer the best pricing. Also, compare pricing at retail and discount consumer outlets.

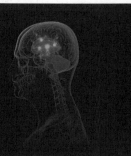

KEY CONCEPT

Most sports medicine budgets are tight and require the use of creative measures to make ends meet.

- Review past purchase orders and training-room treatment logs. This should reveal a purchasing pattern that will be useful for future orders.

- Before ordering new, untried products, ask for free samples so that staff can evaluate their usefulness before spending precious and limited budget money.

- Many supplies have a limited shelf life and thus need to be ordered frequently during the course of the year.

Medical Kits

A well-stocked, functional **medical kit** enables prompt and adequate treatment of athletes (Figure 3–8). It requires a portable storage container for medical supplies such as bandages, gauze, antiseptics, ice packs, gloves, and so on. The Medical Kit Supply List box later in this chapter outlines the equipment typically found in a medical kit.

Medical kits come in many sizes, from the fanny packs worn by athletic trainers to large kits that require wheels for transport. Fanny packs

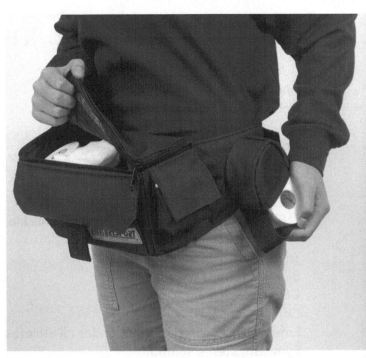

Figure 3–9 Fanny packs allow the certified athletic trainer to bring needed supplies conveniently to the game site or athletic field.

that can be worn in the field allow the mobility needed to take supplies directly to the athlete on the playing field (Figure 3–9). Fanny packs come in different sizes and configurations, so trainers can choose one that best meets their needs.

Medical kits come in both soft-sided and hard-shell models. Soft-sided kits are lighter and more mobile than their hard-sided counterparts. The major drawback to the soft-sided kit is its longevity and relatively smaller size. It is important that the head athletic trainer take into account the intended use and functionality of the kits to be purchased. A medical kit used for football would probably be different from one used for basketball.

GAME SITE EQUIPMENT Many pieces of equipment will be needed and used both in the training room and at various game and practice sites—for example, having crutches at each practice or game site, as well as available in the training room (Figure 3–10). This requires duplicate orders.

All equipment should be inspected daily to ensure that it is in proper working order. The following discussion describes the types of equipment that could be needed at both practice and game sites.

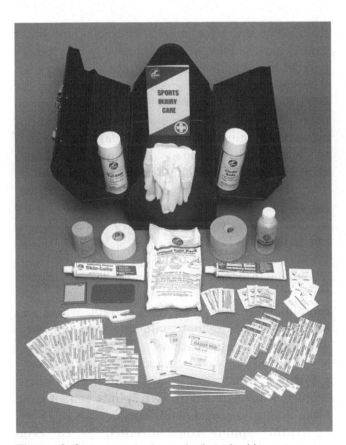

Figure 3–8 Appropriately stocked medical kit.

MEDICAL KIT SUPPLY LIST

Adhesive tape (1", 1 ½")
Analgesics
Antibacterial/antiseptic cream
Antimicrobial hand wipes
Applicators, cotton-tip
Bandage scissors or tape cutters
    Bandages
    Butterfly or steri-strip
    Plastic adhesive type (regular, large, knuckle,
      fingertip)
Triangular
Biohazard bags
Cold pack, instant
Contact lens kit
Emergency contact information for all athletes
Eyewash, sterile solution
Foot powder
Gauze pads, sterile (3×3, 4×4 inches)

Gloves, latex
Heel cups
Hydrogen peroxide
Mirror with plastic holder
Moleskin
Mouth shield or CPR protector
Pencil and paper
Plastic bags for ice
Roller gauze
Saline solution/eyewash
Scissors (bandage, heavy duty)
Skin lubricant or petroleum jelly
Sling or triangular bandage
Tape adherent
Thermometer
Tongue depressors
Underwrap
Wraps, elastic (2", 4", 6")

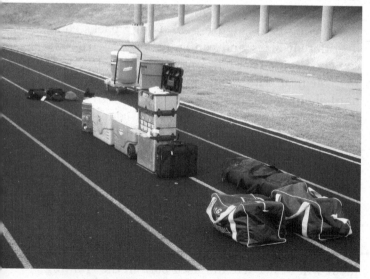

Figure 3–10 Various types of equipment should be on hand at practices and at game sites.

VACUUM SPLINTS AND GENERAL SPLINTING MATERIAL
One of the most popular and easy-to-use products on the market today for splinting an injured extremity is the *vacuum splint*. Vacuum splints, which have been in use in Europe since the 1970s, and offer versatility and adaptability that is hard to beat when compared to traditional, padded-board splints or air splints.

Vacuum splints operate by extracting air from the splint. They contain thousands of small, polystyrene beads that mold and model the splint around the injured body part. They are made of nylon and can be molded to accommodate a bent arm, leg, or dislocation (Figure 3–11). As air is extracted (a process that takes just seconds), thousands of beads gently conform to the injury without exerting unnecessary pressure or impairing circulation.

Air splints work on the opposite principle: air is pumped into the splint instead of being extracted from it. Air splints increase the pressure surrounding an injury site. Air splints, which are made of vinyl, are not malleable and will work only for in-line applications.

Padded wooden or cardboard splints allow splinting of extremities with in-line fractures (Figure 3–12). Padded wooden splints cannot mold around an injury or dislocation.

SAM® splints were invented by Dr. Sam Scheinberg in 1985. It is a flexible, moldable splint

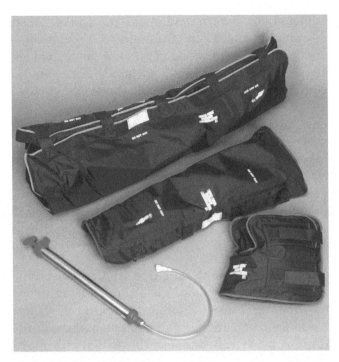

Figure 3–11 Various vacuum splints.

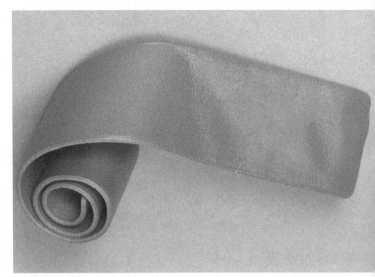

Figure 3–13 SAM® splint.

that can be used for a variety of applications (Figure 3–13). Its lightweight, compact size allows easy storage and portability. It can immobilize almost any bone in the body, including in the neck.

Also on the market today are a variety of plastic, articulated splints that allow the caregiver to adjust the splint to accommodate a variety of different angles and situations (Figure 3–14). Articulated splints work well, but can be awkward when dealing with athletes in a wide range of sizes.

Fingers are among the most commonly fractured body parts. Splinting material designed for

fingers offers good, safe support. Every training room and medical kit should contain an assortment of finger splints. The material used for finger splints is often padded aluminum or plastic strips (Figure 3–15). Several companies manufacture these splints, so certified athletic trainers will need to find the brand and type that best fits their preferences and needs.

CRUTCHES Crutches allow mobility when it is important that the patient bear little or no weight on an injured hip, knee, leg, or ankle. Crutches come in two basic designs: traditional, and the new HOPE crutch (Figure 3–16). The former can be

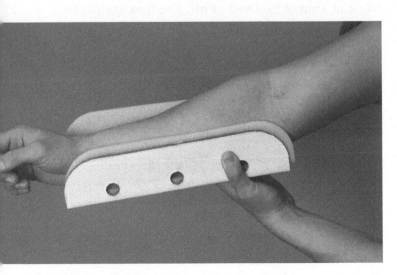

Figure 3–12 Padded wooden board splint.

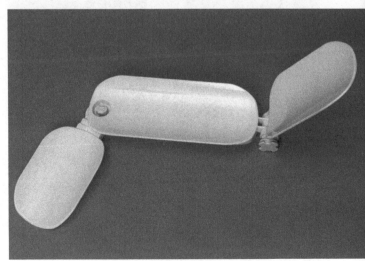

Figure 3–14 Plastic articulated splint.

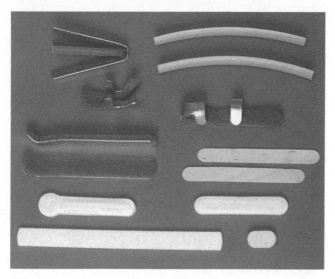

Figure 3–15 Various finger splints.

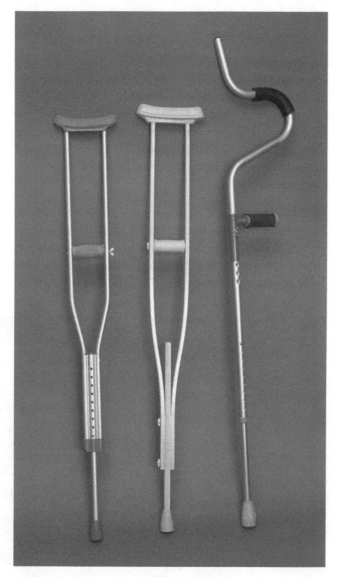

Figure 3–16 Various styles of crutches.

adjusted for length and hand placement. Most are manufactured out of aluminum, though some are still made of wood. Crutches have padded supports for the armpit and hands. Each end is equipped with a nonslip rubber foot.

The HOPE crutch was developed as an alternate to the traditional crutch, which has been used since the Middle Ages. The HOPE crutch takes a different approach that allows users to comfortably use the crutch without sore armpits and decreases the risk of falls because of balance problems. The HOPE crutch also lets the user walk comfortably, using less energy than with traditional crutches.

Proper Adjustment and Use of Crutches It is important to know how to use and adjust crutches to avoid problems created by improper usage. Aside from causing fatigue and frustration, ill-fitting crutches can damage the axillary (armpit) nerves.

The tops of the crutches should be two finger-widths below the armpits. Wrists should be straight, and elbows bent approximately 30 degrees. Crutch tips should be approximately two inches in front of the feet and six inches outside (Figure 3–17). The user's weight should be supported on the palms of the hands, on the handgrips. Do not rest all the weight on the arm pads. The added pressure on nerves and blood vessels in the armpits can cause temporary numbness in the hands and arms. It is important for a crutch user to wear well-fitting, low-heeled shoes with nonslip soles.

The three-point gait is used when one leg is weak or cannot be used at all. The first step is to

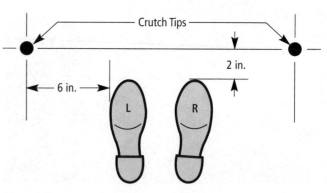

Figure 3–17 Proper adjustment and positioning of crutches.

move the crutches and injured leg 12 to 15 inches ahead of the good leg. Then swing the good leg about 12 to 15 inches ahead of the crutches. Bearing weight on the good leg, move the crutches to the beginning position. Walking on crutches is easier and faster if the injured leg moves simultaneously and in rhythm with the crutches.

To go up stairs, weight is supported on the handgrips while the good leg is moved up one step. Bearing body weight on the good leg, move the crutches and the injured leg up to the same step. To go down stairs, reverse the order and move the crutches and the injured leg first. While the good leg on the upper step supports the weight, place the crutches at the back of the lower step. Bearing weight on the handgrips, move the good leg to the same step. Do not put the crutches or the foot of the good leg at the edge of the step; it is easy to lose one's balance and fall.

If the stairway has a handrail, use that for safer support instead of one of the crutches. The sequence for going up or down stairs is the same: Place the weight normally put on one of the crutches on the handrail instead. Carry the unused crutch perpendicular to the crutch being used, or hold both crutches upright and use them as one. Remember, with curbs or stairs "the good go up; the bad go down."

General First-Aid Supplies, Equipment, and Modalities

Certified athletic trainers use a wide variety of products in their training rooms and offsite facilities. These products fall into four categories: consumable supplies, nonconsumable supplies, miscellaneous equipment, and therapeutic modalities.

CONSUMABLE SUPPLIES Consumable supplies used in the training room are too numerous to list. Most training-room facilities have, at minimum, the items listed in the accompanying box.

NONCONSUMABLE SUPPLIES Nonconsumable supplies, whether used in the training room or loaned to the athlete, can be reused and will last for a considerable period. Examples of nonconsumable supplies include:

- Blankets
- Braces (ankle, elbow, knee, shoulder)

- CPR devices
- Crutches
- Diagnostic instruments
- Penlights
- Scissors, sharps, tweezers, nail clippers
- Slings
- Splints

MISCELLANEOUS EQUIPMENT Miscellaneous equipment includes items such as refrigerators, ice machines, tables, benches, carts, desks, and computers. Most central training rooms have exercise equipment and various rehabilitation items at their disposal. Stretchers, immobilizers, and neck collars should be in all training-room facilities.

THERAPEUTIC MODALITIES *Therapeutic modalities* are various methods and mechanisms used by the training staff to help promote healing and mobility. Chapter 12, "Therapeutic Physical Modalities," discusses this subject in detail.

Some modalities require the permission and supervision of a medical doctor before use by certified athletic trainers. These include ultrasound, e-stim (electrical stimulation), and TENS (Transcutaneous Electrical Nerve Stimulation).

Modalities can be placed into three categories: mechanical, thermal, and electrical:

- **Mechanical modalities** include massage, mobilization, vibration, and manipulation.
- **Thermal modalities** include the various applications of heat (such as the hydrocollator) and cold (such as ice).
- **Electrical modalities** include ultrasound, e-stim, TENS, and other treatments based on the use of electricity.

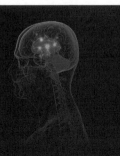

KEY CONCEPT

Three general modalities are used in the central training room: mechanical, thermal, and electrical.

COMMON CONSUMABLE SUPPLIES FOR TRAINING ROOMS

Analgesics
Antiseptics
Applicators, cotton-tip
Bandages
   Absorbent
   Compress
   Plastic adhesive strips, various sizes
   Triangular
Biohazard control
Disinfectants
Dressings
Eye cup
Eye patches
Eyewash/eye care products
Felt
First-aid cream
Foam and padding

Foam rubber
Gauze, sterile and nonsterile
Gloves, latex
Miscellaneous first-aid products
Moleskin
Penlights
Skin lubricant
Soap, disinfecting
Talcum powder
Tape
   Adhesive (1", 2")
   Elastic (1 ½", 2", 3")
Tape adherent
Tongue depressors
Underwrap
Wraps, elastic (3", 4", 6")

WATER AND ITS ADMINISTRATION Of all the supplies the certified athletic trainer must have at a practice or game site, water is the most important. A properly hydrated athlete will perform well and have fewer injuries than an athlete who has neglected water intake.

Numerous water breaks must be scheduled into all practice sessions, regardless of the weather conditions. Needless to say, hot, dry weather will increase the need for and frequency of water and rest breaks. Hydration is addressed in depth in Chapter 25.

Water can be supplied in different ways. Many schools use water bottles, water tables, cups, or pressurized containers to supply water. Regardless of the method, containers must be sterilized each day and before another athlete's use. Unclean water containers can spread disease quickly throughout a team.

The primary goal is to provide athletes an ample supply of fresh, clean, cool water.

OSHA STANDARDS AND THE ATHLETIC TRAINING FACILITY

The **Occupational Safety and Health Administration (OSHA)** has developed federal regulations for employees whose jobs may put them at risk of bloodborne pathogen exposure. See the box

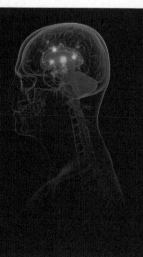

KEY CONCEPT

Equipment and supplies must be well stocked in the medical kits, as well as onsite for games and practices. Common items that are always necessary are bandages, splinting devices, crutches, ice packs, water, and various first-aid equipment.

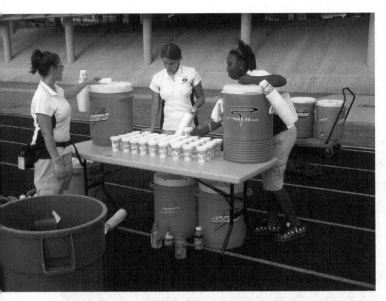

Figure 3–18 Distribution of water is critical to the health and safety of the athlete. Irving High School, Irving Independent School District.

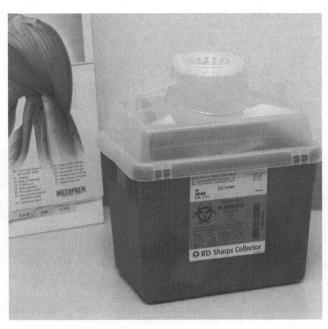

Figure 3–19 Sharps container.

below for common terms used in OSHA guidelines. These regulations must be observed by officials and medical personnel in order to protect everyone involved with sports. OSHA requires each workplace to develop and keep on hand an exposure control plan, which lists and defines staff training, staff duties, documentation of exposure, personal protective equipment, and other items.

OSHA mandates that all employees who are at risk of exposure to bloodborne pathogens be offered hepatitis B vaccinations.

Special containers should be available exclusively for biohazardous waste. These containers should have a labeled, red biohazard bag within for proper waste disposal. The container too must have a red biohazard label. Biohazardous materials include bloodied gauze, bandage strips, and latex gloves. Each facility should also have a red, plastic container for sharps equipment (Figure 3–19). **Sharps equipment** includes scalpel blades, razors, uncapped syringes, and needles.

TERMINOLOGY USED IN OSHA GUIDELINES

- *Bloodborne pathogens* are microorganisms that are present in human blood and can cause disease in humans.

- Contaminated indicates the presence or the reasonably anticipated presence of blood or other potentially infectious materials on an item or surface.

- *A contaminated sharp* is any contaminated object that can penetrate the skin.

- *Other potentially infectious materials* include semen, vaginal secretions, cerebrospinal fluid, synovial fluid, peritoneal fluid, amniotic fluid, saliva, and any body fluid that is contaminated with blood.

- *Standard precautions* is OSHA's approach to infection control.

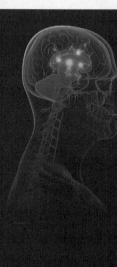

KEY CONCEPT

Federal **OSHA** regulations were put in place for the protection and safety of workers who are at risk of exposure to bloodborne pathogens. **OSHA** mandates:

- That an exposure control plan be on hand
- Training staff about bloodborne pathogens
- Documentation and reporting of all exposures
- That personal protective equipment be available to staff
- That the hepatitis B vaccine be offered to all at-risk staff
- That special containers be used for biohazardous materials and sharps
- That staff follow standard precautions
- That proper disinfection techniques be used to clean tools and work surfaces

Standard Precautions

Standard precautions are strict guidelines, set forth by OSHA, that must be taken to ensure the health and safety of everyone involved in the treatment of athletes:

- Wear vinyl or latex examination gloves when touching biohazardous material such as open skin, blood, bodily fluids, or mucus membranes. Do not reuse gloves!

- Wash hands with soap and hot water immediately after they have been exposed to blood or bodily fluids, even if gloves were worn.

- All surfaces (e.g., counters, tables) must be thoroughly washed after being soiled with blood or bodily fluid. Use a 10% household bleach solution or a commercially available disinfectant.

- Place all used sharps in a special, puncture-resistant sharps container.

- Place all discarded medical waste in a specially labeled biohazardous waste container located in the training room.

- When working outdoors, dispose of medical waste by placing it in a red, plastic biohazard bag and then discarding it in the proper biohazard waste container upon return to the facility.

- Do not allow athletes to share towels that have been contaminated with blood or bodily fluids.

- Put towels and clothing that have been contaminated with blood or bodily fluids into a biohazard bag and place that bag in the laundry basket.

- Be sure all athletes' wounds are well covered before practice and competition.

- If you have an open wound, especially on your hand, avoid providing first-aid care for injuries that involve bleeding or bodily fluids until your wounds are healed. If you must do so, be sure to wear vinyl or latex examination gloves.

Disinfecting Procedures

All equipment, environmental, and work surfaces shall be cleaned and decontaminated after contact with blood or other potentially infectious materials. This should be done after completion of procedures, immediately after a surface has been contaminated, and at the end of the working shift for all surfaces that had the potential to become contaminated. When disinfecting surfaces, use a disinfectant containing a chemical germicide registered with the Environmental Protection Agency. A solution of 10% bleach in water is another approved method. Thoroughly disinfect all surfaces with a clean towel or paper towel. Thoroughly wash all surfaces after treatment of each patient.

Any towel or material that is contaminated with blood or other potentially infectious material is to be considered as HIV/HBV infected and handled as little as possible. (HIV is the human immunodeficiency virus; HBV is the hepatitis B virus.) Contaminated laundry shall be placed and transported in labeled, red biohazard bags.

For cleaning spills:

- Use standard precautions.
- Dispose of any sharps present in a sharps container.
- Contain the spill. If the spill is small, use an absorbing pad (like a paper towel) to absorb it. If large, use absorbing powder (like cornstarch) to absorb it.
- Dispose of the absorbed material by placing it in a labeled biohazardous waste container.
- Decontaminate using a disinfectant over the entire spill area.

- Remove soiled protective equipment and place it in a labeled biohazardous waste container.
- Daily cleaning procedures include:
- Clean all surfaces (e.g., tables, counters, exercise equipment) by coating the surfaces with disinfectant spray.
- Wipe surfaces with a clean, dry towel. Tables and all high-use surfaces should be cleaned after each treatment or use.
- Whirlpool cleaning: Wet the inside of the whirlpool with water. Wet a towel with whirlpool disinfectant. Clean the sides, floor, and agitator with the towel. Rinse the inside of the whirlpool with cold water, then dry with a clean towel.
- Instruments: Wash hands before handling instruments. Place instruments in an instrument tray filled with an approved instrument cleaning solution for 10 minutes. Remove, clean with warm water, dry, and store properly.
- Wash hands.

CONCLUSION

The central training room is a multipurpose facility designed to help athletes with their medical needs. These facilities should be located within the athletic complex and must accommodate both male and female athletes.

A properly designed training room will be large enough to handle all athletes' needs. This facility should be equipped to handle many different uses every day. The optimum training facility will have specific guidelines that athletes and staff must follow. A well-run, well-managed facility is an invaluable asset to any athletic program.

REVIEW QUESTIONS

1. What are the important components of a central training room?
2. Explain the important guidelines and specifications for operation of the central training room.
3. Why is the telephone an important safety item in the training room? What special guidelines should be followed as to its use?
4. Describe the different medical kits in use today.
5. There are two different types of crutches on the market today. Explain the differences between them.
6. How do you properly adjust crutches?
7. Explain the difference between consumable and nonconsumable supplies.
8. Why is it important to carefully track athletic training supplies used?

9. Explain the difference between mechanical, thermal, and electrical modalities.

10. Explain HIPAA and how it relates to athletic training.

11. Summarize the OSHA requirements that pertain to the central training room and athletic facility.

PROJECTS AND ACTIVITIES

Ask the director of the central training room in your school what he or she believes are the most important guidelines for athletes receiving treatment.

1. Visit the central training room in your school at the end of the school day. Take notes as to what you observe immediately after school ends and practices begin. (This is about a 30-minute time period.) Put your observations into a short paper, including what you observed that worked well, and any suggestions you have for improvements.

2. Design the optimum central training room for your school. Include a detailed floorplan. Explain each aspect of your facility.

3. Take a complete inventory of your training room. How will you organize the different categories of materials, supplies, and equipment? How will you track your inventory? When will new items have to be ordered?

4. Define each of the following modalities: e-stim, TENS, and ultrasound. Pick one of them and write a three-page paper describing it in more detail.

LEARNING LINK

• Visit the Occupational Safety and Health Administration website (http://www.osha.gob). What does OSHA do? Why is it important?

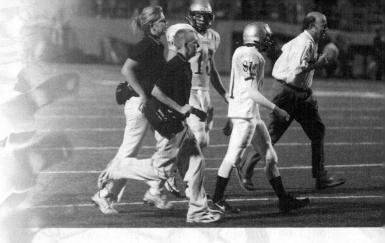

CHAPTER 4

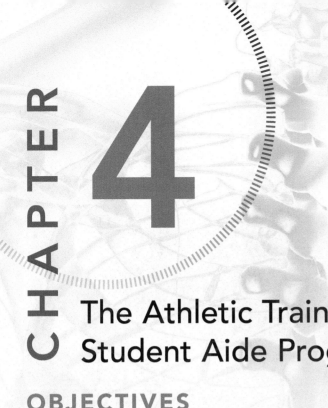

The Athletic Training Student Aide Program

OBJECTIVES

Upon completion of this chapter, the reader should be able to:

- Describe how to organize a sports medicine student aide program
- Describe the role athletic training student aides play in the athletic training program
- List the components of a model athletic training program
- Explain the different funding sources available for implementation of a high school sports medicine program
- List the expectations of an athletic training student aide (ATSA) in a sports medicine program
- Explain the responsibilities of ATSAs in a sports medicine program
- Describe how an athletic training student aide program is evaluated

KEY TERM

athletic training student aide (ATSA) *A student interested in a career in sports medicine and athletic training who begins training and studying the field as an assistant to the athletic director in a high school sports medicine program.*

ATHLETIC TRAINING STUDENT AIDES (ATSAs)

Athletic training student aides (ATSAs) are a very important component in a successful high school or college athletic training program (Figure 4–1). An ATSA program benefits students by allowing them to gain knowledge and skills necessary for a career in the health care industry. ATSAs not only acquire valuable experience in a clinical setting, but also enable the sports medicine director to spend more time addressing the needs of the entire program. An ATSA program benefits the certified athletic trainer by freeing up more administrative time.

Many years ago, the role of the ATSA fell upon the shoulders of a manager or assistant coach. Schools that had the luxury of having a certified athletic trainer on staff usually relied solely on this individual ATC to do everything from making ice to filling out accident report forms. Most high schools had no medical coverage other than what the coaches learned in first aid and CPR. Assistant coaches were commonly asked to take on the role of trainer and team doctor. This arrangement created a conflict of interest and also forced coaches to step out of their field of expertise.

In the mid-1980s, high schools across America began to develop athletic training programs with students in mind. It quickly became clear that high school students were a great resource in the training room and were highly motivated to learn about sports medicine and athletic training.

Today, sports medicine programs are gaining widespread popularity and are taught throughout the United States. Students are integral to the sports medicine team. Well-trained student aides can assist the certified athletic trainer in most aspects of the athletic training program.

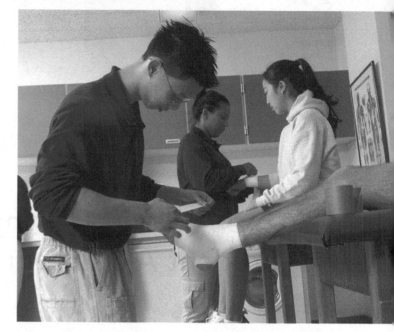

Figure 4–1 ATSAs are valuable members of the athletic training team.

ORGANIZING A FIRST-CLASS PROGRAM

The ultimate success of an athletic training program hinges on the ability of the certified athletic trainer to develop, maintain, and promote an environment that provides appropriate prevention, assessment, treatment, and rehabilitation of athletic injuries to the student athletes at each particular school site. The certified athletic trainer is responsible for the organization and design of the entire athletic training program. The design of the program has to be specific, with outcomes clearly defined for both coaches and school administrators.

KEY CONCEPT

ATSAs gain valuable experience in a clinical setting and enable the sports medicine director to focus more time addressing the needs of the entire program.

FUN FACTS

Numerous summer camps and student aide workshops are active throughout the United States each year. Also, many college athletic training programs offer summer camps for high school students interested in entering the field. Both beginners and advanced students can attend summer training camps.

Coaches, too, should be involved in the design and direction of the program. They must be comfortable with the certified athletic trainer and understand that an athletic training program will not only free up more time for the coaching staff, but also enable their athletes to be cared for properly. Many coaches greatly fear that the certified athletic trainer will unnecessarily keep athletes out of practice or games. Keeping the lines of communication open among coaches, the athletic training staff, athletes, and parents goes a long way toward alleviating this fear. Most coaches understand that a healthy athlete translates to more success, so there should be little resistance.

As the program gains in popularity and credibility, coaches will wonder how they ever managed without it. According to Stephen Bunt, Sports Medicine Program Director at Irving High School Texas, "For coaches, the secondary school sports medicine program removes them from involvement in providing care and making decisions regarding athletic injuries for which they are not trained. The certified athletic trainer takes on this responsibility and also provides an integral component in assisting coaches with the development of young athletes." Figure 4–2 illustrates the lines of communication important to the success of the athletic training program.

Program Staff

The head certified athletic trainer is normally in charge of developing the athletic health care program. This person is usually considered the program coordinator or director. The staff includes all members of the athletic health care team: certified athletic trainers, athletic training student aides, therapists, allied health professionals, supervisors, and coordinators of the athletic health care system.

The program director determines how many ATSAs are required in the program, as well as their training and educational requirements (Figure 4–3). The recruitment and screening of applicants is important to the overall success of the athletic training student aide program. The number of students in the program should be determined by need. Having too few or too many students will create problems, with students being either overworked or bored by having too few responsibilities. The size of the school, number of sports to be covered, and overall objectives are the determining factors.

PROGRAM FUNDING

There are many ways to fund a sports medicine program. Sources include state Career and Technical Education (CTE) dollars, basic education funds,

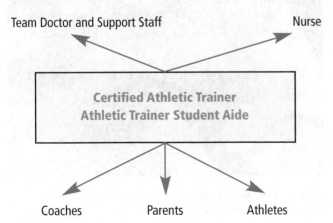

Figure 4–2 Lines of communication critical to the success of the athletic training program.

Team Doctor and Support Staff — Nurse

Certified Athletic Trainer
Athletic Trainer Student Aide

Coaches — Parents — Athletes

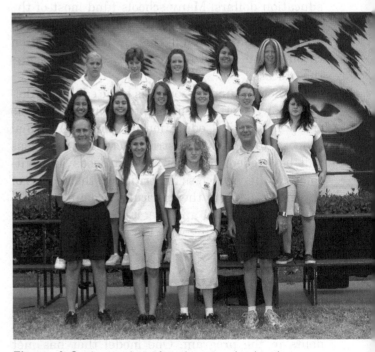

Figure 4–3 The number of students involved in the athletic training student aide program is determined by the athletic director and will vary based on the size of the school's athletic programs. Pictured is Irving High School Sports Medicine Program, Irving, Texas.

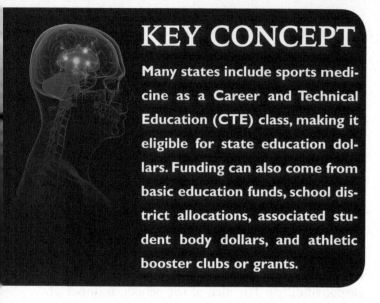

KEY CONCEPT

Many states include sports medicine as a Career and Technical Education (CTE) class, making it eligible for state education dollars. Funding can also come from basic education funds, school district allocations, associated student body dollars, and athletic booster clubs or grants.

school district allocations, associated student-body dollars, athletic booster clubs, and grants, to name a few. Funding will determine if the ATSA program moves beyond the design stage.

One major source of funding for sports medicine programs today is CTE funding. Many states consider sports medicine a career pathway class, which makes such programs eligible for state CTE education dollars. Many schools fund most of the expense of sports medicine, including the program director's salary, through this method. Application through the school district CTE director begins the process.

Another funding source is basic education dollars. Many sports medicine programs offer course credit in physical education or science. A formal proposal to the school district to create a new class will be needed. Specificity as to needs and outcomes of this new class are critical to the success of the proposal. Once the curriculum committee and the school district approve it, the class can be scheduled by working with the principal on site.

A MODEL PROGRAM

The success of a student training program depends on the curriculum and involvement of the students in the program. One model that has met with success establishes a three-year program for grades 10, 11, and 12. Sports medicine is taught

the last two periods of the school day. Students who wish to enter this program must commit to both class periods for all three years prior to being selected for the program.

The first-class period is designated lab science. Students learn the basics of advanced first aid and CPR, athletic training, anatomy, physiology, kinesiology, biomechanics, and sport psychology. Many other disciplines are addressed as well. The curriculum for this class expands as students advance from sophomore to senior year. During the last period, students are in the training room, working with athletes. This is the practical session of the program, where students actually practice what they have learned in previous classroom work (Figure 4–4).

Students who work as athletic training student aides must always be supervised by a certified athletic trainer. As their knowledge grows, they can be given more responsibilities. It is also

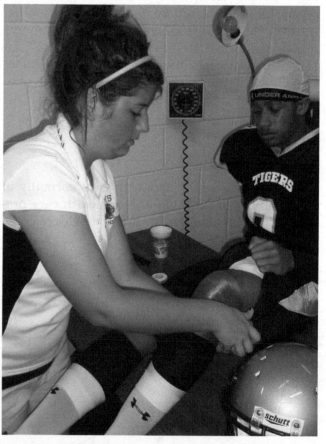

Figure 4–4 ATSAs will learn skills such as taping in the practical portion of the course.

STUDENT EXPECTATIONS

To meet program expectations, students need to be:

- Highly motivated
- Willing to make a long-term commitment to the program
- Successful academically
- On time

- Able to work well with others
- Self-starters
- Willing to do more than asked
- Positive role models

important to note that many states have specific regulatory guidelines that describe the limitations and responsibilities of ATSAs. Not all state guidelines are the same. The following is an example of how they might look for a three-year high school:

First-year students work as apprentices, learning from certified athletic trainers and second-and third-year students. Second-year students take on more leadership roles, with third-year students assuming the role of "head ATSAs." Head ATSAs are in charge of all their sport's organizational needs. They set the training schedule one week in advance, making sure coverage is provided for all practices and contests. All paperwork is completed and checked before being given to the program director for approval. Being able to communicate with the medical staff, coaches, athletes, and parents is important for ATSAs.

Retaining students in the program will be no problem, as long as they are kept involved. It is crucial that students who have been properly trained take an active role. This means actually allowing them to access and treat minor injuries, though always under the direct supervision of the certified athletic trainer. Program directors who insist on doing everything themselves and prevent students from demonstrating what they have learned will have great difficulty retaining and recruiting students. Students must have ownership in "their" program.

One of the most rewarding aspects of teaching a sports medicine class is preparing students for college. Students who graduate from the sports medicine program will be better prepared for post–high school studies. Students' expectations and career goals will be better served by a program that helps them achieve their career objectives.

EXPECTATIONS AND RESPONSIBILITIES OF THE ATSA

Student and program expectations should be set high. Creating expectations with students will generate buy-in. When everyone has a say in how the program will operate, expectations will be easily achieved. The accompanying box describes the expectations required to become an ATSA.

Athletic training student aides have many responsibilities within the athletic training program. The accompanying box describes typical responsibilities assigned to the ATSA.

As students matriculate through the program, head ATSAs are awarded additional responsibilities, as described in the next box. All head ATSAs are under the direct supervision of the certified athletic trainer for all aspects of these additional responsibilities.

Additional Responsibilities of the Head ATSA

- Oversight for all aspects of his or her sport
- Set the training schedule one week in advance

RESPONSIBILITIES OF THE ATSA

- Stock first-aid kit
- Check equipment
- Stock ice chest
- Fill water bottles
- Check injury list from previous practice or game
- Communicate with certified athletic trainer and coaches
- Help with the treatment of injuries and taping (under direct supervision)

- Clean training room prior to leaving for practice or game, and afterward
- Update supply list
- Check out equipment
- Maintain proper training room atmosphere
- Review season with staff and program director
- Have fun!

- Conduct weekly meetings with first-and second-year students
- Communicate expectations to his or her staff (first- and second-year students)
- Communicate daily with coaching staff
- Communicate directly with program director
- Communicate with parents and administration as needed
- Check that all paperwork is completed
- Complete a final report at the end of the season

Daily Duties

Daily duties include setting a good example and representing the program in a positive manner. This means being well groomed and wearing proper attire or a uniform. Suggestive clothing and poor personal hygiene are not conducive to success in a training program. ATSAs must be aware that, just as athletes have required dress codes, so too does the athletic training staff. Proper appearance and behavior demonstrate pride in the program and dedication to the athletic department.

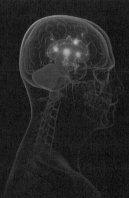

KEY CONCEPT

Expectations of athletic training student aides and the athletic training director are high. ATSAs should be motivated, in good academic standing, able to make and carry through on commitments, and positive role models. Some daily responsibilities of the ATSAs are to maintain equipment and supplies; maintain the training room; communicate with athletes, the certified athletic trainer, and coaches; and assist in the care and treatment of injuries under the supervision of the certified athletic trainer.

Another duty of the ATSA is to be active during practices and games. It is crucial to be visible and to closely follow each and every practice and game. Murphy's Law suggests that the moment one relaxes and stops paying attention, an injury will occur. Everyone at some time finds this to be true. Besides causing embarrassment, such a lapse can put the ATSA's credibility at stake.

The Training Schedule

Many factors must be taken into account when scheduling ATSAs. Today's students are busier than ever; most will be taking advanced courses and have jobs. Transportation to and from practices and games will challenge any program director. This is one of the reasons for scheduling one week in advance. When creating the schedule, flexibility is important. Once a schedule has been set, however, only emergencies should alter it. ATSAs must understand that the training schedule is no different than a schedule for a job. A commitment must be made. See Figure 4–5 for a sample schedule.

Incentives and Awards

All the hours and hard work put in by ATSAs must yield more than intrinsic rewards only. Examples of ways to recognize the dedication of ATSAs are:

- ATSA of the month
- ATSA of the year
- 500 club for attaining 500 hours of training in a year
- School letters
- Recognition at end-of-season banquets
- Pages dedicated to the program in the school's yearbook

EVALUATION OF THE ATSA PROGRAM

Evaluation of the entire program should be ongoing throughout the year. Evaluations are most useful when changes can be made periodically during the year. Successful programs continue to evolve only through self-reflection and outside evaluation.

BOY'S BASEBALL

Monday	Tuesday	Wednesday	Thursday	Friday	Saturday	Sunday
1 Melissa Kelli	2 John Kelli	3 Melissa Scott	4 Scott John	5 Melissa John	6 Kelli Scott	7
8 John Kelli	9 Varsity Game M, K J, S JV Game	10 Melissa John	11 Varsity Game M, S K, J JV Game	12 Melissa Scott	13 Varsity Game M, J S, K JV Game	14
15	16	17	18	19	20	21
22	23	24	25	26	27	28
29	30	31				

Head ATSA
Melissa
ATSAs
John
Kelli
Scott

Practices and games should be scheduled one to two weeks in advance. A similar schedule should be created for each sport.

Figure 4–5 Sample schedule for ATSAs.

Evaluations must be approached as a win–win situation. Constructive evaluation encourages learning and helps the program run more efficiently. Evaluations should be made in these areas:

- Individual ATSAs
- Head ATSA
- Overall sport season
- Coaches' evaluations of their ATSAs and the entire athletic training program
- End-of-year evaluation
- Evaluation of program director

Evaluations are most effective when followed up with a personal meeting.

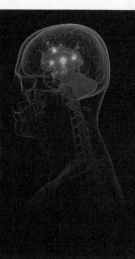

KEY CONCEPT

Evaluations are most useful when changes can be made periodically during the year. Evaluations should be made in the following areas: individual ATSAs, overall sport season, end-of-year evaluation, and evaluation of the program director.

CONCLUSION

The athletic training student aide (ASTA) program can be a huge asset to any athletic training program. When deciding how to implement a program, carefully analyze all of its aspects. The more organized the program is from the beginning, the more successful it will become. A strong ATSA program enables the program director to use his or her time more efficiently. It also helps to ensure that athletes have proper care before, during, and after practices and games. Students will learn skills that will prepare them for college and their eventual careers.

REVIEW QUESTIONS

1. What is an athletic training student aide?
2. What should a certified athletic trainer consider when organizing a student aide program?
3. How does the athletic training program director determine how many ATSAs are needed?
4. List the various sources for funding a sports medicine program.
5. What are the program expectations of a student aspiring to be an ATSA?
6. What responsibilities do ATSAs have in the athletic training program?
7. What are some ways in which an athletic training program can be evaluated?

PROJECTS AND ACTIVITIES

1. If your school has a certified athletic trainer, meet with him or her and discuss the athletic training student aide program. What information do you feel was most important and relevant to your school? If you do not have a sports medicine program at your school, find one in your area that does and report your findings to the class.
2. You were just hired to organize a sports medicine program at a local high school. What steps would you take first? How would you know if your program is successful?

LEARNING LINKS

- The following high schools have athletic training student aide programs. Visit their websites and look for information related to their programs. How do they differ from your own program?

  Issaquah High School: (https://sites.google.com/site/ihssportsmed/home)

  Venice High School: (https://venicesportsmed.org/)

- Wylie High School: (http://www.wylieisd.net)

  Heritage High School: (http://www.edline.net/pages/HeritageHS/Advanced_Academics/Sports) Medicine_Academy

  Irving High School: (http://www.irvingisd.net/tigersportsmed/home.html)

- Visit the athletic training association website for your state. What are the guidelines and regulations for athletic training student aide programs?

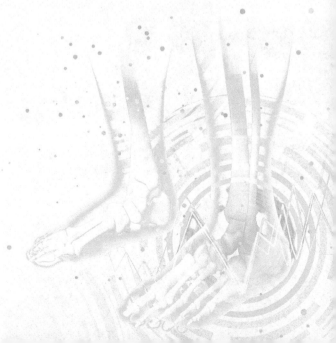

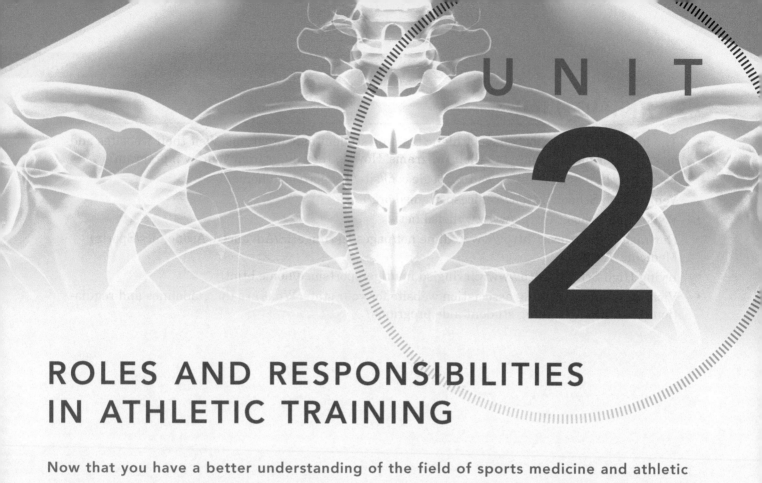

UNIT 2

ROLES AND RESPONSIBILITIES IN ATHLETIC TRAINING

Now that you have a better understanding of the field of sports medicine and athletic training, you are ready to begin to learn about the roles and responsibilities of the professionals in the field. This unit addresses emergency planning, preseason conditioning, nutrition, sport psychology, assessment and evaluation of sports injuries, therapeutic modalities, and taping and wrapping procedures. These topics form the foundation of what you will need to know to help the athlete prepare and stay healthy.

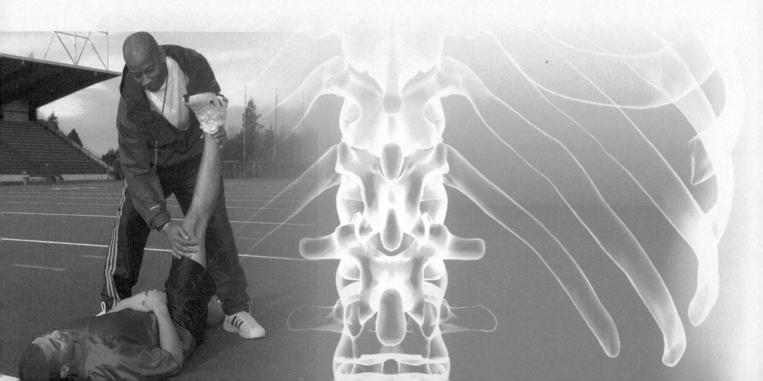

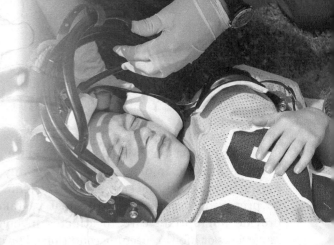

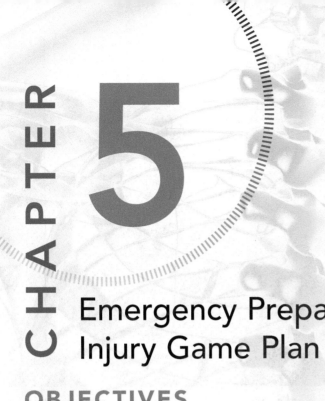

Emergency Preparedness: Injury Game Plan

OBJECTIVES

Upon completion of this chapter, the reader should be able to:

- Define emergency preparedness
- Discuss the importance of a written emergency action plan
- List the components of the emergency plan
- State the roles of everyone involved in an athletic emergency
- Identify how to activate the EMS system
- Identify the difference between defined medical emergencies and nonemergencies
- Describe why emergency medical cards are important

KEY TERMS

defined medical emergency *A medical illness or traumatic injury that has the potential to be life-threatening or progress to a life-threatening event in the absence of treatment.*

emergency action plan (EAP) *A formal document outlining the steps to be taken in the event of a medical crisis or disaster.*

emergency medical service (EMS) system *The response system in a particular area that is called upon in the event of a medical crisis or traumatic injury. This usually consists of personnel trained in basic or advanced life support, and an ambulance or equipped emergency vehicle to transport them and the injured victim to a hospital emergency room.*

emergency preparedness *Being properly equipped and trained for any medical crisis or disaster.*

nonemergency *Any medical illness or injury that does not pose a serious threat to life or limb.*

EMERGENCY PREPAREDNESS

Being properly equipped and trained for any medical crisis or disaster is **emergency preparedness**. Because athletic injuries can occur at any time during any activity, the sports medicine team must be prepared. Expedient action must be taken to provide appropriate care to athletes involved in hazardous or life-threatening conditions. The development and implementation of an emergency plan helps ensure the best care is provided.

Each athletic organization has a duty to develop an emergency plan that can be implemented immediately and to provide appropriate health care (care that meets professional standards) to all sports participants. Preparation includes formulation of an emergency plan, proper coverage of events, maintenance of appropriate emergency equipment and supplies, notification and use of appropriate emergency medical personnel, and continuing education in the area of emergency medicine. Through careful pre-participation physical screenings, adequate medical coverage, safe practice and training techniques, and other safety avenues, some potential emergencies can also be averted.

However, accidents and injuries are inherent to sports, and proper preparation on behalf of the sports medicine team will enable appropriate management of each emergency situation.

THE EMERGENCY ACTION PLAN

Dealing with injuries without a written plan is a recipe for disaster. Programs that have well-thought-out, written action plans can deal with

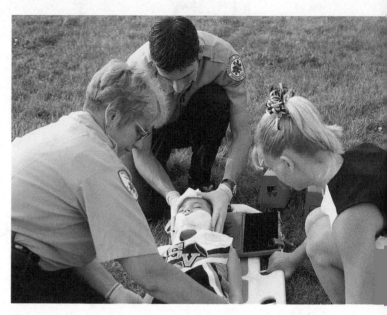

Figure 5–1 When an injury occurs, it is important to follow the emergency action plan.

injuries in a systematic, logical manner that avoids missteps and mistakes. The lack of such a plan can lead to inadequate or inappropriate treatment of injuries (Figure 5–1).

The written **emergency action plan (EAP)** should be customized to fit the needs of the organization. The EAP should specify the program's needs within four basic categories: emergency personnel, emergency communication, emergency equipment, and transportation. A wealth of information that can help in designing a plan for an athletic program is available online. Visit the websites listed in the box on page 57 to view the EAPs developed by these universities and organizations.

The sports medicine staff at the University of Georgia, under the direction of Ron Courson,

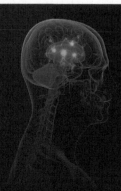

KEY CONCEPT

Athletic organizations have a duty to develop an emergency plan that can be implemented immediately, and to provide appropriate health care to all sports participants.

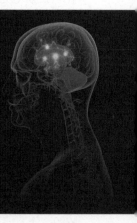

KEY CONCEPT

A written emergency action plan is important because it sets out a systematic approach to be followed in an emergency. This helps personnel avoid mistakes and prevents inadequate treatment.

developed a template for a complete emergency action plan. It can be used in the creation of an emergency plan for any athletic program, at any level. The format of Courson's template is the basis of the framework for the discussion in this chapter.

Emergency Personnel

The EAP should clearly outline the roles of emergency personnel who are on the scene of a medical crisis. Generally the first responder is a member of the athletic training staff. The athletic training staff—members of which should be available at all practices, competitions, and training events—is to be, at a minimum, trained in CPR and first aid. All members of the athletic training staff are responsible for knowing and being able to implement the emergency action plan.

Each member of the athletic training staff should be assigned specific roles to play in the event of an emergency. The most important role is providing immediate care to the injured athlete. This should be done by the most qualified member of the athletic training staff on the scene, usually the head athletic trainer or team physician. Other members of the staff should be assigned to locate and obtain all emergency equipment needed at the scene (Figure 5–2). Emergency team members must know what equipment is needed and where to find it efficiently. These duties are usually assigned to the coach or athletic training student

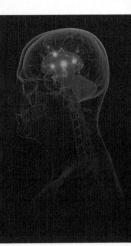

KEY CONCEPT

An emergency action plan should be tailored to the program for which it is written. It should outline the program's needs in terms of emergency personnel, emergency communication, emergency equipment, and transportation.

aides. One member of the athletic staff on scene should be assigned to activate the **emergency medical service (EMS) system** as early as possible. The emergency medical service system is a national medical response protocol designed to address minor and major medical emergencies. EMS is typically activated by calling 911 on any immediately available phone. Some remote areas of the country may not be served by 911 coverage. In this case, it is important to call the local police department. This is especially crucial if emergency medical service is not already present at the sporting event. The individual assigned to this task must be able to clearly and calmly communicate the situation over the telephone, and he or

EMERGENCY ACTION PLAN INTERNET RESOURCES

- California Institute of Technology, Emergency Action Plan: www.safety.caltech.edu/documents/38-emergency_action_plan_template.doc
  - Millersville University, Athletic Training Emergency Action Plan: http://www.millersville.edu/athletictraining/emergency.php
  - University of Northern Iowa, Guidelines for Health and Safety and Emergency Action https://coe.uni.edu/sites/default/files/wysiwyg/ats_pp_handbook_2013_0.pdf
- Emergency Action Plan Template, developed by Lewis Payton, Auburn University, Alabama: http://www.cdc.gov/niosh/docs/2004-101/emrgact/emrgact1.html
  - Emergency Action Plan (EAP): https://usm.maine.edu/sites/default/files/nursing/EAPSONandPresOffice.pdf

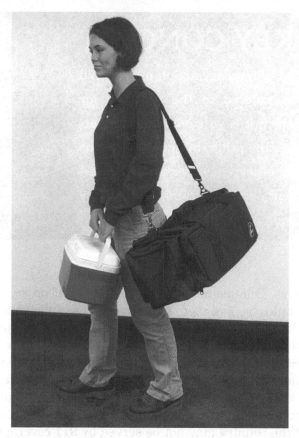

Figure 5–2 At least one member of the athletic training staff should be responsible for bringing the appropriate equipment to the game site or knowing where to quickly retrieve it if the need arises.

she must be familiar with the venue in order to provide proper directions. Once the EMS arrives, someone must be available to direct them to the scene. This individual should be able to enter any locked areas or facilities.

Emergency Communication

Good working relationships between the athletic training staff and emergency medical personnel go a long way toward ensuring the best care for an injured athlete. These relationships should be established long before an emergency occurs. This builds rapport and clarifies the roles of the athletic training staff and the EMS providers in the event of an emergency.

Athletic training staff on the scene must have access to a working phone. Before each event, the communication system should be checked to ensure that it is in proper working order. A backup plan should be in place in case the primary communication system is inoperable.

A procedure should be in place for clearly communicating the situation to the EMS providers after activation of the EMS system (Figure 5–3). It is important to relay to the EMS the name, address, and phone number of the caller; the number of athletes injured; the condition of the injured; care and treatment being provided at the scene by the athletic training staff; accurate directions to the scene; and any other information requested by the dispatcher.

Emergency Equipment

If the equipment needed to deal with an emergency is stored miles away from the site of the crisis, it will do the athletic training staff and the

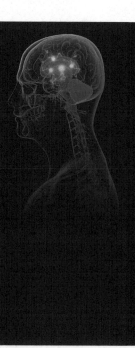

KEY CONCEPT

The athletic training staff should have clearly defined roles in an emergency situation. These roles should encompass immediate care of the athlete, retrieval of emergency equipment, activation of the **EMS** system, and direction of **EMS** to the scene.

KEY CONCEPT

When activating **EMS**, the following information must be readily available: name, address, and phone number of the caller; number of athletes injured; condition of the injured; care and treatment being provided at the scene by the athletic training staff; accurate directions to the scene; and any other information requested by the dispatcher.

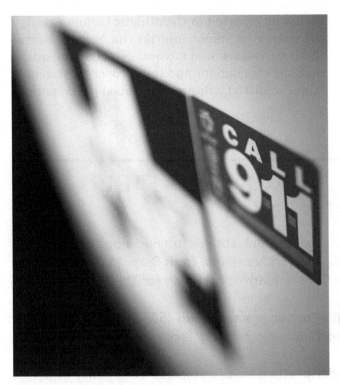

Figure 5–3 To activate EMS, dial 911 (if available in your area) and clearly communicate the situation in a calm, collected ordered tone. Courtesy of PhotoDisc

IDENTIFYING A MEDICAL EMERGENCY

Defined medical emergencies consist of breathing cessation, severe bleeding, no pulse, concussion with loss of consciousness, neck or spinal injury, fractures, dislocations, eye injuries, severe asthma attack, heat-related illness, or any injury causing signs of shock. Shock, which is defined as collapse of the cardiovascular system, is a precursor to death. A complete guide to the assessment and evaluation of athletic injuries is included in Chapter 11.

DID YOU KNOW? The "Golden Hour" is accepted as a national standard in trauma care. This phrase recognizes that, in order to assure the best possible outcome, an injury victim has 60 minutes from the time of initial injury to being admitted to the trauma center for care.

FUN FACTS According to the National Center for Catastrophic Sports Injury Research, high school football accounted for the greatest number of direct catastrophic injuries of all fall sports; it is followed by wrestling for winter sports, and baseball in the spring.

injured athlete no good. All equipment that might be necessary for an emergency must be readily accessible, in good working condition, and checked before each event or competition. Individuals providing care to athletes must be knowledgeable in the purpose and application of the equipment on hand.

Transportation

EMS providers, and an ambulance, should be on standby at any event where there is a high risk of traumatic injury. This will lessen the response time for EMS and ensure that the injured athlete receives timely, proper care. Consideration must be given to the level of experience of the EMS providers available, their qualifications, and the sophistication of equipment available on the ambulance. An onsite ambulance should have clear access to the event so that it can enter and exit the site without delay. Athletes with unstable injuries should never be transported in a vehicle that is not appropriately equipped to deal with emergencies. The box on page 60 shows a completed EAP for a particular sports venue.

KEY CONCEPT The difference between a defined medical emergency and a non-emergency is the threat of loss of limb or life. Any injury, no matter how minor, should be reported to the certified athletic trainer.

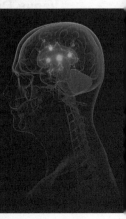

Nonemergencies consist of all other injuries that do not threaten life or limb. These include abrasions, minor cuts, strains, sprains, minor concussions without loss of consciousness, contusions, and so on. All injuries, no matter how minor, should be reported to the athletic training staff. If left untreated, minor injuries can become serious and require advanced medical care. It is important that athletes understand that proper treatment of minor injuries facilitates continued participation.

EMERGENCY PLAN: TRACK AND FIELD STADIUM VENUE

Emergency Personnel: certified athletic trainer and student athletic trainer aides onsite for practice and competition; additional sports medicine staff accessible from Butts-Mehre athletic training facility (adjacent to track) and Stegeman Coliseum athletic training facility (across street from track)

Emergency Communication: fixed telephone line under practice shed (555-5555); additional fixed telephone lines accessible from Butts-Mehre athletic training facility adjacent to track (555-5550 and 555-5555)

Emergency Equipment: supplies maintained under practice shed; additional emergency equipment (AED, trauma kit, splint kit, spine board) accessible from Butts-Mehre athletic training facility adjacent to track

Roles of First Responders

1. Immediate care of the injured or ill student-athlete.
2. Emergency equipment retrieval.
3. Activation of emergency medical system (EMS).
   a. 911 call (provide name, address, telephone number; number of individuals injured; condition of injured; first-aid treatment; specific directions; other information as requested).
   b. notify campus police at 555-5555.
4. Direction of EMS to scene.
   a. open appropriate gates.
   b. designate individual to "flag down" EMS and direct to scene.
   c. scene control: limit scene to first-aid providers and move bystanders away from area.

Venue Directions: Track and field stadium is located on Lumpkin Street (cross street Pinecrest) adjacent to Butts-Mehre Hall. Three gates provide access to track:

1. Lumpkin Street (most direct route): directly across from Catholic Student Center.
2. Smith Street: opens to artificial turf practice field adjacent to track; accesses practice field drive to track.
3. Rutherford Street: opens directly to practice field drive to track; gate must be activated from outside by 5-digit security code or opened by personnel from inside (either by 5-digit security code or trip switch in storage building adjacent to gate).

(*continues*)

(continued)

Venue Map

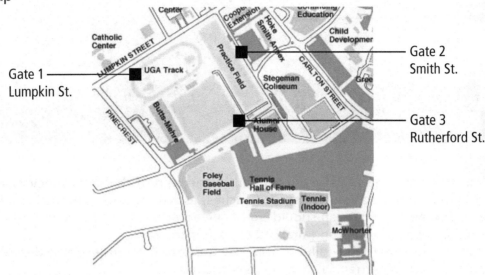

Phone numbers changed from original.

Courtesy of Ron Courson, Director of Sports Medicine, University of Georgia.

EMERGENCY MEDICAL CARDS

Each athlete must have an up-to-date emergency information profile on record. This information is used by athletic trainers and EMS personnel to contact the athlete's nearest relative or guardian if an injury occurs. It also contains important medical information that could be useful in case of an emergency. Hospital preference, family doctor's phone numbers, and parental permission to treat and transport are other important elements of the emergency medical card. Emergency medical cards contain confidential information and should not be left out where others can view them.

CONCLUSION

Emergency preparedness is the central element of a superior sports medicine program. Emergencies become manageable when everyone involved understands his or her role and works as a team.

The emergency preparedness team consists of everyone involved in athletics: certified athletic trainers, athletic training student aides, support medical staff, EMS, coaches, athletes, and (if needed) bystanders.

The emergency plan must be documented and agreed upon by all parties, including the local emergency medical services personnel. Practice makes perfect. An emergency plan that has never been set into action will encounter challenges. It is important to hold practice sessions at least once a year to familiarize everyone involved with the process.

The importance of being properly prepared when athletic emergencies arise cannot be overstated. An athlete's survival may depend on well-trained, well-prepared athletic health care providers.

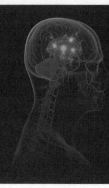

KEY CONCEPT

Emergency medical cards are valuable to the athletic training staff because they place all important contact information at their fingertips. Emergency medical cards also permit the athletic training staff to treat, and provide access to emergency care for, an injured minor athlete in the event the parents or guardians are unavailable.

It is prudent to encourage athletic department ownership of the emergency plan by involving the athletic administration and sport coaches, as well as sports medicine personnel, in its development. The emergency plan should be reviewed at least once a year with all athletic personnel, in conjunction with CPR and first-aid refresher training.

As important as the emergency plan is, it is also important to understand the difference between defined medical emergencies and nonemergencies.

Emergency medical cards should be on the sideline of every practice and game. No athlete should be allowed to participate without an emergency card on hand.

REVIEW QUESTIONS

1. What is meant by emergency preparedness?
2. What is the importance of having a written emergency action plan?
3. Define the four basic components of the emergency plan discussed in this chapter.
4. What are the roles of emergency personnel?
5. How is the EMS system activated in your school or facility?
6. List the defined medical emergencies described in this chapter.
7. What are nonemergencies?
8. Why is it important to have emergency medical cards at every practice and game?

PROJECTS AND ACTIVITIES

1. Review the emergency action plan for your school. What are its primary components? When was the plan written and last revised? Is there a separate, written plan for athletic emergencies?
2. Create a detailed map of each sports venue located on school grounds. This map should easily direct EMS personnel to the site. Include in your map any access doors/gates, as well as any special instructions that might be needed.

LEARNING LINKS

* Please see the Emergency Action Plan Internet Resources box earlier in this chapter for a list of colleges and programs that have EAPs.
* Visit http://www.nata.org and read the NATA position statement on planning for emergencies at athletic events.
* Visit the website of your local EMS agency and search for information on responses to athletic events.

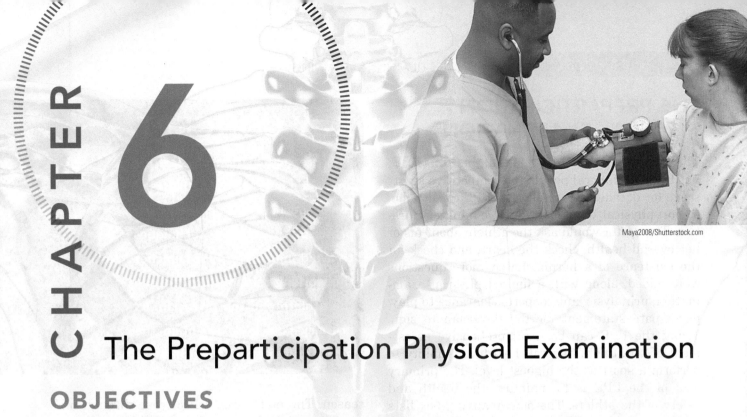
Maya2008/Shutterstock.com

CHAPTER 6

The Preparticipation Physical Examination

OBJECTIVES

Upon completion of this chapter, the reader should be able to:

- Discuss the needs and overall goals of the preparticipation physical examination
- Distinguish between office-based and station-based exams
- List the components of the preparticipation physical examination
- Describe the clearance process for athletic examinations
- Discuss confidentiality concerns with recordkeeping

KEY TERMS

clearance *Permission granted by a physician, based on an athlete's physical examination, to participate in a sporting event.*

office-based preparticipation physical examination *A complete health screening done by the athlete's family physician.*

preparticipation physical examination (PPE) *A comprehensive assessment of an athlete's overall health and ability to perform a sport at the highest level. This examination emphasizes the areas of greatest concern in sports participation and identifies problem areas in the athlete's history.*

station-based preparticipation examination *Screening of the athlete by several different specialists who are responsible for specific aspects of the exam—such as medical history; height, weight, and vital signs; physical examination; and medical clearance.*

THE PREPARTICIPATION PHYSICAL EXAMINATION

The **preparticipation physical examination (PPE)** has been an integral part of the competitive sports scene for decades. Originally, the PPE consisted of a short physical, often less than five minutes' duration. The doctor would ask the athlete about his or her overall health, check the heart, and check for the existence of a hernia. Later, more questions were added, along with a limited physical examination, urinalysis, and a sports clearance to play/participate statement for the physician to sign. Today, the PPE can be a comprehensive assessment of an athlete's overall health and ability to perform a sport at the highest level. The primary goal of the PPE is to maintain the health and safety of the athlete. The accompanying box lists all the goals of the PPE.

Timing of the Preparticipation Physical Examination

The PPE should take place a minimum of six weeks prior to the beginning of the athlete's sport

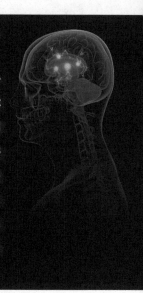

KEY CONCEPT

The preparticipation physical examination helps identify athletes at risk of specific types of injuries and prescribe preventive techniques to avoid injury. The PPE launches the working relationship between the athlete and the physician. Its primary goal is to maintain the health and safety of the athlete.

season. The end of the school year through mid-summer offers the best timing. Athletes who are found to have musculoskeletal problems will then have time for rehabilitation and a strengthening regimen before they begin their seasons. Any athlete who is rehabilitating over the summer must be reevaluated before receiving full clearance to participate.

GOALS OF THE PREPARTICIPATION PHYSICAL EXAMINATION

- Determination of the general health of the athlete
- Disclosure of defects that may limit participation
- Detection of conditions that may predispose the athlete to injury
- Determination of optimal level of performance
- Classification of the athlete according to individual qualifications
- Fulfillment of legal and insurance requirements
- Evaluation of the level of maturation of younger athletes
- Evaluation of fitness and performance for possible improvement prior to participation

- Provision of opportunities to compete for students with specific health issues that may preclude a blanket approval (for instance, an athlete with diabetes can still participate but needs access to medical services and may have to take special precautions)
- Provisions of opportunity to counsel youths regarding personal health issues
- Entry of the athlete into the local sports medicine environment, thereby establishing a doctor-patient relationship

Source: McKeag, D. B.; Sallis, R. E. (2000). "Factors at play in the athletic pre-participation examination." *American Family Physician*, 61, 2683–2690, 2696–2698.

The two most common settings for performance of the PPE are the doctor's office or a station-based environment. Each has its own advantages.

Station-Based Preparticipation Examination

The **station-based preparticipation examination** involves several different specialists in the examination process. Athletes move from one station (specialist) to another. Each specialist is responsible for one aspect of the examination.

Stations include medical history and basic measurements of blood pressure, height, weight, and eyesight. Specialists are responsible for specific examinations in their areas and often include family physicians, orthopedic specialists, physical therapists, athletic trainers, podiatrists, and pediatricians. An example is an orthopedic surgeon examining joints for stability and checking past injuries to joints and the skeletal system. Physical therapists are responsible for strength assessment, and podiatrists look for possible problems involving the feet. This team approach allows a complete assessment of the athlete prior to participation.

FUN FACTS

According to the *Pediatric Annals* (Krowchuk, 1997), 78% of teenagers get their only physical examination through sports physicals.

The stations used in preparticipation physical examinations differ with almost every program. Table 6–1 presents an overview of required and optional stations, and identifies the appropriate personnel for each station.

Station-based examinations offer many advantages over traditional, office-based physicals. These include low cost and the ability to examine many athletes in the same setting. Another major advantage is that the athlete will see several different sports medicine specialists throughout the exam process. A disadvantage can be the difficulty of recruiting volunteer physicians, therapists, and other sports medicine personnel. Finding a facility to handle a station-based examination can also be a challenge.

Table 6–1 Required and Optional Stations and Appropriate Personnel	
REQUIRED STATIONS	**APPROPRIATE PERSONNEL**
Sign-in, height, weight, vital signs, vision	Performed by ancillary personnel (nurse, athletic trainer, or physical therapist)
History review	Must be performed by physician
Physical examination (both medical and orthopedic)	Must be performed by physician
Medical clearance	Must be performed by physician
OPTIONAL STATIONS	**APPROPRIATE PERSONNEL**
Nutrition assessment	Dietitian
Dental exam	Dentist
Orthopedic examination (musculoskeletal)	Physician
Flexibility	Athletic trainer or physical therapist
Body composition	Physiologist, physical therapist
Strength	Trainer, coach, therapist, physiologist
Speed, agility, power, balance, endurance	Trainer, coach, physiologist

Adapted from: Matheson, Gordon O. (1998). "Pre-participation screening of athletes." *Journal of the American Medical Association, 279* (22), 1829–1830.

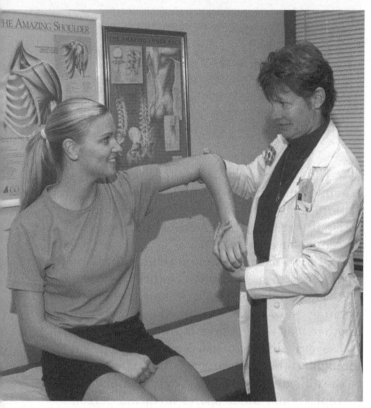

Figure 6–1 The athlete's family physician performs a complete assessment in the office-based physical examination.

Office-Based Preparticipation Physical Examination

The **office-based preparticipation physical examination** is done in the traditional doctor's office (Figure 6–1). The athlete's family physician usually has the patient's complete medical history as a basis for the examination. The quiet setting allows the doctor to discuss multiple health issues with the patient. The patient's immunization history can be reviewed and updated as needed.

COMPONENTS OF THE PREPARTICIPATION PHYSICAL EXAMINATION

The medical history is the cornerstone of any medical evaluation. A complete history will identify approximately 75% of problems affecting athletes. To assure the accuracy of the information to be gathered, the athlete and parents should complete the history section together prior to the examination. Parents or guardians should be actively involved in the athlete's evaluation.

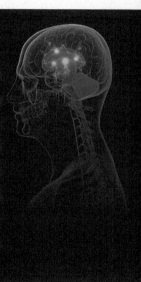

KEY CONCEPT

In a station-based setting, the athlete is evaluated by many physicians or specialists, each responsible for one aspect of the complete physical evaluation. In an office-based setting, the athlete's family physician completes a thorough evaluation of the athlete's physical status.

The recommended baseline history includes the following general information:

- Medical conditions and diseases
- Surgeries
- Hospitalizations
- Medications (prescription, over-the-counter, supplements)
- Allergies (medications, insects, environmental)
- Immunization status
- Menstrual history
- Pulmonary status
- Neurological status
- Musculoskeletal status
- Injuries or illness since last exam

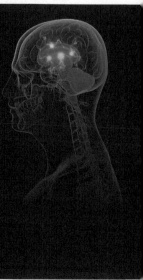

KEY CONCEPT

The components of the preparticipation physical examination include baseline medical history; height, weight, blood pressure; assessment of eyes, ears, nose, and throat; and evaluation of the heart, neurological assessment, abdomen, genitalia (males only), skin, and musculoskeletal system.

The PPE is a screening tool that emphasizes the areas of greatest concern in sports participation and factors identified as problems in the athlete's history. Therefore, the recommended standard components of the PPE include height, weight, pulse, blood pressure, eyes, ear/nose/throat, heart, abdomen, neurological status, genitalia (males only), skin, and musculoskeletal. Figure 6–2A–C shows the qualifying physical examination form used by the Minnesota State High School League. It was developed by their sports medicine advisory committee and is reprinted with permission.

CLEARANCE FOR PARTICIPATION IN SPORTS

The most important and difficult decision in the PPE is determining whether an athlete should be cleared for sports participation. **Clearance** can be divided into three categories:

1. Unrestricted clearance.
2. Clearance after completion of further evaluation or rehabilitation.
3. No clearance for certain types of sports or for all sports.

When an abnormality or condition is found that may limit an athlete's participation or predispose him or her to further injury, the physician must consider the following questions:

- Does the problem place the athlete at increased risk of injury?
- Is another participant placed at risk of injury because of the problem?

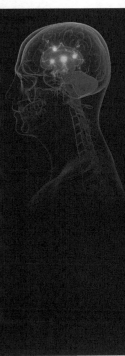

KEY CONCEPT

The physician must consider any potential problems that may put the athlete at risk of injury, and compare those with the potential risks involved in the athlete's sport of choice. Based on this analysis, the physician must determine if the athlete is able to compete fully, able to compete only after training and rehabilitation, or unable to compete because of being at high risk.

- Can the athlete safely participate with treatment?
- Can limited participation be allowed while treatment is being completed?
- If clearance is denied for only certain sports or sports categories, in what activities can the athlete safely participate?

To aid in this decision, sports are classified based on degree or level of contact and strenuousness. Contact or collision sports put the athlete at high risk of traumatic injuries involving force. Limited-contact sports put the athlete at some risk of traumatic injuries. In noncontact sports, the athlete has a low risk of traumatic injury as a result of force. Table 6–2 highlights the sports classified in each category.

RECORDKEEPING

After the preparticipation examination has concluded. and the examination forms have been completed and signed by the physician, the next, crucial step is managing the resulting information. Information gathered through the PPE must be made available to coaches, trainers, and the athletic director.

Valuable information will go to waste if the athletic staff does not have access to it.

DID YOU KNOW? Sudden death in people younger than 35, often due to undiscovered heart defects or overlooked heart abnormalities, is rare. When these sudden deaths occur, it is often during physical activity, such as playing a sport, and more often occurs in males than in females. (Mayo Clinic, 2017.)

Revised 4/18/18

COPY this Clearance Form for the student to return to the school.   KEEP the complete document   in the student's medical record.

2018-2019 SPORTS QUALIFYING PHYSICAL EXAMINATION CLEARANCE FORM
Minnesota State High School League

Student Name: _____   Birth Date: _____   Age: ____   Gender: M / F
Address: _____
Home Telephone: _____ - _____ - _____   Mobile Telephone _____ - _____ - _____
School: _____   Grade: _____   Sports: _____

I certify that the above student has been medically evaluated and is deemed to be physically fit to: (Check Only One Box)

☐ (1) Participate in all school interscholastic activities without restrictions.
☐ (2) Participate in any activity not crossed out below.

Sport Classification Based on Contact		
Collision Contact Sports	Limited Contact Sports	Non-contact Sports
Basketball Cheerleading Diving Football Gymnastics Ice Hockey Lacrosse Alpine Skiing Soccer Wrestling	Baseball Field Events: ❖ High Jump ❖ Pole Vault Floor Hockey Nordic Skiing Softball Volleyball	Badminton Bowling Cross Country Running Dance Team Field Events: ❖ Discus ❖ Shot Put Golf Swimming Tennis Track

Sport Classification Based on Intensity & Strenuousness			
III. High (>50% MVC)	Field Events: ❖ Discus ❖ Shot Put Gymnastics*†	Alpine Skiing*† Wrestling*	
II. Moderate (20-50% MVC)	Diving*†	Dance Team Football* Field Events: ❖ High Jump ❖ Pole Vault*† Synchronized Swimming† Track — Sprints	Basketball* Ice Hockey* Lacrosse* Nordic Skiing — Freestyle Track — Middle Distance Swimming†
I. Low (<20% MVC)	Bowling Golf	Baseball* Cheerleading Floor Hockey Softball* Volleyball	Badminton Cross Country Running Nordic Skiing — Classical Soccer* Tennis Track — Long Distance
	A. Low (<40% Max O₂)	B. Moderate (40-70% Max O₂)	C. High (>70% Max O₂)

Increasing Static Component (vertical axis)

Increasing Dynamic Component → → → →

☐ (3) Requires further evaluation before a final recommendation can be made.
Additional recommendations for the school or parents: _____
_____
_____

☐ (4) Not cleared for: ☐ All Sports
                          ☐ Specific Sports _____
Reason: _____
_____

Sport Classification Based on Intensity & Strenuousness: This classification is based on peak static and dynamic components achieved during competition. It should be noted, however, that higher values may be reached during training. The increasing dynamic component is defined in terms of the estimated percent of maximal oxygen uptake (MaxO₂) achieved and results in an increasing cardiac output. The increasing static component is related to the estimated percent of maximal voluntary contraction (MVC) reached and results in an increasing blood pressure load. The lowest total cardiovascular demands (cardiac output and blood pressure) are shown in lightest shading and the highest in darkest shading. The graduated shading in between depicts low moderate, moderate, and high moderate total cardiovascular demands. *Danger of bodily collision. †Increased risk if syncope occurs. Reprinted with permission from: Maron BJ, Zipes DP. 36th Bethesda Conference: eligibility recommendations for competitive athletes with cardiovascular abnormalities. *J Am Coll Cardiol.* 2005; 45(8):1317–1375.

I have examined the above named student and completed the Sports Qualifying Physical Exam as required by the Minnesota State High School League. A copy of the physical exam is on record in my office and can be made available to the school at the request of the parents.

Attending Provider Signature _____   Date of Exam _____
Print Provider Name: _____
Office/Clinic Name _____
City, State, Zip Code _____   Address: _____
Office Telephone: _____ - _____ - _____   E-Mail Address: _____

IMMUNIZATIONS [Tdap; meningococcal (MCV4, 1-2 doses); HPV (3 doses); MMR (2 doses); hep B (3 doses); hep A (2 doses); varicella (2 doses or history of disease); polio (3-4 doses); influenza (annual)]
☐ Up-to-date (see attached school documentation)   ☐ Not reviewed at this visit
IMMUNIZATIONS GIVEN TODAY: _____

EMERGENCY INFORMATION
Allergies _____
Other Information _____
Emergency Contact: _____   Relationship _____
Telephone: (H) _____ - _____ - _____ (W) _____ - _____ - _____ (C) _____ - _____ - _____
Personal Provider _____   Office Telephone _____ - _____ - _____

This form is valid for 3 calendar years from above date with a normal Annual Health Questionnaire.
FOR SCHOOL ADMINISTRATION USE: ☐ [Year 2 Normal]   ☐ [Year 3 Normal]

Reference: Preparticipation Physical Evaluation (4th Edition): AAFP, AAP, ACSM, AMSSM, AOSSM, AOASM; 2010.

Figure 6–2A Sports Qualifying Physical Examination (page 1). Courtesy of Minnesota State High School League (www.MSHSL.org).

2018-2019 SPORTS QUALIFYING PHYSICAL HISTORY FORM
Minnesota State High School League

Student Name: _____   Birth Date: _____   Date of Exam: _____

History

Circle Question Number (1.) of questions for which the answer is unknown.   Circle Y for Yes or N for No

GENERAL QUESTIONS
1. Has a doctor ever denied or restricted your participation in sports for any reason or told you to give up sports? .... Y / N
2. Do you have an ongoing medical condition (like diabetes, asthma, anemia, infections)? .... Y / N
3. Are you currently taking any prescription or nonprescription (over-the-counter) medicines or pills? .... Y / N
   List: _____
4. Do you have allergies to medicines, pollens, foods, or stinging insects? .... Y / N
5. Have you ever spent the night in a hospital? .... Y / N
6. Have you ever had surgery? .... Y / N

HEART HEALTH QUESTIONS ABOUT YOU
7. Have you ever passed out or nearly passed out DURING exercise? .... Y / N
8. Have you ever passed out or nearly passed out AFTER exercise? .... Y / N
9. Have you ever had discomfort, pain, tightness, or pressure in your chest during exercise? .... Y / N
10. Does your heart race or skip beats (irregular beats) during exercise? .... Y / N
11. Has a doctor ever told you that you have? (circle):
    High blood pressure   A heart murmur   High cholesterol   A heart infection   Rheumatic fever   Kawasaki's Disease
12. Has a doctor ever ordered a test for your heart? (for example, ECG/EKG, echocardiogram, stress test) .... Y / N
13. Do you get lightheaded or feel more short of breath than expected during exercise? .... Y / N
14. Have you ever had an unexplained seizure? .... Y / N
15. Do you get more tired or short of breath more quickly than your friends during exercise? .... Y / N

HEART HEALTH QUESTIONS ABOUT YOUR FAMILY
16. Has any family member or relative died of heart problems or had an unexpected or unexplained sudden death before age 50 (including unexplained drowning or unexplained car accident)? .... Y / N
17. Does anyone in your family have hypertrophic cardiomyopathy, Marfan syndrome, arrhythmogenic right ventricular cardiomyopathy, long QT syndrome, short QT syndrome, Brugada syndrome, or catecholaminergic polymorphic ventricular tachycardia? .... Y / N
18. Does anyone in your family have a heart problem, pacemaker, or implanted defibrillator? .... Y / N
19. Has anyone in your family had unexplained fainting, unexplained seizures, or near drowning? .... Y / N

BONE AND JOINT QUESTIONS
20. Have you ever had an injury, like a sprain, muscle or ligament tear or tendonitis that caused you to miss a practice or game? .... Y / N
21. Have you had any broken or fractured bones or dislocated joints? .... Y / N
22. Have you ever had an injury that required x-rays, MRI, CT scan, injections, therapy, a brace, a cast, or crutches? .... Y / N
23. Have you ever had a stress fracture? .... Y / N
24. Have you ever been told that you have or have you had an x-ray for neck instability or atlantoaxial instability? (Down syndrome or dwarfism) .... Y / N
25. Do you regularly use a brace, orthotics or other assistive device? .... Y / N
26. Do you have a bone, muscle, or joint injury that bothers you? .... Y / N
27. Do any of your joints become painful, swollen, feel warm, or look red? .... Y / N
28. Do you have any history of juvenile arthritis or connective tissue disease? .... Y / N

MEDICAL QUESTIONS
29. Has a doctor ever told you that you have asthma or allergies? .... Y / N
30. Do you cough, wheeze, experience chest tightness, or have difficulty breathing during or after exercise? .... Y / N
31. Is there anyone in your family who has asthma? .... Y / N
32. Have you ever used an inhaler or taken asthma medicine? .... Y / N
33. Do you develop a rash or hives when you exercise? .... Y / N
34. Were you born without or are you missing a kidney, an eye, a testicle (males), or any other organ? .... Y / N
35. Do you have groin pain or a painful bulge or hernia in the groin area? .... Y / N
36. Have you had infectious mononucleosis (mono) within the last month? .... Y / N
37. Do you have any rashes, pressure sores, or other skin problems? .... Y / N
38. Have you had a herpes or MRSA skin infection? .... Y / N
39. Have you ever had a head injury or concussion? .... Y / N
40. Have you ever had a hit or blow to the head that caused confusion prolonged headache, or memory problems? .... Y / N
41. Do you have a history of seizure disorder? .... Y / N
42. Do you have headaches with exercise? .... Y / N
43. Have you ever had numbness, tingling, or weakness in your arms or legs after being hit or falling? .... Y / N
44. Have you ever been unable to move your arms or legs after being hit or falling? .... Y / N
45. Have you ever become ill while exercising in the heat? .... Y / N
46. Do you get frequent muscle cramps when exercising? .... Y / N
47. Do you or someone in your family have sickle cell trait or disease? .... Y / N
48. Have you had any problems with your eyes or vision? .... Y / N
49. Have you had any eye injuries? .... Y / N
50. Do you wear glasses or contact lenses? .... Y / N
51. Do you wear protective eyewear, such as goggles or a face shield? .... Y / N
52. Do you worry about your weight? .... Y / N
53. Are you trying to or has anyone recommended that you gain or lose weight? .... Y / N
54. Are you on a special diet or do you avoid certain types of foods? .... Y / N
55. Have you ever had an eating disorder? .... Y / N
56. Do you have any concerns that you would like to discuss with a doctor? .... Y / N

FEMALES ONLY
57. Have you ever had a menstrual period? .... Y / N
58. How old were you when you had your first menstrual period? _____
59. How many menstrual periods have you had in the last year? _____

Notes: _____

I do not know of any existing physical or additional health reason that would preclude participation in sports. I certify that the answers to the above questions are true and accurate and I approve participation in athletic activities.

_____   _____   _____
Parent or Legal Guardian Signature   Student-Athlete Signature   Date

Figure 6–2B Sports Qualifying Physical Examination (page 2). Courtesy of Minnesota State High Scool League (www.MSHSL.org).

Revised 4/18/18

2018-2019 SPORTS QUALIFYING PHYSICAL EXAMINATION FORM
Minnesota State High School League

Student Name: _____ Birth Date: _____ Age:____ Gender: M / F

Follow -Up Questions About More Sensitive Issues:
1. Do you feel stressed out or under a lot of pressure?
2. Do you ever feel so sad or hopeless that you stop doing some of your usual activities for more than a few days?
3. Do you feel safe?
4. Have you ever tried cigarette, cigar, or pipe smoking, even 1 or 2 puffs? Do you currently smoke?
5. During the past 30 days, did you use chewing tobacco, snuff, or dip?
6. During the past 30 days, have you had any alcohols, even just one?
7. Have you ever taken steroid pills or shots without a doctor's prescription?
8. Have you ever taken any medications or supplements to help you gain or lose weight or improve your performance?
9. Question "Risk Behaviors" like guns, seatbelts, unprotected sex, domestic violence, drugs, and others.
Notes About Follow -Up Questions:
_____
_____
_____

MEDICAL EXAM

Height_____ Weight_____ BMI (optional) _____ % Body fat (optional) _____ Arm Span_____
Pulse _____ BP _____/_____ (_____/_____)
Vision: R 20/____ L 20/____ Corrected: Y / N Contacts: Y / N Hearing: R____ L____ (Audiogram or confrontation)

Exam	Normal	Abnormal Notes	Initials*
Appearance	Y / N		
No Marfan stigmata (kyphoscoliosis, high-arched palate, pectus excavatum, arachnodactyly, arm span > height, hyperlaxity, myopia, MVP, aortic insufficiency)	Y / N		
HEENT	Y / N		
Eyes	Y / N		
Fundoscopic	Y / N		
Pupils	Equal / Unequal		
Hearing	Y / N		
Cardiovascular	Y / N		
No Murmurs (standing, supine, +/- Valsalva)	Y / N		
PMI location			
Pulses (simultaneous femoral & radial)	Y / N		
Lungs	Y / N		
Abdomen	Y / N		
Tanner Staging (optional)	I II III IV V		
Skin (No HSV, MRSA, Tinea corporis)	Y / N		
Musculoskeletal			
Neck	Y / N		
Back	Y / N		
Shoulder/Arm	Y / N		
Elbow/Forearm	Y / N		
Wrist/Hand/Fingers	Y / N		
Hip/Thigh	Y / N		
Knee	Y / N		
Leg/Ankle	Y / N		
Foot/Toes	Y / N		
Functional (Single Leg Hop or Squat, Box Drop)	Y / N		

* Required Only if Multiple Examiners

Notes: _____
_____
_____
_____

Assessment: ☐ Cleared for sports without restriction ☐ Restricted participation (see Clearance Form)
Plan: *Immunizations:* ☐ Up-to-Date ☐ Recommend Annual Flu Shot (Especially for Asthma & winter athletes) ☐ Consider HPV series
☐ Immunize if needed (Tdap, meningococcal MCV4, (1-2 doses), 3 HPV, 2 MMR, 3 hep B, 2 hep A, 3-4 Polio, 2 varicella or history of disease)
Health Maintenance: ☐ Lifestyle, health, and safety counseling ☐ Discussed dental care and mouthguard use
☐ Discussed Lead and TB exposure – (Testing indicated / not indicated) ☐ Eye Refraction if indicated

Provider Signature:_____ Date: _____

Figure 6–2C Sports Qualifying Physical Examination (page 3). Courtesy of Minnesota State High Scool League (www.MSHSL.org).

Minnesota State High School League
2018-2019 PI ADAPTED ATHLETICS MEDICAL ELIGIBILITY FORM Addendum
(Use only for Adapted Athletics - PI Division)

The MSHSL has competitive interscholastic Physically Impaired (PI) competition. Students who are deemed fit to participate in competitive athletics from a MSHSL sports qualifying exam should meet the criteria below to participate in Adapted Athletics – PI Division.

The MSHSL Adapted Athletics PI Division program is specifically intended for students with physical impairments who have medical clearance to compete in competitive athletics. A student is eligible to compete in the PI Division with one of the following criteria:

The student must have a diagnosed and documented impairment specified from one of the two sections below:
(Must be diagnosed and documented by a Physician's Assistant, and/or Advanced Practice Nurse.)

1. _____ Neuromuscular   _____ Postural/Skeletal   _____ Traumatic

    _____ Growth   _____ Neurological Impairment

    Which: _____ affects Motor Function   _____ modifies Gait Patterns

    (Optional) _____ Requires the use of prosthesis or mobility device, including but not limited to canes, crutches, walker or wheelchair.

2. _____ Cardio/Respiratory Impairment that is deemed safe for competitive athletics, but limits the intensity and duration of physical exertion such that sustained activity for over five minutes at 60% of maximum heart rate for age results in physical distress in spite of appropriate management of the health condition.

    (NOTE:) A condition that can be appropriately managed with appropriate medications that eliminate physical or health endurance limitations WILL NOT be considered eligible for adapted athletics   .

Specific exclusions to PI competition:

The following health conditions, <u>without coexisting physical impairments as outlined above</u>, do not qualify the student to participate in the PI Division even though some of the conditions below may be considered Health Impairments by an individual's physician, a student's school, or government agency. This list is not all-inclusive and the conditions are examples of non-qualifying health conditions; other health conditions that are not listed below may also be non-qualifying for participation in the PI Division.

Attention Deficit Disorder (ADD), Attention Deficit Hyperactive Disorder (ADHD), Emotional Behavioral Disorder (EBD), Autism spectrum disorders (including Asperger's Syndrome), Tourette's Syndrome, Neurofibromatosis, Asthma, Reactive Airway Disease (RAD), Bronchopulmonary Dysplasia (BPD), Blindness, Deafness, Obesity, Depression, Generalized Anxiety Disorder, Seizure Disorder, or other similar disorders.

Student Name _____

Provider (PRINT) _____

Provider (SIGNATURE) _____

Date of Exam _____

Figure 6–2C *(continued)*

Table 6–2 Classification of Sports by Contact

CONTACT OR COLLISION	LIMITED-CONTACT	NONCONTACT
Basketball	Baseball	Archery
Boxing	Bicycling	Badminton
Diving	Cheerleading	Body building
Field hockey	Fencing	Bowling
Football, tackle	Field events	Crew or rowing
Ice hockey	High jump	Dancing
Lacrosse	Pole vault	Discus
Martial arts	Football, flag	Javelin
Rodeo	Gymnastics	Shot put
Rugby	Handball	Golf
Ski jumping	Horseback riding	Running
Soccer	Racquetball	Swimming
Team handball	Ice skating	Table tennis
Water polo	Cross-country	Tennis
Wrestling	Skateboarding	Track
	Snowboarding	Weight lifting
	Softball	
	Squash	
	Volleyball	
	Windsurfing or surfing	

For example, suppose an athlete has been identified as having weak, inflexible hamstrings. This condition might not preclude the athlete from gaining full clearance for sports, but might later be the cause of an injury. Coaches and trainers can identify athletes with conditions such as this and work over the off-season to strengthen certain muscle groups, thereby dramatically reducing the risk of injury. Another example is the athlete who is allergic to bee stings. If the coach has no prior knowledge of this condition, the athlete could be at medical risk if stung.

All information contained on the PPE form must be kept strictly confidential. These forms should be secured in the athletic director's office or the athletic trainer's office under lock and key. Coaches should be encouraged to review this information during the course of the school year. All PPE forms should be kept for a minimum of seven years after the athlete graduates or leaves the school. This legal requirement minimizes risk to the school district or university.

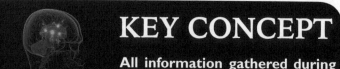

KEY CONCEPT

All information gathered during the PPE must be kept strictly confidential.

CONCLUSION

The preparticipation physical examination has evolved over the past few decades to become a comprehensive approach to the medical assessment of athletes, conducted by an array of sports medicine specialists who are concerned with the athlete's health and well-being. The PPE should be a preseason evaluation, thus allowing time for the athlete to correct any deficiencies noted during the exam. It can be either office based or station based; each has its own advantages. The station-based exam is often hampered by the difficulty of recruiting volunteer physicians, therapists, and other sports medicine personnel. Finding a facility to handle a station-based examination might also be a concern. When all concerns are addressed, the station-based PPE can be a wonderful tool for the assessment of athletes.

Determining clearance for participation is the most important result of any PPE. Physicians must take into account their findings from the exam, as well as the sport or activity in which the athlete desires to participate. After taking all factors into consideration, the physician will either give unrestricted clearance, clearance after completion of further evaluation or rehabilitation, or no clearance for certain sports or all sports.

The ultimate goal of the PPE is to allow athletes to compete safely. With advanced screening, it is hoped that sudden death in young athletes can be avoided.

REVIEW QUESTIONS

1. How has the preparticipation physical examination changed over the past few decades?
2. List five goals of the PPE.
3. What are the benefits of the station-based and office-based PPE?
4. What are some of the challenges of the station-based PPE?
5. What are the five components of the PPE?
6. What is the overall goal of the PPE?
7. Why is determining clearance for participation sometimes a difficult decision for physicians?
8. Why is it important to keep information gathered in the PPE confidential?

PROJECTS AND ACTIVITIES

1. Does your school use an office-based or station-based preparticipation physical examination? Ask your athletic director what other schools in your area use. Report your findings.
2. Contact someone involved in administering a station-based PPE in your area. (This may be your school.) Ask that person what advantages a station-based system has over the traditional office visit. Write down your findings and report them to the class.
3. How are records maintained at your school? Who has access to them? How long are they kept before being destroyed?

LEARNING LINKS

- Many online resources discuss the evolution of the preparticipation physical examination for the athlete. If you are interested in learning more about the research and recommendations being made for the preparticipation physical examination, use a search engine such as Google and enter the keywords "preparticipation physical examination in sports."

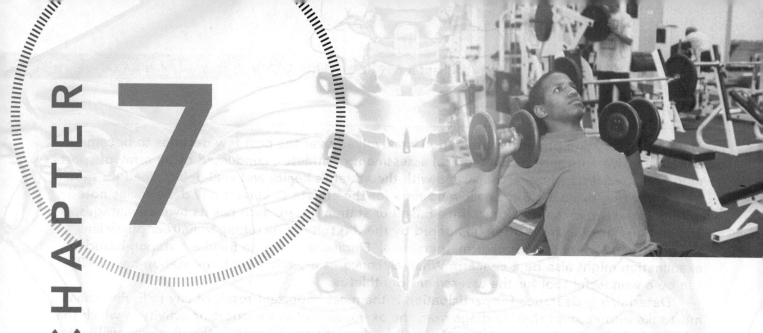

CHAPTER 7

Prehabilitation and Preseason Conditioning

OBJECTIVES

Upon completion of this chapter, the reader should be able to:

- Discuss how prehabilitation can decrease the chance of injury
- Explain how preseason conditioning helps the body adapt to the demands placed upon it
- Describe isometric, dynamic, and isokinetic exercise, and how they are used in a conditioning program
- Compare and contrast manual resistance training, circuit training, and special, individualized programs
- Describe the science behind progressive resistance exercise
- Explain the components of stretching and flexibility programs and how they relate to an overall fitness program
- Explain the benefits of cardiorespiratory conditioning
- Explain the importance of special individualized fitness programs

KEY TERMS

adaptation *The systematic application of exercise stress sufficient to stimulate muscle fatigue, but not so severe that breakdown and injury occur.*

atrophy *Weakness and wasting away of muscle tissue.*

ballistic stretching *A rhythmical, bouncing action that stretches the muscles a little further each time. Once a popular technique, this form of stretching is rarely used today. Especially when the muscles are cold, ballistic stretching was responsible for increased injuries.*

cardiorespiratory conditioning *An activity that puts an increased demand on the lungs, heart, and other body systems; also known as aerobic or endurance training.*

KEY TERMS CONTINUED

circuit training *The use of 6 to 10 strength exercises completed one right after another; each exercise is done by performing a specific number of repetitions or for a specific period of time before moving to the next exercise.*

dynamic (isotonic) exercise *An activity that causes the muscle to contract and shorten.*

fast-twitch fiber *Fiber in a motor unit that produces quick and forceful contractions; these fibers are easily fatigued.*

flexibility *The ability of a joint to move freely through its full range of motion.*

hypertrophy *An increase in the size of muscle tissue.*

isokinetic exercise *A type of exercise in which a machine controls the speed of contraction within the range of motion.*

isometric exercise *An activity that causes tension in the muscle to increase but does not cause the muscle to shorten.*

manual resistance training *A form of dynamic exercise accomplished utilizing a training partner.*

motor unit *A motor nerve plus all the muscle fibers it stimulates.*

overload *Progressive overwork of muscles, at a controlled, increased rate, to achieve consistent gains in strength.*

prehabilitation *Trying to prevent injuries before they occur, through a preventative management program.*

preseason conditioning *A program, beginning six to eight weeks prior to sports participation, that allows the body to gradually adapt to the demands to be placed on it.*

progressive resistance exercise *A type of training in which muscles are worked until they reach their capacity; once the athlete is able to maintain that capacity, the workload on the muscle is increased to further build strength and endurance.*

proprioceptive neuromuscular facilitation (PNF) *A combined relaxing and contracting of the muscles; an initial isometric contraction against maximum resistance is held at the end of the range of motion, followed by relaxation and passive stretching.*

rehabilitation *The process of restoring function through programmed exercise, to enable a return to competition.*

reversibility *The process of muscle atrophy due to disuse, immobilization, or starvation; leads to decreased strength and muscle mass.*

slow-twitch fiber *Fiber in a motor unit that requires a long period of time to generate force; these fibers are resistant to fatigue.*

specificity *The ability of particular muscle groups to respond to targeted training, so that increased strength is gained in that muscle group only.*

static stretching *A gradual, slow stretching of the muscle through the entire range of motion, then holding the position for 20 to 30 seconds.*

stretching *Moving the joints beyond the normal range of motion.*

PREHABILITATION

Most people have heard the term **rehabilitation**, meaning a programmed exercise program designed to return an athlete to fitness and competition after an injury has occurred. **Prehabilitation** attempts to prevent injuries before they occur, through a preventative management program. Addressing early on the concerns or deficits recognized by the athlete's family physician or other sports medicine specialists prior to sports participation enables the athlete to participate with a greater chance of success and lower incidence of injury.

Each year in the United States, approximately 45.7 million children and teenagers participate in organized sports (Sports and Fitness Industry Association, 2016)). Children and adolescents are becoming more involved in sports at earlier ages and with higher levels of intensity. The Centers for Disease Control and Prevention estimates that one-half of all sports injuries in children are preventable with proper education and use of protective equipment.

These statistics make it clear that a personalized prehabilitation program designed to address the total body, as well as sport-specific needs, should be an integral component of any athlete's fitness program.

PRESEASON CONDITIONING

Whenever athletes start a fitness program, or return from an extended hiatus, their bodies need time to adjust to new stresses and demands. The terms **preseason conditioning** and prehabilitation are similar, yet each has a slightly different focus. Preseason conditioning works on developing the athlete in the off-season. Athletes can work on overall conditioning as well as concentrating on specific weaknesses.

Athletes must train hard and long to excel in sports. A preseason conditioning program, beginning six to eight weeks prior to sports participation, allows the body to gradually adapt to the demands to be placed on it. Doing too much, too soon, at too high an intensity, denies the body to opportunity to adapt effectively and therefore increases the risk of injury.

Sports medicine physicians, certified athletic trainers, and qualified youth coaches should prescribe a preseason conditioning program and provide athletes with information on the type, frequency, intensity, and duration of training. Sharing this information with parents can be helpful, as they can reinforce the importance of preseason conditioning at home.

There are many different approaches to conditioning. After the athlete has set his or her goals for the conditioning program, select exercises can be tailored to fit those needs.

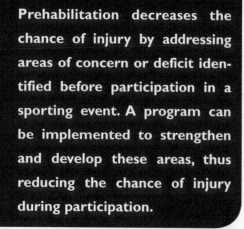

KEY CONCEPT

Prehabilitation decreases the chance of injury by addressing areas of concern or deficit identified before participation in a sporting event. A program can be implemented to strengthen and develop these areas, thus reducing the chance of injury during participation.

KEY CONCEPT

Preseason conditioning allows athletes to gradually build up to the level of activity that will be expected of them on the playing field. By starting slowly, the body is able to adjust to new demands. Once the body has accommodated, the athlete can increase the intensity of the conditioning. Thus, by working incrementally to adjust the body, the athlete prepares for the demands of the season.

STRENGTH TRAINING

Strength training is a highly adaptive process whereby the body changes in response to increased training loads. **Adaptation** is the whole purpose of strength training. Adaptation requires a systematic application of exercise stress. The stress should be sufficient to stimulate muscle fatigue, but not so severe that breakdown and injury occur.

Periodization is the careful planning of specific performance goals spread out over a period of time, generally a year; whereas the exercise program can be tailored to meet specific objectives during preseason, in-season and postseason.

Skeletal muscle is highly adaptable. If a muscle is worked beyond its normal limits, it adapts and becomes larger, or **hypertrophies**. In doing so, the muscle improves in strength, allowing it to accommodate an increased workload. The reverse is also true: If a muscle is worked less than normal, it **atrophies**, or becomes smaller, and therefore cannot accommodate the workload it once did.

The purpose of **progressive resistance exercise** is to allow the body to adapt to the increased demands placed upon it by training. The nature of the muscles adapting must always be considered when designing the training program. Factors that determine the rate and type of strength gains include overload, specificity, reversibility, and individual differences.

Overload

Muscles increase in strength and size when they are forced to contract at tensions close to maximum. Muscles must be **overloaded** to improve strength and power. If consistent gains in strength are to occur, muscles must be overloaded at a progressively increased rate.

Muscular tension must be attained at an adequate intensity and duration for optimal development of strength. Studies have found that the ideal number of repetitions is between four and eight. These repetitions should be done in multiple *sets* of three or more. Strength gains diminish when either fewer or greater numbers of repetitions are used. It is important to include proper rest intervals between sets. This allows the muscles to recover from exertion and prepare for the next work interval. The optimal period of rest between sets has not been scientifically determined.

Specificity

Muscles adapt specifically to the nature of the work performed. This is known as **specificity**. If the leg muscles are exercised, they hypertrophy, whereas the muscles of the shoulders remain the same. A football player who wants to increase leg strength will have to work the leg muscles.

When muscles contract, they recruit different types of **motor units** to carry out the contraction. There are two different muscle fiber types (motor units). Each has different characteristics while con-

KEY CONCEPT

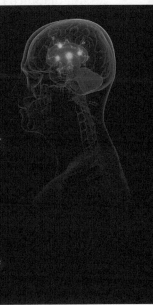

- **Manual resistance training is done with a partner. The partner adds resistance to a lift, allowing the muscles to fatigue, and then releases enough resistance so the lifter can finish the range of motion.**

- **Circuit training uses 6 to 10 strength exercises, completed one after another and performed for a specified number of repetitions or time period.**

- **Athletes may choose to work with a personal trainer to develop an individualized training program that allows them to meet specific goals. A variety of exercise types can be used.**

These techniques can be used alone or in conjunction. The goals of the athlete determine the types of exercises needed to meet those goals.

tracting. **Slow-twitch fibers** are relatively fatigue-resistant; **fast-twitch fibers** can contract more rapidly and forcefully, but also fatigue rapidly.

The low-threshold slow-twitch fibers are recruited for low-intensity activities such as jogging (and for that matter, most tasks of human motion). However, for high-speed or high-intensity activities, such as sprinting or weight lifting, the fast-twitch motor units are engaged.

The amount of training that occurs in a muscle fiber is determined by the extent to which it is recruited. High-repetition, low-intensity exercise, such as distance running, uses mainly slow-twitch fibers. Low-repetition, high-intensity activity, such as weight training, causes hypertrophy of fast-twitch fibers, though there will also be some changes to the lower threshold slow-twitch fibers. The training program should be structured to produce the desired training effect.

Increases in strength are very specific to the type of exercise, even when the same muscle groups are used. Specific motor units are recruited for specific tasks. If a person uses weight training to improve strength for another activity, the exercises should mimic the desired movements of that activity as closely as possible. Likewise, when one is attempting to increase strength after an injury or surgery, rehabilitation should include muscle movements that are as close as possible to those made in normal activities.

Muscle fiber type appears to play an important role in determining success in some sports. Successful distance runners have a high proportion of slow-twitch muscles (the percentage of slow-twitch fibers is closely related to maximum oxygen consumption). Sprinters have a predominance of fast-twitch muscles. Several studies have shown that large numbers of fast-twitch fibers are a prerequisite for success in progressive resistance training.

Not all sports have preferred fiber characteristics. For example, world-class shot-putters show surprisingly diverse muscle fiber composition. In these athletes, larger muscle fibers, rather than percent of fiber type, account for excellent performance. There are differences in the relative percentage of fast-twitch fibers in explosive-strength athletes. Having a high percentage of fast-twitch fibers is not necessarily critical for success. Many strength athletes have a higher fast-to-slow twitch fiber ratio than sedentary persons or endurance athletes. Individual differences in training intensity and technique can make up for deficiencies in the relative percentage of fast-twitch fibers in these athletes.

Training programs designed to stimulate both strength and endurance have been found to interfere with gains in strength. Strength athletes may inhibit their ability to gain strength by participating in vigorous endurance activities. Muscles may be unable to adapt optimally to both forms of exercise.

Reversibility

Muscles will atrophy through disuse, immobilization, and starvation. Disuse leads to a decrease in strength and muscle mass, a process called **reversibility**.

Fast-twitch and slow-twitch fibers do not atrophy at the same rate. If a joint is immobilized as a result of an injury, the slow-twitch fibers will atrophy faster. After immobilization, it is important to undertake a program of strength and endurance exercises that allow the atrophied muscle fibers to regain their pre-injury strength.

Individual Differences

As with other forms of exercise, people vary in the rate at which they gain strength. Some of these differences can be attributed to the relative predominance of fast- and slow-twitch motor units in muscles. Usually, endurance athletes have more slow-twitch fibers (Figure 7–1a) in their active muscles. Strength athletes have more fast-twitch fibers (Figure 7–1b). Intense, progressive, resistance training mainly enlarges fast-twitch fibers. People who have more fast-twitch fibers will tend to gain strength faster than those who do not. Fast-twitch fibers tend to be stronger than other fiber types, so people who have more of them tend to be stronger and have greater potential for strength gains.

Several studies have shown that fiber composition is genetically determined (Fahey, 1998). Genetics is not the sole determinant of individual differences in strength, though genetics exert a strong influence on the ability to gain strength. A good training program can make up for genetic deficiencies.

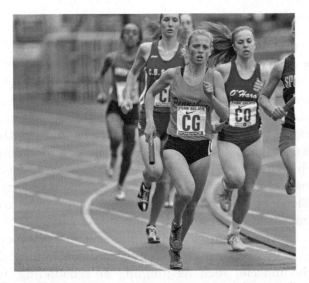

Figure 7–1A Endurance athletes have more slow-twitch fibers in their active muscles. Aspen Photo/Shutterstock.com

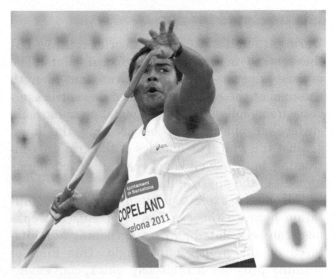

Figure 7–1B Strength athletes have more fast-twitch fibers. Maxisport/Shutterstock.com

KEY CONCEPT

Progressive resistance training allows the body to adapt to the demands placed on it through training. Four factors determine the rate and type of strength gain:

1. **Overload**, the overwork of muscles at tensions close to their maximum.

2. **Specificity**, the targeting of a particular muscle group to improve and gain strength in that muscle group alone.

3. **Reversibility**, the characteristic of muscles that causes decreases in strength and mass with disuse.

4. **Individual differences**, which account for an individual's ability to strengthen certain muscles at a particular rate. Genetics have a strong influence on strength gain.

STRENGTH TRAINING EXERCISES

A variety of exercises and techniques can be used to build up strength based on the principles of progressive resistance training. The athlete should work with the certified athletic trainer or a personal trainer to determine the goals of the strength training program and the exercises and techniques that will best meet those goals.

FUN FACTS

Strength training is not just for youngsters and athletes. Seniors involved in strength training age better and stay healthier. Seniors who strength-train are less likely to suffer serious injuries when they fall, and to recover from injuries sooner than seniors who are not as physically active.

Isometric Exercise

During **isometric exercises**, muscles contract but there is no motion in the affected joints. The muscle fibers maintain a constant length throughout the entire contraction. Isometric exercises are usually performed against an immovable surface or object, such as pressing the hand against the wall. The muscles of the arm are contracting, but the wall is not reacting or moving as a result of the physical effort.

Isometric exercise is often used for rehabilitation because the exact area of muscle weakness can be isolated and strengthening administered at the proper joint angle. This kind of training provides a relatively quick, convenient method for overloading and strengthening muscles without the need for special equipment and with little chance of injury. Static exercise improves strength but also increases blood pressure quickly. People with circulation problems and high blood pressure should avoid strenuous isometric exercises.

Dynamic Exercise

Dynamic (isotonic) exercise differs from isometric exercise in that there is movement of the joint during the muscle contraction. Weight training with dumbbells and barbells is a classic example. As the weight is lifted throughout the range of motion, the muscle shortens and lengthens (Figure 7–2A and B). Calisthenics, including chin-ups, push-ups, and sit-ups, are isotonic exercises that use body weight as the resistance force. Blood circulation, strength, and endurance are improved by these continuous movements.

Another form of dynamic exercise, plyometrics, involves rapid stretching and contracting of the muscle, such as jumping or rebounding, to increase muscle power.

Manual Resistance Training

Manual resistance training is a form of dynamic exercise that is accomplished with a training partner. The training partner assists by adding

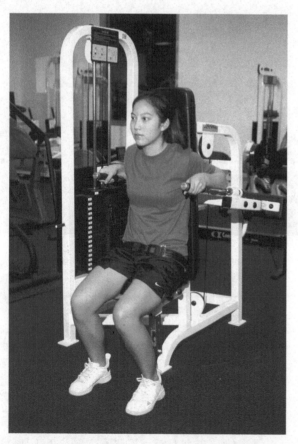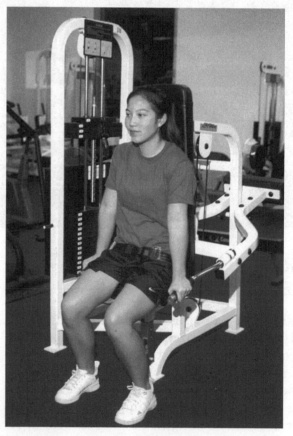

Figure 7–2A–B Dynamic exercise works muscle groups through the range of motion.

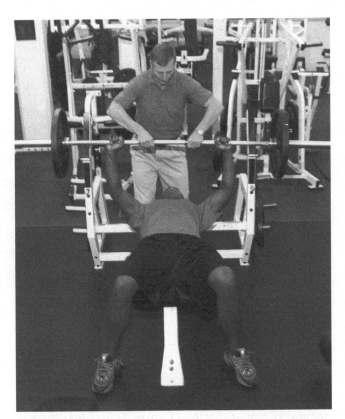

Figure 7–3 The training partner, or spotter, adds enough resistance to allow the lifter to fatigue the muscles, then releases enough resistance so that the lift can be completed.

resistance to the lift as the lifter works the muscles through the full range of motion (Figure 7–3). The training partner, or spotter, adds enough resistance to allow the lifter to fatigue the muscles, then releases enough resistance so that the lift can be completed.

Advantages of manual resistance training are:

- It requires minimal equipment.
- The spotter can help control technique.
- Workouts can be completed in less than 30 minutes.
- Training can occur anywhere.

The disadvantages are that a spotter is required, and both lifter and spotter must be trained to keep the exercise safe and effective.

Isokinetic Exercise

Isokinetic exercise uses machines that control the speed of contraction within the range of motion. Isokinetic exercise attempts to combine the best features of isometrics and weight training. It provides muscular overload at a constant, preset speed while the muscle mobilizes its force through the full range of motion. For example, when an isokinetic stationary bicycle is set at 90 revolutions per minute, no matter how hard and fast the workout the isokinetic properties of the bicycle will allow the cyclist to complete only 90 revolutions per minute. Machines such as the Cybex and Biodex provide isokinetic results; they are generally used by physical therapists and not readily available to the general population.

KEY CONCEPT

- In isometric exercise, the muscles maintain a constant length throughout the contraction. This type of exercise targets an exact area of weakness due to an injury.
- In dynamic isotonic or isotonic exercise, there is movement of the joint during muscle contraction. This type of exercise helps improve blood circulation, strength, and endurance.
- Isokinetic exercises use machines to control the speed of the contraction within a range of motion. These exercises provide muscle overload at a constant, preset speed and full range of motion.

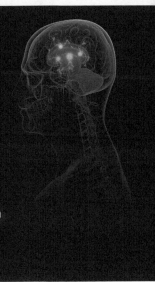

Circuit Training

Circuit training, an excellent way to improve strength and stamina, utilizes 6 to 10 strength exercises that are completed as a circuit, one exercise after another (Figure 7–4). Each exercise on the circuit is performed for a specified number of repetitions or a specific period of time before moving on to the next exercise. Each exercise is separated by a brief, timed rest interval. If more than one circuit is to be completed, the circuits will be separated by a longer rest period. The total number of circuits performed varies depending on the athlete's training level. Another type of exercise similar to circuit training is **interval training**, which is an aerobic-based workout. You choose your aerobic exercise and add intervals of increased speed or resistance. For example, during a brisk walk, add a 1- to 2-minute sprint, then return to your brisk walking for an equal amount of time.

In **Farlek training** the athlete runs fast for a period of time, slows down for a period of time, and speeds up again. For beginners it can be walking, jogging, and walking again. As endurance and cardiovascular conditioning improves, the intervals between the speed workout and resting period increase. Eventually the athlete would strive toward **continuous training**, where the rest interval is eliminated.

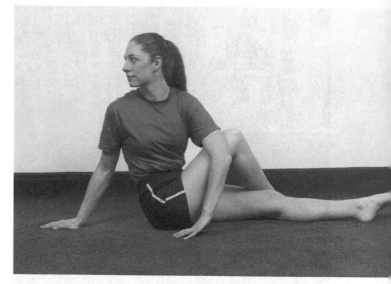

Figure 7–5 The athlete is able to increase muscle length as a result of stretching.

Stretching and Flexibility

Stretching means moving the joints beyond the normal range of motion (Figure 7–5). **Flexibility** is the ability of a joint to move freely through its full range of motion (Figure 7–6).

Stretching is useful for both injury prevention and injury treatment. One of the benefits of stretching is that the athlete increases muscle length. This leads to an increased range of movement—meaning the limbs and joints can move further before they suffer an injury.

Before doing stretching exercises, the athlete should warm up. Warming up is an essential component of stretching. Warming up increases the

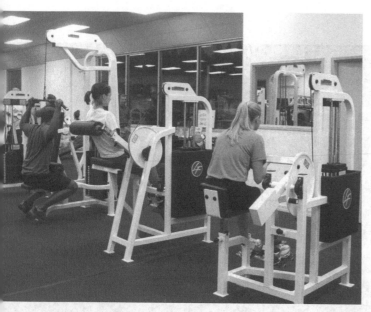

Figure 7–4 Circuit training utilizes 6 to 10 strength exercises that are completed as a circuit, one exercise after another.

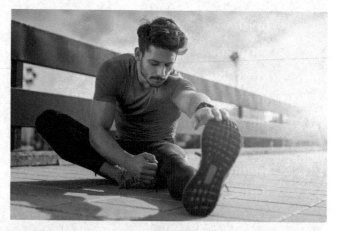

Figure 7–6 Greater flexibility allows the joint to move further before an injury occurs. Ivanko80/Shutterstock.com

heart rate, blood pressure, and respiratory rate, which in turn increases the delivery of oxygen and nutrients to the muscles. This allows the muscles to prepare for strenuous activity. For most activities, the warm up period should be nonstrenuous but still cause the athlete to begin to perspire. It is known that:

- An active person tends to be more flexible than an inactive person.
- Females tend to be more flexible than males.
- Older people tend to be less flexible than younger people.
- Flexibility is as important as muscular strength and endurance.
- To achieve flexibility in a joint, the surrounding muscles must be stretched.

There are three basic types of stretching: static, ballistic, and proprioceptive neuromuscular facilitation.

Static Stretching

Static stretching is a gradual stretching of a muscle through the muscle's entire range of motion. This proceeds slowly, until a pulling sensation occurs. This position should be held for 20 to 30 seconds. Stretching should not be painful; if it is, injury may occur.

Ballistic Stretching

Ballistic stretching was popular a couple of decades ago. This method of stretching involves a rhythmical, bouncing action. Ballistic stretching was done 10 to 15 times, stretching the muscles a little further each time. This method has fallen out of favor as a result of an increased incidence of injury. It was found that the bouncing action activates the stretch reflex, resulting in small muscle tears, soreness, and sometimes injury.

Proprioceptive Neuromuscular Facilitation

Proprioceptive neuromuscular facilitation (PNF) involves a combination of contraction and relaxation of the muscles. *Proprioceptive* refers to stimuli originating in muscles, tendons, and other internal tissues. *Neuromuscular* pertains to muscles and nerves. *Facilitation* is the hastening or enhancement of any natural process. This method requires an initial isometric contraction against maximum resistance at the end of the range of motion. This position is typically held for six seconds, followed by relaxation and a passive stretch. This is repeated several times. PNF is designed to be done with a qualified assistant. Table 7–1 illustrates the advantages and disadvantages of flexibility training.

CARDIORESPIRATORY CONDITIONING

Cardiorespiratory conditioning, also known as *aerobic* or *endurance training*, refers to activities that put an increased demand on the lungs, heart, and other body systems. Aerobic training can improve performance in all types of sports and activities.

Cardiorespiratory conditioning uses large muscle groups for activities such as walking, jogging, swimming, cross-country skiing, or cycling. Team sports such as soccer and water polo are excellent for aerobic conditioning. The goal of aerobic conditioning is to train the heart and other muscles to use oxygen more efficiently. Improved efficiency of the cardiovascular system allows the person to exercise for longer periods of time, therefore improving the overall fitness level.

Muscular endurance is the ability of muscles to sustain high-intensity, aerobic exercise. An example is a weightlifter who has trained to complete 20 bench presses at 150 pounds in 60 seconds. Cardiorespiratory endurance relates to the whole

KEY CONCEPT

Stretching and flexibility decrease the risk of injury. Stretching allows the athlete to actually lengthen the muscles, resulting in an increased range of motion. Therefore, joints and limbs can move further before they suffer an injury.

Table 7–1   Advantages and Disadvantages of Flexibility Training

TYPE	ADVANTAGES	DISADVANTAGES
Static	Safest form of stretching	Takes longer to complete
Ballistic	Good for dynamic flexibility	Increased chance of injury
		Increased chance of soreness
		Reduces static range of motion
PNF	Allows for greater reflex inhibition, greater stretch	Need for a trained assistant
	Increased neuromuscular response by stimulating neural proprioceptors	Relying on assistant could increase chance of injury

body's ability to sustain prolonged, rhythmical exercise. An example of this is a cross-country runner completing a five-mile run.

The body adapts to prolonged cardiovascular exercise in many different ways. The heart increases in size, thereby increasing pumping volume. Because the size of the heart increases (as does any muscle with increased exercise), the resting heart rate decreases. This also contributes to a decrease in blood pressure.

The lungs, too, adapt to aerobic conditioning. A well-conditioned athlete is able to increase the amount of air exchanged (lung volume), providing more efficient oxygen transfer to the blood. This allows the athlete to work, condition, and compete at a higher level. Cardiorespiratory conditioning has also been proven to increase resting metabolism.

Cardiovascular Testing

Several tests are used to quantify cardiovascular fitness, including the VO2 max, Harvard Step Test, Twelve-Minute Run Test, and the Borg Scale.

The VO2 max test measures the volume of oxygen used during one minute of maximum exertion. The data gained helps determine the potential for endurance athletes.

The Harvard Step Test helps to measure a person's aerobic fitness. The test utilizes a step 20 inches high. The person steps up and down at a rate of 30 completed steps per minute, for

5 minutes or until exhaustion. A rating system evaluates overall cardiovascular fitness.

In the Twelve-Minute Run Test the person runs or walks as far as possible in 12 minutes. An increase in the distance covered indicates an increased level of fitness.

The Borg Scale utilizes a simple method of rating perceived exertion (RPE). This scale allows coaches and athletic trainers to gauge an athlete's intensity in training and competition.

For more information on these four fitness tests, check out the Learning Links section at the end of this chapter.

The design of an aerobic conditioning program should take into account several factors, to account for individual differences. These factors include beginning fitness level, age, sex, and physical limitations. In order to maximize its physiological benefit, the training program must be carefully contoured to the athlete's individual needs.

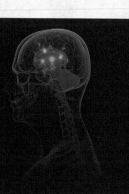

KEY CONCEPT

Cardiorespiratory training conditions the heart and other muscles to use oxygen more efficiently. This allows the athlete to perform for longer periods of time.

Additional benefits of cardiovascular conditioning include:

- Reduced fatigue
- Improved self-confidence
- Improved muscle strength and tone
- Increased endurance
- Reduced stress levels
- Reduced body fat
- Improved overall physical and mental health

An aerobic conditioning program starts with a checkup by the family doctor, who assesses the individual's overall health to assure that there are no physical limitations on beginning a conditioning program.

SPECIAL, INDIVIDUALIZED PROGRAMS

Athletes who desire personalized assistance with their training program can contact a variety of individuals or organizations. The cost of a personal trainer depends on the type of program desired and the amount of time devoted to personalized instruction. Personal trainers can assist in strength training, cardiovascular fitness, speed, and endurance work, as well as help with body composition. Personal trainers should have the proven knowledge and expertise to set up a personal training program, or be certified by one of the following associations:

- The National Federation of Professional Trainers (NFPT)
- National Strength and Conditioning Association
- The International Sport Sciences Association (ISSA)
- The American College of Sports Medicine (ACSM)

Personal trainers can set up programs to meet an athlete's objectives in a safe, controlled manner (Figure 7–7). Referrals are very important. Just because a person has a certification does not mean that he or she is the best choice. The athlete should "comparison shop" to find a personal trainer to fit his or her needs.

Certified athletic trainers are allied health professionals with considerable knowledge of anatomy and physiology. They get involved in setting up personalized programs for athletes and are an excellent resource for training needs. Certified athletic trainers can be found at many high schools and most colleges and universities.

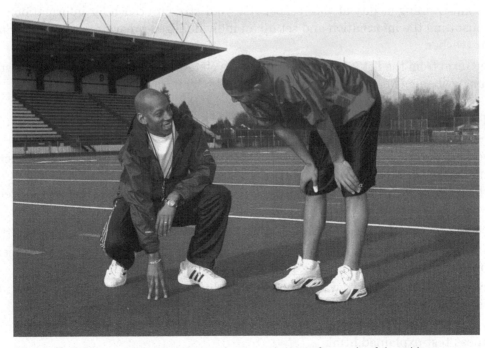

Figure 7–7 Personal trainers tailor workouts to the specific needs of the athlete.

CONCLUSION

Trying to prevent injuries before they occur is known as prehabilitation. Personalized programs designed to address the total body, as well as sport-specific needs, are an integral component of the total athletic fitness program.

There are many different ways to achieve fitness. The use of isometric, dynamic, and isokinetic exercises allows the athlete to develop a program tailored to fit his or her needs.

Stretching and flexibility are important components of fitness. A well-thought-out stretching and flexibility program helps with injury prevention and treatment.

REVIEW QUESTIONS

How can prehabilitation reduce the chance of injury once the season begins?

1. Describe the elements of a well-rounded preseason conditioning program.

2. Give three examples of isometric, dynamic, and isokinetic exercise. Develop a chart comparing manual resistance training, circuit training, and special, individualized programs.

3. What is the importance of having a personal trainer help you achieve your conditioning goals?

4. In a one-page paper, explain the science of progressive resistance exercise.

5. Stretching and flexibility exercises are important components to a fitness program. Why?

6. Explain the differences between static, ballistic, and PNF stretching.

7. Describe the benefits of cardiorespiratory training.

PROJECTS AND ACTIVITIES

1. Interview three athletes from different sports in your school. How do their preseason conditioning programs differ?

2. Call, e-mail, or write to a college or professional athlete that you admire. Ask how he or she prepares in the off-season (prehabilitation) for the sport. Share this information with your class.

3. Visit the weight-training facility at your school. Ask your strength coach for information on circuit training. Consulting the information and set up an individualized program for yourself. Submit your plan to your teacher.

4. Pick the key term from the list at the beginning of the chapter that interests you the most. Research this term and write a one-page paper explaining it and why it interests you.

LEARNING LINKS

1. Visit the websites for the National Federation of Professional Trainers (http://www.nfpt.com), the International Sport Sciences Association (http://www.issaonline.com), and the American College of Sports Medicine (http://www.acsm.org). How do their requirements for personal trainer certification differ? How are they similar?

2. Cardiovascular fitness testing
   - VO2 max: https://med.virginia.edu/exercise-physiology-core-laboratory/fitness-assessment-for-community-members-2/vo2-max-testing/.
   - Harvard Step Test: https://www.health.harvard.edu/staying-healthy/aerobic-fitness-test-the-step-method.
   - Twelve-Minute Run: http://www.fitday.com/fitness-articles/fitness/cardio/the-cooper-12-minute-run-fitness-test-explained.html.
   - Borg Scale: https://www.hsph.harvard.edu/nutritionsource/borg-scale/.

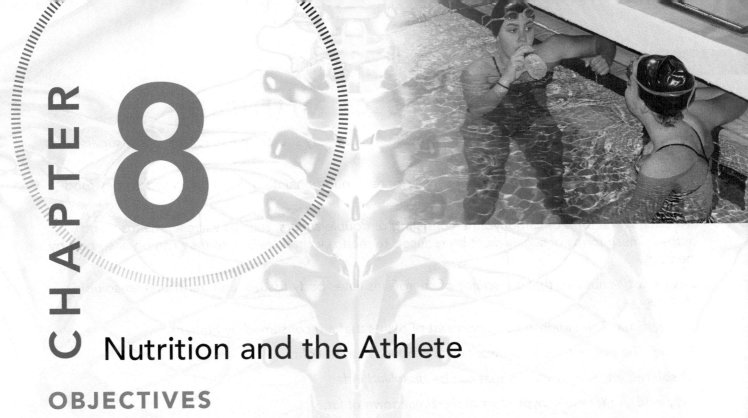

CHAPTER 8

Nutrition and the Athlete

OBJECTIVES

Upon completion of this chapter, the reader should be able to:

- Explain how good nutritional habits lead to increased athletic performance and good health
- Discuss the relationship of energy to food
- Describe the seven food components and their importance to nutrition
- Explain the importance of vitamins and minerals to a sound diet
- Explain why the food guide pyramid was developed
- Define daily values
- Compare and contrast the five food pyramids outlined in the chapter
- Define nutritional quackery
- Discuss proper weight control
- Discuss the underlying reasons for eating disorders
- Describe the importance of special diets and athletic performance
- Explain what an ideal weight for athletes should be

KEY TERMS

anorexia nervosa *A psychophysiological disorder characterized by an abnormal fear of becoming obese, a distorted self-image, persistent unwillingness to eat, and severe weight loss.*

body mass index (BMI) *The medical standard used to define obesity.*

bulimia *An eating disorder characterized by episodic binge eating, followed by feelings of guilt, depression, and self-condemnation.*

calorie *The energy needed to raise the temperature of one gram of water from 14.5° to 15.5°C.*

KEY TERMS CONTINUED

carbohydrate *An essential nutrient that provides the primary source of fuel for the body; sugars and starches.*

Daily Value (DV) *The percentage per serving of each nutritional item listed on a modern-day food label; based on a daily intake of 2,000 calories.*

disaccharide *A form of carbohydrate consisting of double sugars, such as sucrose, maltose, and lactose. These forms of sugars must be reduced to monosaccharides before they can be absorbed by the body.*

dietary fat *A nutrient that is a source of energy, insulates body tissues, and transports fat-soluble vitamins.*

dietary fiber *The indigestible component of plants that are consumed by humans.*

energy *The power used to do work or to produce heat or light.*

fat-soluble vitamin *A vitamin that can be dissolved in fat.*

fatty acid *A metabolic byproduct of the breakdown of fat.*

female athlete triad *A collection of symptoms seen in female athletes, consisting of disordered eating, amenorrhea, and osteoporosis (bone loss).*

Food Guide Pyramid *An outline for making food selections based on the government's dietary guidelines.*

insulin *A hormone produced in the pancreas that lowers the level of glucose in the blood by stimulating cells to store excess glucose.*

manorexia *An eating disorder in men.*

mineral *An inorganic substance that participates in many biochemical and physiological processes required for the growth, maintenance, repair, and health of tissues and bones.*

monosaccharide *The simplest form of carbohydrate, consisting of sugars that cannot be further reduced by the body, such as glucose, fructose, and galactose.*

monounsafurated fatty acid *Fats that do not contain high levels of hydrogen in combination with carbon atoms; these types of fats are found mainly in vegetable, olive, and peanut oils.*

nutrition *The process by which a living organism assimilates food and uses it for growth and replacement of tissues; the science or study that deals with food and nourishment.*

polysaccharide *A form of complex carbohydrate containing combinations of monosaccharides such as starch, cellulose, and glycogen.*

polyunsaturated fatty acid *Fats that contain only limited amounts of hydrogen attached to carbon atoms; found mainly in some forms of vegetable oils and seafood.*

protein *An essential nutrient that contains nitrogen and helps the body grow, build, and repair tissue.*

saturated fatty acid *Fats that contain the maximum number of hydrogen atoms attached to carbon atoms; these types of fats are found mainly in animal sources.*

trans fatty acid *A type of fat that is produced through the process of hydrogenation found mainly in processed foods such as margarine and snack foods.*

vitamin *A complex, organic substance that the body needs in small amounts.*

water-soluble vitamin *A vitamin that can be dissolved in water.*

NUTRITION

Nutrition can be defined as the process by which a living organism assimilates food and uses it for growth and replacement of tissues. It also refers to the field of science or study that deals with food and nourishment.

Athletic performance can be attributed in part to a full understanding of nutritional principles. Proper nutrition can reduce the likelihood of injury and propel the athlete to perform at a higher level. It is important that athletes understand the difference between fads and nutritional science.

ENERGY

Energy is the power used to do work, or to produce heat or light. Energy cannot be created or destroyed, but it can be changed from one form to another. For example, when coal burns, the energy stored in the chemical form in the coal is converted to heat and light.

Energy emanates from the sun, and in that form is called *solar energy*. Living plants convert solar energy to chemical energy by the process of *photosynthesis* (Figure 8–1). This chemical energy is used to make such substances as protein, carbohydrates, and fat, all of which provide energy.

FUN FACTS

March is National Nutrition Month! This is a national information and education campaign sponsored by the American Dietetic Association.

KEY CONCEPT

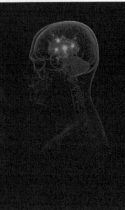

Athletic performance can be enhanced by a full understanding of nutritional principles. An athlete who follows a proper diet will have fewer injuries and perform at a higher level.

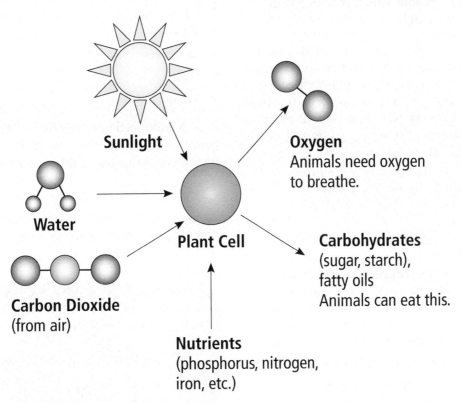

Figure 8–1 The process of photosynthesis.

DID YOU KNOW?

Good nutrition enhances appearance and is commonly exemplified by shiny hair, clear skin, clear eyes, erect posture, alert expression, and firm flesh on well-developed bone structures. Good nutrition aids emotional adjustment, provides stamina, and promotes a healthy appetite. It also helps establish regular sleep and elimination habits.

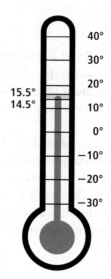

Figure 8–2 A calorie is the energy needed to raise the temperature of one gram of water from 14.5° to 15.5°C.

Animals cannot use solar energy directly, but do use the chemical energy contained in plants or other animals. They can oxidize carbohydrate, fat, and protein (and alcohol) to produce energy, carbon dioxide, and water. The energy is needed:

- To maintain body functions (e.g., to breathe, to keep the heart beating, to keep the body warm, and to carry out all the other functions that maintain life)
- For active movement (e.g., muscle contraction)
- For growth and repair, which requires that new tissues be made

The use of energy nearly always generates heat.

In nutrition, energy is measured as calories. A **calorie** (cal) is defined as the energy needed to raise the temperature of 1 gram of water from 14.5° to 15.5° Celsius (C) (Figure 8–2). People use large amounts of energy, so nutritionists use large units. One kilocalorie (kcal) equals 1,000 calories. To make things simple, nutritionists calculate kcals as one calorie; for example, a 2,000-calories diet really consists of 2,000,000 calories.

The number of kcals in food is the food's energy value. Energy values vary a great deal because they are determined by the types and amounts of nutrients each food contains. For example:

- Carbohydrate = 4 calories per gram
- Protein   = 4 calories per gram
- Fat   = 9 calories per gram
- Alcohol   = 7 calories per gram

FOOD COMPONENTS

The human body must have a balanced diet consisting of the following seven food components or nutrients:

- Carbohydrates
- Proteins
- Fats
- Vitamins
- Minerals
- Water
- Fiber

A balanced combination of these seven components nurtures the growth, repair, and maintenance of all tissues within the human body.

Carbohydrates

Carbohydrates are the body's primary source of fuel (glucose) for energy. This family of substances includes simple carbohydrates (sugars) and

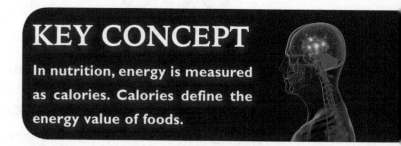

KEY CONCEPT

In nutrition, energy is measured as calories. Calories define the energy value of foods.

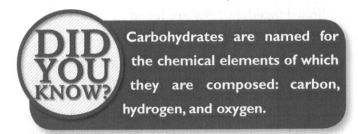

Carbohydrates are named for the chemical elements of which they are composed: carbon, hydrogen, and oxygen.

complex carbohydrates (starches). Though both types end up as glucose, foods that are high in complex carbohydrates, such as grains and vegetables, usually supply a good-health bonus of vitamins, minerals, and fiber as well (Figure 8–3). Simple carbohydrates, from candy, cake, table sugar, syrups, sweetened cereals, and other sources of concentrated sugar, contribute "empty" calories that provide energy but no nutrients.

Before carbohydrates can be used by the body, they must be broken down in the intestines by digestive enzymes into simple sugars: glucose,

fructose (fruit sugar), and galactose (a component of milk sugar). Some glucose is used immediately for energy; the rest is stored in the liver, muscles, and fat cells in the form of glycogen and fat for future use. (Fructose and galactose, however, must first be converted by the liver to glucose.) After a meal, the hormone **insulin**, which is produced in the pancreas, lowers the level of glucose in the blood by stimulating body cells to take up and store excess glucose. When a person's blood sugar is low—say, before breakfast or after exercise—another pancreatic hormone, glucagon, stimulates the conversion of liver glycogen back to glucose, preparing it to be returned to the bloodstream.

When a person has diabetes, a shortage or absence of insulin prevents glucose from moving into the cells. Insulin also plays an important role in preventing an excessive release of glucose from the liver between meals. Eating sugar does not cause the disease—individuals with diabetes have to watch

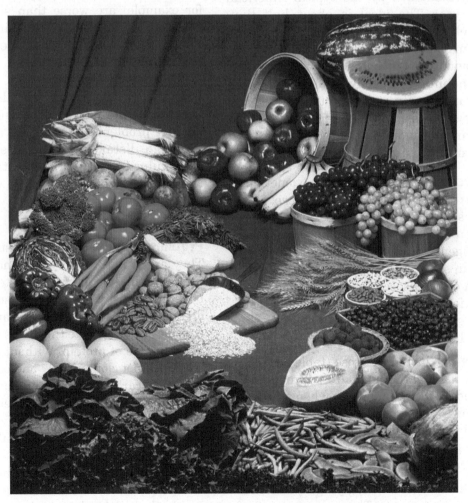

Figure 8–3 Fruits, vegetables, grains, and some dairy products are good sources of carbohydrates. Courtesy of the Agricultural Research Service, USDA

their total carbohydrate intake, rather than the type consumed. Eating sugary foods, however, is an easy way to overload the carbohydrate allotment.

In planning a diet, nutritionists recommend that 45 to 50% of daily calories come from carbohydrate sources, with the bulk of these calories supplied by complex carbohydrates. As stated earlier, 1 gram of carbohydrate equals 4 calories. This means a daily diet should contain at least:

- Six servings of grains such as bread, pasta, cereal, or rice

- Three servings of vegetables

- Two servings of fruit

It is estimated that American adults get about 20% of their daily calories from sugar. In a 2,000-calorie diet, that equals about 400 calories (100 grams)—the equivalent of 25 teaspoons of sugar daily. That amounts to about 130 pounds of sugar being consumed by the typical American adult each year. The ideal is about half that: approximately 10% of total calories, or 200 calories (50 grams) on a 2,000-calorie-a-day diet.

The obvious way to cut back on refined sugar is to limit the intake of candy, cake, cookies, pies, ice cream, and other sweets, and to avoid adding table sugar to foods and beverages. But eliminating sugar is not always so easy, because it comes in many forms:

- **Monosaccharides** include glucose (sometimes called dextrose), fructose, and galactose; all have the same number and types of atoms, but each has a different arrangement. The different arrangements of atoms account for the differences in sweetness. Glucose (one of the two sugars in every disaccharide) is mildly sweet; fructose (found in fruits and honey) is intensely sweet; galactose (a component of milk sugar) is hardly sweet at all.

- **Disaccharides** include sucrose (table sugar), lactose (milk sugar), and maltose (produced in plants and in the human body when starch breaks down). They are all pairs of two monosaccharides: sucrose is glucose and fructose; lactose is glucose and galactose; and maltose is two molecules of glucose.

- **Polysaccharides** (starches, glycogen, and cellulose) do not taste sweet. They are composed of hundreds, even thousands, of glucose molecules

linked together. They are found in foods such as potatoes, rice, and dried beans.

For purposes of overall health, all sugars are created equal. Honey, fructose, sucrose, corn syrup, maple syrup, and molasses are no better (or worse) than refined white sugar. They are absorbed differently, but all sugars eventually break down in the body and end up as glucose. Although refined white sugar has been blamed for an endless array of health problems (including hypoglycemia or low blood sugar, depression, yeast infections, and hyperactivity), there is no hard evidence to back up these claims. Sugar, however, does play a role in tooth decay; bacteria in the mouth break down sugar and produce an acid that erodes tooth enamel. However, the sugar that contributes to tooth decay can just as easily come from the breakdown of starchy foods, such as bread and potatoes, as it can from candy bars. Sugary foods that stay in the mouth (soft drinks and fruit drinks sipped throughout the day, for example) are worse than sugar added to the morning coffee. Regular brushing and flossing to remove sugar before any damage occurs is essential to a healthy mouth.

Sugar can contribute to obesity, which is linked to many diseases and disorders including heart disease, high blood pressure, diabetes, gallbladder problems, joint stress, and some cancers. Although dietary fat is often singled out as the main culprit in weight gain, eating too many calories from any source will cause weight gain.

Proteins

Proteins form the body's main structural elements. They are found in every cell and tissue. The body uses proteins for growth, and to build and repair bone, muscles, connective tissue, skin, internal organs, and blood. Hormones, antibodies, and the enzymes that regulate the body's chemical reactions are all made of protein. Without the right proteins, blood will not clot properly and cuts will not heal. If available carbohydrates and fat cannot meet an individual's energy needs, proteins will be broken down and used as a source of emergency energy. Each gram of protein equals 4 calories of energy.

Each protein is a large, complex molecule made up of a string of building blocks called *amino acids*. The 20 amino acids required by the body can be linked in thousands of different ways to form thousands of different proteins, each with a

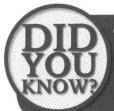

unique function in the body. The amino acids manufactured in the liver, and those derived from the breakdown of the proteins we eat, are absorbed into the bloodstream and taken up by cells and tissues to build new proteins as needed.

The body cannot use food protein directly, even though the amino acids in food and in the body are the same. Digestive enzymes break down ingested protein into shorter amino acid chains (polypeptides and then peptides) and finally into individual amino acids. The amino acids then enter the bloodstream and travel to the cells, where they are incorporated into the necessary proteins.

The quality of a food protein is measured in part by its amino acid content. There are two types: 9 of the 20 amino acids required by human beings are considered *essential* because they come only from the diet; the other 11 are considered *nonessential* because the body can make them. A *complete protein* contains all the essential amino acids in amounts the body needs. Animal proteins from eggs, meat, fish, poultry, cheese, and milk are generally complete. Plant proteins from fruits, vegetables, grains, and beans are usually low in one or more essential amino acid and are considered incomplete. A well-balanced vegetarian diet, however, can provide the body with all the needed amino acids.

The average adult's daily recommended allowance for protein is 0.8 grams (g) of protein for each kilogram (kg) of body weight. To determine this requirement, divide body weight by 2.2 (the number of pounds per kilogram), then multiply that by 0.8 (g of protein for each kg of body weight).

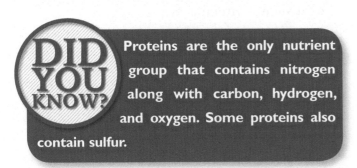

Fat

Dietary fat is required to carry out a number of functions. It is a carrier of fat-soluble vitamins and provides certain essential fatty acids. Fat is also an important source of energy and is used interchangeably with protein and carbohydrates. Each gram of fat contains a little more than twice the calories (9) of carbohydrates and protein. Fats occur naturally in food and play an important role in nutrition. Fats and oils provide a concentrated source of energy for the body. Fats are used to store energy in the body, insulate body tissues, and transport fat-soluble vitamins through the blood.

Not all fats and oils are created equal. Fats and oils are composed of basic units called **fatty acids**. Each type of fat or oil is a mixture of different fatty acids. Because overall fat intake is associated with obesity, cancer, and heart disease risk, it is a good idea to limit your intake of all three kinds of fats:

- **Saturated fatty acids** are found chiefly in animal sources such as meat, poultry, whole or reduced-fat milk, and butter. Some vegetable oils, like coconut, palm kernel oil, and palm oil, are saturated. Saturated fats are usually solid at room temperature. A diet high in saturated fats has been associated with increased risk of cancer and heart disease.

- **Monounsaturated fatty acids** are found mainly in vegetable oils such as canola, olive, and peanut oils. They are liquid at room temperature. Monounsaturated fats and polyunsaturated (found in vegetable oil, corn oil, and safflower oil) are less closely linked to disease unless they are altered during processing by hydrogenation into trans fatty acids.

- **Polyunsaturated fatty acids** are found mainly in vegetable oils such as safflower, sunflower, corn, flaxseed, and canola oils. Polyunsaturated fats are the main fats found in seafood. They are liquid or soft at room temperature. Specific polyunsaturated fatty acids, such as linoleic acid and alpha-linoleic acid, are *essential fatty acids* necessary for cell structure and making hormones. Essential fatty acids must be obtained from foods.

- **Trans fatty acids** are formed when vegetable oils are processed into margarine or shortening.

Sources of trans fats in the diet include snack foods and baked goods made with "partially hydrogenated vegetable oil" or "vegetable shortening." Trans fatty acids also occur naturally in some animal products such as dairy products.

Current dietary standards recommend that no more than 10% of one's total daily calories come from saturated fats, and that total fat intake be no more than 30% of one's total daily calories. Experts give the following tips to reduce the amount of fat in the diet:

- Limit the amount of red meat consumed.
- Choose low-fat or no-fat varieties of milk and cheese.
- Remove the skin of chicken and turkey before eating.
- Snack on pretzels instead of potato chips.
- Decrease or eliminate fried foods, butter, and margarine from the diet.
- Cook with small amounts of olive oil instead of butter, to cut your saturated fat intake.

Read food labels to see exactly how much fat is in foods (Figure 8–4). If the number of "fat calories" is more than 30% of total calories per serving, the food should be considered high-fat.

Vitamins

Vitamins are complex, organic substances that the body needs in small amounts, measured in milligrams (mg) or micrograms (mcg). A *milligram* is one thousandth of a gram. A *microgram* is one thousandth of a milligram or one-millionth of a gram. These small amounts are essential to proper health. Most vitamins cannot be manufactured by the body and must be provided by the diet.

Vitamins have a variety of different functions in the body. If the body lacks sufficient amounts of vitamins, certain symptoms will appear. These symptoms can develop into a deficiency disease.

Vitamins are grouped into two categories: fat-soluble and water-soluble.

Fat-soluble vitamins are found in foods such as meats, liver, dairy products, eggs, and leafy green vegetables. These vitamins are stored in the body's fat reserves and released as the body needs

Nutrition Facts		
Serving Size 1/2 cup (114g)		
Servings Per Container 4		
Amount Per Serving		
Calories 90		Calories from Fat 30
		% Daily Value
Total Fat 3g		**5%**
Saturated Fat 0g		**0%**
Cholesterol 0mg		**0%**
Sodium 300mg		**13%**
Total Carbohydrate 13g		**4%**
Dietary Fiber 3g		**12%**
Sugars 3g		
Protein 3g		

Vitamin A	80%	•	Vitamin C	60%
Calcium	4%	•	Iron	4%

• Percent Daily Values are based on a 2,000 calorie diet. Your daily values may be higher or lower depending on your calorie needs:

		Calories	2,000	2,500
Total Fat	Less than		65g	80g
Sat Fat	Less than		20g	25g
Cholesterol	Less than		300mg	300mg
Sodium	Less than		2,400mg	2,400mg
Total Carbohydrate			300g	375g
Fiber			25g	30g

Calories per gram:
Fat 9   •   Carbohydrate 4   •   Protein 4

Figure 8–4 Food labels contain important information about the nutritive value of the foods. Courtesy of the FDA

them. Large doses of these vitamins have the potential to cause toxicity.

Table 8–1 lists fat-soluble vitamins, food sources, functions, and signs of deficiency in each. The fat-soluble vitamins are:

- Vitamin A (retinol)
- Vitamin D (calciferol)
- Vitamin E (tocopherol)
- Vitamin K_1 (phytonadione)
- Vitamin K_2 (menaquinones)
- Vitamin K_3 (menadione)

Table 8–1 Fat-Soluble Vitamins

NAME	FOOD SOURCES	FUNCTIONS	DEFICIENCY/TOXICITY

Vitamin A (retinol)	Animal
	  Liver
	  Whole milk
	  Butter
	  Cream
	  Cod liver oil
	Plants
	  Dark green leafy
	    vegetables
	  Deep yellow or
	    orange fruit
	  Fortified margarine
		Maintenance of vision
		  in dim light
		Maintenance of mucous
		  membranes and
		  healthy skin
		Growth and development
		  of bones
		Reproduction
		Healthy immune system
			Deficiency
			  Night blindness
			  Xerophthalmia
			  Respiratory infections
			  Bone growth ceases
			Toxicity
			  Birth defects
			  Bone pain
			  Anorexia
			  Enlargement of liver

Vitamin D (calciferol)	Animal
	  Eggs
	  Liver
	  Fortified milk
	  Fortified margarine
	  Oily fish
	Plant
	  None
	Sunlight
		Regulation of
		  absorption
		  of calcium and
		  phosphorus
		Building and
		  maintenance
		  of normal bones
		  and teeth
		Prevention of tetany
			Deficiency
			  Rickets
			  Osteomalacia
			  Osteoporosis
			  Poorly developed teeth
			    and bones
			  Muscle spasms
			Toxicity
			  Kidney stones
			  Calcification of
			    soft tissues

Vitamin E (tocopherol)	Animal
	  None
	Plant
	  Green and leafy
	    vegetables
	  Margarines
	  Salad dressing
	  Wheat germ and
	    wheat germ oils
	  Vegetable oils
	  Nuts
		Antioxidant
		Considered essential
		  for protection of cell
		  structure, especially
		  of red blood cells
			Deficiency
			  Destruction of red blood
			    cells
			Toxicity

Vitamin K	Animal
	  Liver
	  Milk
	Plant
	  Green and leafy
	    vegetables
	  Cabbage, broccoli
		Blood clotting	Deficiency
			  Prolonged blood
			    clotting/ hemorrhaging
			Toxicity
			  Hemolytic anemia
			  Interferes with
			    anticlotting
			    medications

Water-soluble vitamins are found in foods such as whole-grain cereals, leafy green vegetables, fruits, and legumes. Vitamin B_{12} is present only in meat and dairy foods. These vitamins are not stored to any great extent in the body and must be replenished regularly. When taken in excess, these vitamins are excreted by the body in the urine. Table 8–2 lists the water-soluble vitamins, food sources, functions, and signs of deficiency. The water-soluble vitamins are:

- Folic acid
- Nicotinic acid (niacin) and nicotinamide (niacinamide)

- Vitamin B_1 (thiamine hydrochloride)
- Vitamin B_2 (riboflavin)
- Vitamin B_6 (pyridoxine hydrochloride)
- Vitamin B_{12} (cyanocobalamin)
- Vitamin C (ascorbic acid)

Minerals

Minerals are inorganic substances that are active in many biochemical and physiological processes necessary for proper growth, development, and health. If the body requires more than 100 milligrams of an inorganic substance each day, it is labeled a

Table 8–2 Water-Soluble Vitamins

NAME	FOOD SOURCES	FUNCTIONS	DEFICIENCY/TOXICITY

Thiamin (vitamin B_1)	Animal
	  Lean pork
	  Beef
	  Liver
	  Eggs
	  Fish
	Plant
	  Whole and
	    enriched grains
	    Legumes
	    Brewer's yeast
		Metabolism of
		  carbohydrates and
		  some amino acids
		Maintains normal
		  appetite and
		  functioning of
		  nervous system
			Deficiency
			  Gastrointestinal tract,
			    nervous system, and
			    cardiovascular system
			    problems
			  Beriberi
			Toxicity
			  None

Riboflavin (vitamin B_2)	Animal
	  Liver, kidney, heart
	  Milk
	  Cheese
	Plant
	  Green, leafy
	    vegetables
	  Cereals
	  Enriched bread
		Aids release of energy
		  from food
		Health of the mouth
		  tissue
		Healthy eyes
			Deficiency
			  Cheilosis
			  Eye sensitivity
			  Dermatitis
			Glossitis
			  Photophobia
			Toxicity
			  None

Niacin (nicotinic acid)	Animal
	  Milk
	  Eggs
	  Fish
	  Poultry
	Plant
	  Enriched breads
	    and cereals
		Energy metabolism
		Healthy skin and
		  nervous and
		  digestive systems
			Deficiency
			  Pellagra-dermatitis,
			    dementia, diarrhea
			Toxicity
			  Vasodilation of blood
			    vessels

(continues)

Table 8–2 Water-Soluble Vitamins (*continued*)

NAME	FOOD SOURCES	FUNCTIONS	DEFICIENCY/TOXICITY

Pyridoxine (vitamin B$_6$)	Animal
	  Pork
	  Fish
	  Poultry
	  Liver, kidney
	  Milk
	  Eggs
	Plant
	  Whole-grain cereals
	  Legumes
		Conversion of tryptophan to niacin
		Release of glucose from glycogen
		Protein metabolism and synthesis of nonessential amino acids
			Deficiency
			  Cheilosis
			  Glossitis
			  Dermatitis
			  Confusion
			  Depression
			  Irritability
			Toxicity
			  Depression
			  Nerve damage

Vitamin B$_{12}$ (cobalamin)	Animal
	  Seafood
	  Poultry
	  Liver, kidney
	  Muscle meats
	  Eggs
	  Milk
	  Cheese
	Plant
	  None
		Synthesis of red blood cells
		Maintenance of myelin sheaths
		Treatment of pernicious anemia
		Folate metabolism
			Deficiency
			  Degeneration of myelin sheaths
			  Pernicious anemia
			  Sore mouth and tongue
			  Anorexia
			  Neurological disorders
			Toxicity
			  None

Folate (folic acid)	Animal
	  Liver
	Plant
	  Leafy green vegetables
	  Spinach
	  Legumes
	  Seeds
	  Broccoli
	  Cereal fortified with folate
	  Fruit
		Synthesis of RBCs
		Synthesis of DNA
			Deficiency
			  Anemia
			  Glossitis
			  Neural tube defects such as anencephaly and spina bifida
			Toxicity
			  Could mask a B$_{12}$ deficiency

Biotin	Animal
	  Milk
	  Liver and kidney
	  Egg yolks
	Plant
	  Legumes
	  Brewer's yeast
	  Soy flour
	  Cereals
	  Fruit
		Coenzyme in carbohydrate and amino acid metabolism
		Niacin synthesis from tryptophan
			Deficiency
			  Dermatitis
			  Nausea
			  Anorexia
			  Depression
			  Hair loss
			Toxicity
			  None

(*continues*)

Table 8–2 Water-Soluble Vitamins (*continued*)

NAME	FOOD SOURCES	FUNCTIONS	DEFICIENCY/TOXICITY

Pantothenic Acid	Animal
	  Eggs
	  Liver
	  Salmon
	  Poultry
		Metabolism of carbohydrates, lipids, and proteins	Deficiency
			  Rare: burning feet syndrome; vomiting; fatigue

	Plant
	  Mushrooms
	  Cauliflower
	  Peanuts
	  Brewer's yeast
		Synthesis of fatty acids, cholesterol, steroid hormones	Toxicity
			  None

Vitamin C (ascorbic acid)	Animal
	  None
	Plants
	  All citrus fruits
	  Broccoli
	  Melons
	  Strawberries
	  Tomatoes
	  Brussels sprouts
	  Potatoes
	  Cabbage
	  Green peppers
		Prevention of scurvy
		Formation of collagen
		Healing of wounds
		Release of stress hormones
		Absorption of iron
		Antioxidant
		Resistance to infection
			Deficiency
			  Scurvy
			  Muscle cramps
			  Ulcerated gums
			  Tendency to bruise easily
			Toxicity
			  Raised uric acid level
			  Hemolytic anemia
			  Kidney stones
			  Rebound scurvy

mineral. If the body requires less than 100 milligrams a day, the substance is considered a trace element.

Many minerals are essential parts of enzymes. They also help regulate many physiological functions, including:

- Transporting oxygen to each of the body's 60 trillion cells
- Providing the stimulus for muscles to contract
- Guaranteeing normal function of the central nervous system

Minerals are required for the growth, maintenance, repair, and health of tissue and bone.

FUN FACTS
Vitamins are lost during food processing because they are easily destroyed by light, air, heat, and water. Vitamin loss can be avoided by eating foods that are fresh and by properly preparing foods to minimize the loss. For example, use as little water as possible to prepare vegetables; keep the pan covered; and heat them only briefly.

FUN FACTS
The elements oxygen, carbon, nitrogen, and hydrogen make up 96% of body weight. All remaining elements are minerals that make up only 4% of body weight.

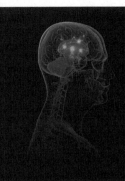

KEY CONCEPT

Vitamins are essential to helping the body use energy taken in as food. Minerals are necessary to repair and maintain tissue and bone.

Some, such as selenium, effect this by forming antioxidant enzymes.

Most minerals are widely distributed in foods (Table 8–3). Of all essential minerals, only a few may be deficient in a typical diet. Even so, there are exceptions. Iron deficiency is common in infants, children, and pregnant women. Zinc and copper deficiencies occur fairly frequently as well. However, severe mineral deficiency is unusual in the Western world.

Table 8–3   Major Minerals

NAME	FOOD SOURCES	FUNCTIONS	DEFICIENCY/TOXICITY

Calcium (Ca⁺⁺)	Milk, cheese
	Sardines
	Salmon
	Some dark green, leafy vegetables
		Development of bones and teeth
		Transmission of nerve impulses
		Blood clotting
		Normal heart action
		Normal muscle activity
			Deficiency
			  Osteoporosis
			  Osteomalacia
			  Rickets
			  Tetany
			  Retarded growth
			  Poor tooth and bone formation

Phosphorus (P)	Milk, cheese
	Lean meat
	Poultry
	Fish
	Whole grain cereals
	Legumes
	Nuts
		Development of bones and teeth
		Maintenance of normal acid-base balance of the blood
		Constituent of all body cells
		Necessary for effectiveness of some vitamins
		Metabolism of carbohydrates, fats, and proteins
			Deficiency
			  Poor tooth and bone formation
			  Weakness
			  Anorexia
			  General malaise

Potassium (K)	Oranges, bananas
	Dried fruits
	Vegetables
	Legumes
	Milk
	Cereals
	Meat
		Contraction of muscles
		Maintenance of fluid balance
		Transmission of nerve impulses
		Osmosis
		Regular heart rhythm
		Cell metabolism
			Deficiency
			  Hypokalemia
			  Muscle weakness
			  Confusion
			  Abnormal heartbeat
			Toxicity
			  Hyperkalemia

(continues)

Table 8–3   Major Minerals (*continued*)

NAME	FOOD SOURCES	FUNCTIONS	DEFICIENCY/TOXICITY

Sodium (Na+)	Table salt
	Beef, eggs
	Poultry
	Milk, cheese
		Maintenance of fluid
		  balance
		Transmission of nerve
		  impulses
		Osmosis
		Acid-base balance
		Regulation of muscle
		  and nerve irritability
			Deficiency
			  Nausea
			  Exhaustion
			  Muscle cramps
			Toxicity
			  Increase in blood
			    pressure
			  Edema

Chloride (Cl–)	Table salt
	Eggs
	Seafood
	Milk
		Gastric acidity
		Regulation of osmotic
		  pressure
		Osmosis
		Fluid balance
		Acid-base balance
		  Formation of
		  hydrochloric acid
			Deficiency
			  Imbalance in gastric
			    acidity
			  Imbalance in blood pH
			  Nausea
			  Exhaustion

Magnesium (Mg++)	Green, leafy
	  vegetables
	Whole grains
	Avocados
		Synthesis of ATP
		Transmission of nerve
		  impulses
		Activation of metabolic
		  enzymes
			Deficiency
			Normally unknown
			  Mental, emotional, and
			    muscle disorders

	Nuts
	Milk
	Legumes
	Bananas
		Constituent of bones,
		  muscles, and red blood
		  cells
		Necessary for healthy
		  muscles and nerves	

Sulfur (S)	Eggs
	Poultry
	Fish
		Maintenance of protein
		  structure
		For building hair, nails,
		  and all body tissues
		Constituent of all body
		  cells
			Unknown

Iron (Fe+)	Muscle meats
	Poultry
	Shellfish
	Liver
	Legumes
	Dried fruits
		Transports oxygen and
		  carbon dioxide
		Component of
		  hemoglobin and
		  myoglobin
			Deficiency
			  Iron deficiency anemia
			    characterized by
			    weakness, dizziness, loss
			    of weight, and pallor

(*continues*)

Table 8–3 Major Minerals (*continued*)

NAME	FOOD SOURCES	FUNCTIONS	DEFICIENCY/TOXICITY
	Whole grain or enriched breads and cereals Dark green and leafy vegetables Molasses	Component of cellular enzymes essential for energy production	Toxicity Hemochromatosis (genetic) Can be fatal to children May contribute to heart disease Injure liver
Iodine (I⁻)	Iodized salt Seafood	Regulation of basal metabolic rate	Deficiency Goiter Cretinism Myxedema
Zinc (Zn⁺)	Seafood, especially oysters Liver Eggs Milk Wheat bran Legumes	Formation of collagen Component of insulin Component of many vital enzymes Wound healing Taste acuity Essential for growth Immune reactions	Deficiency Dwarfism, hypogonadism, anemia Loss of appetite Skin changes Impaired wound healing Decreased taste acuity
Selenium (Se⁻)	Seafood Kidney Liver Muscle meats Grains	Constituent of most body tissue Needed for fat metabolism Antioxidant functions	Deficiency Unclear, but related to Keshan disease Muscle weakness Toxicity Vomiting Loss of hair and nails Skin lesions
Copper (Cu⁺)	Liver Shellfish, oysters Legumes Nuts Whole grains	Essential for formation of hemoglobin and red blood cells Component of enzymes Wound healing Needed metabolically for the release of energy	Deficiency Anemia Bone disease Disturbed growth and metabolism Toxicity Vomiting; diarrhea Wilson's disease (genetic)
Manganese (Mn⁺)	Whole grains Nuts Fruits Tea	Component of enzymes Bone formation Metabolic processes	Deficiency Unknown Toxicity Possible brain disease

(*continues*)

Table 8–3   Major Minerals (*continued*)

NAME	FOOD SOURCES	FUNCTIONS	DEFICIENCY/TOXICITY

Fluoride (F⁻)	Fluoridated water
	Seafood
		Increases resistance to
		   tooth decay
		Component of bones
		   and teeth
			Deficiency
			   Tooth decay
			   Possibly osteoporosis
			Toxicity
			   Discoloration of teeth
			   (mottling)

Chromium
(Cr)
	Meat
	Vegetable oil
	Whole grain cereal
	   and nuts
	Yeast
		Associated with glucose
		   and lipid metabolism
			Deficiency
			   Possibly disturbances of
			   glucose metabolism

Molybdenum
(Mo)
	Dark green, leafy
	   vegetables
	Liver
	Cereal
	Legumes
		Enzyme functioning
		Metabolism
			Deficiency
			   Unknown
			Toxicity
			   Inhibition of copper
			   absorption

Water

Water is the most important, yet an often neglected, nutrient. Without it we cannot exist; when it is limited, our bodies suffer. A fluid loss of just 2 to 3% of body weight will impair performance (Figure 8–5). Fluid loss of 7 to 10% can be fatal. The kidneys play an important role in conserving and excreting water.

Blood circulates throughout the body, carrying nutrients and energy to cells. Water in the bloodstream helps regulate body temperature, transport nutrients, eliminate toxins and waste products, and maintain proper metabolism.

On average, the body will lose approximately seven glasses of water each day. An active individual will lose a much greater amount. We lose water by way of sweat, urine, and bowel movements. We actually lose water every time we exhale.

To maintain proper hydration, drink six to eight glasses of fluids each day, more when active. Thirst is not always a good indicator of the need for fluid replacement. When working out or being physically active, it is a good idea to pre-hydrate by drinking a glass or two of fluids within an hour of exercise. This helps the body to cope with

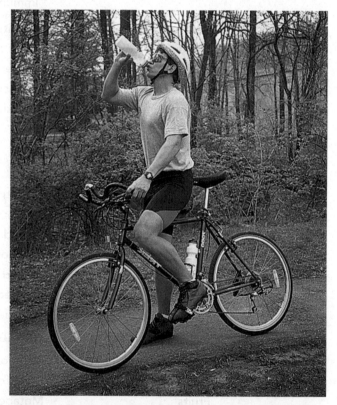

Figure 8–5 Preventing dehydration is an important element of proper nutrition. A fluid loss of just 2 to 3% of body weight will impair performance.

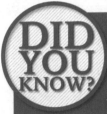

FUN FACTS
A person can live about 8 days without food, but only a few days without water.

immediate water loss due to perspiration and increased metabolism. After the activity ceases, it is important to drink as much as possible to replace fluid loss.

As important as water intake is before and after activity, it is essential to drink water at intervals *during* activity. Restricting water intake during a practice or game is dangerous and also hampers performance. Coaches once believed that restricting water from athletes during a practice or game would toughen them up. This old-school thinking had many tragic results. Most coaches today understand the need for fluid replacement and know that a well-hydrated athlete will perform at a higher level and be healthier.

DID YOU KNOW? The sensation of thirst often lags behind the body's need for water, especially in children, the elderly, athletes, and persons who are ill.

SPORTS DRINKS Today's sports drinks contain sugar, minerals such as potassium and sodium, and water. In terms of ingredients, little distinguishes the major brands of sports drinks; they are nearly identical in nutritional content. Some brands have additional vitamins or sodium. At least one brand contains *ephedra* (ma huang), a powerful herbal stimulant that can cause nervousness, insomnia, nausea, spikes in blood pressure, and even heart attack and stroke. It also works to suppress the sweat mechanism while the athlete is exercising. This can cause a rapid rise in body temperature, leading to hyperthermia. Avoid any sports drink or supplement containing this ingredient.

Sports drinks can help with long, hard workouts that exceed one hour. During these workouts, the body needs carbohydrates and water. Added sodium and potassium will do little good unless the athlete sweats profusely for more than four hours. Water works as well as anything else if exercise lasts less than one hour. The real value of sports beverages lies in the carbohydrates, sugars, and other energy compounds that help feed the muscles and delay fatigue.

Dietary Fiber

Dietary fiber is the indigestible component of plant material that humans consume. Fiber is found in all plant foods such as grains, beans, lentils, fruits, and vegetables. Even though the

KEY CONCEPT

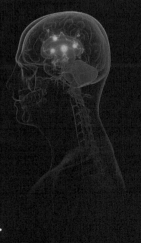

Each food component plays an important role in maintaining health:

- Carbohydrates are the body's primary source of fuel for energy.
- Proteins are necessary for growth and to repair and build tissues.
- Fats store energy, insulate body tissues, and transport fat-soluble vitamins through the bloodstream.
- Vitamins do not provide energy, but are needed to help utilize the energy from other nutrients.
- Minerals are necessary for growth, maintenance, and repair of tissue and bone.
- Water is the most important nutrient.
- Fiber aids in maintaining the health of the digestive tract.

nutritional component of fiber is not essential, it keeps the digestive tract running smoothly.

There are two types of fiber: soluble and insoluble. *Soluble fiber* is found in fruits, oats, barley, legumes, and psyllium seed. It dissolves in fluids in the large intestine and helps to lower cholesterol levels, which may reduce the risk of coronary heart disease. *Insoluble fiber* is found in some fruits and vegetables, whole grains, and wheat bran. This type of fiber does not dissolve in the fluids of the large intestine, but instead soaks up water to add bulk. This helps prevent constipation by making it easier for the intestines to eliminate waste.

The National Academy of Medicine advises the following daily recommendations for adults:

	AGE 50 AND YOUNGER	AGE 51 AND OLDER
Men	38 grams	30 grams
Women	25 grams	21 grams

There is no daily reference value (DRV) for fiber. It is suggested that the diet include approximately 25 grams of fiber each day. Table 8–4 highlights the fiber found in common foods.

Table 8–4   Fiber Content in Popular Foods

FOODS HIGH IN INSOLUBLE FIBER	SERVING SIZE	GRAMS
Banana	1 small	0.7
Bran cereal (100%)	1/2 cup	9.7
Broccoli	1 cup	4.0
Carrot	1 medium	2.3
Peas	1/2 cup cooked	3.2
Popcorn	3 cups	2.0
Potato, baked with skin	1 medium	3.6
Prunes	1 cup cooked	14
Raisin bran cereals	3/4 cup	4.8
Spinach	1/2 cup cooked	2.0
Whole-wheat bread	1 slice	1.9
FOODS HIGH IN INSOLUBLE FIBER	SERVING SIZE	GRAMS
Apple	1 medium	3.0
Banana	1 small	0.6
Broccoli	1/2 cup cooked	1.6
Lentils, cooked	1/2 cup	3.7
Oat bran	1/3 cup	4.9
Pear	1 medium	4.3
Peas	1/2 cup cooked	2.0
Popcorn	3 cups	0.8
Strawberries	1 cup	3.9

DAILY VALUES

In 1973, the United States Food and Drug Administration introduced the Recommended Daily Allowances (RDAs) as reference values for vitamins, minerals, and protein in voluntary nutrition labeling. In 1994, the RDA table was replaced with the **Daily Value (DV)** guide to help consumers use food label information in planning their overall diet. Table 8–5 outlines daily values for the nutrients we require.

The DVs are actually two sets of reference values for nutrients: Daily Reference Values (DRVs), based on the National Academy of Sciences' 1998 Recommended Dietary Allowances, and Dietary Reference Intakes (DRIs). In food labeling the government uses the Daily Value. The change from RDAs to DVs is the government's effort to help the public recognize and comprehend nutrition information easily, and understand its significance in a healthy daily diet.

DRVs for the energy-producing nutrients (fat, carbohydrate, protein, and fiber) are based on the number of calories consumed per day. For labeling purposes, 2,000 calories has been established as the reference for calculating percent Daily Values. This makes it easier for consumers to calculate their individual nutrient needs. DRVs

Table 8–5 United States Food and Drug Administration Daily Values

DAILY REFERENCE VALUES (DRVs)		DIETARY REFERENCE INTAKES (DRIs)	
Food Component	DRV	Nutrient	Amount
Fat	65 g	Vitamin A	5,000 International Units (IU)
Saturated fatty acids	20 g	Vitamin C	60 mg
Cholesterol	300 mg	Thiamin	1.5 mg
Total carbohydrate	300 g	Riboflavin	1.7 mg
Fiber	25 g	Niacin	20 mg
Sodium	2,300 mg	Calcium	1.0 g
Potassium	3,500 mg	Iron	18 mg
Protein*	50 g	Vitamin D	400 IU
		Vitamin E	30 IU
		Vitamin B_6	2.0 mg
		Folic acid	0.4 mg
		Vitamin B_{12}	6 micrograms (mcg)
		Phosphorus	1.0 g
		Iodine	150 mcg
		Magnesium	400 mg
		Zinc	15 mg
		Copper	2 mg
		Biotin	0.3 mg
		Pantothenic acid	10 mg

*DRV for protein does not apply to certain populations. Dietary Reference Intake (DRI) for protein has been established for these groups: children 1 to 4 years, 16 g; infants under 1 year, 14 g; pregnant women, 60 g; nursing mothers, 65 g.

for the energy-producing nutrients are always calculated as follows:

- Fat based on 30% of calories
- Saturated fat based on 10% of calories
- Carbohydrate based on 60% of calories
- Protein based on 10% of calories (the DRV for protein applies only to adults and children over the age of four; DRIs for protein for special groups have been established)
- Fiber based on 11.5 grams of fiber per 1,000 calories

Thus, someone who consumes 3,000 calories a day—a teenage boy, for example—would have a recommended fat intake of 100 grams or less per day:

$$0.30 \times 3,000 = 900$$

900 (calories) ÷ 9 (calories per gram of fat) = 100 grams

The DRVs for cholesterol, sodium, and potassium, which do not contribute calories, remain the same regardless of calorie level.

Because of the links between certain nutrients and certain diseases, DRVs for some nutrients represent the uppermost limit that is considered desirable. Eating too much fat or cholesterol, for example, has been linked to an increased risk of heart disease. Too much sodium can raise the risk of high blood pressure in some people. Therefore, labels show DVs for fats and sodium as follows:

- Total fat: less than 65 grams
- Saturated fat: less than 20 grams
- Cholesterol: less than 300 milligrams
- Sodium: less than 2,400 milligrams

FOOD GUIDE PYRAMID

The **Food Guide Pyramid** was designed by the United States Department of Agriculture (USDA) and supported by the Department of Health and Human Services (HHS) as an easy way to educate people about food, nutrition, and exercise choices. It was redesigned in 2005, and later modified in January, 2018 (Figure 8–6) to visually engage people of all ages in nutrition and exercise choices.

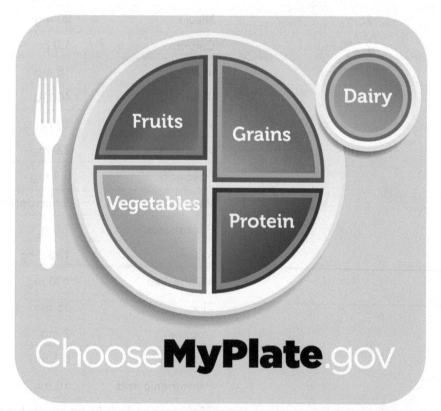

Figure 8–6 MyPlate Dietary Guidelines, 2018. United States Department of Agriculture. Courtesy of the USDA

The current design is a representation of the importance of each food group in staying healthy. The color scheme represents the different food groups organized upon a plate. The primary focus is that all food and beverage choices matter, with an emphasis on variety, amount, and nutritional content.

The 2015–2020 Dietary Guidelines also emphasize that choice matters.

A focus on making healthy food and beverage choices from all five food groups, including fruits, vegetables, grains, protein foods, and dairy to get the nutrients you need.

Choosing an eating style low in saturated fat, sodium, and added sugars.

Making small changes to create a healthier eating style. This includes making half your plate fruits and vegetables, focusing on whole fruits, varying your vegetable selection, making half your grains whole grains, eating low-fat and fat-free dairy, varying your protein intake, and eating and drinking the right amount.

Overall, the American diet is too high in fat. Following the USDA guidelines will help maintain a diet low in total fat and saturated fat. This reduces the chances of getting certain diseases associated with a high-fat diet.

The following guidelines were developed jointly by the USDA and HHS in 2005, and were modified for their 2015-2020 dietary guidelines. These guidelines are considered the latest, most up-to-date advice from nutrition scientists for Americans age two and over:

- Consume a variety of nutrient-dense foods and beverages within the basic food groups
- Limit the intake of saturated and trans fats, cholesterol, added sugars, salt, and alcohol
- Meet recommended intakes within energy needs by adopting a balanced eating pattern
- Maintain body weight in a healthy range
- Engage in regular physical activity and reduce sedentary activities (60–90 minutes daily)
- Consume a sufficient amount of fruits and vegetables while staying within energy needs
- Consume three or more ounces of whole grain products each day
- Consume three cups of fat-free or low-fat milk or equivalent milk products each day

- Consume less than 10% of calories from saturated fatty acids and added sugars.
- Choose and prepare foods and beverages with little added sugars or sweeteners
- Consume less than 2300 milligrams of sodium (approximately 1 tsp of salt) per day
- Aim for a healthy weight.
- Let the food pyramid guide your food choices.
- Choose a variety of grains daily, especially whole grains.
- Choose a variety of fruits and vegetables daily.
- Keep food safe to eat.
- Choose a diet that is low in saturated fat and cholesterol and moderate in total fat.
- Choose beverages and foods to moderate your intake of sugars.
- Choose and prepare foods with less salt.
- If you drink alcoholic beverages, do so in moderation.

Each culture has its own nutritional standards for healthful living. To devise food guidance systems appropriate for each nation, many countries have applied research regarding their national food supplies, food consumption patterns, nutrition status, and nutritional standards toward development of individual food guides. For instance, the U.S. Food Guide Pyramid is firmly based on USDA research as to the types of foods Americans consume, the nutrient composition of those foods, and their relation to the individual's nutrient needs. In some food guides, the presence of indigenous foods and particular dietary patterns resulting from different geographical conditions and cultural heritages have also been considered. It is well known that various cultures have different food options, food preferences, dietary patterns, and cultural definitions of foods. The food pyramids in Figures 8–7 through 8–9 are included for comparison.

The Mediterranean diet delivers as much as 40% of total daily calories from fat, yet the associated incidence of cardiovascular diseases is significantly decreased. Because it is a monosaturated fatty acid, olive oil does not have the same cholesterol-raising effect of saturated fats. Olive oil is also a good source of antioxidants. Eating fish a few times per week benefits Mediterranean

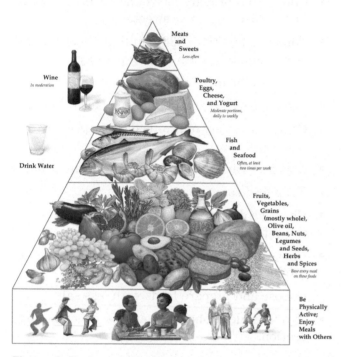

Figure 8–7 The Mediterranean Diet Pyramid. Oldways Preservation and Exchange Trust, http://www.oldwayspt.org

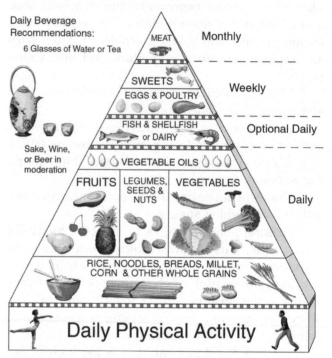

Figure 8–8 The Asian Diet Pyramid. Oldways Preservation and Exchange Trust, http://www.oldwayspt.org

people by increasing their intake of omega-3 fatty acids, which other developed societies usually do not consume adequately.

The Asian Diet Pyramid emphasizes a wide base of rice, rice products, noodles, breads, and grains, preferably whole-grain and minimally processed foods, topped by another large band of fruits, vegetables, legumes, nuts, and seeds. Physical exercise, a small amount of vegetable oil, and moderate consumption of plant-based beverages (including tea, especially black and green, sake, beer, and wine) also are recommended daily. Small daily servings of dairy products (low-fat) or fish are optional; sweets, eggs, and poultry are recommended no more than weekly, and red meat no more than monthly.

The Latin American diet places poultry, meats, and eggs near the top of the pyramid. It also recommends that beans, nuts, vegetables, and fruit be consumed at every meal. Daily physical activity is another important component of overall fitness.

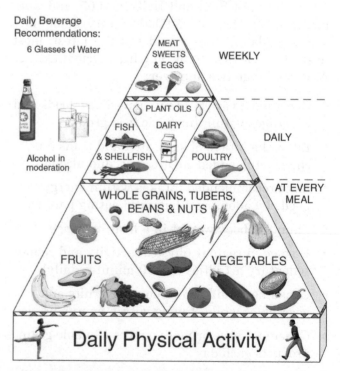

Figure 8–9 The Latin Diet Pyramid. Oldways Preservation and Exchange Trust, http://www.oldwayspt.org

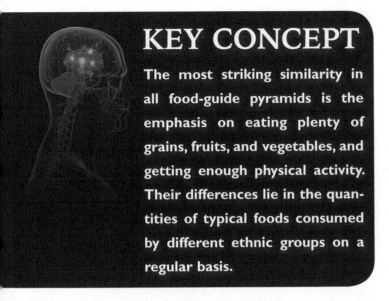

KEY CONCEPT

The most striking similarity in all food-guide pyramids is the emphasis on eating plenty of grains, fruits, and vegetables, and getting enough physical activity. Their differences lie in the quantities of typical foods consumed by different ethnic groups on a regular basis.

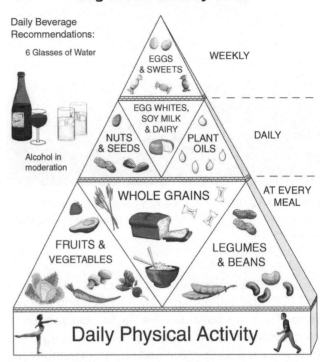

Figure 8–10 The Vegetarian Diet Pyramid. Oldways Preservation and Exchange Trust, http://www.oldwayspt.org

Note the similarities and differences in the diets from these three regions of the world and the food pyramid of the United States. The Mediterranean, Asian, and Latin American diets emphasize cultural eating patterns and include a more limited range of foods. Another major difference is that these pyramids utilize more plant-based proteins (those from legumes, soybeans, nuts, and seeds) than those found in meat, poultry, eggs, and dairy products. Similarities include an emphasis on eating plenty of grain products, vegetables, and fruit. Physical activity is another common aspect of all food guide pyramids

The vegetarian diet is also popular (Figure 8–10). According to the American Dietetic Association, planned vegetarian diets are healthful, nutritionally adequate, and provide health benefits in the prevention and treatment of certain diseases.

FOOD GROUPS There are six food groups in the USDA food pyramid:

- Breads, cereals, rice, and pasta
- Vegetables
- Fruit
- Meat, poultry, and fish
- Milk products
- Fats, oils, and sweets

BREADS, CEREALS, RICE, AND PASTA Eat at least three ounces of breads, cereals, rice, and pasta each day (Figure 8–11). These foods provide

complex carbohydrates (starches), which are an important source of energy, especially in low-fat diets. They also provide vitamins, minerals, and fiber.

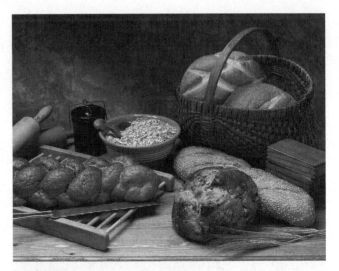

Figure 8–11 These foods provide complex carbohydrates (starches), which are an important source of energy, especially in low-fat diets. They also provide vitamins, minerals, and fiber. Courtesy of Wheat Foods Council

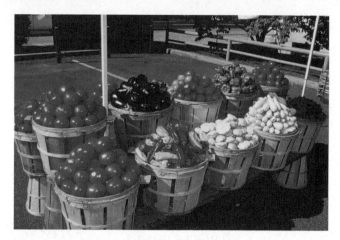

Figure 8–12 Vegetables are rich in vitamins A and C, folate, and minerals such as iron and magnesium. Courtesy of USDA

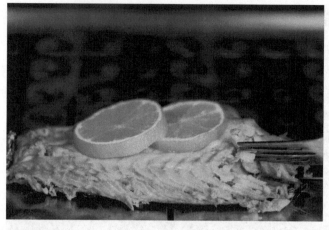

Figure 8–14 Two to three servings from the meat, poultry, and fish food group should be consumed each day. Courtesy of USDA

VEGETABLES Vegetables are rich in vitamins A and C, folate, and minerals such as iron and magnesium. They are naturally low in fat and provide a good source of fiber (Figure 8–12). It is suggested that you eat darker green and orange vegetables, as well as more dry beans and peas. The number of servings each day depends upon age, sex, and physical activity.

FRUIT Fruit and 100-percent fruit juices abound in vitamins A and C and potassium (Figure 8–13). They are low in fat and sodium. It is suggested that 1½ to 2 cups of fruit be consumed each day.

MEAT, POULTRY, AND FISH The food group that includes meat, poultry, and fish is abundant in protein, B vitamins, iron, and zinc (Figure 8–14). Other foods in this group—dry beans, eggs, and nuts—are similar to meats in supplying protein and most vitamins and minerals. Consume five to six ounces from this food group daily.

MILK PRODUCTS Milk products provide protein, vitamins, and minerals, and are an excellent source of calcium (Figure 8–15). The Food Guide Pyramid recommends three cups from this group daily. Women who are pregnant or breastfeeding should add at least one more serving.

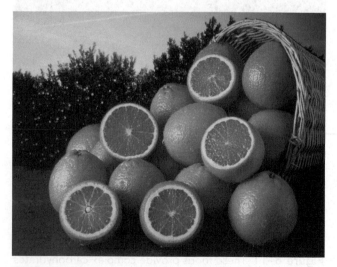

Figure 8–13 Fruits provide vitamins A and C, potassium, magnesium, iron, and carbohydrates, including dietary fiber. Courtesy of USDA

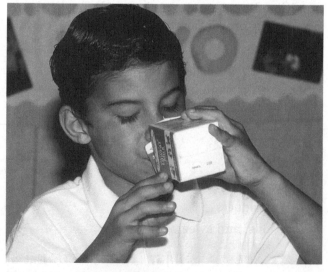

Figure 8–15 Milk continues to be an important source of nutrition for school-age children.

FATS, OILS, AND SWEETS Being listed at the top of the food pyramid is not an honor. Consumption of items in this food group should be limited, even though some nutrients found here are important to good health. The USDA recommendation is to use these foods sparingly.

NUTRITIONAL QUACKERY

Many athletes seek out "magic" supplements that will give them an edge over their competitors. As a result, they become susceptible to nutritional quackery. Most athletes would love an alternative to hard work and training. Nutritional quackery is successful because individuals and companies prey on emotions and misinformation.

New dietary supplements are marketed each day. These products are often developed and sold without any supporting scientific research on benefits or harmful side effects. The Food and Drug Administration treats dietary supplements as foods. Therefore, these products are not evaluated for safety and effectiveness.

Individuals and companies promote false or unproven nutritional supplements or products with the aim of making money. They prey on the innocent, unsuspecting athlete who is eager for an edge. If their claims appear too good to be true, they probably are false.

Before taking any product, the athlete should consult with someone who has nutritional training. It may save money, disappointment, and the athlete's health. The best protection against nutritional quackery is to be an informed consumer.

MAKING THE WEIGHT

One of the most important aspects of fitness and athletic performance is controlling weight. Proper weight management enhances good health and athletic performance. This goes back to the earlier discussion of nutrition: A properly conditioned athlete is also one who takes proper nutrition seriously.

One pound of fat equals 3,500 calories. Most active men and women require about 2,200 calories a day. Some active men may need 2,800 calories. High-endurance athletes will require considerably more.

Being overweight or underweight is the result of eating more or fewer calories, respectively, than the person needs. The person's food choices, along with exercise, determine body weight.

Gaining Weight

The objective of gaining weight is to increase lean body mass. *Lean body mass* is muscle, as opposed to body fat. It takes about 2,500 calories to gain one pound of lean body mass and 3,500 calories to gain one pound of fat. Lean body mass cannot be increased by the use of vitamins, foods, or supplements. It is possible to gain one or two pounds per week, providing that a weight training program is central to the program. Without a weight training program and increased energy expenditure, excess caloric intake will be converted to fat.

Losing Weight

There are three ways to lose weight:

- Restricting caloric intake (dieting)
- Exercise
- Restricting caloric intake *and* exercise

Dieting alone is the most difficult means of losing weight. Long-term weight control through dieting alone is successful only 2% of the time. In dieting, 35 to 45 % of the weight decrease is from lean body tissue. The minimum caloric intake for a female should not go below 1,000 to 1,200 calories per day. A male's intake should not drop below 1,200 to 1,400 calories per day.

Weight loss through exercise may result in increased cardiorespiratory endurance, as well as gains in strength and increased flexibility. These are all positive for the athlete's overall health. Using exercise as the sole means of losing weight will probably have the same limited results as dieting alone.

The best approach to losing weight and keeping it off is to combine exercise with a moderate diet. A moderate increase in activity, coupled with a moderate decrease in caloric intake, will cause the body to burn fat reserves and thereby lose weight. A weight loss of one to two pounds each week is considered healthy. Weight loss of more than two pounds a week may be partially the result of dehydration.

It is always important to check with the family doctor before beginning any weight loss or gain program.

EATING DISORDERS

Eating disorders are extreme expressions of food and weight issues experienced by many individuals, particularly girls and women. They include anorexia nervosa, bulimia nervosa, and binge eating. These disorders are very dangerous behaviors that result in health problems.

Participants in sports that emphasize appearance and a lean body are at higher risk for developing disordered eating behavior. Many female athletes who engage in harmful methods of weight control suffer from amenorrhea and bone loss. *Amenorrhea* is the abnormal suppression or absence of menstruation.

According to a 2007 Harvard University study, 25 % of all the athletes with eating disorder behavior are male. The term now associated with this condition is **manorexia**. The symptoms of anorexia and bulimia are similar for men and women, but the underlying cause can be quite different. A common issue for men is having been overweight as a child and teased about it.

One particular issue with male disordered eating concerns the sport of wrestling, which has several different weight classifications. These classifications require the athlete to make the weight limit or forfeit the match (Figure 8–16). This encourages extreme weight-loss measures aimed at losing a few pounds as quickly as possible. These athletes often wear rubber suits while exercising, chew gum and spit excess saliva into a cup, fast, and drink no fluids. These methods of losing weight are unhealthy, and sometimes deadly. It is imperative that coaches and parents monitor these athletes carefully so that they do not "make weight" at the risk of their health.

The Female Athlete Triad

In 1992, the American College of Sports Medicine termed a collection of symptoms diagnosed in female athletes the **female athlete triad**. The triad consists of eating disorder, amenorrhea, and osteoporosis (bone loss). The triad is especially prevalent in sports that emphasize the aesthetic of leanness, such as gymnastics, figure skating, diving, and dance (Figure 8–18). It is also seen in sports such as swimming and running, where leanness is thought to yield a competitive edge.

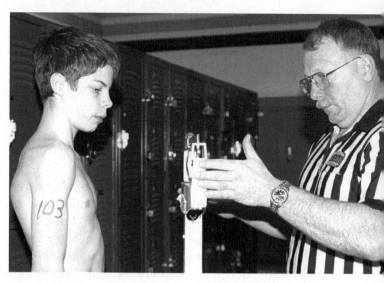

Figure 8–16 Athletes, like this wrestler, who consistently try to lose weight through starvation and dehydration run the risk of serious health problems. Courtesy of Mark Dickerson, Action Sports Photography

The National Institute of Mental Health reports that 2.7% of teens ages 13 to 18 struggle with an eating disorder.

Because the triad may result in irreversible bone loss and death, early detection is important. Signs and symptoms include eating alone, trips to the bathroom during or after meals, use of laxatives, fatigue, anemia, depression, and eroded tooth enamel from frequent vomiting.

Treatment of the female athlete triad involves education, nutrition, determining contributing factors, and care from a medical specialist trained in disordered eating. Fifty percent of teenage girls and 30% of teenage boys use unhealthy weight control behaviors such as skipping meals, fasting, smoking cigarettes, vomiting, and taking laxatives to control their weight.

Girls and women often experiment with these different ways to lose weight:

- Diuretics
- Laxatives
- Self-induced vomiting
- Diet pills
- Serious overexercise

All of these methods can have dangerous side effects. Understanding the female athlete triad, and the importance of proper nutrition and a positive body image, is imperative for coaches, athletic

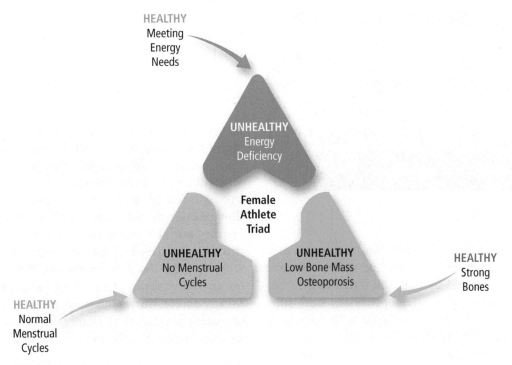

Figure 8–17 The Female Athlete Triad Model.

trainers, parents, and athletes. The following suggestions for coaches and trainers can help:

- Avoid weighing athletes and obtaining body composition data.
- Observe meals to check for disordered eating patterns.

- Encourage a snack period midway through practice to replenish energy.
- Provide mandatory seminars by a qualified nutritionist on the importance of a balanced diet for athletic performance.

Anorexia Nervosa

Anorexia nervosa is a psychophysiological disorder, usually occurring in young women, that is characterized by an abnormal fear of becoming obese, a distorted self-image, a persistent unwillingness to eat, and severe weight loss. It is often accompanied by self-induced vomiting, excessive exercise, malnutrition, amenorrhea, and other physiological changes. As many as 4% of individuals diagnosed with anorexia nervosa will die from this disorder. Signs and symptoms include substantial weight loss (at least 15% of a person's normal body weight), loss of appetite, loss of menstruation, fatigue and dizziness, constipation, and abdominal pains. The person may feel cold to the touch even in warm weather. Physical dangers associated with anorexia nervosa include starvation (as the body begins to use its own tissue for energy), dehydration, muscle and cartilage deterioration, osteoporosis, irregular or abnormally slow heart rate, and heart failure.

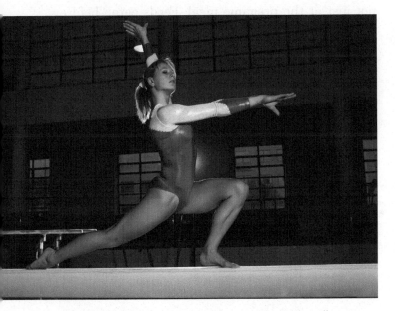

Figure 8–18 The female athlete triad is especially prevalent in sports that emphasize the aesthetic of leanness, such as gymnastics, figure skating, diving, and dance. I T A L O/Shutterstock.com

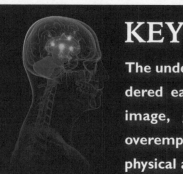

KEY CONCEPT

The underlying reasons for disordered eating are distorted self-image, guilt, depression, and overemphasis on leanness and physical appearance.

Bulimia

Bulimia is an eating disorder, common especially among young women of normal or nearly normal weight, characterized by episodic binge eating followed by feelings of guilt, depression, and self-condemnation. It is often associated with measures taken to prevent weight gain such as self-induced vomiting, the use of laxatives, dieting, or fasting. Signs and symptoms include fluctuations in weight, often from one extreme to the other (underweight to overweight); dental cavities caused by stomach acid regurgitation during vomiting; dehydration, fatigue and dizziness, constipation and abdominal pains, swelling of the salivary glands (leading to "chipmunk cheek," enlarged cheeks or jowls); and irregular or absent menstruation. Physical dangers associated with bulimia include stomach ulceration, bowel damage, inflammation and occasionally tearing of the esophagus, laxative addiction, tingling in the hands and feet, and electrolyte imbalances, which can lead to heart failure.

Bigorexia

Bigorexia, known as muscle dysmorphia, is a disorder that causes a person to obsess about being too small or inadequate. These individuals work out constantly to obtain a large muscle mass. This disorder is consistent with obsessive compulsive disorder (OCD).

SPECIAL DIETS

Many special diets on the market today promise significant weight loss, while claiming to be safe and healthy. Many offer incredible weight loss without calorie limitation or exercise. Many require taking a few pills each day or consuming a special diet powder mixed with water or fruit juice. Some require a diet high in protein and low in carbohydrates; others eating cabbage soup, using hypnosis, wraps . . . the list goes on and on. Before embarking on any special diet, the athlete should talk with a family doctor, nutritionist, certified athletic trainer, or health professional. Good health is too important to risk on potentially dangerous diets.

Pregame Meal

Before competition—sometimes several days prior—many athletes begin a special diet that limits protein intake and concentrates on carbohydrates. Athletes believe that a pregame meal will give them the energy they need to compete. However, the energy for the game actually comes from muscle glycogen stores that are built up by consuming high-carbohydrate meals every day, not just at the pregame meal. Foods eaten before the game supplement muscle glycogen stores. The pregame meal also helps to prevent a low blood sugar level, with its symptoms of light-headedness, fatigue, and low concentration; all of these can interfere with performance.

The pregame meal should be eaten approximately three to four hours before the game. Food should be high in carbohydrates and fluids. Grain

SAMPLE PREGAME MEAL

1 to 2 cups pasta with 1 1/2 cups tomato meat sauce
Bread
Milk (low-fat or skim)
Orange juice
Oatmeal raisin cookie
Water

products, vegetables, and fruit are the best choices for a pregame meal, because they are digested quickly and are readily available for fuel. Protein intake should be moderate, as protein takes longer to digest than carbohydrates. High-fat foods stay in the stomach the longest and may feel heavy and uncomfortable for the athlete. Restrict sugary foods. Sweets can cause rapid swings in blood sugar levels and result in low blood sugar and less energy. Avoid foods and drinks that contain caffeine. Caffeine stimulates the body to increase urine output, which can contribute to dehydration, and a full bladder can be very uncomfortable. The accompanying box is an example of a pregame meal.

If there is not enough time for a pregame meal, then a small carbohydrate snack—such as whole-wheat bread with peanut butter and banana, juice, and water—can be consumed one to two hours prior to the game.

CALCULATING "IDEAL" WEIGHT FOR ATHLETES

Various charts and indexes calculate the proper weight for people of all ages. One calculation, **body mass index (BMI)**, is a reliable indicator of total body fat, which is related to the risk of disease and death. The score is valid for both men and women, but it does have these limits:

- It may overestimate body fat in athletes and others who have a muscular build.
- It may underestimate body fat in older persons and others who have lost muscle mass.

To determine BMI, weight in pounds is divided by height in inches, then divided again by height in inches and multiplied by 703:

BMI = weight in pounds ÷ height in inches ÷ height in inches × 703

Example: A person weighing 210 pounds who is 6 feet tall would calculate BMI as follows:

210 pounds ÷ 72 inches ÷ 72 inches × 703 = 28.5

As outlined in Table 8–6:

- Normal weight = BMI of 18.5–24.9
- Overweight = BMI of 25–29.9
- Obesity = BMI of 30 or greater

Additional Methods of Weight Calculations

One traditional method of calculating ideal weight is the use of a height chart (Table 8–7). Height/weight charts are useful for comparing individuals of the same age and gender. Such charts are based on a national average.

Use of hydrostatic weighing, where the athlete is submerged in water to determine body composition (body fat to lean muscle), is considered an accurate way to measure body fat percentage. The athlete is first weighed on land and then in the water. Since muscle weighs more than fat, the differential between dry and wet weight will determine body fat percentage. This method is usually reserved for universities; however, several companies offer this service.

Weight calipers provide a quick snapshot of one's body fat percentage (see Figures 8–19 and 8–20). Because there are many ways errors can be made utilizing these devices, they should be used to track progress toward your overall goal, not a specific body fat percentage. Body fat calipers measure skinfolds to determine how much subcutaneous fat a person has.

Bod Pod® Composition Testing is one of the newer methods being utilized in trying to determine an accurate assessment of body fat percentage to lean muscle mass. This device utilizes air displacement to determine body composition in adults and children. The test takes about 5 minutes and a computer prints out the results. The error ratio is said to be less than 3%. These devices are widely available in medical clinics and some fitness facilities.

Table 8–6 Body Mass Index

ARE YOU AT A HEALTHY WEIGHT?

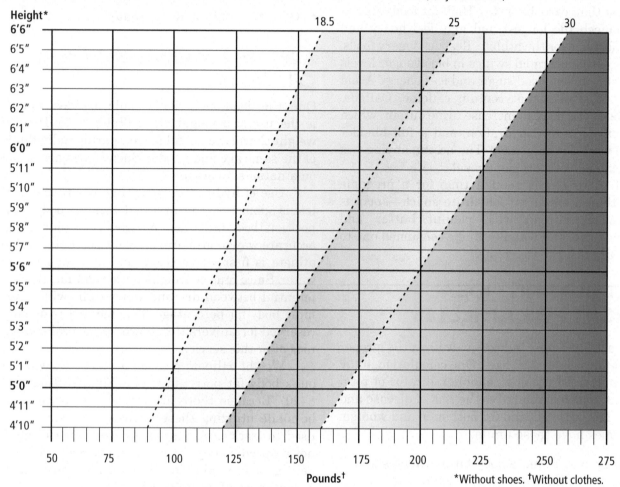

BMI measures weight in relation to height. The BMI ranges shown above are for adults. They are not exact ranges of healthy and unhealthy weights. However, they show that health risk increases at higher levels of overweight and obesity. Even within the healthy BMI range, weight gains can carry health risks for adults.

Directions: Find your weight on the bottom of the graph. Go straight up from that point until you come to the line that matches your height. Then find your weight group.

Healthy Weight: BMI from 18.5 up to 25 refers to healthy weight.

Overweight: BMI from 25 up to 30 refers to overweight.

Obese: BMI 30 or higher refers to obesity. Obese persons are also overweight.

Source: *Report of the Dietary Guidelines Advisory Committee on the Dietary Guidelines for Americans*, 2000.

Table 8–7	Weight Chart

WHAT IS YOUR IDEAL WEIGHT?

MEN		WOMEN	
Height	Weight (in pounds)	Height	Weight (in pounds)
5'2"	115–121	4'11"	93–100
5'3"	120–129	5'0"	98–102
5'4"	125–137	5'1"	103–106
5'5"	130–145	5'2"	106–112
5'6"	135–153	5'3"	109–118
5'7"	140–161	5'4"	112–124
5'8"	145–169	5'5"	115–130
5'9"	150–177	5'6"	118–136
5'10"	155–185	5'7"	121–142
5'11"	160–193	5'8"	124–148
6'0"	165–201	5'9"	127–153
6'1"	170–209	5'10"	130–158
6'2"	175–217	5'11"	133–163
6'3"	180–225	6'0"	136–168

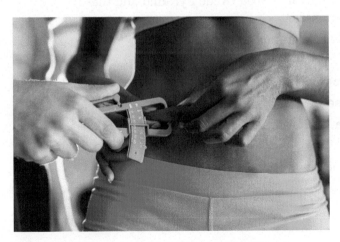

Figure 8–19 Body calipers come in many different designs. They should be used to track progress, not exact body composition. Myvisuals/Shutterstock.com

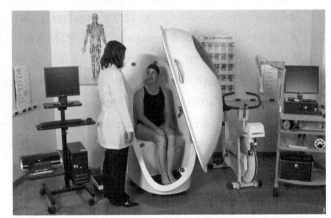

Figure 8–20 Body calipers come in many different designs. They should be used to track progress, not exact body composition. Photo courtesy of Cosmed USA, Inc. Concord, CA

CONCLUSION

Athletic performance can be attributed in part to a sound understanding of nutritional principles. Proper nutrition reduces the likelihood of injury and allows the athlete to perform at a higher level. Understanding the principles of good nutrition helps the athlete make informed choices.

An eating disorder is an extreme expression of food and weight issues experienced by many individuals, particularly girls and women. Eating disorders include anorexia nervosa, bulimia nervosa, and binge eating. These disorders cause very dangerous behaviors that result in health problems.

As athletes become aware of the nutritional components of their diet, they face fewer problems associated with poor nutrition.

REVIEW QUESTIONS

1. Explain how good nutritional habits lead to increased athletic performance and good health.
2. Explain how energy is used to maintain body functions.
3. Briefly describe the seven food components and nutrients.
4. What is insulin? How is it used by the body?
5. A person requires 2,800 kilocalories each day to maintain weight. How many true calories is this?
6. Why is it important to control your weight?
7. How can you limit the amount of fat in your diet?
8. What are vitamins? Why are they important for the body?
9. What is the difference between fat-soluble and water-soluble vitamins?
10. How much water will your body naturally lose each day?
11. What are DRVs, and how are they calculated?
12. Why was the Food Guide Pyramid developed?
13. What are the differences and similarities between the USDA Food Guide Pyramid and the Mediterranean, Asian, and Latin American diet pyramids?
14. What are the six food groups in the USDA Food Guide Pyramid?
15. What is nutritional quackery?
16. Describe the importance of special diets on athletic performance.
17. List some methods that girls and women use to lose weight.
18. What are the dangers of anorexia nervosa, bulimia, and bigorexia?
19. What percentage of males have disordered eating?
20. How do you calculate BMI? Calculate your BMI, showing your work.

PROJECTS AND ACTIVITIES

1. Track your entire dietary intake for one day, including water. List the quantities of the foods and drinks you consume as accurately as possible. After compiling your list, determine the amount of each food component that you consumed during the day. How does your list compare with the DRVs developed by the National Academy of Sciences?

2. Create a food pyramid typical of the types of foods teenagers eat today.

3. Develop an ad campaign on nutrition targeted at elementary school students.

4. Take a trip to your local nutrition store. Bring back three ads promising fast, easy programs to lose weight. Are they scientifically proven? If so, what is the science used to support their claims? (i.e., on what research do they base the claims?)

5. Talk with gymnastics and wrestling coaches about problems with eating disorders. Do they see such problems in their athletes? What are they doing to educate their athletes about these concerns?

LEARNING LINKS

- Visit the following websites for more nutrition knowledge:
  - American Dietetic Association: http://www.diabetes.org/
  - British Nutrition Foundation: http://www.nutrition.org.uk/
  - Harvard Medical School's Consumer Health Information: http://www.health.harvard.edu/
  - American Society for Nutrition: http://www.nutrition.org
  - Information for consumers on food and health nutrition: http://www.nutrition.gov
- Visit the Gatorade Sports Science Institute for information regarding nutrition and athletics: http://www.gssiweb.com
- Learn more about the Food Guide Pyramid and Dietary Guidelines for Americans. Visit the National Agriculture Library, of the United States Department of Agriculture Food and Nutrition Information Center: http://www.nal.usda.gov/fnic/
- For more information about eating disorders, check out http://www.anred.com and http://www.anred.com.

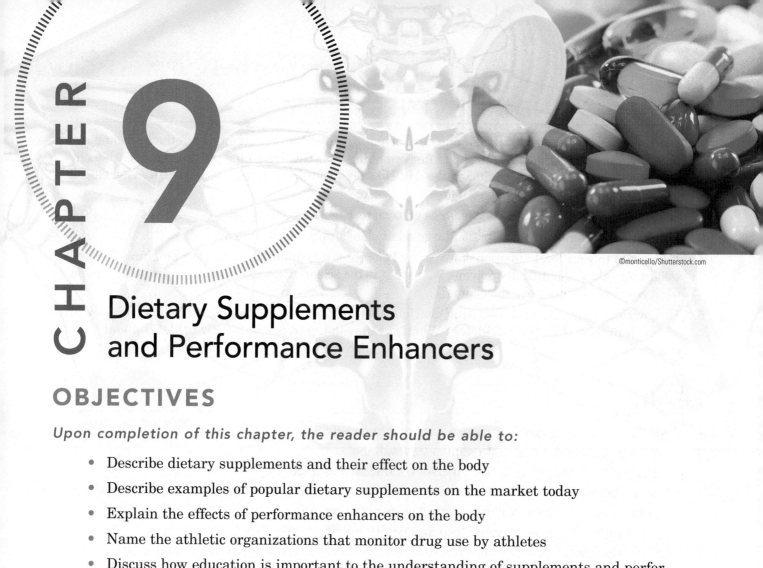

CHAPTER 9

Dietary Supplements and Performance Enhancers

OBJECTIVES

Upon completion of this chapter, the reader should be able to:

- Describe dietary supplements and their effect on the body
- Describe examples of popular dietary supplements on the market today
- Explain the effects of performance enhancers on the body
- Name the athletic organizations that monitor drug use by athletes
- Discuss how education is important to the understanding of supplements and performance enhancers
- Explain the athletic code of ethics

KEY TERMS

anabolic steroids *Substances that are used to enhance metabolism and thus act to build up the body tissues.*

anabolic-androgenic steroids *Manmade substances related to male sex hormones that are used to build muscle and enhance masculine characteristics.*

androstenedione *A steroid produced naturally in both men and women that can change or enhance the growth and development of masculine or feminine traits.*

athletic code of ethics *A tool to clarify and distinguish proper practices from those that can be detrimental and harmful.*

caffeine *An alkaloid present in coffee, many soft drinks, and chocolate that acts as a stimulant and is believed to enhance endurance and improve reaction times.*

chondroitin *A naturally occurring substance, found in human and animal cartilage, that is often used as a supplement to treat osteoarthritis.*

creatine monohydrate *An amino acid, found naturally in skeletal muscle, that is stored for quick energy and as a supplement to increase skeletal muscle.*

KEY TERMS CONTINUED

dietary supplement *A product, other than tobacco, intended to enhance the diet, which bears or contains one or more of the following dietary ingredients: vitamins, minerals, amino acids, herbs, and/or other botanicals.*

doping *The unnatural use of any substance or means to gain an unfair edge over the competition.*

ephedra *A substance derived from a shrublike plant; used as a stimulant to boost energy and weight loss.*

ergogenic aid *Any agent that enhances energy utilization, including energy production and efficiency.*

glucosamine *A substance produced naturally in the body; often used as a supplement to maintain cartilage in the joints.*

growth hormone *An ergogenic aid; a supplement of a substance produced naturally by the pituitary gland that works to increase conversion of amino acids into protein.*

medicinal herbs *Plant matter, used in the form of powders, extracts, teas, and/or tablets, believed to have therapeutic benefits.*

POPULAR NUTRITIONAL SUPPLEMENTS

The Dietary Supplement Health and Education Act defines a **dietary supplement** as a product, other than tobacco, intended to enhance the diet, which bears or contains one or more of the following dietary ingredients: vitamins, minerals, amino acids, herbs, and/or other botanical substances. Dietary supplements are available widely through many commercial sources, including health food stores, grocery stores, pharmacies, and by mail. Dietary supplements come in the form of tablets, capsules, powders, geltabs, extracts, liquids, and other formulations as well.

Historically in the United States, the most prevalent type of dietary supplement was a multivitamin/mineral tablet or capsule that was available in pharmacies, whether by prescription or over the counter (OTC). Supplements containing strictly herbal preparations were less widely distributed. Today, a wide array of supplement products exists. They include vitamins, minerals, other nutrients, and botanical supplements, as well as ingredients and extracts of animal and plant origin.

Vitamins

Recall from Chapter 8 that vitamins are organic (carbon-containing) compounds that are essential in small amounts for body processes. Vitamins do not provide energy; they enable the body to use the energy provided by fats, carbohydrates, and proteins. Vitamins should not be overused—more is not necessarily better (Figure 9–1). In fact, megadoses can be toxic (poisonous). Normally, a healthy person who eats a balanced diet will obtain all the necessary nutrients, including vitamins.

Vitamins taken in addition to those received through the diet, called *vitamin supplements,* are available in concentrated form in tablets, capsules, and drops. Vitamin concentrates sometimes distinguish between natural or synthetic (manufactured). Some people believe that a meaningful difference exists between the two types, and that

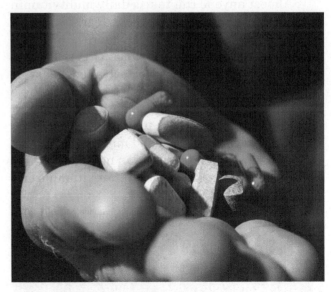

Figure 9–1 Vitamins come in many forms and are usually not necessary for good health. Megadoses can be toxic. Courtesy of Photodisc.

the natural supplements are far superior in quality to the synthetic. However, according to the United States Food and Drug Administration (FDA), the body cannot distinguish between a vitamin of plant or animal origin and one manufactured in a laboratory. Once they have been absorbed by the digestive system, the two types of the same vitamin are chemically identical.

Healthy athletes who eat a variety of foods using the Food Guide Pyramid should be able to obtain all the vitamins needed to maintain good health. However, some people take supplements because they believe that:

- Food no longer contains the right nutrients in adequate quantities.
- Supplements can "bulk up" muscles and enhance athletic performance.
- Vitamins provide needed energy.
- Vitamins and minerals can cure anything, including heart trouble, the common cold, and cancer.

The facts argue otherwise. A balanced diet *does* meet all the nutritional needs of athletes. No amount of vitamins will help to build muscles; only weight training can accomplish that. Only certain diseases caused by vitamin deficiencies (such as beriberi, scurvy, and rickets) can be cured with the help of vitamin supplements. Heart disease, cancer, and the common cold cannot.

Almost anyone can take a daily multivitamin and mineral supplement without fear of toxicity. A megadose, which is 10 or more times the Recommended Dietary Allowance (RDA) Dietary Reference Intake (DRI), to correct a deficiency or to help prevent disease, should be prescribed by a physician. If a multivitamin-mineral is taken as a supplement, it is best not to exceed 100% of the RDA/DRI for each vitamin and mineral. An excess of one vitamin or one mineral can negatively affect the absorption or utilization of other vitamins and minerals. If vitamin supplements are believed to be indispensable, it is essential that a physician or registered dietitian be consulted first.

Minerals

A mineral is an inorganic (non-carbon-containing) element that is necessary for the body to build tissues, regulate body fluids, and assist in various other body functions. Minerals are found in all body tissues. They cannot provide energy, but in their role as body regulators they contribute to the production of energy within the body.

Minerals are found in water and in natural (unprocessed) foods, together with proteins, carbohydrates, fats, and vitamins. Minerals in the soil are absorbed by growing plants. Humans obtain minerals by eating plants grown in mineral-rich soil or by eating animals that have eaten such plants.

Because it is known that minerals are essential to good health, some would-be nutritionists claim that more is better. Ironically, more can be hazardous to health when it comes to minerals. A healthy individual who eats a balanced diet will normally lose some minerals through perspiration and saliva, and will excrete amounts in excess of body needs in urine and feces. However, when concentrated forms of minerals are taken on a regular basis, over a period of time they build up to more than the body can handle, and toxicity develops. An excessive amount of one mineral can sometimes cause a deficiency of another mineral. In addition, excessive amounts of minerals can cause hair loss and changes in the blood, hormones, bones, muscles, blood vessels, and nearly all tissues. Concentrated forms of minerals should be used only on the advice of a physician.

Herbal Supplements

Medicinal herbs are among the world's oldest medicines. Increased use of herbs in recent years is evidence of a public interest in alternatives to conventional medicine (Figure 9–2). Nearly half of all Americans take herbal supplements as a form of medication. This amounts to over $15 billion a year in out-of-pocket expense. According to the *New England Journal of Medicine*, research shows that many patients see no need to inform their physicians of their use of alternative medicines, including herbal supplements (Haller & Benowitz, 2000).

FUN FACTS

Three thousand years ago, the ancient Greeks ate "substances" to improve athletic performance.

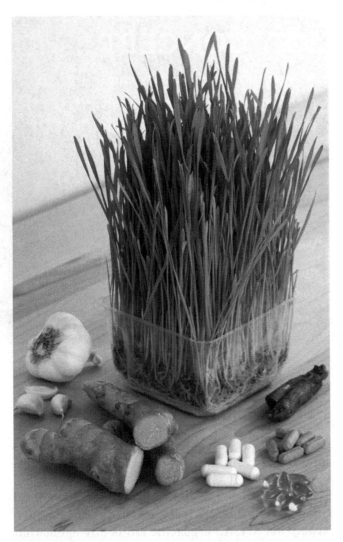

Figure 9–2 Herbal products are considered dietary supplements by the Food and Drug Administration. Courtesy of Photodisc.

A national survey by National Public Radio, the Kaiser Family Foundation, and Harvard's Kennedy School of Government found that over 50% of all Americans believe that dietary supplements other than standard minerals and vitamins are generally good for their health and well-being. About 400 herbs are currently used widely and distributed as capsules, extracts, tablets, and teas. Many of these dietary supplements are safe, but many are not.

Approximately 1,500 botanicals are sold as dietary supplements or traditional ethnic medicines. The FDA considers herbal products to be dietary supplements; therefore, they are not regulated by the FDA, as are traditional drugs. The manufacturers of these products are not required to demonstrate the safety and effectiveness of their products before they are put on the market. In addition, manufacturers do not have to adhere to any of the standard quality controls mandated for drugs. As a result, the composition of herbal products may vary greatly from manufacturer to manufacturer, and even from one batch to another. Under its current regulatory authority, the FDA can remove an herbal supplement from the market only after it has been shown to be unsafe.

New regulations contained within the Federal Food, Drug, and Cosmetic Act that in June 2010 began, giving the FDA the authority to oversee the manufacture of domestic and foreign-made dietary supplements, including herbal supplements. The new regulations aim to improve safety by requiring supplement manufacturers to follow certain manufacturing practices, ensure that supplement labels are exact, and that the product is free of contaminants. The FDA is responsible for monitoring the safety of supplements after they are on the market, and enforcing action against unsafe supplements.

In May 2000, researchers at the University of Arkansas published a study on ephedra supplements sold as decongestants, energy boosters, or diet aids. In half of the samples examined, they found significant differences between the labels and the actual contents, a discrepancy in some cases as much as 20%. One product contained no ephedra alkaloids, whereas at least one sample contained potentially dangerous amounts of ephedra—154% of the label amount. Dr. William J. Gurley, the lead researcher, said that poor

KEY CONCEPT

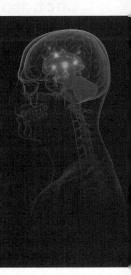

Dietary supplements are products that are believed to enhance the diet. They come in a variety of forms. Their effects on the body vary based on the supplement and the amount used. Megadoses of dietary supplements can be harmful and lead to toxicity.

quality may contribute to the problems associated with safety and efficacy of herbal supplements. Ephedra, for example, has been linked to hundreds of adverse reactions and several deaths (Gurley, Gardiner, & Hubbard, 2000).

The National Institute of Health's National Center for Complementary and Alternative Medicine (NCCAM) is currently studying the safety and effectiveness of a number of herbal remedies. The results of these studies should help clarify who can benefit from these products.

Glucosamine

Glucosamine, which is naturally produced by the human body, is used as a supplement to maintain joint cartilage. It is not usually possible to ingest extra glucosamine through food; most glucosamine tablets are made from shellfish shells. Glucosamine has proven to be an effective treatment for osteoarthritis and aids in the recovery of some sports injuries.

There are three different types of glucosamine: glucosamine sulfate, glucosamine hydrochloride, and N-acetyl-glucosamine. There is some debate as to which type is the most effective.

Side effects may include stomach problems, heartburn, or diarrhea. Labels usually recommended that glucosamine be taken with food. People with histories of heart disease or high blood pressure should consult with their health care providers before starting glucosamine supplements. Glucosamine should not be taken while on heart medications or with insulin.

Chondroitin

Chondroitin is a naturally occurring substance found in human and animal cartilage. Animal tissues are a good source of chondroitin. It has proven abilities to treat osteoarthritis (bone loss), and it has been used to treat psoriasis and cancers, although tests of its effectiveness in treating the latter have proven inconclusive.

Chondroitin appears to be nontoxic, with no contraindications, although anticoagulant users should consult a physician before starting chondroitin supplements. The biggest danger appears to be wasting money on products that claim to contain the substance but actually deliver little or no chondroitin.

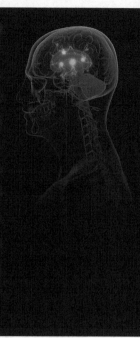

KEY CONCEPT

A vast array of dietary supplements crowd the market today. They consist of vitamins (e.g., vitamin E, vitamin B-complex, and vitamin C); minerals (e.g., zinc, iron, and sodium); herbs (e.g., St. John's Wort, ginko biloba, and ginseng); and other naturally occurring substances (e.g., glucosamine and chondroitin).

PERFORMANCE ENHANCERS

The "win at all cost" mentality in athletics creates an unhealthy incentive of doing whatever is necessary to excel. It is estimated that between 1 and 3 million athletes in the United States have used **anabolic steroids**, which are the most common **ergogenic aid**. An ergogenic aid is any agent that enhances energy utilization, including energy production and efficiency. Thousands of others have experimented with alternative performance enhancers (Figure 9–3).

Anabolic Steroids

Anabolic-androgenic steroids are manmade substances related to male sex hormones. *Anabolic* refers to muscle-building, and *androgenic* refers to increased masculine characteristics. *Steroids* refers to the class of drugs. These drugs are available legally only by prescription, to treat conditions that occur when the body produces abnormally low amounts of testosterone, such as delayed puberty and some types of impotence. They are also used to treat body wasting in patients with AIDS and other diseases that result in loss of lean muscle mass. Abuse of anabolic steroids, however, can lead to serious health problems, some of which are irreversible.

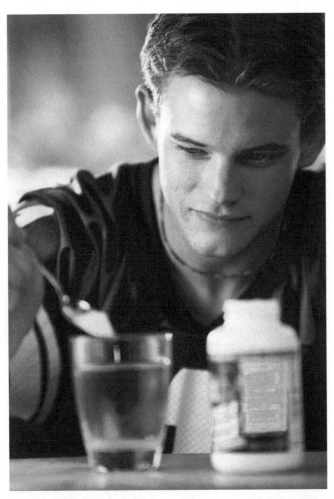

Figure 9–3 Athletes often experiment with performance enhancers in hopes of gaining an edge over their competitors. Courtesy of Photodisc.

Today, athletes and others abuse anabolic steroids in the quest to enhance performance and improve physical appearance. Anabolic steroids are taken orally or injected, typically in cycles of weeks or months (referred to as *cycling),* rather than continuously. Cycling involves taking multiple doses of steroids over a specific period of time, stopping for a period, and starting again. Users often combine several different types of steroids to maximize their effectiveness while minimizing negative effects (referred to as *stacking).*

The major side effects of anabolic steroid abuse include liver tumors and cancer, jaundice (yellowish pigmentation of skin, tissues, and body fluids), fluid retention, high blood pressure, increases in low-density lipoproteins (LDL, or bad cholesterol), and decreases in high-density lipoproteins (HDL, or good cholesterol). Other side effects may include kidney tumors, severe acne, and

trembling. Many gender-specific side effects are associated with these drugs. Many men suffer shrinking of the testicles, reduced sperm count, infertility, baldness, development of breasts, and increased risk of prostate cancer. Women may suffer growth of facial hair, male-pattern baldness, changes in or cessation of the menstrual cycle, enlargement of the clitoris, and a deepened voice. Adolescents' growth may be halted through premature skeletal maturation and accelerated puberty changes, meaning that they risk remaining of short stature for the rest of their lives if they take anabolic steroids before the normal adolescent growth spurt. In addition, people who inject anabolic steroids run the added risk of contracting or transmitting HIV/AIDS, which is potentially fatal, or hepatitis, which causes serious liver damage.

Scientific research also shows that aggression and other psychiatric side effects may result from abuse of anabolic steroids. Many users report feeling good about themselves while on anabolic steroids, but researchers report that extreme mood swings also occur, including manic symptoms leading to violence. Depression often results when the user stops taking steroids, and this may contribute to dependence on anabolic steroids. Researchers also report that users may suffer from paranoid jealousy, extreme irritability, delusions, and impaired judgment stemming from feelings of invincibility (Pope & Katz, 1988).

Some users turn to other drugs to alleviate the negative effects of anabolic steroids. For example, a study of 227 men admitted in 1999 to a private treatment center for dependence on heroin or other opioids (opiates and synthetic narcotics) found that 9.3% had abused anabolic steroids before trying any other illicit drug. Of this population, 86% first used opioids to counteract insomnia and irritability resulting from the anabolic steroids.

The "Monitoring the Future" (MTF) study by the National Institute on Drug Abuse (December 2007) assessed drug use among eighth-, tenth-, and twelfth-graders nationwide annually since 1975. Because of growing professional and public concern over use of anabolic steroids by adolescents and young adults, questions regarding anabolic steroid use were added to the MTF in 1989 to provide a better understanding of the extent of the problem. Lloyd Johnston, principal investigator for the MTF survey, tracked a fairly sharp increase in the use of anabolic steroids by male teens in the late 1990s and early 2000s, with peak levels reached in 1999 among eighth-grade males; in 2000 among tenth-grade males; and in 2001 and 2002 among twelfth-grade males. Since those peak years, the annual prevalence rate has dropped by more than half among the eighth- and tenth-grade males (to 1.1 and 1.7%, respectively), and by 40% among twelfth-grade males (to 2.3% annual prevalence in 2007). Over the past 4-year interval, there has been an increase in the proportion of twelfth-grade males who acknowledge great risk in trying anabolic steroids—which may help to account for the decline in use. There was a sharp drop in 2005 in the perceived availability of these drugs, very likely due to the Anabolic Control Act of 2004, which placed 32 additional steroids into Schedule III and expanded the Drug Enforcement Agency's regulatory and enforcement authority regarding their sale and possession. "While a number of states are considering implementing expensive programs to test student athletes for anabolic steroid use, the problem has been diminishing sharply," Johnston said. "It appears that supply control efforts, in combination with educational efforts, are having the intended effects." Use among females is considerably lower than among males and has been declining since 2002 in the lower grades, and since 2004 in grade 12. In 2007, the annual prevalence of anabolic steroid use for girls ranges from 0.4% in eighth and tenth grades to 0.6% in the twelfth grade. These rates are down by about two-thirds from their recent peak levels.

Most anabolic steroid users are male. Among male students in 2007, use of these substances was reported by 1.5% of eighth-graders, 1.8% of tenth-graders, and 2.2% of twelfth-graders (Table 9–1).

Growth Hormones

Growth hormones are another ergogenic aid used by athletes to gain an edge. Growth hormone, which is produced by the pituitary gland, acts on most organs and tissues in the body. Growth hormone works by increasing the conversion of amino acids into protein. It allows fat to be used as an energy source, sparing muscle glycogen. The adverse effects of growth hormone can include heart disease, impotence, osteoporosis, and death.

Androstenedione

Androstenedione (andro) is a steroid hormone naturally produced in both men and women. Androstenedione produced in the body is converted either to testosterone or to estrogen. Elevated testosterone levels can have masculinizing effects on women; men with increased estrogen levels can experience feminizing effects, such as the growth of breasts. Young people who have elevated levels of either hormone could develop early puberty and premature cessation of bone growth, leading to shorter-than-normal adult height. Androstenedione is also known to set off extreme aggression and mood changes. Other adverse effects of androstenedione include decreased levels of cardiac-protective HDLs and elevated levels of estrogen. This exposes the consumer to potential cardiovascular disease, breast cancer, and pancreatic cancer.

Androstenedione was widely available as a nonprescription nutritional supplement prior to the passage of the Anabolic Steroid Control Act of 2004. That law amended the Controlled Substance

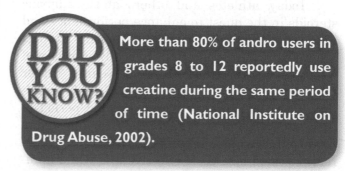

DID YOU KNOW? More than 80% of andro users in grades 8 to 12 reportedly use creatine during the same period of time (National Institute on Drug Abuse, 2002).

Table 9–1 Anabolic Steroid Use by Students, Year 2008 "Monitoring the Future Study"			
	8TH-GRADERS	**10TH-GRADERS**	**12TH-GRADERS**
Ever used	1.5%	1.8%	2.2%
Used in past year	0.8	1.1	1.4
Used in past month	0.4	0.5	1.0

Act to place both anabolic steroids and prohormones on a list of controlled substances, making possession of the banned substances a federal crime. The law took effect on January 20, 2005. On April 11, 2004, the United States FDA banned the sale of andro, citing that the drug posed significant health risks commonly associated with steroids. Androstenedione is banned by the International Olympic Committee (IOC), the National Collegiate Athletic Association (NCAA), most major league sport teams, as well as the United States military.

Caffeine

Many people like **caffeine** because it makes them feel more alert, gives them more energy, improves their mood, and makes them more productive. Studies indicate that some endurance athletes may benefit from ingesting caffeine prior to exercise, but others show that caffeine has no effect at all on endurance performance.

High levels of caffeine can cause sleeplessness, anxiety, headache, upset stomach, and nervousness, as well as dehydration. Caffeine-induced dehydration may actually decrease athletic performance by decreasing the efficiency of the muscles, which are forced to work while being deprived of fluids. These side effects may very well offset any possible benefits.

DID YOU KNOW? The NCAA ban on caffeine applies when its concentration in urine exceeds 15 micrograms per milliliter. This is equal to eight cups of coffee at one sitting, with testing within two to three hours thereafter.

The IOC has banned caffeine over a certain limit. Coffee, tea, chocolate, and colas, as well as performance drinks, and some nonprescription painkillers, contain caffeine. Because caffeine is a common ingredient in foods and drinks, the IOC allows an upper limit. Table 9–2 shows common foods and over-the-counter (OTC) items that contain caffeine.

Creatine Monohydrate

One of the most popular performance enhancers used today is **creatine monohydrate**. Creatine, an amino acid produced in the body by the liver and kidneys (amino acids are the building blocks of protein), is derived from a diet of meat and animal products. It is found naturally in skeletal muscle.

Table 9–2 Caffeine Content of Foods and Drugs		
PRODUCT	SERVING SIZE	CAFFEINE (MG)
OTC Drugs		
NoDoz, maximum strength; Vivarin	1 tablet	200
Excedrin	2 tablets	130
NoDoz, regular strength	1 tablet	100
Anacin	2 tablets	64
Coffees		
Coffee, brewed	8 ounces	135
Coffee, instant	8 ounces	95
Coffee, decaffeinated	8 ounces	5
Teas		
Tea, leaf or bag	8 ounces	50

(continues)

Table 9–2 Caffeine Content of Foods and Drugs (*continued*)

PRODUCT	SERVING SIZE	CAFFEINE (MG)
Soft Drinks		
Mountain Dew	12 ounces	55.5
Surge	12 ounces	52.5
Diet Coke	12 ounces	46.5
Coca-Cola Classic	12 ounces	34.5
Dr. Pepper, regular or diet	12 ounces	42
Sunkist orange soda	12 ounces	42
Pepsi-Cola	12 ounces	37.5
Barqs Root Beer	12 ounces	22.5
7-Up or Diet 7-Up	12 ounces	0
Barqs Diet Root Beer	12 ounces	0
Sprite or Diet Sprite	12 ounces	0
Energy Drinks		
Red Bull	8.3 ounces	80
Monster and Rockstar	16 ounces	160
Wired X505	24 ounces	505
Juices		
Juiced	10 ounces	60
Frozen Desserts		
Ben & Jerry's No Fat Coffee Fudge frozen	1 cup	85
Starbucks coffee ice cream, assorted types	1 cup	40–60
Häagen-Dazs coffee ice cream	1 cup	58
Chocolates or Candies		
Hershey's Special Dark chocolate bar	1 bar (1.5 ounces)	31–58
Häagen-Dazs coffee ice cream	1 cup	
Hershey Bar (milk chocolate)	1 bar (1.5 ounces)	10
Chocolates or Candies		
Hershey's Special Dark chocolate bar	1 bar (1.5 ounces)	31
Hershey Bar (milk chocolate)	1 bar (1.5 ounces)	10
Cocoa or hot chocolate	8 ounces	5

Serving sizes are based on commonly eaten portions, pharmaceutical instructions, or the amount of the leading-selling container size. For example, beverages sold in 16-ounce or half-liter bottles were counted as one serving.

Sources: National Coffee Association; National Soft Drink Association; Tea Council of the USA; information provided by food, beverage, and pharmaceutical companies; Barone & Roberts, 1996.

In the body, creatine is converted into the molecule phosphocreatine, which serves as a storage reservoir for quick energy. Phosphocreatine is especially important in tissues such as the voluntary muscles and the nervous system, which periodically require large amounts of energy.

Athletic use of creatine increased dramatically after a 1992 study showed that high doses of creatine could increase skeletal muscle by 20%. It has become increasingly popular among athletes involved in power sports. Creatine theoretically works by increasing energy production during exercise and enabling athletes to sustain strenuous exercise for a longer period of time.

The beneficial effects of creatine have only been noted in poorly trained athletes, not in elite athletes. An adverse effect of creatine supplementation is weight gain due to increase in cellular water in muscle. Potential side effects include muscle cramping, dehydration, gastrointestinal distress, nausea, and seizures. Creatine may also affect kidney function. The long-term health effects of high doses of creatine are unknown, especially for persons who have liver or kidney problems or diabetes. Creatine supplements may depress the body's own synthesis of the substance, which may not return to normal once the athlete stops taking the supplements.

Creatine is categorized as a food supplement by the FDA and is available over the counter at drugstores and nutrition centers. Although readily accessible, creatine supplements are somewhat expensive, costing as much as $30 to $50 a month.

Ephedra

The terms *ephedrine, ephedra,* and *ma huang* refer to the same substance derived from **ephedra**, a shrublike plant found in desert regions in central Asia and other parts of the world. The dried greens of the plant are used medicinally. Ephedra is a stimulant containing the herbal form of ephedrine, an FDA-regulated drug found in OTC asthma medications.

In the United States, ephedra and ephedrine are sold in health food stores under a variety of brand names. The FDA does not currently regulate ephedrine because it is a dietary supplement protected under the Dietary Supplement Health and Education Act of 1994. Nevertheless, ephedra is banned by the NCAA, the NFL, and the IOC.

Ephedrine is widely used for weight loss, to boost energy, and to enhance athletic performance. Such products also often contain other stimulants such as caffeine. Ephedrine alkaloids are amphetamine-like compounds used in OTC and prescription drugs. They have potentially lethal stimulant effects on the central nervous system and heart, including hypertension (elevated blood pressure), palpitations (rapid heart rate), neuropathy (nerve damage), myopathy (muscle injury), psychosis, stroke, memory loss, heart-rate irregularities, insomnia, nervousness, tremors, seizures, heart attacks, and death.

One illustrative case is that of Baltimore Orioles pitcher Steve Bechler, who died in February 2003 less than 24 hours after taking ephedra. Bechler took three tablets of Xenadrine, an OTC drug whose primary ingredient is ephedra. The 6-foot-2, 239-pound Bechler collapsed at spring training with heatstroke. His body temperature was reported to be 108°F. A Florida medical examiner stated that his death may have been linked to Xenadrine, an ephedra-based diet pill. The FDA issued a warning on the dangers to anyone taking ephedrine-based supplements.

CURRENT IOC, NCAA, AND PROFESSIONAL STANDARDS

The International Olympic Committee Medical Commission was created in 1961 to deal with the increasing problem of **doping** in the sports world. Doping is the unnatural use of any substance or means to gain an unfair edge over the competition. The initial goal of an anti-doping structure was rapidly widened to encompass the following fundamental principles:

- Protection of athletes' health
- Respect for both medical and sport ethics
- Equality for all competing athletes

Today, the IOC has strict rules governing the use and misuse of banned substances. The elimination of doping in sport is a fundamental objective of the Olympic Movement. The Anti-Doping Code, which the entire Olympic Movement must observe, contains the following key points:

- It applies to the Olympic Games, the various championships, and all competitions to which the IOC grants its patronage or support.

- It intends to ensure respect for the main ethical concepts of sport and to protect the health of the athletes.

- It enables appeals to be lodged with the Court of Arbitration for Sport against certain decisions rendered in the course of application of the code.

The National Collegiate Athletic Association (NCAA) has a drug-testing program that mandates urine collection on specific occasions and laboratory analyses for substances on a list of banned-drug classes developed by the NCAA Executive Committee. This list consists of substances generally purported to be performance enhancing and/or potentially harmful to the health and safety of the student-athlete. The drug classes specifically include stimulants (such as amphetamines and cocaine) and anabolic steroids, as well as other drugs. To review the list of banned substances, visit the NCAA's website at http://www.ncaa.org/health-safety; click on "Drug Testing/Banned Substances."

Several professional athletic teams have written policy statements concerning the use of banned substances.

EDUCATION FOR ATHLETES

Athletes need to understand the dangers and risks inherent in the use of dietary supplements and performance enhancers. This understanding comes from education, so programs should be designed to educate athletes at a very young age. Everyone associated with athletics—parents, coaches, teachers, trainers, and athletes—must work together toward this goal.

Organizations that provide a wealth of information on this topic are:

- American College of Sports Medicine
- International Olympic Committee
- National Athletic Trainers Association
- National Collegiate Athletic Association
- National Federation of State High School Associations
- Physician and Sports Medicine
- United States Food and Drug Administration
- United States Anti-Doping Agency (USADA)
- World Anti-Doping Agency

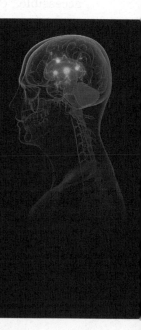

KEY CONCEPT

Athletes use performance enhancers because they believe these substances will improve athletic performance, strength, and endurance. Athletes may experiment with performance enhancers because they are striving, and being pushed, to win—no matter the cost.

KEY CONCEPT

To maintain ethics in athletics and fairness in competition, many organizations have banned the use of performance enhancers and monitor their athletes for use of these substances. The NCAA and the IOC are the two largest organizations monitoring use of performance-enhancing drugs by athletes.

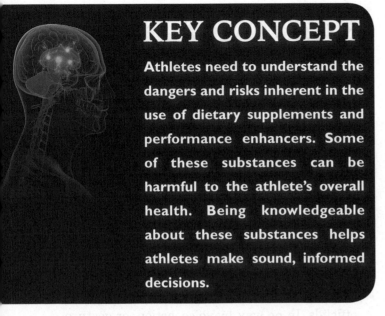

KEY CONCEPT

Athletes need to understand the dangers and risks inherent in the use of dietary supplements and performance enhancers. Some of these substances can be harmful to the athlete's overall health. Being knowledgeable about these substances helps athletes make sound, informed decisions.

ETHICS IN ATHLETICS

The **athletic code of ethics** is an essential tool for protecting and promoting the interests of athletics and the coaching profession. Ethics are the basic principles of proper action. Proper ethics in athletics implies a standard of character that affords confidence and trust. The essential elements of a modern athletic code of ethics are honesty and integrity. Coaches and athletes whose conduct reflects these two characteristics bring credit to the field of athletics and to themselves. Only through such conduct can athletics earn and maintain a rightful place in our educational program and make a full contribution to our way of life.

The code's primary purpose is to clarify and distinguish ethical practices from those that are detrimental and harmful. It also emphasizes the value of athletics in educational institutions, and stresses the contributions of the coaches and athletes within them.

The future of the athletic code of ethics rests in the hands of those engaged in athletics. All members of the athletic community assume obligations and responsibilities in relation to competitors, teams, coaches, and student bodies. These relationships are important in establishing the kind of friendships that count most in athletics.

Proper Conduct and Good Sportsmanship

Proper conduct and good sportsmanship refer to standards such as:

- Treat other persons as you know they should be treated, and as you would wish them to fairly treat you.
- Regard the rules of your game as agreements, the spirit or letter of which you should not evade or break.
- Treat officials and opponents with respect.
- Accept the final decision of any official.
- Honor visiting teams and spectators as your own guests and treat them as such. Likewise, behave as an honored guest when you visit another school.
- Be gracious in victory and defeat.
- Be as cooperative as you are competitive.
- Remember that your actions on and off the field reflect upon you and your school.

Purpose of Athletics in Schools

Athletics exists primarily because it is an important part of the student's full education. As an educational process, athletics and sports serve these purposes:

- To teach and instruct students in the rules, fundamentals, and skills of various individual and team sports, and to provide physical training.
- To provide healthy competition and cooperation within and between schools.
- To develop aspects of good sportsmanship that will enhance each student's education.
- To maintain the spirit of true amateur competition.

Guidelines for Coaches

Coaches should adhere to these principles:

- Coaches shall remember that athletics is a part of each student's education, not a goal in itself.

- Coaches shall assist each student toward developing his or her fullest potential in athletics.

- Coaches shall remember that the behavior of a team can reflect the coach's own manner, attitude, temper, and approach to athletics. Therefore, coaches shall conduct themselves in a way that brings credit to them, their teams, their schools, and their sports.

- Coaches shall be responsible for maintaining objectivity and a sense of balance commensurate with good sportsmanship.

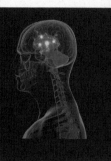

KEY CONCEPT

The athletic code of ethics emphasizes and values honesty, integrity, good sportsmanship, and proper conduct.

Guidelines for Players

Players and athletes should adhere to the following principles:

- Players shall represent themselves and their schools with honor, proper conduct, and good sportsmanship. They shall understand that competitive rivalries are encouraged, but that disrespect for opponents is unsportsmanlike and lessens the value of rivalries. They shall confine the competitiveness of the game to the field, and in particular behave properly on the sidelines and in the locker rooms, both before and after games.

- Players shall comply fully with the rulings of officials. In no way, by voice, action, or gesture, shall they demonstrate their dissatisfaction with any decisions made.

- Players shall adhere to the rules of the school and the athletic department.

CONCLUSION

The use of dietary supplements and performance enhancers is a controversial issue facing athletes of all ages. Substantial research has been done by sports medicine and nutritional experts on this issue. It is widely acknowledged that the use of supplements and enhancers can do more harm than good. Most organizations associated with athletics have banned the use of ergogenic aids.

Athletes need to understand the risks associated with the use of supplements and performance aids. Education can provide athletes, and everyone associated with athletics, the necessary information on dietary supplements and performance enhancers. As long as there are claims of increased performance from using a certain substance, there will always be people willing to give it a try. However, the best and safest way to improve performance is hard work. The rest will take care of itself.

REVIEW QUESTIONS

1. What is a dietary supplement?
2. Why do many people take supplements?
3. List four popular supplements on the market today. What are their benefits and dangers?
4. Give four examples of performance enhancers. What are their benefits and dangers?
5. What athletic organizations monitor drug use by athletes?
6. Why is education an important tool when dealing with issues of supplements and performance enhancers?
7. Why is it important for everyone involved in athletics to observe and follow an athletic code of ethics?

PROJECTS AND ACTIVITIES

1. Talk with two athletes who use nutritional supplements and/or performance enhancers. Ask them why they use the substances, and what benefits they have gained. Have they noticed any side effects? Report your findings to the class, keeping the names of the athletes confidential.

2. Visit your state high school athletic association's website. What information do offer have on supplements and performance enhancers? Do they have a policy statement on this? If so, what does it say?

3. Create an educational poster or ad campaign on the dangers of dietary supplements and performance enhancers.

4. What is the athletic code of ethics for your school?

LEARNING LINKS

*   For information on performance enhancers, visit the websites of the International Olympic Committee http://www.olympic.org, and the National Collegiate Athletic Association (http://www.ncaa.org).

*   Visit the National Institute of Health Office of Dietary Supplements for additional information on a variety of substances: http://dietary-supplements.info.nih.gov/.

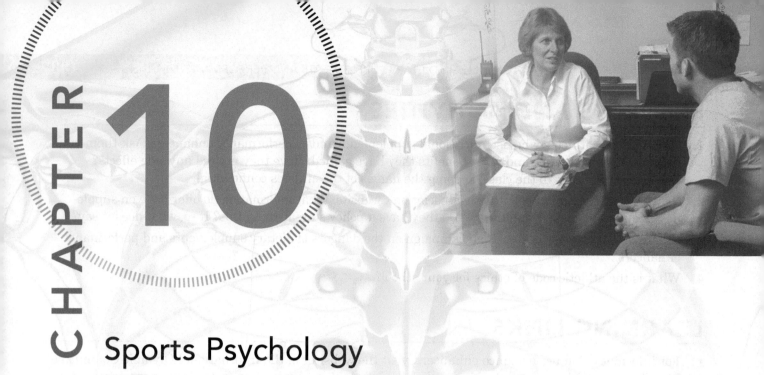

CHAPTER 10

Sports Psychology

OBJECTIVES

Upon completion of this chapter, the reader should be able to:

- Discuss the importance of sports psychology to athletic performance
- Describe how motivation effects performance
- Explain the importance of setting goals
- Explain the difference between imagery and simulation
- Explain the benefits and dangers of stress
- Discuss the dangers of burnout
- Explain how self-confidence improves self-worth
- Describe career opportunities in the field of sports psychology

KEY TERMS

burnout *Mental and physical exhaustion that causes an athlete to drop out of a sport or quit an activity that was once enjoyable.*

goal setting *Identifying clearly defined, specific objectives that are measurable.*

imagery *The process of reviewing and training in the mind only, using visualization.*

motivation *An internal state or condition (need or desire) that serves to activate or energize behavior and give it direction.*

simulation *Making physical training circumstances as close as possible to real competition.*

sports psychology *The study of sport and exercise and the mental (psychological) factors influencing performance.*

stress *A factor that causes awareness, anxiety, focus, or fear. Stress can be either good or bad and have both positive and negative effects.*

SPORTS PSYCHOLOGY

Sports psychology is the study of sport and exercise, and the mental (psychological) factors influencing performance. Sport psychologists apply psychological principles and a number of different techniques to the field of sport and exercise, all aimed at improved performance and positive self-image. The connection of mind, body, and athletic performance is a powerful one. Athletes do so much physical preparation to get an edge on the competition that they often forget about the mental aspects of their sport. It is often said that performance in a sport is 95% mental; however, most of the athlete's time is spent in physical preparation for competition.

Until a couple of decades ago, the general perception was that sport psychologists and consultants dealt only with athletes who had a problem of one kind or another—definitely not the athlete who was healthy and successful. Today, sports psychology has become a booming field in which practitioners guide athletes at all levels to achieve increased success and happiness (Figure 10–1). Sport psychologists can help athletes develop:

- Goals
- Self-confidence
- Motivation

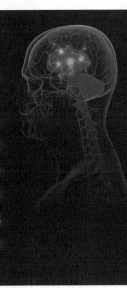

KEY CONCEPT

Sports psychology is a rapidly growing field in which practitioners guide athletes at all levels to achieve increased success and happiness. Sports psychologists can help athletes set goals, boost self-confidence, stay motivated, enhance self-image, and cope with stress and disappointment.

- Positive self-image
- Strategies to cope with stress and disappointment

MOTIVATION

In 1981, Kleinginna and Kleinginna defined **motivation** as an internal state or condition (sometimes described as a need, desire, or want) that serves to activate or energize behavior and give it direction.

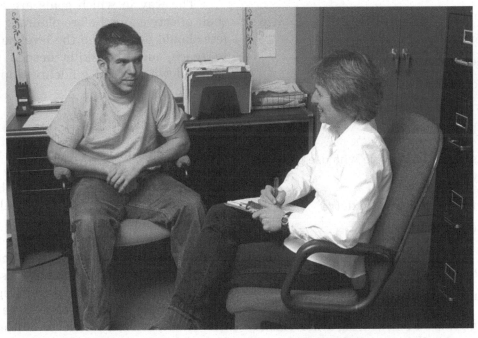

Figure 10–1 Sport psychologists can help athletes improve performance through motivation, goal setting, and development of a positive self-image.

FUN FACTS
Most athletes fatigue mentally before they fatigue physically, because their minds are not as well trained as their bodies.

There are two types of motivation: extrinsic and intrinsic. *Extrinsic* means from the outside. One who is extrinsically motivated is driven by an external reward such as money or praise. Extrinsic motivation is based on the goals, interests, and values of others. *Intrinsic* motivation comes from within. It is behavior for its own sake, rather than for the rewards or outcomes the behavior might reap. Intrinsically motivated behaviors, such as personal achievement, enjoyment, self-confidence, or feeling positive emotions, require no external support or reinforcement.

GOAL SETTING

Goal setting is one of the most powerful motivation techniques. Goal setting encompasses long-term vision and short-term motivation. By setting clearly defined, specific goals, the athlete can measure progress and take pride in the achievement of those goals. With goals in mind, the individual can:

- Achieve more
- Improve performance
- Improve the quality of training
- Increase motivation to achieve at a higher level
- Increase pride and satisfaction in performance
- Improve self-confidence

Research has shown that people who use goal setting effectively:

- Suffer less from stress and anxiety
- Concentrate better
- Show more self-confidence
- Perform better
- Are happier with their performances

By setting goals and measuring achievement, athletes can track their accomplishments and visualize how much more they are capable of

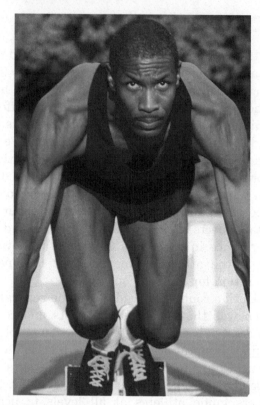

Figure 10–2 The athlete must have confidence and believe that he or she will be able to reach higher, more difficult goals. Courtesy of Photodisc.

attaining. This boosts the athlete's confidence that he or she is able to reach higher, more difficult goals (Figure 10–2).

The way in which goals are set determines their effectiveness. Before planning goals, the athlete should understand the level he or she wishes to reach, and the skills needed to achieve it. The following broad guidelines apply to setting effective goals.

Express Goals Positively

Express goals in ways that allow the athlete to envision success. For example, "By *X* date, I will improve *Y* by 20%" or "I will be able to do *A* by *B* date." Taking small steps, and celebrating each accomplishment, keeps motivation high and the desire to continue strong. Positive reinforcement from friends and colleagues will help when motivation is low. Posters and positive visual reminders also assist in keeping the goal in sight.

It is very difficult to achieve a goal when the athlete secretly believes it cannot be done. Negativity in any form only highlights difficulties and focuses attention on failure.

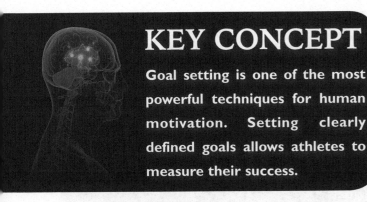

KEY CONCEPT

Goal setting is one of the most powerful techniques for human motivation. Setting clearly defined goals allows athletes to measure their success.

Set Priorities

For the individual striving to attain several goals, set a priority for each. Doing so keeps the athlete from feeling overwhelmed by too many goals and directs attention to the most important goal.

Document Goals

Documenting goals helps to avoid confusion and gives the goals more power. Specific, written goals force the individual focus his or her energy in a specific direction and keep the goal setter from straying off course. Written goals should be displayed and recited each day. Jotting down goals and putting them in a drawer just means they will be forgotten or ignored. A visible list of goals acts as a constant reminder of what remains to be accomplished.

Use Operational Goals

Operational goals are "mini-goals" that help accomplish larger goals a step at a time. An example is an athlete whose goal is to run a mile in 8 minutes. If the starting point is 10 minutes, a weekly operational goal of shaving off 15 seconds allows the athlete to work progressively toward the ultimate goal. If a goal is too large, it can appear that no progress is being made. Incremental goals offer more opportunities for reward. Today's operational goals should be derived from larger goals.

Set Performance Goals, Not Outcome Goals

It is very important that goals be set in such a way that the athlete retains as much control as possible over achievement. There is nothing as dispiriting as failing to achieve a personal goal for reasons beyond an one's control, such as poor judging, bad weather, injury, excellence of other athletes, or just plain bad luck. Goals based on outcomes are extremely vulnerable to occurrences that are beyond the athlete's control.

Instead, base goals on personal performance targets or skills to be acquired. This allows control over achievement of the goals. Assign dates and times to goals so that achievement can be measured. If goals are left to chance, they will only happen by chance. Deadlines help to maintain focus and motivation; both are important to achievement.

Set Specific Goals

Set specific, measurable goals. When all conditions of a measurable goal are achieved, the athlete's confidence will increase, and he or she will be motivated and able to set more difficult goals. If goals are consistently unmet, the athlete will have a basis on which to evaluate the reasons for failure and take appropriate action to improve skills.

Set Goals at the Right Level

Setting goals at the correct level is a skill acquired by practice. Athletes should set goals that are slightly out of their immediate grasp, but not so far that there is no hope of reaching them. No one puts serious effort into achieving a goal that he or she believes is unrealistic. Personal factors such as fatigue, injury, stage in the season, and the like should be taken into account when goals are set. It is best to set goals that raise average performance.

Setting a measurable, attainable goal will help the athlete strive to accomplish it. Setting a goal too high leads only to frustration and possible failure. Conversely, setting low goals can lead to complacency and mediocrity. The old saying, "Only the mediocre are always at their best," applies here. If athletes are not prepared to stretch and work hard, then they are extremely unlikely to achieve anything of any real worth.

Set Short-Term and Long-Term Goals

Goals can be placed into two categories: short term and long term. *Short-term goals* are specific outcomes to be reached within a set period: a day, a week, a month, or perhaps even a few months. Any time period longer than a few months puts the goal into the long-term category. Short-term

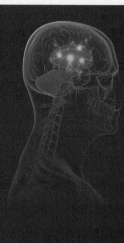

KEY CONCEPT

When setting personal goals, keep the following guidelines in mind:

- **Express goals positively**
- **Set priorities**
- **Document goals**
- **Use operational goals**
- **Set performance goals, not outcome goals**
- **Set specific goals**
- **Set goals at the right level**
- **Set both short-term and long-term goals**

goals should be perceived as immediate and attainable. An example is an athlete who sets a goal to increase the amount she can bench-press by 10 pounds within 3 weeks. This goal specifies the amount of gain and the time frame within which it must be attained.

Long-term goals are those that one strives to reach in the more distant future. To attain these goals, the athlete must work consistently and reach numerous short-term goals along the way. Long-term goals must be documented, reviewed periodically, and reevaluated as needed.

IMAGERY AND SIMULATION

Imagery, a training process done purely within the mind, helps create, modify, or strengthen neurological pathways that are important to muscle coordination. Imagination is the driving force of imagery.

Imagery is based on the important principle that anyone can exercise areas of the brain with stimulus from the imagination rather than from the senses. Imagery allows the athlete to practice and prepare for events and eventualities he or she can never train for in reality. This allows the athlete to pre-experience the achievement of goals.

Practicing with imagery can help "slow down" complex skills so that the athlete can isolate and *feel* the correct component movements of the skills, and thus isolate where problems in technique lie. For example, if a discus thrower is having trouble with the release, he can practice the correct technique over and over again in his

mind. This can be done anywhere, at any time. He can only physically practice throwing the discus a limited amount of time each day. Through the use of imagery, an athlete can move closer to preparing for the "95% mental" part of the game.

Simulation is similar to imagery in that it seeks to improve the quality of training by teaching the brain to cope with circumstances that would not otherwise be encountered until an important competition. Simulation is carried out by making the physical training circumstances as close as possible to the real competition. An example is having training sessions timed or judged, or bringing in spectators to watch the practice performance.

In many ways, simulation is superior to imagery in training because the stresses introduced are more vivid because they exist in reality. However, simulation requires much greater resources of time and effort to set up and

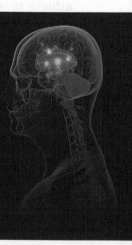

KEY CONCEPT

Imagery allows the athlete to practice mentally and prepare for events and eventualities that he or she can never train for in reality. Simulation emulates the circumstances of competition in practice.

implement, and is less flexible in terms of the range of eventualities that can be approximated.

STRATEGIES TO COPE WITH STRESS AND DISAPPOINTMENT

Stress from athletics takes many forms. A certain amount of stress can be healthy and help to improve performance. Stress can help the athlete increase awareness, maintain a clearer focus, increase motivation, and filter out distractions that could have a negative effect on performance. Too much stress can hinder performance and lead to problems in other areas of life. Some situations that can cause excess stress are discussed here.

Transitional Stress

When an athlete makes a transition between levels in a sport, he or she may experience a great deal of stress from being faced with unknowns. These may include increased competition, new teammates, or simply a change from the level of competition he or she is accustomed to. An example is the highly talented high school athlete who goes to college on an athletic scholarship and fails to live up to his or her potential. Transitional stress in athletes typically occurs when:

- Beginning a new sport
- Going from high school to college
- Changing leagues
- Changing levels of competition
- Going from junior high to high school
- Going from college to professional
- Retiring from athletics

KEY CONCEPT

Too much stress can hinder performance and lead to problems in other areas of life. The proper amount of stress, however, can help improve performance.

Injury

Injury can be devastating to the motivated athlete. Injury prevents the athlete from competing and also sets him or her back in terms of training and performance goals. Understanding that injuries are part of competitive athletics will allow the athlete to modify goals when injuries do occur. Support from other athletes, family, and friends will help the athlete cope with the stress of the injury and its consequences for his or her competitive life.

Burnout

Burnout is both physically and mentally challenging. Pressure to win, along with criticism from coaches, parents, and other teammates, can create excess stress and anxiety (Figure 10–3). **Burnout** manifests as dropping out of a sport and quitting an activity that was once enjoyable. An example is a highly competitive gymnast or swimmer who began the sport very early in life. After a while, the stress of early and late practices, coupled with the lack of a normal social life and pressure from parents and coaches, causes the athlete to quit the

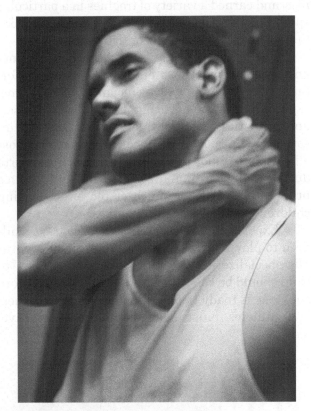

Figure 10–3 Athletes must be able to deal with stress and disappointment. It is important that short-term disappointment not be permitted to translate into long-term failure. Courtesy of Photodisc.

sport. These athletes are usually excellent at their sport, but mentally they simply cannot continue.

According to the *Georgia Tech Sports Medicine & Performance Newsletter* (2000), experts recommend steps adults can take to encourage a healthy interest in sports among young people. As many as 70% of children who participate in youth sports drop out of athletics by the time they are 13 years old. This is true of a variety of sports popular throughout the country. There are several reasons for this drop off in interest among teens. In some cases, children begin participating in sports too soon. They can become frustrated when parents enroll them in highly competitive situations before they fully understand how to play a particular sport.

The Olympics also pose a problem. The games often highlight and promote top athletes, who begin training at young ages. This sometimes sends the message that children must have an early start in a specific sport if they are to excel.

Experts also claim that some young athletes achieve success too early. If by the age of 12 a child has won, lost, traveled, attended awards ceremonies, and earned a variety of trophies in a particular sport, he or she might wonder if there is any point in playing for another four or five years.

There are other causes for concern. Parents and coaches sometimes emphasize sports performance and winning above enjoyment of the game, especially as they get caught up in wins, losses, and statistics. Young athletes who limit themselves to one sport often face early burnout; most elite athletes enjoy participating in multiple sports during their youth, and some teams and leagues practice and play too much or too often, leaving children exhausted or overextended.

Experts instruct parents to encourage children to play multiple sports, and let them eventually specialize in one or two sports they like. No child should be rushed into organized sports before she or he is ready to play. Finally, parents, coaches, and athletes must keep sports in perspective.

Participating in sports should be fun, not a profession or a mission with the goal of earning a college scholarship or professional contract.

Gender differences can lead to stress in athletic involvement. The benefits and positive outcomes of sport involvement for sexes are many. Problems occur when females are involved in sports involving bodily contact and great physical exertion—these activities are characterized as being masculine, and many girls and women see this as too problematic an issue to permit participation. Men and boys who pursue sports and activities that are expressive and artistic in nature (such as ballet and ice dancing) often have to overcome similar barriers.

The European Federation of Sports Psychology makes the following recommendations (1998):

- Organizations should work toward making all sporting opportunities available to all individuals, regardless of gender. This should not be taken to mean that all sporting contests should be mixed; providers of sport and recreation facilities should recognize that there may be occasions when men and women need to participate in single-sex groupings.

- All persons involved with the provision and promotion of sport opportunities should recognize the possible existence of psychological barriers and work toward overcoming them.

- All persons involved with media presentation of sports should work to produce positive images of athletes, regardless of gender.

- Resource allocation in sports should show evidence of gender equity.

- Opportunities for employment and professional development in coaching, management, and sports science should be equally available to all individuals, regardless of gender.

- Organizations should work toward giving all individuals the choice to be coached or advised by someone of their own gender. This includes sport psychology consultants.

- Those involved in sports should recognize that the needs of male and female athletes may differ in some respects and be similar in others.

- Providers of sport should recognize that participation is influenced by the range of activities available, and should make every effort to

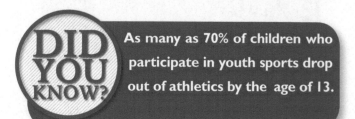

DID YOU KNOW? As many as 70% of children who participate in youth sports drop out of athletics by the age of 13.

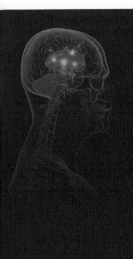

KEY CONCEPT

Burnout can make an athlete who excels in his or her sport turn away from competition and sports altogether. Burnout can be caused by increased pressure to win, beginning a sport too early, not being involved in other activities, and gender differences.

Managing Stress

The negative effects of stress can interfere with judgment and fine motor control. Stress can also cause competition to be seen as a threat rather than a challenge. This may lead the athlete to think negatively and lose self-confidence. The more stress an athlete faces, the more of his or her mental energy it consumes.

One of the best ways to manage stress is through goal setting. Athletes who program their workouts and competitions tend to be better prepared for unforeseen situations. When an unexpected situation does arise, these athletes are more likely to handle it in a positive way. Other ways to handle stress are through meditation, positive thinking, time management, talking with friends, and taking breaks.

The following quiz was designed to be an initial step in understanding and combating the harmful effects of stress on athletic performance. It was developed by Mick G. Mack of the University of Northern Iowa. Answers appear at the end of the chapter.

promote activities that meet the needs of both men and women.

- Research is fundamental and should not be gender blind. It should take into consideration the needs and aspirations of girls and boys, men and women.

STRESS AND ATHLETIC PERFORMANCE QUIZ

All of the questions are to be answered either true or false.

1. Under high levels of stress, athletes typically have a broad attention span. **T or F**
2. The clammy feeling we often get when stressed is caused by our body's natural defense against bleeding to death. **T or F**
3. Elite-level performers have fewer nervous reactions to stress than do nonelite-level performers. **T or F**
4. High levels of stress make it more difficult to think clearly. **T or F**
5. Getting sick to your stomach and throwing up when nervous is your body's way of telling you that you are overstressed. **T or F**
6. Caffeine exaggerates the physical and mental effects of stress. **T or F**
7. The body's stress response, which is commonly referred to as the fight-or-flight response, allows us to do superhuman feats. **T or F**
8. The only time stress is good is when there is no stress. **T or F**
9. Sighing as you exhale is more relaxing than not sighing. **T or F**
10. Under stress, athletes often revert to their most well-learned behaviors. **T or F**

Reprinted with permission of Mick G. Mack of the University of Northern Iowa.

SELF-CONFIDENCE

Self-confidence is one of the most important attributes an athlete can have. It reflects an athlete's assessment of his or her own self-worth, and plays a large part in determining the athlete's happiness throughout life.

Participation in athletics can be enormously positive in improving self-worth, and highly negative in damaging it. When sports are used creatively, with an emphasis on enjoyment, effective goal setting, and monitoring the achievement of goals, self-confidence builds as targets are reached and improvement in performance is noted. Self-confidence allows athletes to take risks because they have enough belief in their own abilities to know that if things do go wrong, they can be put right.

The way in which the athlete approaches self-confidence is important. An underconfident athlete will not take the risks that should be taken. Overconfidence, though, can lead to a decrease in performance because the athlete is not trying hard enough. Overconfidence is confidence that is not based on ability. It may be a result of parents or coaches who try to help without understanding an athlete's abilities; it may be caused by vanity or ego; or it may be caused by positive thinking or imagery that is not backed up by ability. Overconfidence is dangerous because it can lead to situations that the athlete is unable to manage. It can set up the athlete for a serious failure that could devastate self-confidence.

Confidence should be based on observed reality—that is, on the achievement of performance goals. Athletes should be confident that they will perform up to their current abilities. True self-confidence comes from a realistic expectation of success based on well-practiced physical skills, thorough knowledge of the sport, respect for one's own competence, adequate preparation, and good physical conditioning (Figure 10–4). The success attained should be measured by achievement of personal performance goals, not outcome goals such as winning.

When children are compelled to participate in a sport in which they have no interest or aptitude, it can destroy self-confidence. Consistent failure can lead to a lack of self-esteem. Persons who are underconfident commonly suffer from fear of failure (which prevents them from taking risks effectively), self-doubt, lack of concentration, and negative thinking. Use of imagery and effective goal setting will help improve self-confidence and self-image.

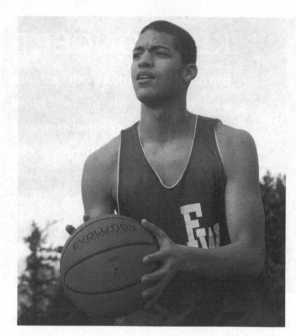

Figure 10–4 Confidence leads to success. Athletes should be confident that they will perform up to their current abilities.

By setting and visualizing measurable goals, achieving them, then setting new goals and achieving them, the athlete builds self-confidence. This increases the chances for success and allows a reasonably accurate assessment of the athlete's real abilities.

CAREERS IN SPORTS PSYCHOLOGY

The world's first sports psychology laboratory was founded by Carl Diem at the Deutsch Sporthochschule in Berlin, Germany, in 1920. In 1925, A. Z. Puni opened a sports psychology laboratory at the Institute of Physical Culture in Leningrad. That same year, Cloman Griffith of the University of Illinois established the first sports psychology laboratory in North America. Griffith had begun research into psychological factors that affect sports performance in 1918, and in 1923 he offered the first course in sports psychology. Griffith was interested in the effects on athletic performance of factors such as reaction time, mental awareness, muscular tension and relaxation, and personality. Due to the financial constraints of the Great Depression, Griffith's laboratory closed in 1932.

In North America, little or no research in sports psychology took place between the closing of Griffith's laboratory and the 1960s. Then, rather quickly, physical education departments in many

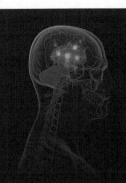

KEY CONCEPT

Sport psychology is a rapidly expanding field with many career opportunities. Careers in sport psychology may be pursued in educational, clinical, or research settings.

institutions began to offer courses in sports psychology, and graduate programs began to appear.

The first scholarly journal devoted to sports psychology, the *International Journal of Sport Psychology,* was established in 1970, followed in 1979 by the *Journal of Sport Psychology.* Increasing interest in conducting sports psychology research in settings outside the laboratory triggered the

formation of the Association for the Advancement of Applied Sport Psychology (AAASP) in 1985, and focused attention more directly on applied psychology in both the health field and sports contexts.

Sports psychology is a very interesting, intriguing field of study. A student of sports psychology can pursue three tracks:

- Educational sports psychology, which emphasizes the teaching, strategies, and mental skills involved in enhancing athletic performance in the field.

- Clinical sports psychology, which treats athletes in a clinical setting.

- Academic sports psychology, which focuses on research and teaching.

For a listing and description of all programs, consult the *Directory of Graduate Programs in Applied Sport Psychology*, available from AASP.

CONCLUSION

Sports psychology is the study of the mental factors influencing performance in sport and exercise. Sports psychologists apply psychological principles and a number of different techniques to the fields of sports and exercise, all aimed at improving performance and building a positive self-image.

Goal setting can help the athlete attain greater success by focusing his or her energy in a positive, measurable way. By setting goals and measuring their achievement, athletes can track what they have accomplished and discover how much they are capable of achieving.

REVIEW QUESTIONS

1. List several techniques that the athlete can use to increase performance and boost positive self-image.
2. Why is motivation an important factor in athletic performance?
3. What are the advantages of goal setting?
4. What guidelines apply to setting effective goals?
5. Compare and contrast imagery and simulation.
6. How can stress be beneficial? Harmful?
7. After taking the stress quiz, what did you learn?
8. What are the dangers of excessive stress?
9. Explain how self-confidence improves self-worth.
10. Why do athletes burn out and leave their sport, especially at a young age?
11. List the three career tracks for a student of sports psychology.

PROJECTS AND ACTIVITIES

1. Find a sports psychologist practicing in your area. Arrange an interview and ask at least these questions:
   a. How did you become interested in this field?
   b. How difficult is it to become a sports psychologist?

   c. What difference do you think you make in the lives of the athletes with whom you work?

   d. What is the most difficult part of your job?

   e. Are career opportunities expanding? Will there be opportunities when I graduate from college?

   f. How much does a sports psychologist earn?

   g. If you had to do it all over again, would you choose this field?

2. Using the information learned in this chapter, establish a personal goal-setting program. You must list both short-term and long-term goals. Use the worksheet at the end of this chapter.

3. Write a two-page paper on the following: How has stress affected your life? What strategies do you use to manage stress in a positive way?

4. You have decided on a career in sports psychology. Research what you need to do to become a sports psychologist.

5. Meet with the coach you admire most and ask how he or she uses sports psychology in motivating athletes. Report back to class.

LEARNING LINKS

- Visit the website http://www.peaksports.com for what this mental game coach has to say about motivation and sports psychology.

- Browse the resources and articles at http://www.topachievement.com and discover some tools and techniques for motivation and goal setting.

- Learn more about careers in sports psychology by visiting the website of the Association for the Advancement of Applied Sport Psychology: http://www.aaasponline.org.

ANSWERS TO STRESS PERFORMANCE TEST

1. False. Under high levels of stress, athletes tend to have a narrow attention span, often referred to as tunnel vision. Attention may also focus on the athlete's internal thought process, which can lead to "choking" under pressure.

2. True. One of the body's physical responses to stress is to divert blood away from the small vessels near the skin. This provides a defense against bleeding to death from wounds, but gives the skin a cold, clammy feeling.

3. False. Elite-level performers have just as many nervous reactions to stress as any other type of performer. However, elite athletes often interpret these reactions as being more positive and beneficial than do other athletes.

4. True. Clear thinking is more difficult in pressure situations. This is why coaches and athletes must constantly practice what they are going to do and how they are going to respond in pressure-packed situations.

5. False. So that more blood will be available to the large muscles of the body in preparation for strenuous physical activity, such as fighting or fleeing, the digestive system shuts down. During this shutdown, the acid in your stomach makes you feel nauseated, which sometimes results in vomiting. This is a normal reaction to stress.

6. True. Caffeine tends to exaggerate the physical and mental effects of stress. Knowing this, coaches and athletes should avoid caffeine products before entering potentially stressful situations.

7. True. Under stress, the body produces adrenalin, which provides a powerful, quick burst of energy that sometimes results in superhuman feats.

8. False. Certain stresses are good. For example, being elevated to the starting team brings additional stress that most athletes would enjoy. Another example of positive stress is physical and mental

training. All athletes are under stress when, during training, they push themselves to the edge so that their bodies will adapt to the demand and get stronger.

9. True. For some reason, letting out an audible sigh as you exhale is very relaxing. A number of additional relaxation techniques also involve breathing exercises.

10. True. In stressful situations, athletes often revert to familiar, comfortable behaviors. This is one reason why athletes should try to learn and perfect new skills and techniques in the off-season.

WHAT ARE YOUR GOALS?

Use the chart below to record your personal, educational, professional, and community goals. Remember to classify goals as either short term (one year or less to accomplish), intermediate-term (one to five years), or long term (more than five years to achieve). You may have more than one goal, or no goals in a particular category.

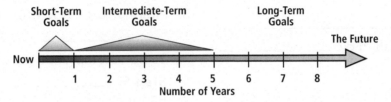

Personal Goals
Short term: _____
_____
_____

Intermediate term: _____
_____
_____

Long term: _____
_____
_____

Educational Goals
Short term: _____
_____
_____

Intermediate term: _____
_____
_____

Long term: _____
_____
_____

Professional Goals
Short term: _____
_____
_____

Intermediate-term: _____
_____
_____

Long term: _____
_____
_____

Community Goals
Short term: _____
_____
_____

Intermediate term: _____
_____
_____

Long term: _____
_____
_____

ACTION PLAN: INTERMEDIATE- OR LONG-TERM GOALS

1. Intermediate- or long-term goal:
_____

To be accomplished by: _____
Step 1: _____
Results needed:
_____

To be accomplished by: _____
Step 2: _____
Results needed:
_____

To be accomplished by: _____
Step 3: _____
Results needed:
_____

To be accomplished by: _____
Step 4: _____
Results needed:
_____

To be accomplished by: _____

2. Intermediate- or long-term goal:
_____

To be accomplished by: _____
Step 1: _____
Results needed:
_____

To be accomplished by: _____
Step 2: _____
Results needed:
_____

To be accomplished by: _____

Step 3: _____
Results needed:
_____

To be accomplished by: _____
Step 4: _____
Results needed:
_____

To be accomplished by: _____

3. Intermediate- or long-term goal:
_____

To be accomplished by: _____
Step 1: _____
Results needed:
_____

To be accomplished by: _____
Step 2: _____
Results needed:
_____

To be accomplished by: _____
Step 3: _____
Results needed:
_____

To be accomplished by: _____
Step 4: _____
Results needed:
_____

To be accomplished by: _____

(Throop & Castellucci, 1999)

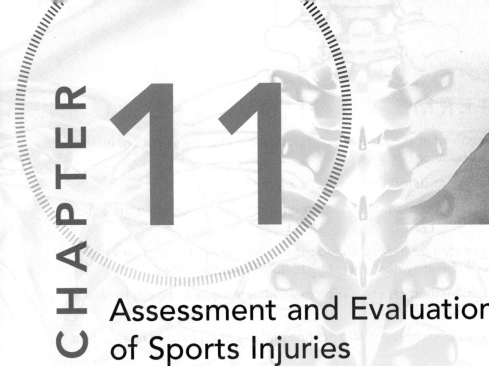

CHAPTER 11

Assessment and Evaluation of Sports Injuries

OBJECTIVES

Upon completion of this chapter, the reader should be able to:

- Explain the difference between assessment, evaluation, and diagnosis of an injury
- Describe the various factors that influence the type and severity of athletic injuries
- Describe the evaluation process of an athletic injury using a systematic approach
- Describe what the acronym CAB stands for
- Explain the different methods and reasons for documenting injuries
- Explain why return-to-play criteria is important in evaluating an injured athlete prior to resuming sports

KEY TERM

active motion *Movement through a range of motion done by the athlete during examination to assess injury.*

AED *Automated electronic defibrillator. Device used to shock heart back into normal rhythm.*

anthropomorphic data *Statistics on size, weight, body structure, gender, strength, and maturity level of an individual.*

assessment *The orderly collection of objective and subjective data on an athlete's health status.*

diagnosis *Using information from assessment and physical evaluation findings to establish the cause and nature of the athlete's injury or disease; made only by a physician or other licensed health care provider.*

functional activity *The level of movement at which the athlete can comfortably work and participate.*

H.O.P.S. *An acronym for the approach to the secondary-injury survey: history, observation, palpation, and special tests.*

ligamentous laxity *Degree of looseness in the ligaments of a joint.*

KEY TERMS CONTINUED

mechanism of force *All energies involved at the time of an impact, including the direction, intensity, duration, activity, and position of the body or body part.*

palpation *Touching during examination to determine extent of injury.*

passive motion *Movement through a range of motion performed by the examiner while the athlete relaxes all muscles.*

primary-injury survey *Assessment of life-threatening emergencies and management of airway, breathing, and circulation. EMS should be activated when threats to life are suspected.*

secondary-injury survey *A thorough, methodical evaluation of an athlete's overall health to reveal additional injuries beyond the initial injury.*

sport-specific activity *Particular types of movement and actions that are needed in or related to a particular sport.*

ASSESSMENT AND EVALUATION OF ATHLETIC INJURIES

The **assessment and evaluation** of athletic injuries are important proficiencies that everyone on the athletic health care team must possess. The certified athletic trainer is often the first person on the scene of an athletic injury and must institute the duty of care expected by the profession. The knowledge and expertise of the certified athletic trainer, which are applied to evaluate injuries immediately after they occur, help in getting the proper aid to the athlete as quickly as possible.

It is important to note that certified athletic trainers can assess and evaluate an injury, but they cannot diagnose. Diagnosis of injuries is the domain of the licensed health care provider, typically the physician. Licensed health care providers who can make diagnoses are often limited by their specialties. Podiatrists can diagnose foot problems. Chiropractors usually base their diagnoses on the relationship of the body's structure to its overall function. Dentists are limited to diagnosing tooth and mouth problems, and optometrists are limited to the problems with the eyes.

Assessment and evaluation consist of the orderly collection of objective and subjective data on an athlete's health status. based on professional knowledge and knowledge of the events that occurred. A **diagnosis** is what the physician or licensed provider states to be the problem,

based on his or her skills, expertise, and medical school training. Even though this sounds like semantics, it is a principle that must be followed closely. The certified athletic trainer must remain within the limits of his or her ability and training and act according to professional ethics. Stepping beyond the scope of practice could constitute negligence and breach of duty.

The physician uses all the information obtained in an evaluation to arrive at a diagnosis of the injury. The certified athletic trainer uses information from the physician to set short- and long-term goals for recovery. Both the physician and the certified athletic trainer work together to create an effective management plan.

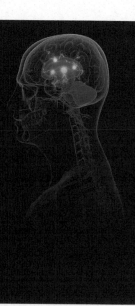

KEY CONCEPT

Assessment and evaluation is the compilation of subjective and objective data related to the presenting signs and symptoms of a particular injury or disease state. Diagnosis is the ability to take that data and make a scientifically based statement specifying the injury or disease process.

FACTORS INFLUENCING ATHLETIC INJURIES

Many factors influence the type and severity of an athletic injury. Some, but not all, factors can be controlled by the athlete. Significant factors include:

- Anthropomorphic status
- Mechanism of force
- Speed
- Protective equipment
- Skill level

Anthropomorphic Data

Anthropomorphic data include the athlete's size, weight, and structure. It also includes gender, strength, and maturity level. These data describe the anthropomorphic status of an individual or situation. For example, compare high school athletes to college athletes. Even if body size and strength are similar at both levels, college athletes have a distinctive advantage in level of maturity. Collegiate athletes, for the most part, are stronger, faster, have mature body structure, and have advanced skill training. Collegiate athletes also enjoy an advanced system of medical care. Cultural awareness is also important, because it pertains to the manner in which an evaluation is conducted. Someone who does not speak the native language would need an interpreter to bridge the communication gap and successfully conduct an evaluation. Other cultural differences must be taken into account as well.

Mechanism of Force

Mechanism of force comprises all forces involved at the time of an impact: the direction of the force, its intensity and duration, the activity being undertaken, and the position of the body or body part at the time of injury. Biomechanical factors must be taken into account as well. An example is a basketball player who falls to the court after trying to rebound the ball. The basic mechanism of force for this occurrence is falling from a height of several feet onto a hardwood floor without any cushioning effect. Other considerations are how the player's body struck the court and whether anyone else was involved or landed on him. These data, along with knowledge of the mechanism of force, enable the medical staff to form a preliminary picture of the injury and its extent.

Speed

Speed influences the type and severity of athletic injuries. The greater the speed of the collision, the greater the chance of injury. As athletes continue to get larger and faster, the types and severity of collision injuries increase. This is why it is not advisable to have athletes of different maturity levels practice or compete against one another. If high school senior and sophomore football players practice contact drills at full speed against each other, the rate and degree of injuries to the sophomores could be expected to be much greater. This goes back to the issue of maturity and skill levels. This is not to say that no sophomore athlete could practice or compete at this level, but to emphasize that coaches need to be very careful not to place immature athletes at risk.

Protective Equipment

Protective equipment can greatly reduce the risk of injury by absorbing and distributing force. Dissipation of force reduces the amount and type of forces absorbed by the body. New materials and better equipment design have helped keep injury levels moderate even as athletes get bigger, faster, and stronger. An example of this is the pole vault (in track and field): The landing pits have undergone several modifications in the past few years to make the sport safer. More padding, along with higher safety standards, will help keep injury rates down.

Skill Level

The skill level of any athlete partially determines the rate and severity of athletic injuries. Beginners are often at greater risk for both minor and major injuries because of their unfamiliarity with or inability to master the basic techniques of the activity or sport. Judgment may also be underdeveloped. Playing within one's ability, and being in control, are important factors in minimizing the risk of injury.

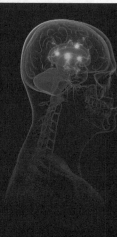

KEY CONCEPT

The type and severity of an injury are determined by factors such as anthropomorphic status, mechanism of force, speed, protective equipment in use, and skill level:

- Anthropomorphic status is based on size, body structure, and maturity level; if large athletes compete against smaller athletes, the chance of injury to the smaller athletes is increased.
- Mechanism of injury is related to the force and energy involved in impact; the greater the force and the more energy behind the force, the more serious the injury.
- Speed is a factor because the faster the body is moving, the greater is the force needed to stop; more force increases the severity of injury.
- Protective equipment, designed to absorb and distribute force, as well as to provide added strength to certain areas of the body, prevents or lessens the severity of injury.
- Athletes performing at higher skill levels have a reduced risk of severe injuries, because of their increased knowledge of basic skill sets.

RECOGNITION AND EVALUATION

Certified athletic trainers are trained to recognize when an injury has occurred, determine its severity, and apply proper evaluation procedures and treatment protocols. *Recognition of injuries* is the process whereby the certified athletic trainer determines the probable cause and mechanism of injury. This determination may be based on direct observation or second-hand accounts.

It is vital to obtain consent prior to any contact with the person. There are two types of consent, informed consent and implied consent. Informed consent is permission given by the injured or ailing person. Implied consent is assumed if the person cannot verbally give permission to help with the ailment or injury. An example would be an unconscious person unable to respond. Young children, even though they may refuse help, can be helped because it is reasonable

to assume that their age prohibits them from making a proper decision. It is also assumed under these circumstances that the child's parents would want you to help their child in need of medical attention. Failure to obtain consent can put one in legal jeopardy.

When evaluating emergencies, it is important to control life-threatening conditions first, and to activate emergency medical services (EMS) when needed. If in doubt, activate EMS. This is called the *primary-injury survey*. Next comes the management of non-life-threatening injuries, the *secondary-injury survey*.

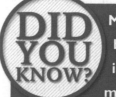

DID YOU KNOW? More than 70% of all cardiac and breathing emergencies occur in the home when a family member is present and available to help the victim.

Primary-Injury Survey

A **primary-injury survey** means determining whether serious or life-threatening injuries exist. It includes the basic CABs of assessing *c*irculation, *a*irway, and *b*reathing:

> *Circulation*—Check for signs of circulation such as breathing, coughing, or movement in response to the breaths. If the victim has no signs of circulation, start chest compressions. Adults require 30 chest compressions for every 2 rescue breaths.
>
> *Airway*—Open the victim's airway by tilting the head back and lifting the chin, if no spinal or neck injury is suspected (Figure 11–1). If spinal injury is a possibility, use the jaw-thrust technique (Figure 11–2).
>
> *Breathing*—Listen, look, and feel for signs of breathing. If the victim is not breathing, give two breaths and check for signs of circulation.

Immediate response and appropriate care are crucial for the survival of the athlete who has sustained a potentially life-threatening injury.

Cardiopulmonary Resuscitation

Coronary heart disease is responsible for an estimated 610,000 deaths in the United States each year (Centers for Disease Control and Prevention (CDC), 2015). High-quality bystander cardiopulmonary resuscitation (CPR) can double or triple survival rates from cardiac arrest. What follows is a brief description of CPR: It is *not* a certification. CPR should not be performed based solely on reading this text. Only individuals properly trained and certified should apply CPR. Again, this is merely a brief description of what is involved, and is not intended to provide proper training. Although the Good Samaritan law protects most helpers from legal actions brought against them, it does not apply if the helper performs procedures for which he or she is not properly trained. This could be considered malpractice.

Health care providers risk exposure to communicable diseases, such as HIV and the hepatitis B virus, through contact with bodily fluids. OSHA's standard precautions policy states that if workers will be exposed to blood or bodily fluids, they should use personal protective equipment such as latex gloves, protective eyewear, and gowns, and should use barriers if they have to perform rescue breathing.

The American Heart Association CPR guidelines, revised in 2015 and updated in 2018, recommend the following:

- Rescuers should phone 911 for an unresponsive victim before beginning CPR.

- If alone with an unresponsive infant or child, give about five cycles of compressions and ventilations (about two minutes) before leaving the child to phone 911.

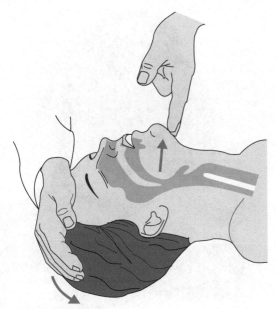

Figure 11–1 The head tilt/chin lift maneuver opens the airway of an unconscious person. It should be used only if there is no suspicion of spinal injury. If a spinal injury is suspected, in-line stabilization is important; supporting the head/neck in a spine neutral position until advanced medical care is present.

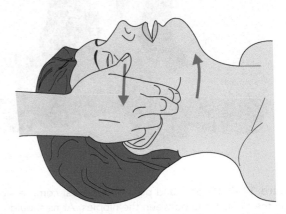

Figure 11–2 The jaw-thrust maneuver also opens the airway and is used when there is reason to suspect spinal injury.

- Begin chest compressions. Push hard and fast, trying not to interrupt compression rate. Compression rate should be 100 to 120 compressions per minute. Compression depth should be at least 2 inches, but no more than 2.4 inches (see Figure 11–3).

- The compression-to-ventilation ratio for all victims is 30:2, with a compression rate of 100 to 120 compressions per minute

- For children, use one or both hands to perform chest compressions at the nipple line; for infants, compress with two fingers on the breastbone just below the nipple line. Compression rate is still 100 to 120 compressions per minute.

- Chest-compression-only CPR is recommended only when the rescuer is unwilling or unable to perform mouth-to-mouth rescue breathing.

- Do not try to open the airway using a jaw thrust for injured victims. Use the head tilt/chin lift for all victims.

- Take a normal (not deep) breath before giving a rescue breath to a victim.

- Utilizing the head tilt-chin life method, give two rescue breaths, each over one second (see Figure 11–4). Each rescue breath should cause the chest to rise.

- If the victim's chest does not rise when the first rescue breath is delivered, perform the head tilt/chin lift again before giving the second breath.

- If the victim begins to breath normally but remains unresponsive, place the victim in the recovery position and monitor his or her breathing until help arrives.

- Continue until help arrives or you are too tired to continue.

Automated Electronic Defibrillator (AED)

An **automated electronic defibrillator** (AED) is a device about the size of this textbook that analyzes the heart's rhythm for any abnormalities

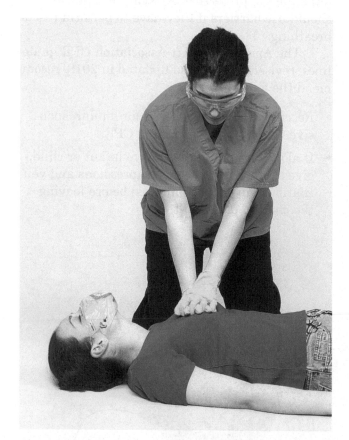

Figure 11–3 Proper hand position for chest compressions is on the breastbone between the nipples. Arms should remain in an extended, locked position with the shoulders over the victim's chest.

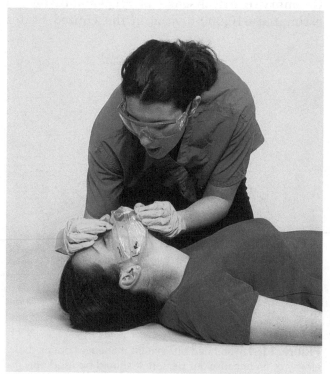

Figure 11–4 When performing CPR, pinch the victim's nose, lift the chin, and cover the chin and nose with your mouth to provide breaths.

and, if necessary, directs the rescuer to deliver an electrical shock to the victim. This shock, called defibrillation, may help the heart to reestablish an effective rhythm. AEDs are easy to operate and use voice prompts to instruct the rescuer. Once the machine is turned on, the rescuer will be prompted to apply two electrodes provided with the AED to the victim's chest. Once applied, the AED will begin to monitor the victim's heart rhythm. If a "shockable" rhythm is detected, the machine will charge itself and instruct the rescuer to stand clear of the victim and to press the shock button.

Communities with comprehensive AED programs that include CPR and AED training for rescuers have achieved survival rates of nearly 40% for cardiac arrest victims (*New England Journal of Medicine*, 2011). It is estimated that

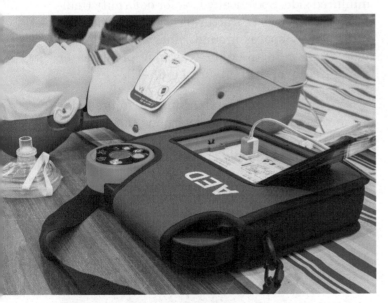

Figure 11–5 Automated electronic defibrillator (AED). Reprinted with permission from the American National Red Cross. All rights reserved in all countries. narin phapnam/ Shutterstock.com.

one-fourth of all heart attack victims' lives can be saved using this device.

AEDs can be found in corporate offices, shopping malls, airports, sports stadiums, schools, community centers, and other places where large groups of people gather and the risk of a sudden cardiac arrest incident is present. The number of devices in communities will grow as more and more people begin to understand the importance of AEDs and AED training. Only persons trained to use AEDs can utilize the device. Training has become widespread and available where first aid and CPR are taught.

Secondary-Injury Survey

A **secondary-injury survey** is a thorough, methodical evaluation of an athlete's overall health. Secondary-injury surveys may reveal additional injuries beyond the initial injury. A thorough evaluation of an athlete should use a systematic approach. The **H.O.P.S.** (history observation, palpation, and special tests) evaluation format is discussed in this section, along with additional methods of evaluating injury.

Be Thorough

Take your time and be thorough; look beyond the obvious! A complete examination decreases the likelihood of overlooking important details. Rule out the most serious injuries first. Be alert, calm, conservative, and safe. Certified athletic trainers run the risk of overlooking additional injuries if they are pressed to return an athlete to competition. The well-being of the athlete always comes first.

Gather a History

Obtain a history immediately. Do not touch the individual until *all* related questions have been answered. Question individuals who witnessed the incident:

1. What happened? Body part injured; description of injury.
2. When did the injury occur?
3. What factors influenced the injury?
   - Position of body and injured area at time of injury. Weight-bearing or non-weight-bearing? (Weight-bearing refers to the injured part having sustained the weight of the athlete during the injury event.)

- Activity at time of injury (from question 1, "What happened?"). Collision or contact?

- Speed at time of injury—velocity or acceleration?

- Direction of force?

- Intensity and duration of force?

- Results of force—twisting, hyperextension, hyperflexion?

4. Was a sound heard? By the individual or anyone else? Quality of sound: pop, snap, rip?

5. Where is pain located now? Where was it located at the time of injury? Ask the athlete to point to where the pain is located.

6. Pain characteristics: sharp or dull/achy? Stabbing, throbbing? Constant, cramping, intermittent? Painful at rest or only with use of injured body part? How intense is the pain? One method of assessing pain is to ask the athlete to rate, on a scale of 1 to 10, how badly it hurts. The following scale can be used in pain assessment:

0	=	No pain
1–3	=	Minimal pain
4–6	=	Moderate pain
7–9	=	Severe pain
10	=	Emergency-room pain

7. Is neurological function intact? Numbness, pins-and-needles prickling, muscle weakness, paralysis, burning sensation?

8. Is there any instability? A sense that something isn't working right? "If I let you, would you be able to use the injured body part now?" [*Do not have the person use it*—merely ask the question.]

9. Prior history of injury to this body part?

Expose the Injury

Expose the injured part, removing tape if necessary (if it is appropriate to complete the physical examination). If the examination requires the removal of a jersey or pants by cutting, use scissors to do so. Cutting along the seams will allow later repair. The injury must be exposed to observe the extent of damage.

It is important to do this while preserving the utmost modesty. It is one thing to take off a shoe and sock, and another to remove a jersey, especially from a female athlete. If this is necessary, the certified athletic trainer should shield the athlete from the view of contestants and spectators. Clothing removal and the examination should be done in a locker room or private area if at all possible. It is always good practice to have a member of the training staff who is the same sex as the injured athlete in attendance for all examinations.

Perform a Physical Examination

Perform the physical examination by first comparing the injured and uninjured sides. Start one joint above the injured area and go one joint below. If the forces that caused the injury were great enough, there could be additional injuries above and below the main injury.

OBSERVATION Compare the injured side to the uninjured side. Specifically look for deformity (indicating dislocation or fracture), swelling (especially in the hollow spaces around joints), bleeding, and color changes in the skin (vascular problems or bruising/ecchymoses) (Figure 11–6A–C).

PALPATION Palpation is touching the injured athlete during examination to determine the extent of the injury. Examine the uninjured side first. Be sure to palpate (touch) firmly enough to produce pain if

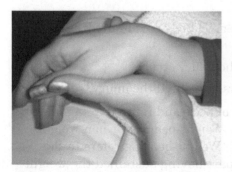
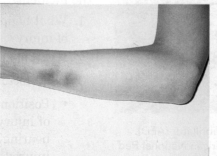
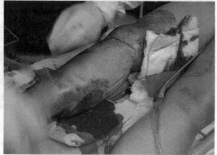

Figure 11–6 Use skills of observation to detect (A) deformity, (B) bruising, and (C) bleeding, and uncover any additional injuries. Photos courtesy of Dr. Deborah Funk, Albany Medical Center

it is present; palpating too lightly may result in missing a significant injury. On the uninjured side, the pressure should feel firm and slightly unpleasant, but not painful. During palpation, observe the athlete's face for signs of wincing (Figure 11–7). Palpate one joint above the injured area and continue to one joint below. During palpation, be sure to feel the bones, ligaments, and muscles/tendons.

ACTIVE MOTION **Active motion** is movement done by the athlete. Have the athlete move the injured body part through the full range of motion: up and down, in and out, and rotating. Permit the individual to tolerate some discomfort while attempting this. Refusal or inability to move through the full range of motion suggests a significant injury.

PASSIVE MOTION **Passive motion** is movement through a range of motion performed by the examiner while the athlete relaxes all muscles. The examiner supports the individual's injured body part and moves it through the range of motion, noting location and type of pain (Figure 11–8).

STRENGTH To test for strength, begin isometrically without resistance, then continue through the range of motion against resistance. Ask the athlete to contract the injured muscle, or the

muscles around the injured joint, without moving the bones. Compare to the uninjured side for size and firmness of muscle mass. Note any visible defects in the injured muscle. Palpate for knots or lumps in the injured muscle.

STABILITY Stability tests investigate **ligamentous laxity**. The athlete must relax all muscles around the injured joint to obtain a satisfactory evaluation. This is a stress test for ligaments. Support the injured body part at the far end of the distal bones of the joint (e.g., for the knee, support the leg just above the ankle, at the distal part of tibia). Use the other hand to stress the ligament at the affected joint line.

With all of the athlete's muscles relaxed, put enough pressure through the joint to cause stretching of the ligament fibers. Some laxity is normal. An acute grade I sprain will involve a few torn fibers that will make this maneuver painful, but not show any ligamentous laxity (looseness) compared to the uninjured side. An acute grade II sprain will produce both pain and increased ligamentous laxity; there will, however, be an endpoint (where movement stops). The movement of the joint will stop as the ligament is fully stretched. In a grade III sprain, there may or may not be pain, but there will be complete instability of the joint, with such marked looseness that the joint can be dislocated; hence,

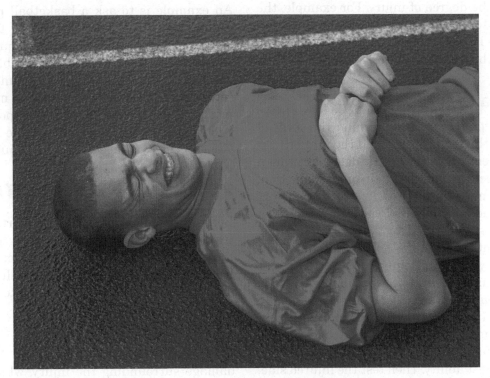

Figure 11–7 When palpating an injured body area, watch the victim's face for grimacing.

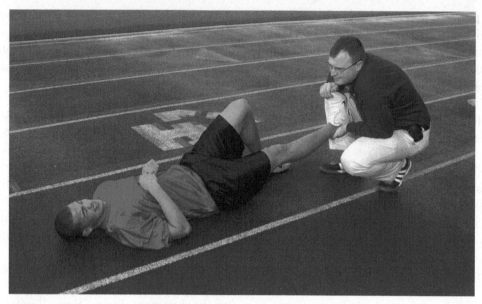

Figure 11–8 In passive motion, the certified athletic trainer assesses an injury by moving a body part through the range of motion while the athlete keeps the muscles relaxed.

there is no end point as a result of pressure. A grade III sprain or complete tear of the ligament will require prompt referral to an orthopedic surgeon for repair. A prior grade II sprain will show some laxity but no pain with this stress test.

SPECIAL EXAMINATIONS

Special tests and examinations may be necessary to establish the degree of injury. For example, the Lachman Anterior Drawer Test for the knee can establish the integrity of the anterior cruciate ligament (see Chapter 18, Figure 18-18).

Functional Activity

Functional activity tests determine the level of activity the athlete may resume. If the injured athlete has passed the various tests, demonstrating a normal inspection, minimal pain upon palpation, full range of motion, full muscle strength against resistance, and joint stability (no pain or marked laxity to stress compared to the uninjured side), the certified athletic trainer must determine what level of activity to permit during treatment. Instruct the injured athlete to stand, walk, hop, jog, sprint, cut, and twist, one after another, to demonstrate the ability to perform normally and pain-free compared to the uninjured side. Always ask the individual to test the uninjured side first to his or her best ability. Then test the injured side.

This will make any difference between the two sides more obvious.

Sport-Specific Activity

Testing for **sport-specific activity** determines if it is safe to resume the activities of a particular sport. Ask the athlete to demonstrate the specific maneuvers and actions of that sport to determine if he or she can do them normally and painlessly. An example is to ask a basketball player who is coming back from an ankle injury to sprint, cut, jump, and back-pedal. These are required skills for the sport, and the athlete must be able to complete these activities at full speed and intensity before returning to play. In some cases, it may be appropriate to use taping or other supportive devices before conducting these tests. Table 11–1 reviews steps in the evaluation of sports injuries.

RETURN-TO-PLAY CRITERIA

Before the team physician or certified athletic trainer clears an athlete to return to sports, several criteria must be met: full strength, freedom from pain, ability to perform the skills of the sport, and emotional readiness to return to competition.

Full Strength

After an injury occurs, there will be soft-tissue damage surrounding the injury, which can affect

KEY CONCEPT

A systematic approach to injury assessment and evaluation will ensure that no injuries go undiscovered. The approach should be the same each and every time an injury is encountered, so that the manner in which injury is assessed and evaluated becomes routine. First, obtain a history; then observe for swelling, deformities, and bleeding; continue by palpating the injury; and finally perform any special tests to determine the extent of the injury.

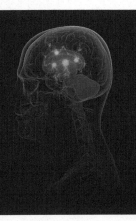

Table 11–1 Understanding Injuries: Common Steps in Evaluation, Treatment/Rehabilitation, and Return-to-Play Criteria

STEP	EVALUATION	TREATMENT/ REHABILITATION	RETURN-TO-PLAY CRITERIA
1. History	History		
2. Observation— looking	Swelling (and deformity, alignment, vascular integrity)	Control of swelling a. RICE—rest, ice, compression, elevation b. Support—splints, slings, crutches c. Anti-inflammatories*—after bleeding stops	Little or no swelling
3. Palpation— feeling	Pain (and neurological function, skin temperature, swelling)	Control of pain a. Rest b. Splints, slings, casts c. Analgesics as needed	Little or no pain
4. Range of motion	Range of motion— pain-free	Restore full range of motion— pain-free	Full range of motion— pain-free
5. Strength of muscles	Resisted strength— pain-free	Restore strength compared to uninjured side	Full strength—equal to (or greater than) the uninjured side
6. Stability of joints	Ligament integrity/ laxity Joint stability	Restore stability, as needed, as follows: a. Surgery as indicated b. Extra muscle strength—to compensate for loss of ligamentous stability	No instability during functional activity or sport-specific activity. Taping or use of a brace may help to achieve this criterion, in addition to surgery or extra muscle strength.

(continues)

Table 11–1 Understanding Injuries: Common Steps in Evaluation, Treatment/Rehabilitation, and Return-to-Play Criteria, *continued*

STEP	EVALUATION	TREATMENT/ REHABILITATION	RETURN-TO-PLAY CRITERIA
7. Functional activity	Functional activity (examples: hopping, jumping, running, cutting, twisting— other general athletic activities)	Restore functional activity for injured part. Maintain general body conditioning/fitness a. Aerobic capacity b. Muscle strength and endurance c. Flexibility	Full functional activity, using the injured body part AND whole body normally and painlessly
8. Sport-specific activity	Sport-specific activity	Restore sport-specific activity	Sport-specific activity— normally and painlessly

*Taken only with doctor's direction.

Reprinted with permission of Stephen G. Rice, M.D.

muscles, ligaments, tendons, and support tissue. Before an athlete can return to practice or competition, these tissues must be healed. Muscle atrophy (reduced muscle mass) is common with athletic injuries. Proper rehabilitation is needed because all muscles supporting the injury must be at 100% of pre-injury strength prior to return to play.

Free from Pain

An athlete in pain is at risk for a significant injury. A mild amount of soreness is not the same as pain. Athletes may experience mild soreness after returning to their sport from an injury. True pain is an indication that an injury has not completely healed. An athlete meets this criterion if there is no pain during the return-to-play performance tests.

Skill Performance Tests

To be certain the athlete is ready to return to sports, a series of performance tests will be necessary. These tests are designed to simulate the actual skills required for the sport. Performance tests should begin at a low level of intensity and gradually increase until the athlete is performing at game speed. If at any time the athlete is not able to perform one of the tests, she is not ready to return to the sport. Tests may include sprinting, jumping, cutting, back-pedaling, pushing

(football), and so on. The certified athletic trainer should be familiar with the given sport and its demands on the athlete, in order devise appropriate skill performance tests.

Emotional Readiness

Even though an athlete has recovered physically from an injury, he or she may not have recovered emotionally. It is important for the certified athletic trainer or sport psychologist to counsel the athlete before he or she returns to the sport. This will help the athlete work through any hesitation about returning to play after sustaining an injury. Athletes who have had significant injuries will be

DID YOU KNOW? Approximately 55% of athletic injuries occur to the knee. The shoulder is the joint next most frequently injured in sports, accounting for approximately 20% of sports injuries. The elbow is the third most frequently injured joint; it factors in approximately 7% of sports injuries.

more prone to emotional distress upon return to the sport. This may cause them to hesitate and perform at a lower level than before the injury. Athletes who do not perform at 100% will also be prone to new injuries. It is always important to ask the athlete if he or she is ready to return. An athlete who is hesitant or does not feel ready should not be allowed to return. The certified athletic trainer needs to pay careful attention to all athletes returning from injuries to make accurate assessments

DOCUMENTING INJURIES

Documenting athletic injuries is important for many reasons, perhaps most importantly for follow-up care. Injuries require immediate care and recognition, as well as a plan to completely heal and rehabilitate the athlete. Having injuries well documented, with follow-up care clearly written and followed, is essential for the total health of the athlete. This also helps to keep athletes from "falling through the cracks" and going without the care they require.

Detailed records of all injuries will create a database for the sports medicine program director. This information can be used to create a profile of injuries by sport, which enables the program director to recognize trends by injury type or occurrence. This information can be shared with the coaching staff, which may implement strengthening and stretching programs to target the specific concern. The result may be lower injury rates.

Careful, accurate records are also beneficial in case a lawsuit is filed claiming negligence or malpractice. Recording the specific time and type of treatment, as well as the person administering treatment, is important to the overall professionalism of the recordkeeping system. Many recordkeeping programs on the market today can help the training staff input and manage data.

There are many formats for reporting injuries. Many training facilities use the following:

- SOAP notes
- Daily sideline injury reports
- Training-room treatment logs
- Daily red-cross lists
- Athlete medical referral forms

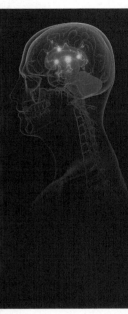

KEY CONCEPT

Meticulously documenting injuries, with follow-up care clearly written and followed, is essential to the total health of the athlete. A wide variety of tools and methods are used to document the care the athlete is receiving. The certified athletic trainer will determine which tools to use in the program.

SOAP Notes

SOAP notes refers to a particular format of recording information regarding treatment procedures. This method combines information provided by the athlete and the examiner's observations. Documentation of acute athletic injury can be effectively accomplished through a system designed to record subjective and objective findings and to document the immediate and future treatment plan for the athlete—subjective, objective, assessment, and plan (SOAP):

- *Subjective.* This component incorporates the subjective statements made by the injured athlete. Chronicling the event is designed to elicit the athlete's subjective impressions relating to the time, mechanism, and site of injury. The type and course of the pain and the degree of disability experienced by the athlete are also noteworthy.

- *Objective.* Objective findings include the certified athletic trainer's visual inspection, palpation, and assessment of active, passive, and resistive motion. Results of any special testing should also

FUN FACTS

Did you know that more injuries occur in practice than in games?

be noted here. The objective report also includes assessment of posture, presence of deformity or swelling, and location of point tenderness. Limitations on active motion, and pain arising or disappearing during passive or resistive motion, should be noted. Finally, the results of tests for joint stability or apprehension are also included.

- *Assessment.* Assessment of the injury is the certified athletic trainer's professional judgment and impression as to the nature and extent of injury. Although the exact nature of the injury is not always known initially, information pertaining to suspected site and anatomical structures involved is appropriate. A judgment of severity may be included, but is not essential at the time of acute injury evaluation.

- *Plan.* The plan should include the first-aid treatment rendered to the athlete and the sports therapist's intentions as to disposition. Disposition (what is done next) may include referral for more definitive evaluation or simply application of a splint, wrap, or

crutches and a request to report for revaluation the next day. If the injury is of a more chronic nature, it would be appropriate for the examiner to include treatment and therapeutic exercise in the plan. An example of SOAP notes appears in the accompanying box.

Daily Sideline Injury Report

The daily sideline injury report tracks every athlete who participates in a sport (Figure 11–9). It allows the training and coaching staff to follow every athlete every day throughout the season. Coaches can clearly see if an athlete has been injured and missed practice, or if the athlete can practice on a limited basis. The data can later be analyzed by computer to reveal injury patterns.

Training-Room Treatment Log

The training-room treatment log is filled out by certified athletic trainers as they treat athletes (Figure 11–10). The requisite information is the

SOAP NOTES

Scenario
A cyclist [name] reports left-sided low back pain along her iliac crest since crashing and landing on her left shoulder and back while on a training ride on [date]. She rates her pain 7/10.

Subjective
A 21-year-old competitive cyclist reports that she has been experiencing intense, left-sided low back pain along her iliac crest since crashing and landing on her left shoulder and back while on a training ride on [date].

Objective
The patient is point tender to palpation along the posterior iliac crest, with increased pain noted while actively bending to the left. All trunk motion is limited, but extension and passive flexion cause pain. Strength was not tested due to pain. Circulation and neurological status were within normal limits. Mild swelling and discoloration were observed over the left posterior iliac crest.

Assessment
Strain or contusion of the left quadratus lumborum.

Plan
An ice bag was applied for 20 minutes to control pain, swelling, and spasm. As the pain and swelling subside, gentle stretching will be instituted, followed by strengthening and gradual return to activity as tolerated.

DAILY INJURY REPORT

SCHOOL ___WILSON HIGH___ MONTH ___DECEMBER___ YEAR _____

SPORT ___WRESTLING, V.___ COACH ___JOHN JAMES___

ROSTER NUMBER

ROSTER	DAY OF WEEK: T	W	Th	F	Sa	Su	M	T	W	Th	F	Sa	Su	M	T	W	Th	F	Sa	Su	M	T	W	Th	F	Sa	Su	M	T	W	Th	INJURY TYPE AND PART OF BODY INJURED
DATE	1	2	3	4	5	6	7	8	9	10	11	12	13	14	15	16	17	18	19	20	21	22	23	24	25	26	27	28	29	30	31	
PRACTICE = P; GAME = G	P	P	P	G	-	-	P	G	P	P	G	-	-	P	G	P	P	P	G	-	-	P	G	P	P	G	-	-	P	P	P	
Bob Arnold																																
Jerry Brooks		S	S				S																									
Hal Cannon						S																										
Jeff Davidson										X	X																					Sprain R Ankle
Al East									N	I	I			I	I	L	L															
Mike Fredrich																																
George Gillespie																					X	X	X									Strain L Hamstring
Steve Harris			I*	I*			L*																									
Wayne Jones																						N	S	S	S							Flu
Charlie King									N	L	L																					Contusion L Forearm
Pat Long		N	I	I	I																											
Jim Murray																						T										Sprain R Wrist
Bill Newton																		X	X	X												
Larry Post																																
Dick Ross															N		R	I	I		R	I	L					L				Strain L Gastric
Bruce Storey																																
Mark Tunney																					N	I	O									Fracture R Elbow
Dave Vinson				N				I	I	L	L																					
Barry Watkins																	R	I	I		I	I	I	I								Concussion
Max Young																																

I = Injured (prior to practice)—did not practice at all.
S = Sick or Ill; did not practice at all.
X = Did not practice for other reasons (personal, disciplinary, cut practice, etc.).
L = Limited practice (no cutting, no contact, etc.).
n = New Injury; began practice full go, got hurt, had to stop.
R = Reinjury to same body part; began full go, got hurt, stopped.

LEGEND:

NL = New Injury; began practice full go, got hurt, returned on limited basis.
RL = Reinjury; began practice full go, got hurt, returned on limited basis.
NS = New Sickness; began full go, got sick, had to stop.
* = Any injury that occurred unrelated to game or practice should be noted by adding * after N, NL, I, R, or L.
T = Terminated or quit for non-injury related reason; enter T in the box for the day after the last participation.
R = Reinjury to same body part; began full go, got hurt, stopped.

Figure 11–9 Daily sideline injury report.

Daily Treatment Log

Date _____   Page _____ of _____

Name	Area	Time In	Time Out	STATUS	SPORT	Bag	Cup	Cryocuff	Immersion	Whirlpool	Contrast	Hydrocollator	Betadine Soak	Whirlpool	Diathermy	Paraffin	Ultrasound	E-Stim	Interferential	Compression	Balance/Proprioception	Passive	Active	Act. Assisted	Isometric	Isotonic	PNF	Static Stretch	PNF	Upper Body	Lower Body

Column groups: Ice (Bag, Cup, Cryocuff, Immersion, Whirlpool, Contrast), Heat (Hydrocollator, Betadine Soak, Whirlpool, Diathermy, Paraffin, Ultrasound), ROM (E-Stim, Interferential, Compression, Balance/Proprioception, Passive, Active, Act. Assisted), Strength (Isometric, Isotonic, PNF), Flex (Static Stretch, PNF), CV (Upper Body, Lower Body)

Rows numbered 1–24.

Status: 1. Athlete, 2. Private Patients, 3. Students, 4. Faculty/Staff, 5. High School Athletes

Sport: 1. Football, 2. Baseball, 3. Softball, 4. (W) Basketball, 5. (M) Basketball, 6. Volleyball, 7. Cross Country, 8. Rodeo, 9. Cheer, 10. Dance, 11. Other

Figure 11–10 Training-room treatment log.

athlete's name, the date, injury/complaint, treatment given, and a column to check for follow-up care, if needed. Everyone who has been taped, wrapped, iced, and so on should be documented. This information is also helpful in creating budgets, tracking inventory, and showing the need for athletic health care services.

Daily Red-Cross List

A daily red-cross list informs coaches of the status of athletes from one practice to another. This form tells the coaching staff that the athlete is either to have no practice (Ø), limited participation (L), or return to full practice and competition (R)

(Figure 11–11). After the athlete returns to full practice and competition, his or her name is taken off the list. This procedure is especially useful for sports that have large rosters. Using a duplicate form allows both the training and coaching staff to retain copies.

Athlete Medical Referral Form

A medical referral form, which the athlete takes to the doctor from the certified athletic trainer, allows accurate communication between the training staff and the physician's office (Figure 11–12). The physician can then respond with instructions on how to manage the athlete's injury.

DAILY RED-CROSS LIST

DATE: _____ SPORT: _____

★★

Athlete's Name	Assessment	ø	L	R	Description of Limitation
1.					
2.					
3.					
4.					
5.					
6.					
7.					
8.					
9.					
10.					

ø = no activity   L = limited activity   R = return to full activity

Figure 11–11 Daily red-cross list.

ATHLETE MEDICAL REFERRAL

ATHLETE _____   CLASS _____   DATE _____

SPORT _____

Dear Doctor: The athlete above must present to the school officials written permission from the physician to resume participation
in both athletics and physical education classes. Thank you.

SIGNS, SYMPTOMS AND IMMEDIATE CARE GIVEN:

_____

_____

_____

_____

SUSPECTED INJURY / ILLNESS _____

OCCASION: _____ Game _____ Practice _____ PE _____ Other: _____ Parent Contacted: Yes _____ No _____

_____ (From) _____ (To) _____

SPECIFIC DIAGNOSIS   PERIOD OF RESTRICTIONS

(Check all that are applicable)		Physical Education (Check One)
TREATMENT	**REHABILITATION**	☐ Regular
_____ None Required	_____ None required	
_____ No Weight Bearing	_____ Active Stretching	☐ Regular – Minor Restrictions _____
_____ Crutches	_____ Passive Stretching	_____
_____ Ice Packs	_____ R.O.M. Exercises	_____
_____ Cold Whirlpool	_____ Isometrics	_____
_____ Warm Whirlpool	_____ Manual Resistance	_____
_____ Ice Massage	_____ Progressive Resistance	_____
_____ Hydrocollator Hot Pack	_____ Isotonic/Isokinetic	
_____ Massage	_____ Orthotron Program	
_____ Contrast Baths	_____ Bicycle	**SPECIFIC INSTRUCTIONS FOR ATHLETICS**
_____ Protective Taping	_____ Swimming	_____
_____ Protective Padding	_____ Slideboard	_____
_____ Ultrasound		_____
_____ EMS		_____
_____ No Contact		_____
_____ Limited Contact		_____
_____ Running/Jogging Only		_____
_____ Dummy Drills Only		_____
_____ Full Contact		_____
_____ Other:		_____

Frequency _____ x per day for _____ weeks

Physician's Name Printed _____   Physician's Signature _____   Date _____   Phone No. _____

Figure 11–12 Athlete medical referral form.

CONCLUSION

Athletic injuries are inevitable as long as we enjoy competitive athletics. The care and treatment of athletic injuries constitute an important aspect of a sports medicine program. Certified athletic trainers complete assessments of athletic injuries and write referrals to the family physician. Physicians then diagnose the injury and prescribe a treatment plan for the sports medicine team to execute. Prompt assessment and follow-up will enable the athlete to return to practice or competition much faster.

Writing out and archiving accurate records helps to keep athletes from being overlooked or foregoing needed treatment. A reliable recordkeeping system tracks athletes and allows planning for their future care. Recordkeeping also allows injury data to be shared with coaches and helps in inventory planning for the next year. A comprehensive recordkeeping system will be valuable if a lawsuit is filed for negligence or malpractice.

REVIEW QUESTIONS

1. Explain the difference between an assessment, an evaluation, and a diagnosis.
2. How can anthropomorphic status influence the type and severity of an athletic injury?
3. Explain the difference between a primary- and secondary-injury survey.
4. When an athlete is injured, what questions would you ask to find out about prior injury history?
5. Give one example each of active and passive motion.
6. How do you test for a sport-specific activity?
7. Why is it a good idea to document injuries?
8. Explain three different types of recordkeeping. Why should injuries be documented and athletes tracked?
9. What does the acronym CAB stand for?
10. What does the acronym SOAP stand for?
11. Explain what an athlete may go through emotionally upon return to play from a significant injury.

PROJECTS AND ACTIVITIES

1. Make an appointment to see the certified athletic trainer at your school. Explain that you are on a fact-finding mission, exploring different types of recordkeeping. Ask for sample copies of the formats and forms. Share them with the class.
2. Meet with the staff of a local physical therapy clinic in your area. Ask them what types of recordkeeping they do. If they can give you some sample copies, compare and contrast the difference between your school's recordkeeping and that of the physical therapists.
3. Scenario: You are covering a girls' basketball game as an athletic training student aide. You see one of the girls come down on the side of another player's foot, inverting her ankle. She is in a lot of pain, and says she heard a "pop." Write down all the steps you would take in evaluating her ankle injury.

LEARNING LINKS

- Visit the website for the National Athletic Trainers Association (http://www.nata.org) and search for information on assessing and documenting injuries.

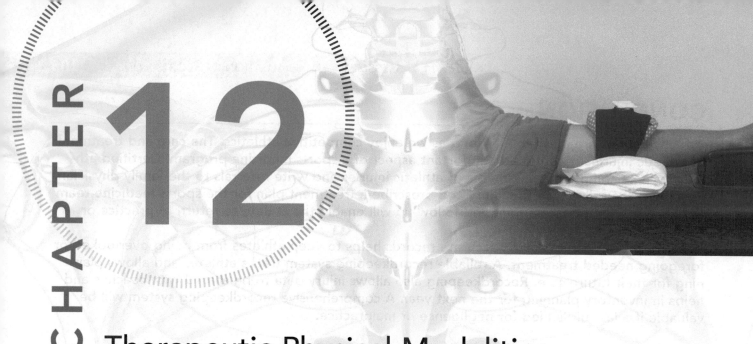

CHAPTER 12

Therapeutic Physical Modalities

OBJECTIVES

Upon completion of this chapter, the reader should be able to:

- Explain the use and effectiveness of physical modalities
- Describe the various thermal modalities and their applications
- Explain and describe the use of therapeutic ultrasound
- Explain and describe the use of electrical modalities

KEY TERMS

coupling agent *A cream or gel, applied to an area before ultrasound treatment, that provides a medium for sonic waves to penetrate the skin.*

cryotherapy *The therapeutic use of cooling agents.*

electrical stimulation (e-stim) *Use of electrical impulses to produce muscle contractions by stimulating the motor nerves.*

hydrocollator *A stainless-steel container filled with hot water that is used to heat moist packs for superficial heat therapy.*

hydrotherapy *A form of superficial heating that uses agitated, heated water in a specially designed piece of equipment.*

ice massage *The technique of rubbing ice over the injured area.*

modalities *Treatment of injuries, including heating, cooling, and mechanical/electrical methods.*

transcutaneous electrical nerve stimulation (TENS) *Use of electrical impulses to reduce pain by stimulating the sensory and pain-signaling nerves.*

ultrasound (US) *Therapeutic deep heating that uses high-frequency soundwaves; also called ultrasonic diathermy.*

whirlpool *A stainless-steel or fiberglass tub with an attached turbine.*

THERAPEUTIC PHYSICAL MODALITIES

Therapeutic physical **modalities** are the various heating, cooling, and mechanical/electrical methods of treatment used on the human body. Physical modalities include hot and cold treatments, therapeutic ultrasound, and various electrical modalities.

Effective application of physical modalities is an important aspect of athletic training and the appropriate care of athletes. Modalities are used adjunctively (that is, in addition to other treatments) for management of many sports injuries. These include the therapeutic use of cold, heat, sound, and electricity to induce a therapeutic (healing) effect.

Modalities are utilized to relieve pain, reduce or prevent swelling, decrease spasm, and promote healing. When used properly, they minimize time lost from athletic participation and shorten recovery time. It is very important for the certified athletic trainer to understand when application of a physical modality is or is not warranted. If the modality is used improperly, the condition being treated may worsen. Another important decision the certified athletic trainer must make is determining the correct modality to use, or whether to use one at all.

Therapeutic use of heat and cold are the two most common treatments in sports medicine. In general, only cold is used in the acute stages of an injury. The combination of cold and heat, or heat alone, may be utilized in the subacute, healing, or chronic stages.

THERMAL MODALITIES

Thermal modalities are treatments that use thermal agents—cold and heat applications—to create a therapeutic effect on the body. These modalities include cryotherapy (use of cold) and use of heating agents. Cryotherapy modalities include ice packs, ice massage, cold water compression, ice baths, and hydrotherapy. Some of the various heating agents employed are hydrocollator packs, hydrotherapy, contrast therapy, and ultrasound diathermy. Thermal agents can be applied via many different methods. Following are descriptions of the most common thermal modalities used by certified athletic trainers across the country today. However, it is important to know that numerous other modalities are also used.

Cryotherapy

Cryotherapy is the therapeutic use of cooling agents delivered by several alternate means. It is the most widely used thermal modality in sports medicine. Cooling agents such as cold packs, cold bucket baths, and ice massage are used in pain management and edema (swelling). They are effective in decreasing muscle guarding and spasm.

Once cold is delivered to tissues, a number of things happen. When localized cooling is used, the anticipated physiological responses are initial vasoconstriction (constriction of blood vessels), reduction of tissue metabolism, decrease in nerve conduction velocity (the speed at which nerves conduct messages to the brain), reduction of muscle spasm, secondary vasodilatation, and an increase in muscle strength after treatment. If the cold application is left in place too long, the body may actually move more, rather than less, blood to the area, thereby having a counterproductive effect.

Cold, the modality of choice for acute injuries, should be applied following almost all musculo-

KEY CONCEPT

Effective application of physical modalities is an important aspect of athletic training and the appropriate care of athletes. Hot and cold treatments, ultrasound, and various electrical modalities can be used to reduce swelling, decrease spasm, and promote healing.

FUN FACTS

Cold decreases feeling in an area by reducing the ability of the nerve endings to conduct impulses.

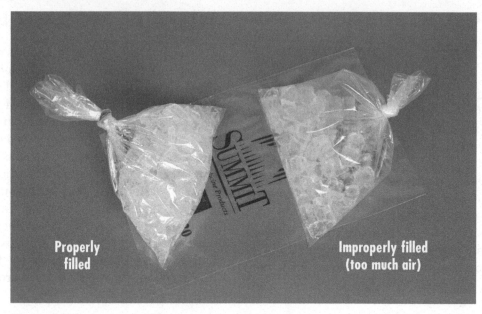

Figure 12–1 A properly filled ice bag contains very little air. Air in the bag does not allow the ice bag to mold to the area needed.

skeletal traumas. The sooner after an injury that cold is used, the better. Application of heat to an acute trauma may exacerbate the condition. For any flare-ups of a preexisting condition, the use of a cooling agent is a first line of approach. Cold treatment should be applied for a maximum of 20 minutes at a time. After the treatment has concluded, a minimum of two hours should elapse prior to reapplication. Cooling modalities should be applied three to four times a day—a reasonable goal, even for busy athletes.

Ice Packs

Ice packs are effectively used for local areas of concern such as an acute ankle sprain. They can be made quickly and are economical. Plastic bags filled with small ice cubes or crushed ice are preferred by most certified athletic trainers because they are more comfortable for the athlete. Once the ice bag is full, remove the air and tie it shut (Figure 12–1). Too much air in the bag allows the ice to slide around, making it difficult to hold the bag in place.

Reusable, commercially manufactured gel packs, which must be stored in a freezer, are also available. They are appropriate for clinical settings but not for sideline treatments. One advantage of a gel pack is that it comfortably molds to the body part, whereas ice chunks in an ice pack can be uncomfortable. Another, more expensive alternative is a chemical-activated cold pack. This

product is activated by striking or squeezing the pack, which mixes the contents to begin a chemical reaction that turns pack cold. It can be used only once, then must be discarded.

An ice pack can be secured to an athlete's body by placing it under the clothing, wrapping it with an elastic bandage, or using a commercially available plastic wrap to secure the ice to the injured area (Figure 12–2).

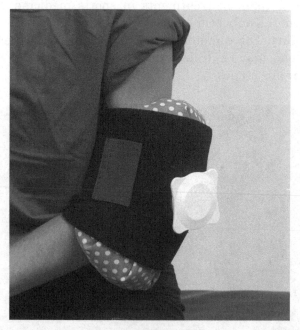

Figure 12–2 Commercial ice bags with wraps are available. The only disadvantage is their relatively high cost.

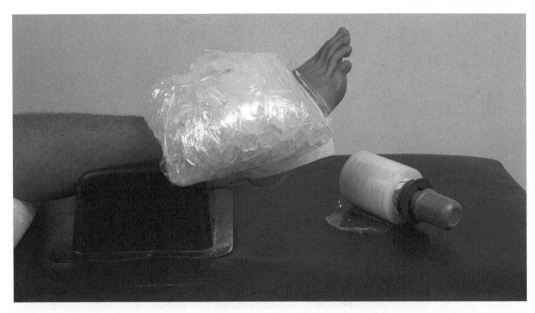

Figure 12–3 Disposable ice bags are inexpensive and work well in all environments.

It is important to elevate the extremity during ice-pack treatment (Figure 12–3). Application time is typically 15 to 20 minutes, and should not exceed 20 minutes.

A thin cloth barrier should always be placed between the cold pack and the skin. Most current cryotherapy techniques are not likely to cause tissue damage, but improper use of chemical ice packs or ice bags can freeze the skin. This causes additional injury to the athlete.

Inspect the body part after application for any adverse reaction. Some athletes are very sensitive to cold treatment and may break out in a rash. Discontinue treatment if this occurs. An alternative approach for these athletes is to add more layers of cloth so that the cooling effect is more gradual.

At home, a bag of frozen peas, frozen corn, or gel packs covered with a cloth barrier can substitute for an ice pack. If these are not available, a sealable sandwich bag filled with crushed ice makes a convenient ice pack.

Ice Massage

Ice massage is used for localized problems such as tennis elbow or shin splints. Ice massage is performed in several ways. Simply holding an ice cube in a washcloth during application is a basic technique. Water can be frozen in a foam or paper cup, which is then peeled off to expose the ice. (Reusable plastic cups are also available for this purpose.)

Briskly rubbing ice over the injured area produces the desired cold effect (Figure 12–4). A towel should be draped around and under the treated area to catch the water dripping from melted ice.

One advantage of ice massage over cold packs is that this process takes only about five minutes, compared to 10 to 15 minutes for a cold pack. Ice massage can be performed conveniently at home.

Cold-Water Compression

Several systems have been developed to apply cold and compression simultaneously, one being a commercial sleeve containing an internal water bladder. These are manufactured in several shapes to accommodate different body parts, such as the shoulder, knee, or ankle. The sleeve is secured around the injury and connected to a container filled with ice water. When the container is raised, gravity forces cold water into the sleeve, providing cooling and comfortable compression. The higher the container is placed, the greater the amount of pressure that will be applied. Treatment time for this therapy is 15 to 20 minutes. Machines equipped with a pump to circulate cold water into the sleeve are also available (Figure 12–5).

Ice Baths

Immersion of a hand or ankle in a bucket of ice water is a convenient cooling method. It is easy to

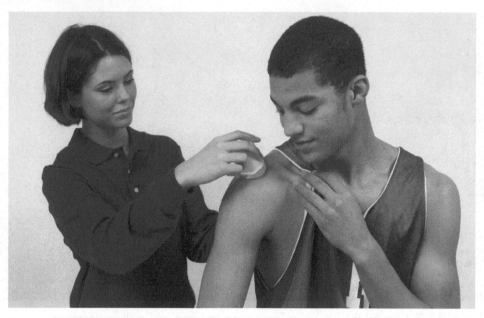

Figure 12–4 Ice massage is an effective way to use localized cold therapy. Ice cups are inexpensive and easy to use.

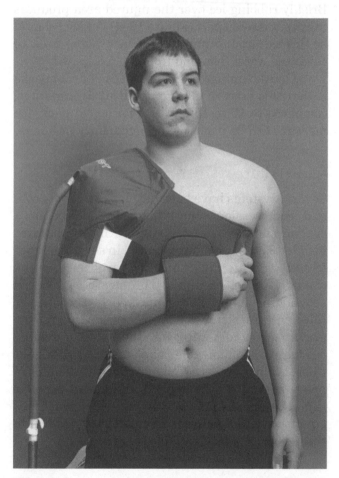

Figure 12–5 Cold compression therapy utilizes both cold and compression to help alleviate inflammation and swelling. Compression units are expensive but very effective.

do and allows complete, uniform coverage of the area receiving therapy. One advantage of this therapy is that the athlete can perform movement exercises during immersion. Because cold has an anesthetizing effect on the body, the athlete will be able to exercise with less discomfort. Begin this therapy by filling a bucket large enough to contain the body part, about two-thirds full. Add ice to lower the water temperature to between 55°F to 64°F. The body part being treated will be uncovered. Typical treatment time is approximately 10 minutes. The athlete receiving this treatment may feel the following sensations, in this order:

- Cold: 0 to 3 minutes into treatment
- Burning: 3 to 5 minutes into treatment
- Aching: 5 to 8 minutes into treatment
- Numbness: 8 to 10 minutes into treatment

These sensations are the body's normal reaction to cold immersion therapy. Ice baths can be done conveniently at home.

Contraindications and Precautions

Cryotherapy should be used with caution on persons who have thermoregulatory problems, sensory deficits, hypersensitivity to cold, impaired circulation, heart disease, and malignant tissue. Always monitor the injured person's reactions to cold applications, and do not maintain an application for longer than the recommended time.

Heating Agents

Physiological responses to heat application are the result of therapeutic heating of tissues. Heat is applied either superficially, for effects that are basically skin deep, or with a modality that is capable of heating tissues up to a few inches beneath the skin. Appropriately heating tissues has several beneficial effects including reduced pain, promotion of healing, increased range of motion, and muscle relaxation.

Localized, vigorous heating has a significant effect on blood flow, producing substantially increased vasodilatation. A localized increase in temperature increases metabolic rate, capillary pressure and flow, clearance of metabolites, and oxygenation of tissue. These basic physiologic responses occur as a result of local inflammation, caused by the body's effort to initiate healing. Because the body responds naturally to acute inflammation and trauma, vigorous, local heating is only appropriate when such natural responses have subsided. When augmentation of these responses is desired to promote healing in a subacute or chronic state, heat is utilized.

Hydrocollator Packs

Hydrocollator packs, moist hot packs that are used for superficial heating, are kept warm in a heated stainless-steel container filled with hot water in the range of 60°C to 90°C (Figure 12–6). They are manufactured in a variety of shapes and sizes, are easy to apply, and are cost effective. The warm moisture is very soothing.

Once the packs are removed from the water, they should be covered with insulated coverings as recommended by the manufacturer. Hot packs should be left in place for only 10 to 20 minutes. Longer application times may result in adverse reactions, including burns.

The covered packs are placed over the affected body area, where they either rest in place or are secured with an elastic wrap. In some situations, the athlete may lie on the pack, but never allow an individual to fall asleep on one. Care must be

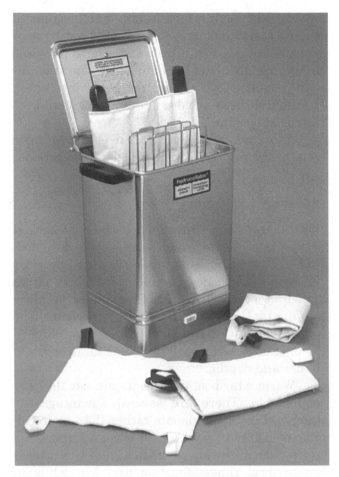

Figure 12–6 Hydrocollators use specially designed heat packs to administer long-term warmth. Heat packs will remain warm for up to 30 minutes.

taken in this situation; because the heat is trapped and accumulates, it could potentially result in a burn. Instruct the athlete that the hot pack should be comfortably warm. If it proves to be too hot, remove it and inspect the body part for abnormal reaction. Add additional layers of insulating towels or another hot pack cover.

Electrical heating pads or bean bags heated in a microwave oven may be used at home. The same application guidelines apply to home heating agents: apply at a comfortable warm temperature for 10 to 20 minutes.

Contraindications/Precautions

Prior to the use of heat, the certified athletic trainer must assess the condition being treated and the injury status. Heat is typically not used until 48 to 72 hours after injury. Heat dilates the vessels and could cause additional bleeding if healing is not adequate. Heat should not be used in acute states, with athletes who have impaired circulation, in areas of diminished sensation, or with athletes who may be heat intolerant. It should also be avoided in areas susceptible to increased bleeding.

As with cold applications, it is important to monitor the injured athlete for adverse reactions.

Hydrotherapy

Hydrotherapy is a form of superficial heating that uses agitated, heated water in a specially designed **whirlpool**, typically a stainless-steel or fiberglass tub with an attached turbine; the turbine mixes air with water, which then flows under pressure into the tank of water to produce turbulence. The water temperature can be regulated depending on the diagnosis. Whirlpool tubs come in a variety of shapes and depths.

Warm whirlpool treatments are usually very comfortable. There are several advantages to using whirlpool treatments rather than hydrocollator packs. With a whirlpool bath, a larger area on an extremity can be treated, and the athlete can perform range-of-motion exercises while in the whirlpool. Disadvantages of the whirlpool include the extra time and effort needed to fill and clean the whirlpool, clinic space for the whirlpool, equipment expense, and the fact that the body part being treated cannot be elevated.

Fill the whirlpool with water at the desired temperature (typically 35°C to 40°C or 95°F to 104°F) to about eight inches from the top of the tank. Immerse the part to be treated so that it is fully covered with water. Turn on the turbine and adjust the amount of desired agitation of the water. Treatment time is 10 to 20 minutes.

Contrast Therapy

Contrast therapy uses alternating hot and cold water baths to the ankle, foot, hand, or elbow. It may be used in the subacute stage of an injury (that is, 48 to 72 hours after the injury incurs), to help reduce swelling, reduce pain, and increase range of motion. Contraindications include impaired circulation as a result of diabetes, vascular disease, and tendency to hemorrhage.

This form of therapy requires two containers large enough to accommodate the body part to be treated. Fill the "hot" container with water at a temperature between 38°C to 44°C (102°F to 110°F), and the "cold" container with water at a temperature between 10°C to 18°C (50°F to 66°F).

There are several formulas for performing contrast baths. One commonly used 20-minute treatment has the body part to be treated alternately immersed in the containers, following this schedule:

HOT	COLD
4 minutes	1 minute
4 minutes	1 minute
4 minutes	1 minute
4 minutes	1 minute

It is always advisable to end the treatment with a cold bath. This helps keep swelling and inflammation to a minimum.

Ultrasound

The technical term for this therapeutic deep-heating modality is *ultrasonic diathermy*, or *through heat*. It is commonly referred to as **ultrasound (US)**. This modality should not be confused with a different type of ultrasound that is used in medicine to produce internal body images (of a fetus, for example). Ultrasound should not be used over fluid-filled cavities, the eyes, heart, uterus, testes, growth plates, fracture sites, artificial joints, or herniated discs. Ultrasound is not recommended during the acute stage of an injury, because the heat generated could cause damage.

Therapeutic ultrasound is capable of affecting tissues at depths up to five centimeters (cm). Ultrasound is a very high-frequency soundwave that is absorbed by tissues high in protein content. Such tissues include tendons, ligaments, joint capsules, and (to a lesser degree) muscle tissue. Some of the soundwave is absorbed by bone tissue, and the remainder is reflected off.

The soundwave can be produced either as a continuous, uninterrupted flow or in a pulsed mode. Continuous ultrasound is a form of energy that is transformed to deep heat within the targeted tissue. In a pulsed mode, the fraction of time

KEY CONCEPT

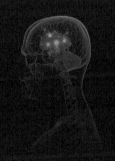

- Cryotherapy is the use of cooling agents to manage pain and edema, and to decrease muscle spasms.
- Ice packs are effective in the treatment of local areas. The area of concern should be elevated, and cold applied for 15 to 20 minutes.
- Ice massage is also used for local areas. Ice should be rubbed briskly over the injured area for about five minutes.
- Cold-water compression is a technique in which cold water and pressure are simultaneously applied to the injured area for 15 to 20 minutes.
- Ice baths involve immersion of the affected area in a bucket of cold water (temperature of 55°F to 64°F). Movement exercises can also be done during an ice bath.
- Hydrocollator packs are used for superficial heating and should be applied for 10 to 20 minutes.
- Hydrotherapy, a form of superficial heating in which the affected area is immersed in hot, turbulent water, should be applied for 10 to 20 minutes.
- Contrast therapy is the alternating use of cold baths and hot baths for specified time periods.

when the ultrasound beam is flowing during one pulse is called the *duty cycle*. The duty cycle is measured as a percent. Continuous ultrasound is measured as 100%, whereas a pulsed-mode duty cycle could be 20%. Low-intensity, or pulsed, ultrasound (0.1 to 0.2 W/cm² pulsed in 20% duty cycle) has nonthermal effects that have been shown to facilitate tissue repair in humans. Table 12–1 highlights some ultrasound parameters.

The highest frequency soundwave a human can hear is around 18,000 to 20,000 cycles

KEY CONCEPT

Continuous ultrasound is a form of energy that is transformed to deep heat within the targeted tissue. It facilitates tissue repair in humans.

Table 12–1 Sample Ultrasound Parameters

CONDITION	FREQUENCY	DUTY CYCLE
Deep muscle adhesion	1 MHz	100%
Deep bursitis	1 MHz	20%–50%
Superficial scar	3 MHz	100%
Superficial tendonitis	3 MHz	20%–50%

(or waves) per second. One cycle per second is called a *hertz* (Hz). Therapeutic ultrasound used in medicine in the United States is either 1 million cycles per second (or 1 megahertz, 1 MHz) for deep structures (about 2 to 5 cm beneath the surface of the skin), or 3 million cycles per second (3 MHz) for tissues lying just under the skin (Figure 12–7). Therapeutic ultrasound is at a frequency too high to be heard by the human ear.

The ultrasonic beam is created by a vibrating, synthetic crystal housed in a metal shield called the *sound head* or *transducer*. Crystals are available in several sizes, generally 1, 5, and 10 square centimeters. To achieve tissue temperatures at therapeutic levels, the area being treated must be no larger than twice the size of the transducer.

A cream or gel called a **coupling agent** must be applied to the area to be treated. The coupling agent provides a medium by which the sonic waves can penetrate the skin. Moving the sound head (transducer) at a surface speed of about two to four centimeters per second will give the best results. Movement of the transducer should be restricted to an area about twice the size of the transducer (Figure 12–8).

The athlete should be instructed to inform the therapist if the treatment causes any aching pain or if the skin becomes too warm. Stopping

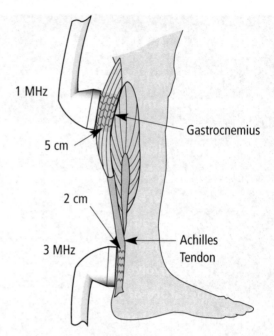

Figure 12–7 Ultrasound at 3 MHz will penetrate up to 2 cm; ultrasound at 1 MHz will penetrate up to 5 cm.

the sound head, moving the transducer too slowly, or setting the power level too high might all cause discomfort. Treatment length is usually 5 to 10 minutes.

Each state has different laws governing the use of electrical therapeutic modalities and

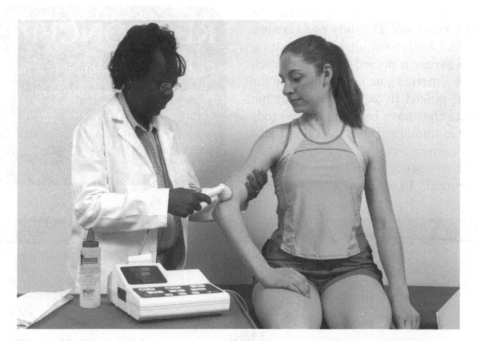

Figure 12–8 Ultrasound diathermy is an effective treatment for many different injuries. Proper training is needed. Protocols must be followed to avoid injury and derive the greatest benefit from this therapy.

who may apply them. In some states, the certified athletic trainer's use of electrical therapeutic modalities is limited to readying the patient for treatment (e.g., applying electrodes, preparing an area for ultrasound treatment); a physical therapist must be on hand to activate the equipment and perform the treatment. In other states, the certified athletic trainer who works in a clinical setting is considered to be on the same level as a physical therapist assistant or aide, and thus might be limited as to modality use.

THERAPEUTIC ELECTRICAL MODALITIES

Therapeutic methods that pass electrical currents through skin into the body have been used for many years. As with any electrical modality, physical therapists and physicians are the primary users. As stated in the preceding section, certified athletic trainers' use of these modalities may be limited by law.

Electrical modalities achieve their effect by stimulating nerve tissue; they do not produce heat or cold. Numerous electrical stimulators have been developed over the years; most use a pulsed, direct current or an alternating current. These units can be divided into two main categories:

- Those that produce muscle contractions and muscle facilitation by electrically stimulating motor nerves (nerves going to muscles) are generally called **electrical stimulation** techniques, or **e-stim**. This use of electricity is also termed neuromuscular stimulation (NMS).
- Those that reduce pain by stimulating sensory and pain-signaling nerves, collectively known as **transcutaneous electrical nerve stimulation (TENS)** (transcutaneous means through the skin).

Electrical Stimulation Therapy

Electrical stimulation is commonly used in physical therapy and has proven effective for many purposes, including increasing range of motion, increasing muscle strength, reeducating muscles, improving muscle tone, enhancing function,

DID YOU KNOW? The median annual earnings of physical therapists was $85,400 in 2016. The lowest 10% earned less than $58,190. The highest 10% earned more than $122,130. Median annual earnings in the industries employing the largest numbers of physical therapists in 2016 were as follows:

Offices and clinics of medical doctors	$77,980
Home health care services	93,200
Offices of other health practitioners	81,220
Nursing and personal-care facilities	92,960
Hospitals	87,010

controlling pain, accelerating wound healing, and reducing muscle spasm.

The use of electricity to stimulate a peripheral nerve and to cause either a sensory or a motor (movement) response is termed *neuromuscular electrical stimulation (NMES)*. This is the most common type of e-stim. The use of e-stim to improve function is called *functional electrical stimulation (FES)*.

TENS (transcutaneous electrical nerve stimulation) is commonly applied with a portable unit for pain control. Although one of the primary clinical uses of e-stim is pain management, in actuality almost all e-stim units are TENS units, in that they apply a transcutaneous current.

Electric current is applied through a surface electrode pad that is in contact with the external skin surface. When electrical stimulation is used, two electrodes are required to complete the electric circuit. Electrodes are usually placed some distance away from the injury site. The operator of the stimulator unit selects the different parameters to control the type of current being delivered to the athlete. Large stimulators can be used in clinical settings as well as portable home units. Specialized training is a prerequisite before anyone applies electrical modalities.

Contraindications of Electrical Stimulation Use

Electrical stimulation should not be used over the carotid sinus, during pregnancy, in individuals with pacemakers, on people who are sensitive to electricity, or any time active motion is contraindicated. Use under these conditions could cause additional injury.

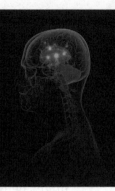

KEY CONCEPT

Electrical modalities achieve their effect by stimulating nerve tissue, not by producing heat or cold. These modalities are used to reduce pain and rehabilitate muscles.

CONCLUSION

The appropriate selection and use of physical therapeutic modalities can have a dramatic beneficial effect on athletic injuries. However, the wrong selection or implementation of a thermal or electrical modality can have an adverse effect. Careful consideration of the nature and stage of the injury is mandatory. If modalities are used at home, it is important that proper instruction be given.

REVIEW QUESTIONS

1. Define physical modality and give examples of its uses.
2. What are the therapeutic effects of thermal modalities?
3. List and explain the different types of cryotherapy.
4. Why is the use of cold important for an acute injury?
5. What are the contraindications of cryotherapy?
6. What is ultrasound diathermy?
7. Explain the difference between pulsed and continuous ultrasound.
8. Why is a coupling agent used with ultrasound therapy?
9. Explain how electrical modalities achieve their effect.
10. What are the two main categories of electrical modalities?

PROJECTS AND ACTIVITIES

1. Create a true-and-false test for this chapter on therapeutic physical modalities. Your test should include questions on all topics covered in this chapter.
2. Make an appointment to visit a physical therapist in your area, and ask to be shown the various physical agents he or she uses with patients. Write a short report on your findings.

LEARNING LINKS

- Visit the websites of the American Physical Therapy Association (http://www.apta.org), NCAA (http://www.ncaa.org), the National Athletic Trainers Association (http://www.nata.org), and other athletic training websites to locate additional information on therapeutic techniques.

CHAPTER 13

Taping and Wrapping

OBJECTIVES

Upon completion of this chapter, the reader should be able to:

- Describe the importance of taping and wrapping in athletics
- Describe the common supplies used in taping and wrapping
- Perform the basic taping and wrapping techniques described in this chapter
- Explain the difference between taping and bracing.

KEY TERMS

circumferential *Around an extremity or body part.*

hypermobility *The ability of a body part to move beyond the normal range of motion.*

hypoallergenic *Reduced potential for causing an allergic reaction.*

prophylactic *Any agent or method that prevents or guards against injury.*

spray adherent *An aerosolized liquid that creates a sticky surface to help underwrap and tape stay in place.*

underwrap *A lightweight foam material used as a base for application of tape; helps to reduce irritation caused by tape.*

TAPING AND WRAPPING IN THE PREVENTION AND TREATMENT OF ATHLETIC INJURIES

Taping and wrapping are important skills for the sports medicine team. They can be used as preventive measures to help an athlete who needs additional protection, or as a treatment for new and healing injuries. Before any tape or wraps are applied, a certified athletic trainer or team physician should complete a full assessment of the athlete's injury. This evaluation provides information that guides the medical staff in the proper selection of taping, wrapping, or bracing. Chapter 11 addresses the assessment and evaluation of sports injuries.

The primary purpose of taping and wrapping is to provide additional support, stability, and compression for the affected body part. Elastic wraps are used for support and compression of a weak or injured area of the body. It is very important to note that prevention of injuries is always the key to success. Properly fitting equipment, as well as properly prepared practice and game sites, will help prevent injuries in the first place.

Supplies Commonly Used in Taping

One of the most important aspects of taping is the selection of proper supplies. This will depend on the number and types of sports played and the frequency of injuries. Numerous manufacturers market tape and supplies. Purchases are based on budget, the medical staff's philosophy regarding taping techniques, and the occurrence of injury. The certified athletic trainer will need to evaluate new supplies that come to market, and their cost-effectiveness.

Several considerations must be taken into account when selecting a new taping supply product:

- Is it better than the product currently being used?
- Is the cost per application comparable?
- Is there more or less waste?
- Does it last as long?
- Does the product have a long shelf life?
- Do athletes like it?
- Does the medical staff like it?

Athletic Tape

Adhesive athletic tape comes in a variety of sizes and colors for a variety of uses. Sizes range from ½ to 6 inches. The size most commonly used is 1½ inches wide and 15 feet long. Athletic tape is **hypoallergenic** (has little tendency to provoke an allergic reaction) and is cotton-backed, with an adhesive designed to withstand temperature changes. Adhesive tape should be stored in a cool, relatively dry environment.

Tearing Athletic Tape

Athletic tape can be torn easily if it is held firmly on each side and pulled away at an angle so that the force breaks the fibers of the fabric. The tear then continues through the fabric until the break is complete. Not all brands of tape are equally easy to tear. With practice, tearing tape will become second nature.

KEY CONCEPT

The primary purpose of taping and wrapping is to provide additional support, stability, and compression for an affected body part. Taping can be used as a preventive measure or as protection for new or healing injuries.

FUN FACTS

A roll of athletic tape is typically 15 yards long. The University of Arizona uses approximately 7,200 rolls of tape for its athletes each year—that's 108,000 yards each year, or more than 61 miles of athletic tape!

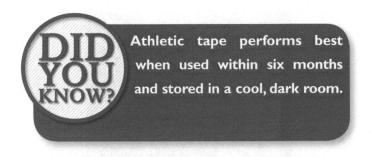

Athletic tape performs best when used within six months and stored in a cool, dark room.

Underwrap

Tape **underwrap** helps to eliminate irritation from repeated taping. Underwrap is made of a light foam material and is typically 2¾ inches wide by 30 yards long. The advantages of underwrap are that it promotes athlete comfort, holds heel and lace pads in place at high-friction areas, and helps keep tape away from the skin of athletes who are allergic to it. The disadvantages of underwrap are the added cost and the fact that underwrap can compromise the stability of the taping. Like athletic tape, underwrap comes in a variety of colors.

Spray Adherent

Spray adherent, which is produced by several manufacturers, is designed to help adhesive tape or underwrap adhere to the skin. The less the tape slips, the more protection and less chafing the athlete will have. Spray adherent is colorless and dries quickly on the skin.

Heel and Lace Pads

Heel and lace pads help prevent pinching and blistering in friction-prone areas. For added protection, a lubricant ointment is placed under the pads. Pads are typically 3 inches by 3 inches by 1/16 inch thick and made of a light foam material.

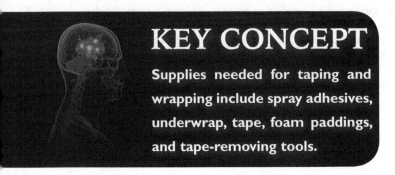

KEY CONCEPT

Supplies needed for taping and wrapping include spray adhesives, underwrap, tape, foam paddings, and tape-removing tools.

Tape-Removing Tools

Tape removal is done using specialized scissors or tape-cutting devices designed to slip under the tape and underwrap, and quickly slice through it with no irritation to the athlete.

PROPHYLACTIC TAPING OF THE ANKLE

Prophylactic (preventive) taping of the ankle is the most common use for athletic tape; whereas an athlete who already has instability of a joint, or needs additional support for a previous injury, would require functional taping and support. Ankle taping is an effective, relatively inexpensive way to add support and protect an athlete from new or additional injury.

Before the ankle is taped, the athlete's foot should be checked for blisters, abrasions, cuts, and athlete's foot (fungal infections). If any of these conditions are noticed, the certified athletic trainer will need to treat them before taping the ankle.

Basic Ankle Taping

There are many different methods of taping an ankle. The method shown and described in Figures 13–1 through 13–18 provides basic support and stability. Additional support or taping to address specific injuries will require additional steps or procedures.

Compression Wrap of the Ankle

When an athlete sprains an ankle, it is necessary to control swelling and inflammation. A compression wrap with a felt horseshoe puts gentle pressure on the areas of the ankle where swelling is likely to occur (Figures 13–19 through 13–21). Elastic wraps should not be applied too tightly. The rule of thumb is not to stretch the elastic wrap to more than half of its elastic capability. Compression wraps can be worn for up to 24 hours, or more if instructed. The acronym RICES—rest, ice, compression, elevation, support—describes the steps in the care of sprains. An athlete who has a compression wrap applied will most likely use crutches to maximize healing.

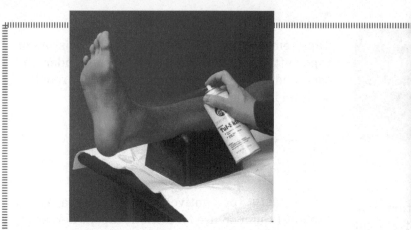

Figure 13–1 After the foot has been inspected for any blisters or other conditions, have the athlete dorsiflex (bring upward) the foot to approximately 90°. The foot should also be in a subtalar neutral position; this means that the foot should not be turned inward or outward. Use a liberal amount of spray adherent over the entire surface to be taped.

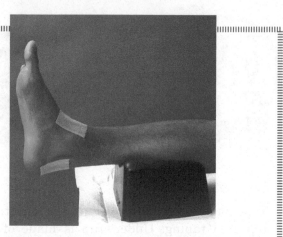

Figure 13–2 Heel and lace pads (with a small amount of lubricant beneath each pad) are placed in the major friction areas. These areas are the top (lace area) of the foot and the back of the heel.

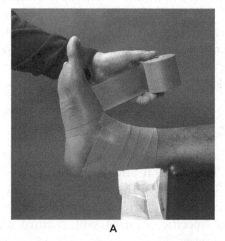
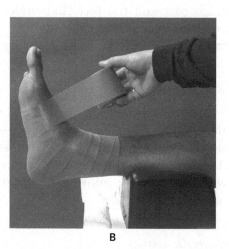

A   B

Figure 13–3A–B Underwrap is applied to the entire area to be taped. Equal tension should be maintained to ensure an even application without large wrinkles or rolls. Rolling from the top or bottom of the roll is a personal preference.

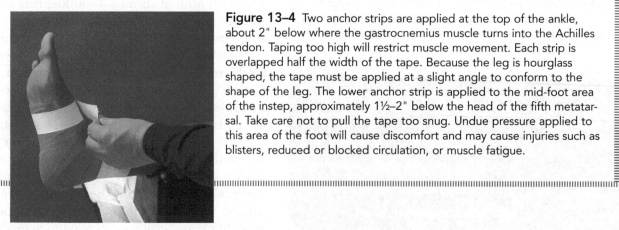

Figure 13–4 Two anchor strips are applied at the top of the ankle, about 2" below where the gastrocnemius muscle turns into the Achilles tendon. Taping too high will restrict muscle movement. Each strip is overlapped half the width of the tape. Because the leg is hourglass shaped, the tape must be applied at a slight angle to conform to the shape of the leg. The lower anchor strip is applied to the mid-foot area of the instep, approximately 1½–2" below the head of the fifth metatarsal. Take care not to pull the tape too snug. Undue pressure applied to this area of the foot will cause discomfort and may cause injuries such as blisters, reduced or blocked circulation, or muscle fatigue.

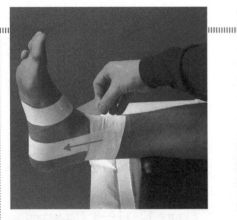

Figure 13–5 Three stirrups are applied around the outside of the ankle. The first stirrup begins on the medial side of the ankle, goes onto the middle of the heel, and continues to the lateral side. Gentle pressure is applied to the tape as it is secured on the lateral side. This pressure helps to keep the ankle everted (pulled slightly outward). Most ankle sprains are inversion (foot rolling inward) injuries, so keeping the foot slightly everted helps to avoid inversion ankle sprains.

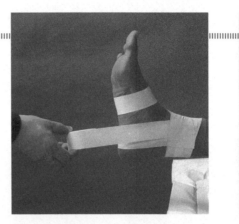

Figure 13–6 Two additional stirrups are added. The first is applied half the width of the tape forward of the first piece, extends down to the heel, and is secured half the width of the tape forward of the first piece on the lateral side. The third stirrup is identical to the second stirrup, except that it is located half the width of the tape behind the first stirrup. Note that all three stirrups must pass over the middle of the heel. If these stirrups are applied forward, to the arch, the athlete will experience discomfort.

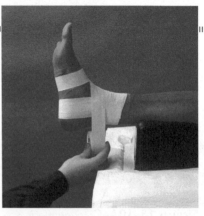

Figure 13–7 Cover strips are applied down the ankle. Cover strips are overlapped by half the width of the tape. The tape must be angled slightly to compensate for the shape of the leg.

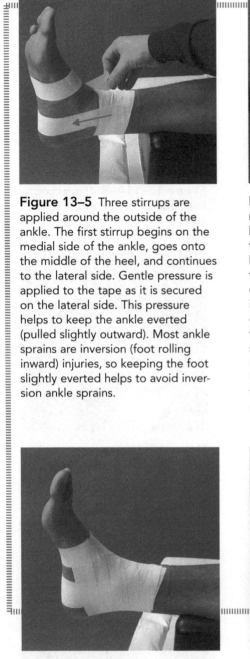

Figure 13–8 Cover strips continue down the entire length of the ankle.

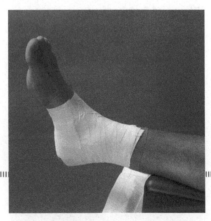

Figure 13–9 The bottom of the foot is wrapped with cover strips. Strips are applied medial to lateral. Again, strips are applied halfway overlapping the previous strip.

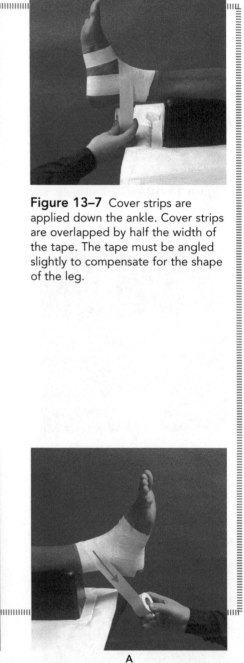

A

Figure 13–10A–C Two heel locks are applied. The first heel lock begins on the lateral side of the ankle, half an inch above the lateral malleolus. This is the only step that begins on the lateral side of the ankle. Taping continues around the heel, under the foot, and finishes approximately 1/2" below the lateral malleolus. Take care to ensure even tension throughout this step, or wrinkles may appear. Heel locks help to keep the ankle from inverting or everting. (*continues*)

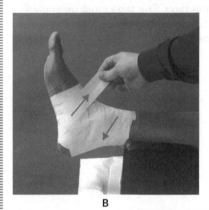
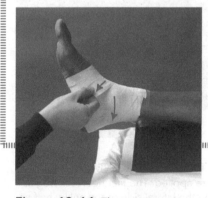

B

Figure 13–10A–C (continued)

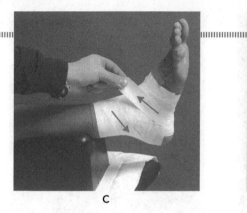

C

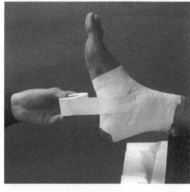

Figure 13–11A–B (continued)

Figure 13–12 The final step is called a *Figure eight*. Tape begins on the medial side of the ankle, just below the medial malleolus.

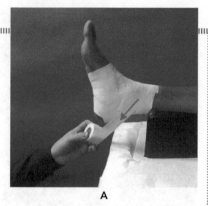

A

Figure 13–11A–B The second heel lock is identical to the first, except that it begins on the medial side of the ankle. (continues)

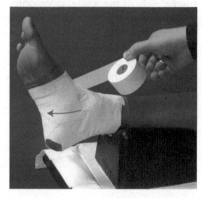

Figure 13–13 The tape comes under the foot and over the top of the ankle.

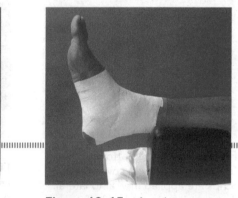

Figure 13–14 The tape continues around the ankle and finishes back on top. This final step also helps to keep the ankle from inverting.

Figure 13–15 After the taping is complete, gently compress the taped ankle. This helps to ensure that the adhesive on the tape sticks well to the other strips. Finally, ask the athlete how it feels, and apply additional support as necessary. A well-taped ankle should show no wrinkles; the taping should be uniform and at the proper tension.

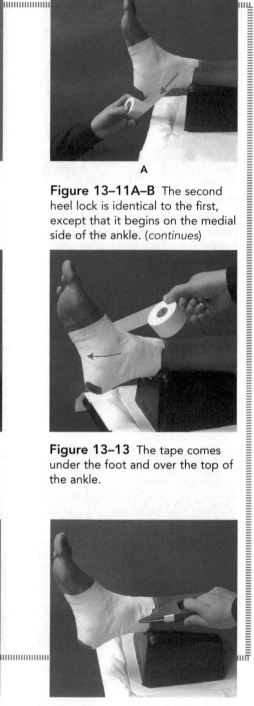

Figure 13–16 Remove the tape, beginning on the medial side of the ankle. A specialized tape cutter makes this task easy and painless for the athlete. A small amount of lubricant applied to the tip of the cutter, next to the skin, allows easy movement along the ankle.

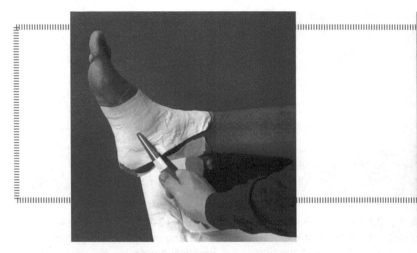

Figure 13–17 The tape is cut vertically down the ankle to the heel. Slight upward pressure on the cutter makes removal easier.

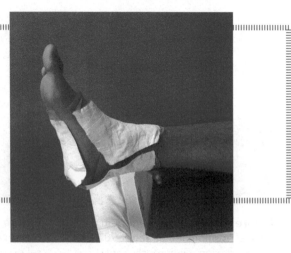

Figure 13–18 The tape is then cut horizontally along the foot. Remove the tape and inspect the foot for any sores or problems.

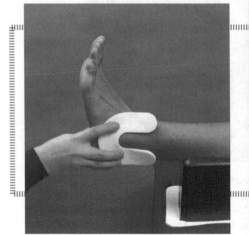

Figure 13–19 The felt horseshoe is placed around the lateral malleolus (inversion sprain). This is the space where most of the swelling and inflammation will occur.

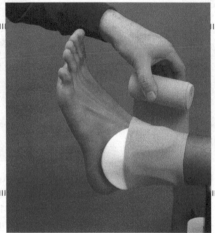

Figure 13–20 Use the elastic wrap to cover the felt horseshoe.

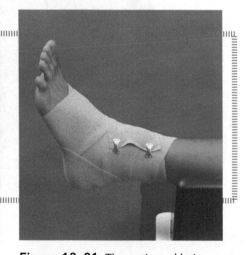

Figure 13–21 The entire ankle is covered to create support and gentle compression. Compression is not so tight that circulation is impaired.

LOW-DYE TAPING

Low-dye taping helps to improve foot biomechanics by keeping the athlete from overpronating (foot rotating inward). Overpronation can cause several problems with the lower leg, including plantar fasciitis, heel pain, shin splints, and stress fractures. If low-dye taping gives significant relief, it is a strong indication that functional orthotics may be appropriate.

Low-dye taping can provide therapeutic relief of functional problems on the initial visit; however, this procedure will not help everyone who overpronates. If the athlete feels no relief after two or three procedures, taping should cease. Also, because low-dye taping is performed on the skin, irritation will occur after the procedure is done several times. Low-dye taping is not a long-term solution, but rather a diagnostic tool for overpronation problems.

Taping techniques are not universal. Figures 13–22 through 13–34 illustrate one method of low-dye taping of the foot.

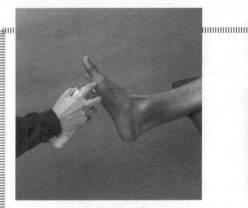

Figure 13–22 Place the foot in a neutral position and at about 90° of dorsiflexion. Generously apply tape adherent around the outside of the foot.

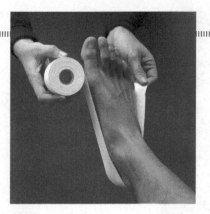

Figure 13–23 Measure the tape so that it reaches from the first metatarsal phalangeal joint (MPJ) to the fifth metatarsal phalangeal joint (big toe to little toe).

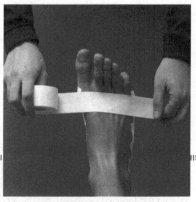

Figure 13–24 Tear the tape down the middle, creating two identical pieces.

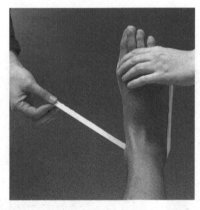

Figure 13–25 Starting at the fifth MPJ, bring the first strip of tape around the heel.

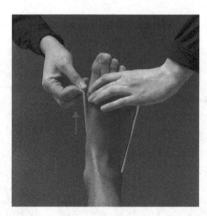

Figure 13–26 Anchor the tape at the first MPJ. While anchoring the tape, turn the foot medially. Repeat steps shown in Figures 13–25 and 13–26 with the second piece of tape (from the strip that was torn down the middle). The second piece is identical to the first.

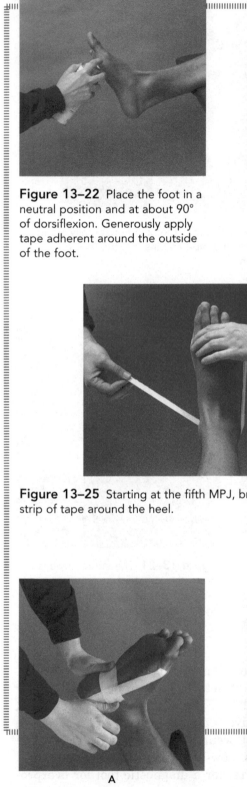

A   B

Figure 13–27A–B Use cover strips, full width, to cover the sole of the foot from the heel to the metatarsals. Tape should overlap by half the width of the tape. It is important that these strips be laid down and not pulled, so that the skin on the bottom of the foot does not wrinkle. The cover strips should extend just above the lateral half strips; they need not go further.

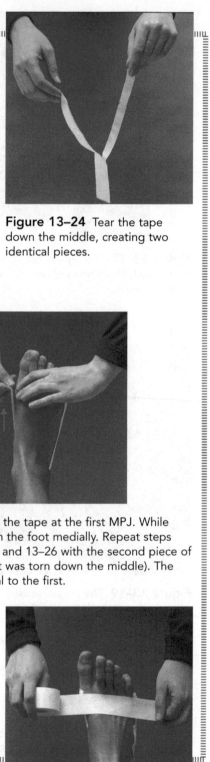

Figure 13–28 Measure a piece of tape twice the width of the forefoot.

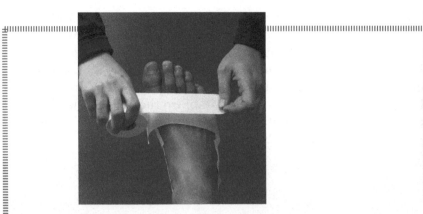

Figure 13–29 Measure another piece of tape the width of the forefoot. This piece of tape is placed in the middle of the last piece measured. The two pieces of tape must be placed adhesive side to adhesive side.

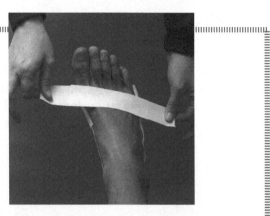

Figure 13–30 Place the tape along the line of the metatarsal phalangeal joints on the top of the forefoot.

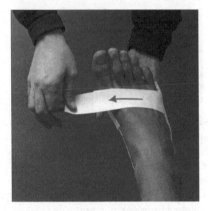

Figure 13–31 Place the tape underneath the forefoot on the lateral side.

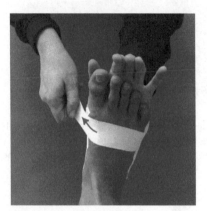

Figure 13–32 Bring the tape across the top of the forefoot. With the heel of your hand pushing the foot upward, place the other end of the tape under the medial side of the foot.

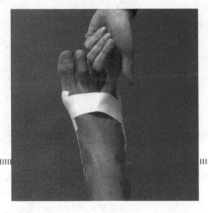

Figure 13–33 When the athlete puts the foot in plantar flexion, a gap should be created on top of the forefoot. This acts as a "break," keeping the athlete from excessively dorsiflexing the foot.

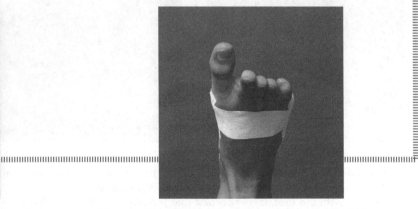

Figure 13–34 When low-dye taping is finished, there should be a gap between the first and second digits.

TURF-TOE TAPING

Turf toe got its name because it occurs frequently in people who play games on artificial surfaces. The shoe grips hard on the surface and sticks, causing body weight to go forward and bend the toe upward. Athletes who wear soft, flexible shoes are more at risk .

Turf toe can occur after a forceful hyperextension (upward bending) of the big toe. When the toe is bent upward, the ligaments and joint capsule can be damaged. Technically, it is called a metatarsal-phalangeal joint (MPJ) sprain. Special taping can help to stabilize the MPJ of the big toe, keeping it from hyperextending. Figures 13–35 through 13–38 illustrate this procedure.

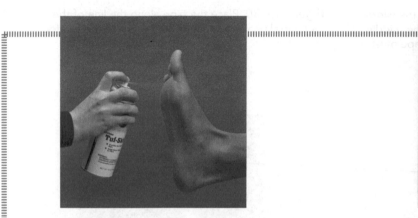

Figure 13–35 Spray tape adherent on the bottom of the foot where the tape will be applied. Spray adherent from the big toe to the heel. See Figure 13–37B.

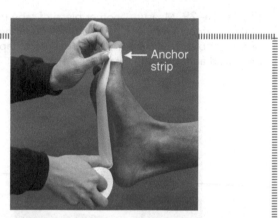

Figure 13–36 After placing an anchor strip around the big toe, measure a length of tape from the anchor on the big toe to the heel. After measuring this piece, tear two more identical pieces of tape. Combine all three pieces to form one triple-strength piece of tape. Moleskin can be used for this purpose because of its added strength. Usually one piece of moleskin is enough.

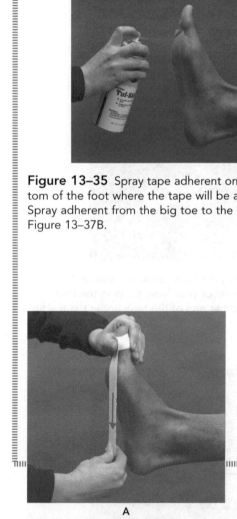

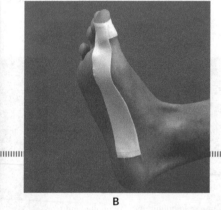

A   B

Figure 13–37A–B After securing the tape at the anchor site, pull down on the tape and attach it under the foot. During this procedure, keep the big toe aligned with the foot. It is important that the big toe not bend after completion of this step.

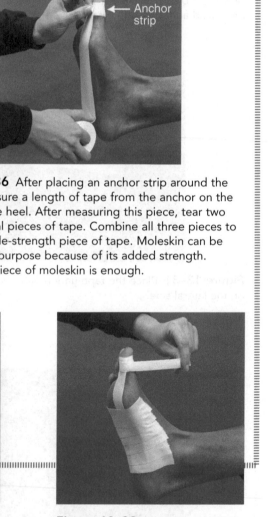

Figure 13–38 Place cover strips under the foot, overlapping by half the width of the tape. The cover strips should cover the entire arch. Secure the tape to the big toe by adding another half-width strip of tape around the big toe. Have the athlete walk around to assure that the taping is effective.

ACHILLES-TENDON TAPING

The Achilles tendon, the largest tendon in the body, joins the gastrocnemius and the soleus muscles in the calcaneus of the lower leg. The gastrocnemius muscle crosses the knee, the ankle, and the subtalar joint. The movement of these joints creates pressure and tension in the Achilles tendon. Like ligaments, tendons are strong, but they are not particularly flexible. They will stretch only so far before they wear, tear, or rupture.

A rupture usually occurs when a force exerted on the tendon is greater than the strength of the tendon. Most ruptures occur from a forceful stretch of the tendon with a contraction of the calf muscles.

Taping the Achilles tendon is an effective method of relieving strain. It also helps to keep the Achilles tendon from overstretching. Achilles tendon taping should be done when a minor strain is suspected. Tears or ruptures of the Achilles tendon must be managed by the team physician and physical therapist. Figures 13–39 through 13–50 illustrate this procedure.

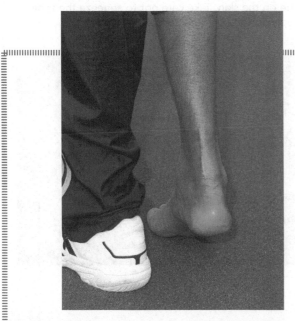

Figure 13–39 This photograph shows a repaired Achilles tendon rupture. This injury occurred during a college basketball game.

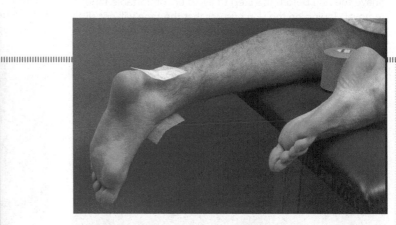

Figure 13–40 Place heel and lace pads as indicated to help reduce friction on these areas.

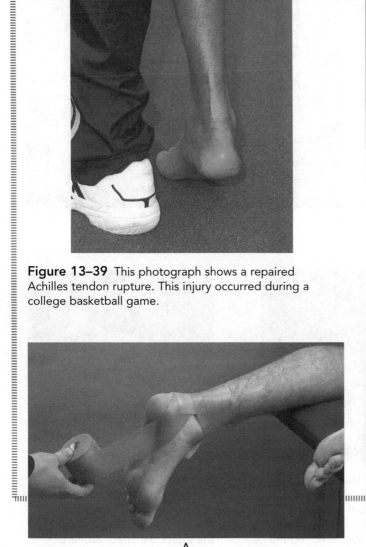

A

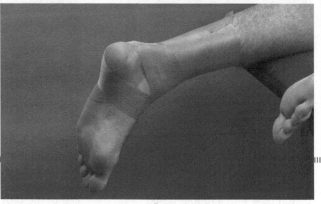

B

Figure 13–41A–B Underwrap is used to cover the areas that will be taped.

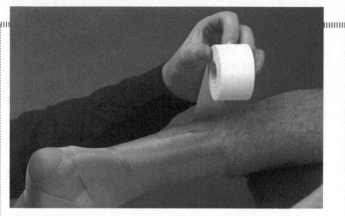

Figure 13–42 The top anchor is placed halfway on the underwrap and halfway on the skin. Two top anchors are used. Shave the skin before this step to avoid uncomfortable tape removal. Taping on the skin ensures that the tape will not slide down the ankle and thus reduce the effect of the procedure.

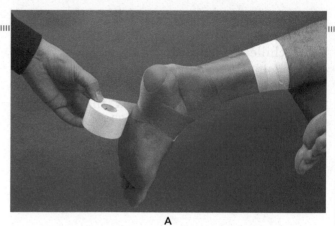

A

Figure 13–43A–C Two bottom anchors are used on the bottom of the foot. Again, half the width of the tape should be on the skin. Take care not to squeeze the foot when applying the bottom anchors. (*continues*)

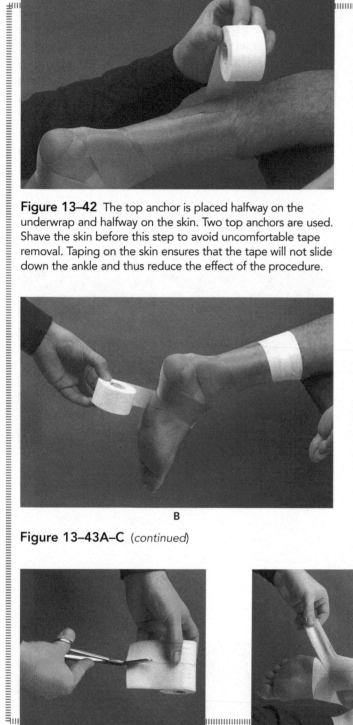

B

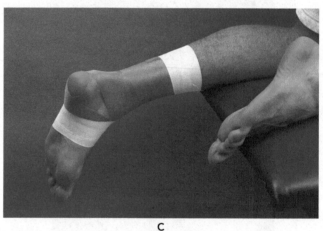

C

Figure 13–43A–C (*continued*)

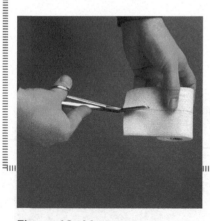

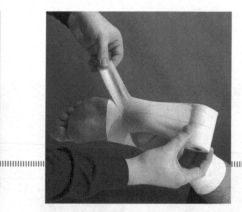

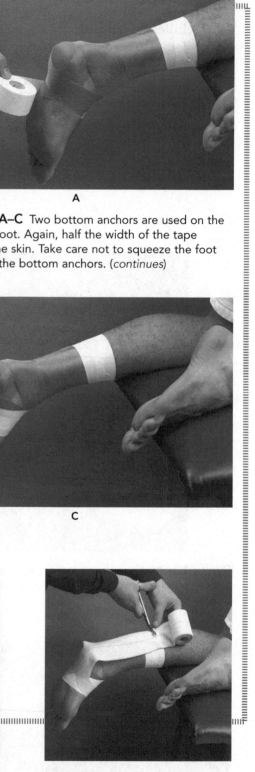

Figure 13–44 Using 3" Elastikon™ (or equivalent) tape, cut down the middle approximately 4". Elastikon™ is a high-strength elastic cotton tape with a rubber-based adhesive. It works well for applications requiring strong support.

Figure 13–45 Using the red line down the middle of the tape as your guide, wrap the cut ends around the foot as shown. The red line of the tape should run up the middle of the heel.

Figure 13–46 The foot should be plantar flexed (pointed down) about 30° from the normal 90°. The tape is measured and cut at the top of the upper anchors.

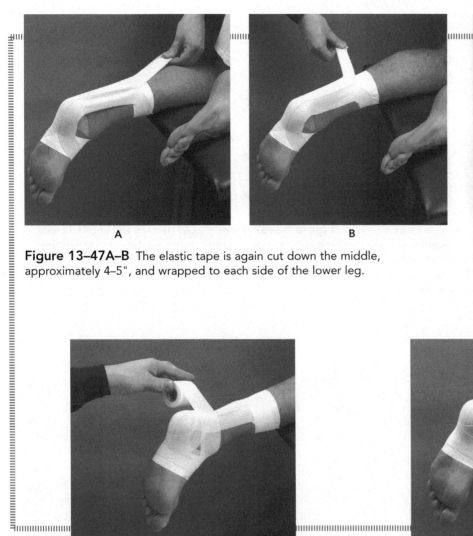

Figure 13–47A–B The elastic tape is again cut down the middle, approximately 4–5", and wrapped to each side of the lower leg.

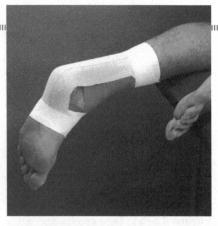

Figure 13–48 Anchors are applied over the cut ends at the top and bottom of the foot. Regular 1½" athletic tape is used here.

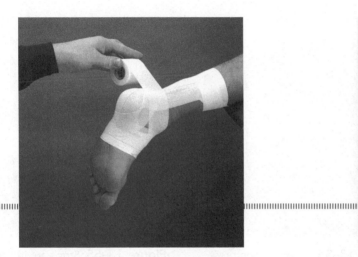

Figure 13–49 Lightweight 2" elastic tape is then used to cover the Elastikon™ tape.

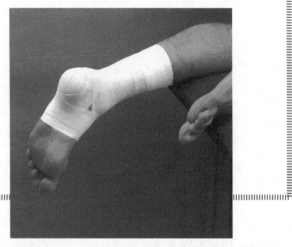

Figure 13–50 The entire ankle and lower leg are wrapped. The back of the heel need not to be wrapped over the Elastikon™. The lightweight elastic tape is used to add gentle compression and help keep the Elastikon™ in place. Be careful not to wrap too tightly, as circulation could be compromised.

SHIN-SPLINT TAPING

Shin splints, more accurately called *medial tibial stress syndrome (MTSS)*, should be properly diagnosed prior to treatment (see Chapter 17 for a detailed description of this condition). One common method for providing relief is to apply **circumferential** elastic taping (i.e., taping around the leg) (Figures 13–51 and 13–52). This method gives gentle compression that relieves some of the discomfort of this condition.

WRIST TAPING

There are numerous products on the market today aimed at wrist support, and many do a good job of adding mild compression with support. To support the wrist even further, taping will be required. Figures 13–53 through 13–56 illustrate basic wrist taping.

Additional support will be needed to prevent hyperextension of the wrist. The steps shown and described in Figures 13–57 through 13–61 are

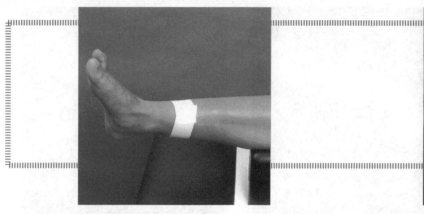

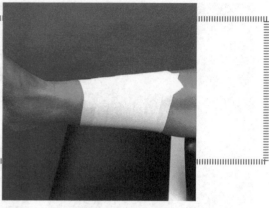

Figure 13–51 Tape can be applied on either bare skin or skin prepared with underwrap. If the application will be applied onto the bare skin, it is important to shave the skin first. The skin should be sprayed with a tape adherent before taping. Tape (either 1½ or 2", elastic or nonelastic) should begin just above the Achilles tendon.

Figure 13–52 Strips should be torn and applied separately. Continue to apply strips (overlapping by half the width of the tape) 6–8" up from the ankle. It is important that these strips not be applied tightly.

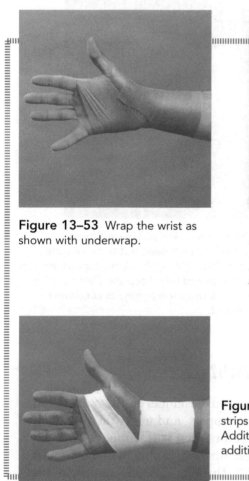

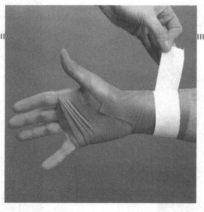

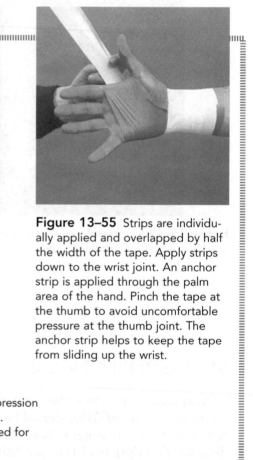

Figure 13–53 Wrap the wrist as shown with underwrap.

Figure 13–54 Cover, or compression, strips are applied starting approximately 3–4" above the wrist. Compression means just moderate tension, not tight.

Figure 13–55 Strips are individually applied and overlapped by half the width of the tape. Apply strips down to the wrist joint. An anchor strip is applied through the palm area of the hand. Pinch the tape at the thumb to avoid uncomfortable pressure at the thumb joint. The anchor strip helps to keep the tape from sliding up the wrist.

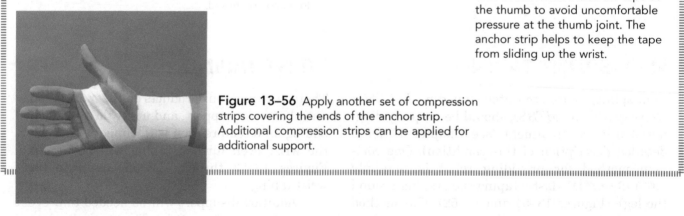

Figure 13–56 Apply another set of compression strips covering the ends of the anchor strip. Additional compression strips can be applied for additional support.

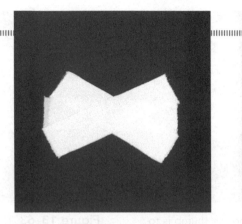

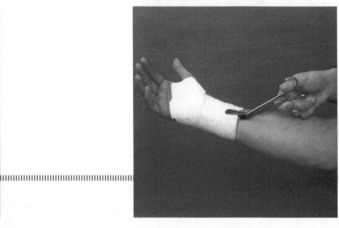

Figure 13–57 Measure the distance from the tape at the arm and the palm.

Figure 13–58 Tear three pieces of tape and create a fan shape as shown. Duplicate this fan and attach the two to each other. This gives a double-strength application.

Figure 13–59 Apply the doubled fan to the wrist. The wrist should be slightly flexed on application. The fan should be exactly in the middle of the wrist.

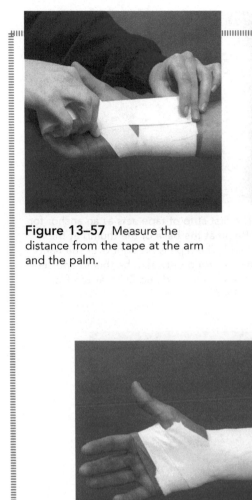

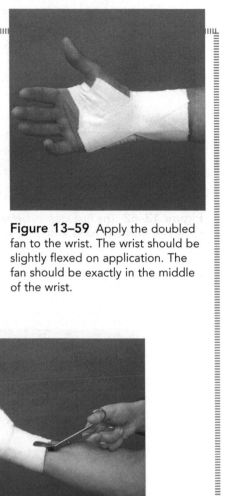

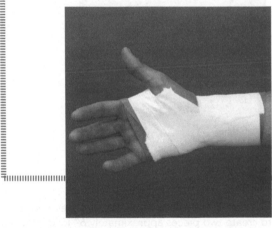

Figure 13–60 Cover the entire fan with cover strips. This will help to add support and keep the athlete from hyperextending the wrist.

Figure 13–61 Removal of tape can be accomplished with tape scissors or by separately unwrapping each piece of tape.

used in conjunction with basic wrist support. Commercial products called orthopedic spica splints provide added support by enclosing metal or plastic within the fabric to limit motion, while allowing the fingers to operate normally. These are also available for the thumb.

THUMB TAPING

If the thumb is bent beyond its normal range of movement (usually backward), damage may occur to the ligaments that support the MPJ joint at the bottom of the thumb (metacarpophalangeal joint).

If the injury is a mild sprain, proper taping will allow safe return to play. Figures 13–62 through 13–69 outline this procedure.

FINGER SUPPORT

Fingers can become sprained and hyperextended. A simple buddy taping procedure creates an anatomical splint to help protect the injury (see Figures 13–70 through 13–72). This is done by taping the injured finger to the adjoining uninjured finger.

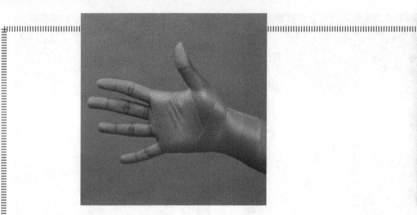

Figure 13–62 The first step in taping the thumb is to cover the wrist and hand with underwrap, as shown.

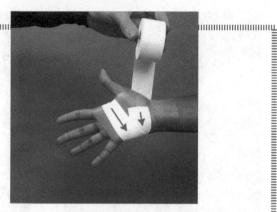

Figure 13–63 The first strip of tape acts as an anchor for additional strips. Begin at the base of the thumb at the palm side of the hand. The tape is brought over the hand and across the palm, passing between the thumb and second finger. Bring the tape around and finish at the first anchor (see Figure 13–68).

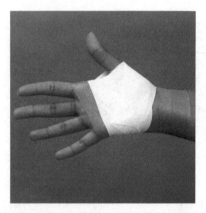

Figure 13–64 Additional cover strips are used as support.

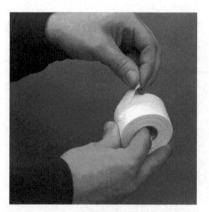

Figure 13–65 Using 1½" adhesive tape, tear a piece down the middle to create two pieces approximately 6" in length.

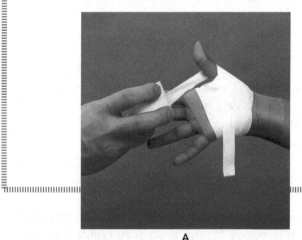

A

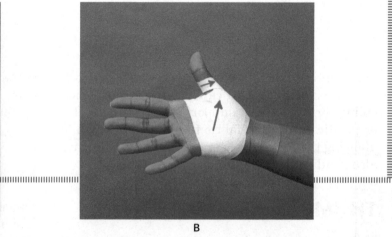

B

Figure 13–66A–B The half-width strips begin at the wrist and wrap around the thumb to the outside of the hand. Do not squeeze the thumb when bringing this tape around the thumb. Do this step twice.

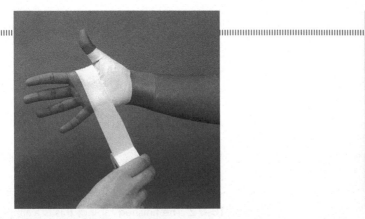

Figure 13–67 The last step is identical to the first. Begin at the base of the thumb at the palm side of the hand. Bring the tape over the hand and across the palm, passing between the thumb and second finger. Bring the tape around and finish at the first anchor.

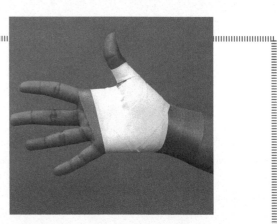

Figure 13–68 The finished taping should be free of wrinkles and have even tension. Additional strips can be applied for more support.

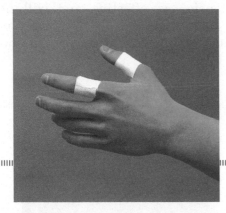

Figure 13–69A A simple method to keep the thumb from hyperextending is to tape the thumb to the adjacent finger. The difference between buddy taping and this procedure is that the normal space between the thumb and adjacent finger is maintained. Begin by using 1" adhesive tape and applying an anchor around the thumb and adjacent finger as shown.

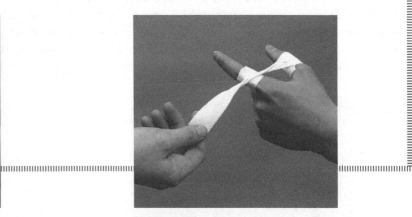

Figure 13–69B Again using 1" tape, wrap the tape around the thumb two times. The tape is then twisted (providing greater strength) and applied to the adjacent finger, wrapping twice.

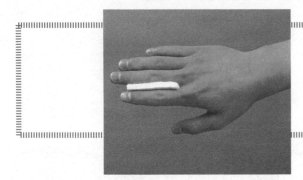

Figure 13–70 A thin piece of foam or felt will provide comfort and protection. The foam or felt should be cut to the width of the finger and the length of the shortest finger. Place the foam or felt between the injured and uninjured fingers.

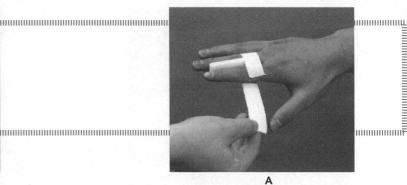

A

Figure 13–71A–B Using ½" or ¾" adhesive tape, wrap around the fingers above and below the joint. Do not wrap tightly, as this will impair circulation. (*continues*)

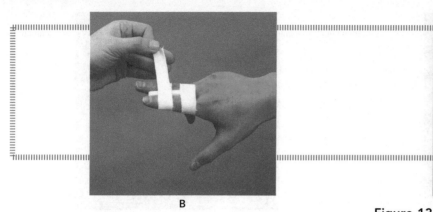

Figure 13–71A–B (*continued*)

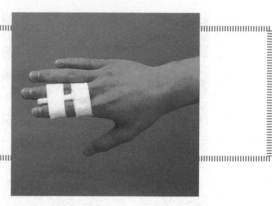

Figure 13–72 The finished taping; this is a simple yet effective way to protect a sprained finger.

ELBOW TAPING

Hyperextension of the elbow is normally the result of falling on an outstretched arm or hand. The impact forces the elbow into an overextended state. Pain will be felt on the inside of the elbow from the stretch of the biceps, and often in the back as a result of "jamming" the bones against one another. Taping the elbow (see Figures 13–73 through 13–80) to prevent hyperextension is effective and will help to prevent **hypermobility** (a body part moving beyond its normal range of motion, as shown in Figures 13–73).

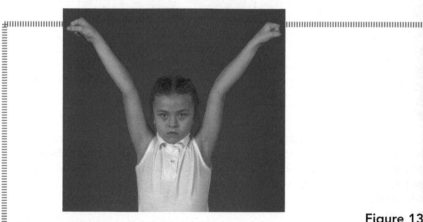

Figure 13–73 Hypermobility at the elbows is an inherited condition. This girl shows a greater mobility than most.

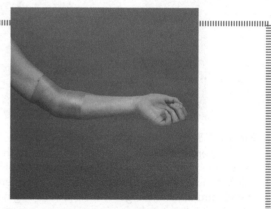

Figure 13–74 Apply underwrap to the elbow as shown. Apply spray adherent liberally 2" above and below the underwrap. Shave skin area if needed.

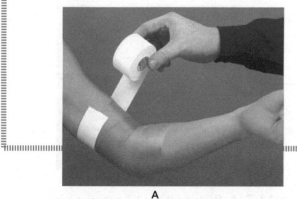

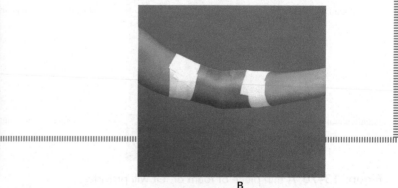

Figure 13–75A–B The athlete will need to keep the arm flexed during this procedure. This will help compensate for tape slippage during practice or competition. Some trial and error will be needed to determine the proper angle of flexion. Tape an anchor strip onto the skin above and below the underwrap. This helps keep the tape from slipping down the arm.

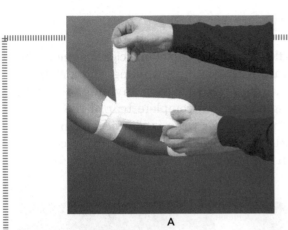

A

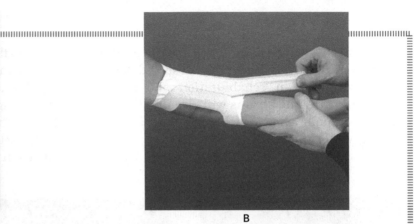

B

Figure 13–76A–B Using 2" or 3" Elastikon™ or similar elastic tape, cut down the middle to create two anchor strips. Wrap these strips around the arm over the initial anchor.

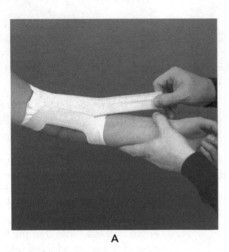

A

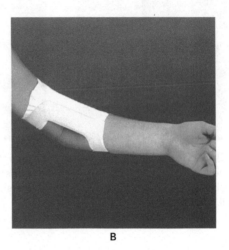

B

Figure 13–77A–B Duplicate this procedure for the bottom of the tape. Stretch the elastic tape to within 90% of its maximum.

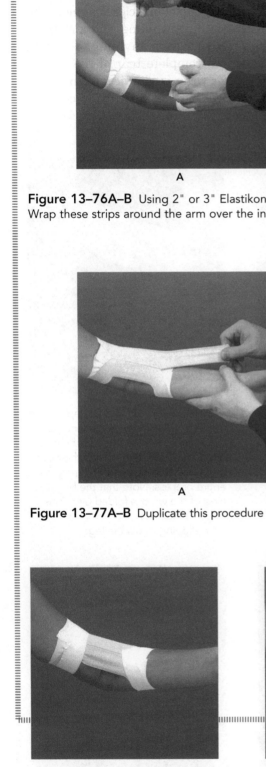

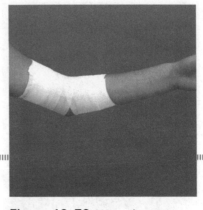

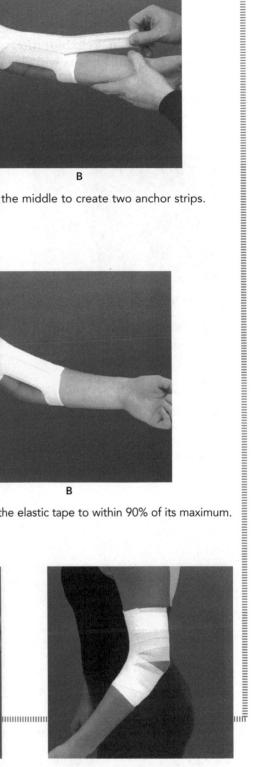

Figure 13–78 Apply cover strips to the top and bottom of the "elastic" anchor strips.

Figure 13–79 Wrap the entire elbow with 2" lightweight elastic tape. It can be one continuous piece of tape. This helps keep the rest of the tape in place and adds stability.

Figure 13–80 The athlete can still practice or perform, knowing that the injury is well stabilized.

GROIN WRAP

Groin strains can be painful and greatly limit participation. A specialized wrap designed for this area will help in rehabilitation and recovery. Athletes with mild strains will also find the wrapping technique shown in Figures 13–81 through 13–88 very helpful.

HIP FLEXOR WRAP

The hip flexors are a group of muscles that move the hip forward when running, walking, and kicking. A hip flexor injury can vary from anything to a slight stretching strain to a complete tear of the muscle tissue. The hip flexor wrap is identical to the groin wrap except that it goes in the opposite direction, as shown in Figures 13–89 through 13–94.

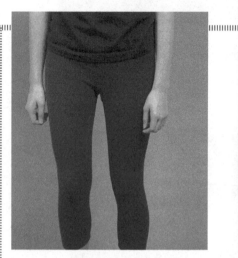

Figure 13–81 The athlete should have the heel of the injured leg elevated about 2". A roll of tape works well.

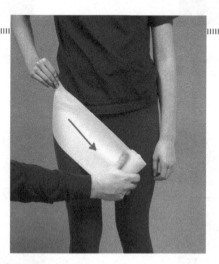

Figure 13–82 Using a 6" double-length elastic wrap, begin at the lateral side of the hip.

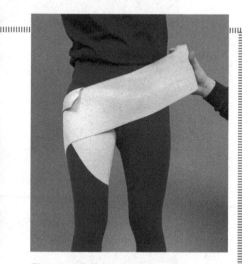

Figure 13–83 Bring the wrap around the leg, close to the crotch, and pull the wrap across the body to the other hip. Extend the wrap to half the maximum stretch of the elastic during the entire process. Note that the beginning of the wrap is folded over. This helps to lock this piece in and keep it from slipping down the leg.

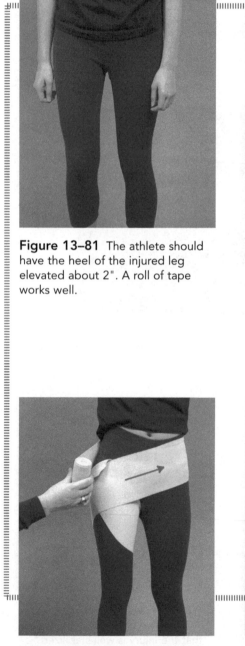

Figure 13–84 Continue the wrap around the back at the waist, and back to where you began.

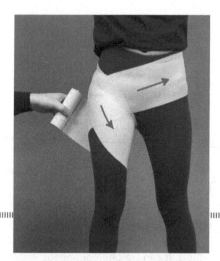

Figure 13–85 Go around the leg, pull, and bring across the body as before.

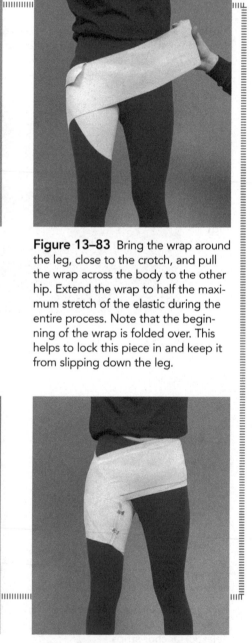

Figure 13–86 Continue this process until you run out of wrap. Secure with two clips.

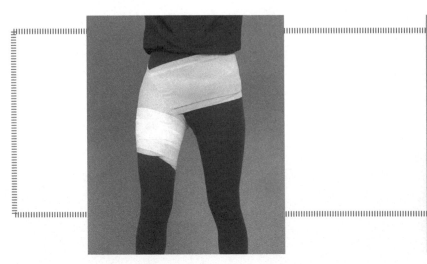

Figure 13–87 Cover the clips with lightweight elastic tape.

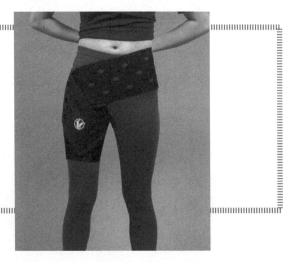

Figure 13–88 Commercial wraps are available.

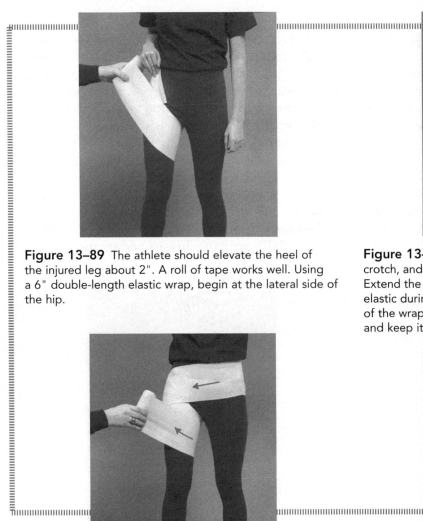

Figure 13–89 The athlete should elevate the heel of the injured leg about 2". A roll of tape works well. Using a 6" double-length elastic wrap, begin at the lateral side of the hip.

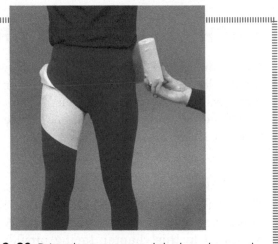

Figure 13–90 Bring the wrap around the leg, close to the crotch, and pull the wrap behind the body to the other hip. Extend the wrap to half of the maximum stretch of the elastic during the entire process. Note that the beginning of the wrap is folded over. This helps to lock this piece in and keep it from slipping down the leg.

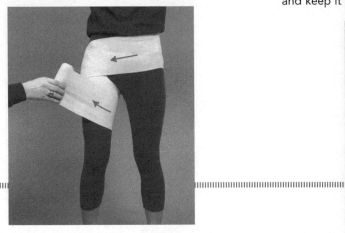

Figure 13–91 Continue the wrap across the front of the body at the waist. The wrap continues around the back of the leg and to the front.

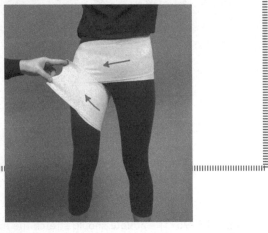

Figure 13–92 Repeat these steps until you run out of wrap. Secure the end of the wrap with clips.

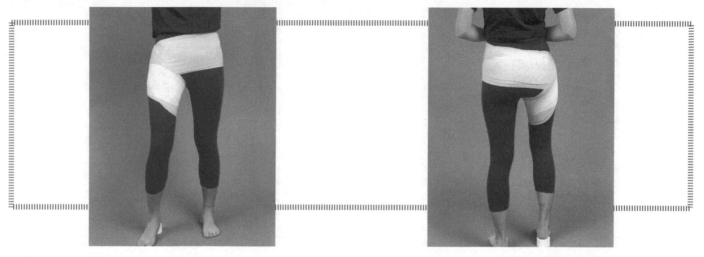

Figure 13–93 Cover the clips with lightweight elastic tape.

Figure 13–94 Back view of the hip flexor wrap.

THIGH COMPRESSION WRAP

When an athlete receives a severe blow to the thigh, bleeding will occur within the muscle. A compression wrap will help control the extent of the bleeding and inflammation. Figures 13–95 through 13–99 illustrate this procedure.

Taping Versus Bracing

There will always be a debate on what is better, taping or buying a commercially produced brace. As stated in this chapter, taping provides a per-

sonal, professionally fitted support to address a specific condition. Bracing can do much the same thing if properly fitted. Advantages of properly fitted braces are savings in cost and time. If an athlete needs to have an ankle taped each time he or she practices or competes, it become costly over time. An ankle brace will more than pay for itself before the season is over. Some areas of the body are very difficult to tape effectively, such as the knee and shoulder. Braces in this instance will do a better job of helping the athlete stay safe. Throughout this book you will find examples of commercially available braces and wraps.

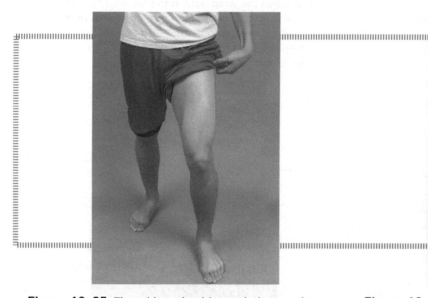

Figure 13–95 The athlete should stretch the muscles gently by bringing the leg forward.

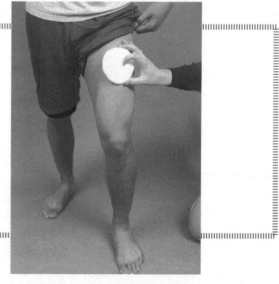

Figure 13–96 Place a compression pad made of felt over the injury site. The compression pad should be 1" greater in diameter than the injury.

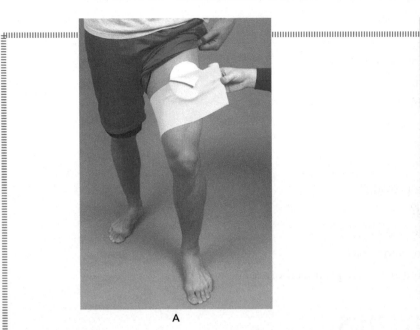
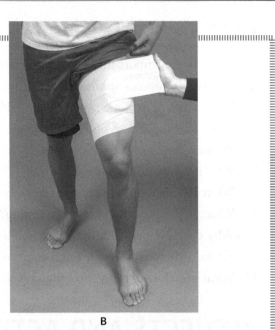

A

B

Figure 13–97A–B Using 4" or 6" elastic wrap, wrap the leg. Pull it tight enough to compress the injury site, but take care not to wrap too tightly (see Figure 13–99). This will be uncomfortable to the athlete at first.

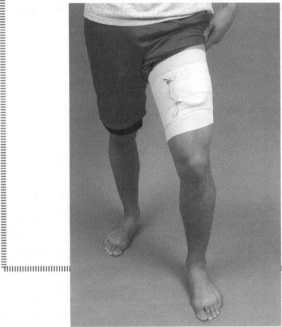

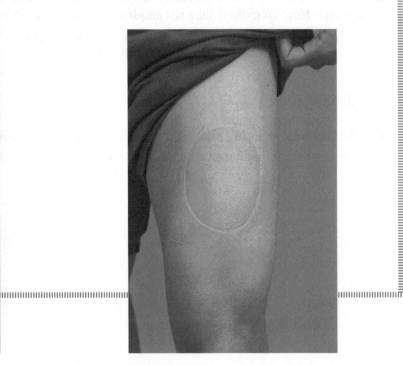

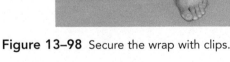

Figure 13–98 Secure the wrap with clips.

Figure 13–99 The compression pad will leave a temporary impression after removal.

CONCLUSION

Taping and wrapping are important skills used by sports medicine professionals. Their primary purpose is to provide additional support, stability, and compression for affected areas of the body. To become proficient in taping and wrapping techniques, the certified athletic trainer must have a good working knowledge of anatomy and biomechanics. Coordination, skill, and practice are also required to master these techniques.

REVIEW QUESTIONS

1. What is the importance of taping and wrapping?
2. List the common supplies used in taping.
3. What sizes of athletic tape are available?
4. What is the purpose of hypoallergenic tape?
5. Explain how to tear athletic tape.
6. Why is spray adherent used?
7. What protection do heel and lace pads provide?
8. What is the purpose of low-dye taping?
9. Why do some people have hypermobile joints?
10. Explain the purpose of a thigh compression wrap
11. What are the advantages of using a commercially produced brace?

PROJECTS AND ACTIVITIES

1. Working with a partner, practice each of the different taping and wrapping procedures described in the chapter. How long did it take to complete each procedure? Was your first attempt successful?
2. Keep a diary of your experience with taping and wrapping. Write a short paper describing your suggestions to a new student just beginning this chapter.

LEARNING LINKS

•   Visit athletic training and sports medicine association websites and search for additional techniques and methods for taping and wrapping.

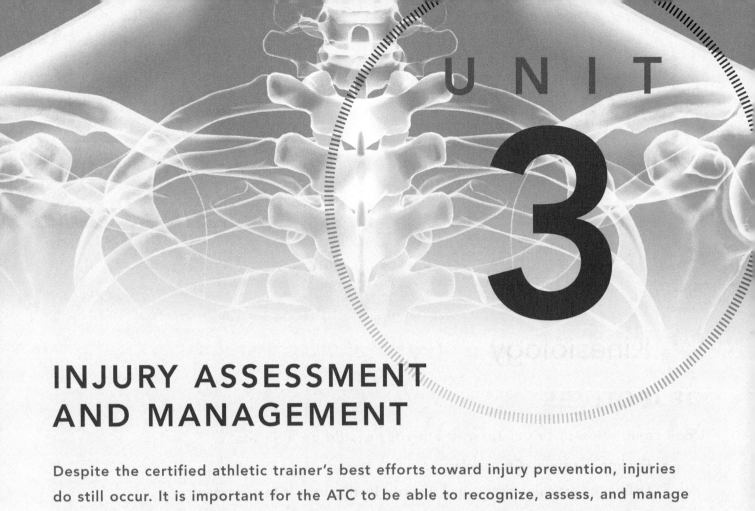

INJURY ASSESSMENT AND MANAGEMENT

Despite the certified athletic trainer's best efforts toward injury prevention, injuries do still occur. It is important for the ATC to be able to recognize, assess, and manage injuries, both when they occur and throughout the process of rehabilitation and return to play. To have a sound understanding of injuries, the ATC must first study anatomy and physiology. The chapters that follow introduce anatomy, physiology, and the injuries most commonly encountered on the athletic field, gymnasium, or sports arena. Techniques used in the initial management and rehabilitation of those injuries are also discussed.

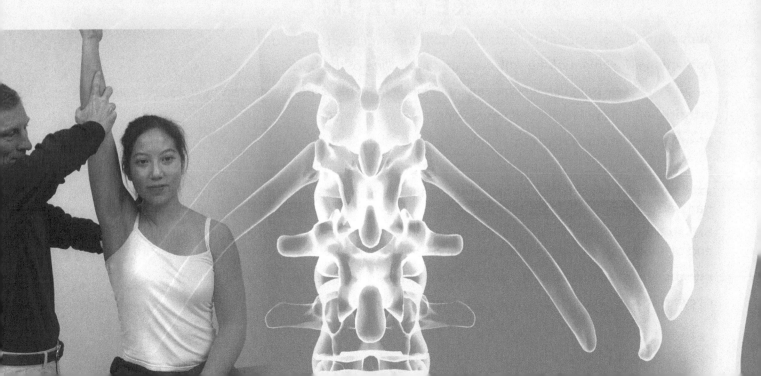

CHAPTER 14

Kinesiology

OBJECTIVES

Upon completion of this chapter, the reader should be able to:

- Explain the study of kinesiology
- Define the articular system and describe its importance to movement
- Define the three classifications of joints
- State the six types of diarthroses joints
- Define the 18 different movements of synovial joints
- Explain the three anatomical planes and their importance to medicine
- Explain the concept of open and closed kinematic chains

KEY TERMS

abduction *Movement of the limbs away from the midline of the body.*

adduction *Movement of the limbs toward the midline of the body.*

amphiarthroses *(singular: amphiarthrosis) Slightly movable joints connected by fibrocartilage.*

arthritis *An inflammation of an entire joint.*

arthrology *The study of joints.*

articular cartilage *Connective tissue covering the ends of long bones.*

axial plane *A horizontal flat surface dividing the body into upper and lower parts; also known as the transverse plane.*

ball-and-socket joints *Freely movable joints in which a rounded end of one bone fits into an indented end of another bone; allows the widest range of motion.*

bursitis *An inflammation of the synovial cavity caused by excessive stress or tension.*

circumduction *Circular movement of the limbs around an axis.*

KEY TERMS CONTINUED

closed kinematic chain *A sequence of action in which the body part farthest from the trunk is fixed during movement.*

concave *A half-circle-shaped indentation to a surface.*

condyloid (ellipsoidal) joints *Freely movable joints that allow bones to move about one another in many different directions, but not to rotate.*

convex *A half-circle-shaped protrusion on a surface.*

coronal plane *A vertical flat surface running from side to side of the body; also known as the frontal plane.*

depression *Movement of a body part downward in a frontal plane.*

diarthroses *(singular: diarthrosis) Freely movable joints; also known as synovial joints.*

dorsiflexion *Movement that flexes the foot.*

elevation *Movement of a body part upward in a frontal plane.*

eversion *Movement of the sole of the foot outward.*

extension *Movement that increases the angle between two bones.*

fibrocartilage *Specialized connective tissue with thick collagen fibers.*

flexion *Movement that decreases the angle between two bones.*

gliding joint *A freely movable joint that allows bones to make a sliding motion.*

gomphoses *(singular: gomphosis) Immovable joints in which a conical process fits into a socket held in place by ligaments.*

gout *An accumulation of uric acid crystals in the joint at the base of the large toe and other joints of the feet.*

hinge joint *A freely movable joint that allows flexion and extension.*

hyperextension *Movement beyond the natural range of motion.*

inversion *Movement of the sole of the foot inward.*

joint articulation *The connecting point of two bones.*

kinesiology *The multidisciplinary study of physical activity or movement; encompasses anatomy, biomechanics, physiology, psychomotor behavior, and social and cultural factors.*

open kinematic chain *A sequence of action in which the body part farthest from the trunk is free during movement.*

opposition *Movement of the thumb to touch each finger.*

osteoarthritis *A degenerative joint disease.*

pivot joint *A freely movable joint in which a bone moves around a central axis, creating rotational movement.*

plantar flexion *Movement that extends the foot.*

primary fibrositis *An inflammation of the fibrous connective tissue in a joint.*

pronation *Movement of the radius and ulna posterior or inferior.*

protraction *Movement of a body part forward in a transverse plane.*

KEY TERMS CONTINUED

retraction *Movement of a body part backward in a transverse plane.*

rheumatic fever *A bacterial infection that can be carried in the blood to the joints.*

rheumatoid arthritis *A connective-tissue disorder resulting in severe inflammation of small joints.*

rotation *Movement of a bone on an axis, toward or away from the body.*

saddle joint *A freely movable joint between two bones with complementary shapes; allows a wide range of motion.*

sagittal plane *A vertical flat surface running from front to back of the body.*

supination *Movement of the radius and ulna anterior or superior.*

sutures *Joints where a thin layer of dense, fibrous connective tissue unites the bones of the skull.*

synarthroses *(singular: synarthrosis) Immovable joints that lack a synovial cavity and are held together by fibrous connective tissue.*

syndesmoses *Slightly movable joints where bones are connected by ligaments.*

synovial fluid *A lubricating substance found in joint cavities.*

synovial joint *Freely movable joint; also known as a diarthrosis.*

synovial membrane *A double layer of connective tissue that lines joint cavities and produces synovial fluid.*

KINESIOLOGY

Kinesiology is the multidisciplinary study of physical activity or movement. It encompasses anatomy, biomechanics, physiology, psychomotor behavior, and various social and cultural factors. The study of kinesiology focuses on exercise stress, movement efficiency, and fitness.

The term is fashioned from two Greek verbs, *kinein* and *logus,* which mean "to move" and "to discourse." Modern phrasing has changed the meaning of the suffix *logus* to "the study of," so that *kinesiology* reads literally as "the study of movement." Kinesiology encompasses both the theory and practice of movement. The study of movement in physical activity has a long history in American higher education, in many institutions dating to the late-nineteenth century. The field of study was primarily oriented to the practice of movement such as physical training and playing sports. The beginning of the study of movement from a disciplinary perspective was a fragmented effort driven by the insight of a few individuals operating as individual scholars, practitioners of medicine, or aspiring academics in universities. Today, these various approaches to the study of movement all come under the single umbrella of kinesiology. This chapter addresses how the body moves by way of its joints and related structures.

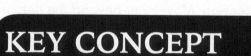

KEY CONCEPT

The study of kinesiology focuses on exercise stress, movement efficiency, and fitness.

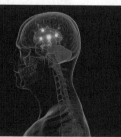

DID YOU KNOW? Careers related to the study of kinesiology include occupational and physical therapy, professional athletics, coaching, athletic training, and even nutrition.

ARTICULAR SYSTEM

The *articular system* is a series of joints that allows movement of the human body. This series of joints, combined with the neuromuscular system, enables locomotion.

When two bones come into contact, they form a **joint articulation**. Joint articulations can be freely movable, as in the knee or hip; slightly movable, as in the pubic symphysis, which moves slightly during childbirth; or immobile, as in the fused sutures of the skull. Many joints are identified by combining the names of the two bones that form the joint. An example is the sternoclavicular joint, which is the articulation between the sternum and the clavicle. The study of joints is called **arthrology**.

CLASSIFICATION OF JOINTS

Joints have two main functions. They allow motion, and at the same time provide stability. They are classified in three different ways:

- Synarthroses, or immovable
- Amphiarthroses, or slightly movable
- Diarthroses, or freely movable

Synarthroses

Synarthroses joints lack a synovial cavity and are held closely together by fibrous connective tissue. Synarthroses are immovable joints in which the

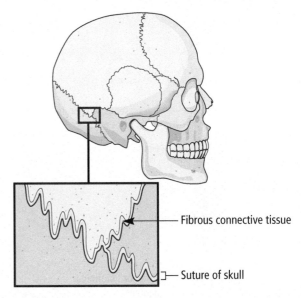

- Fibrous connective tissue

- Suture of skull

Figure 14–1 Sutures.

bones come into very close contact and are separated only by a thin layer of fibrous connective tissue. The sutures in the skull are examples of immovable (synarthric) joints. There are three structural types of synarthroses: sutures, syndesmoses, and gomphoses.

SUTURES In **sutures**, a thin layer of dense, fibrous connective tissue unites the bones of the skull (Figure 14–1). They are immovable and fuse completely by adulthood. Sutures are found only in the skull.

SYNDESMOSES In a **syndesmosis** joint the bones are connected by ligaments. Examples of syndesmoses are the fibula and tibia in the lower leg (Figure 14–2), and the ulna and radius of the arm. These bones move as one when one pronates (turns or rotates the hand or forearm so that the palm faces down or back) and supinates (turns or rotates the hand or forearm so that the palm faces up or forward) the forearm, or rotate the lower leg. These joints offer slight movement and thus are sometimes considered to be amphiarthroses.

GOMPHOSES In **gomphoses** joints a conical process fits into a socket and is held in place by ligaments. An example is a tooth in its alveolus (socket), held in place by the periodontal ligament (Figure 14–3).

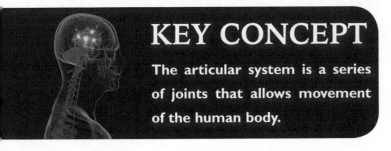

KEY CONCEPT

The articular system is a series of joints that allows movement of the human body.

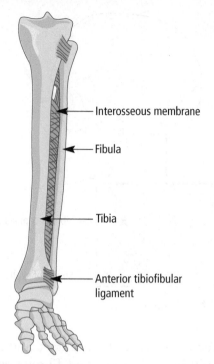

Figure 14–2 Syndesmosis.

Amphiarthroses

Amphiarthroses joints are slightly movable. In this type of joint, the bones are connected by hyaline cartilage or **fibrocartilage**. The connections of the ribs to the sternum are slightly movable joints connected by costal hyaline cartilage. The symphysis pubis is a slightly movable joint in which there is a fibrocartilage pad between the two bones. The joints between the vertebrae are also amphiarthroses (Figure 14–4).

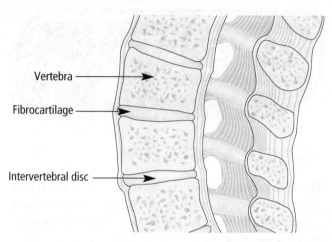

Figure 14–4 Amphiarthrosis.

Diarthroses or Synovial Joints

Most joints in the adult body are **diarthroses**, or freely movable joints in which the ends of the opposing bones are covered with a type of hyaline cartilage, the **articular cartilage**, and are separated by a space called the joint cavity. The components of the joints are enclosed in a dense, fibrous joint capsule. The outer layer of the capsule consists of the ligaments that hold the bones together. The inner layer, the **synovial membrane**, secretes **synovial fluid** into the joint cavity for lubrication. Because all **diarthroses** joints have a synovial membrane, they are sometimes called **synovial joints**.

Each of the six different types of synovial joints allows a different degree of mobility.

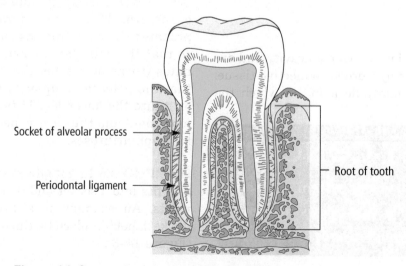

Figure 14–3 Gomphosis.

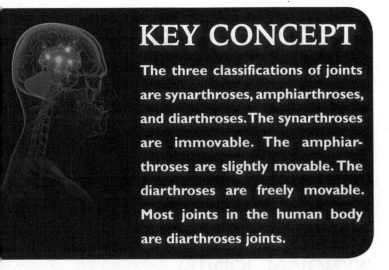

KEY CONCEPT

The three classifications of joints are synarthroses, amphiarthroses, and diarthroses. The synarthroses are immovable. The amphiarthroses are slightly movable. The diarthroses are freely movable. Most joints in the human body are diarthroses joints.

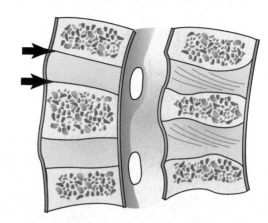

Figure 14–6 Gliding joint.

PIVOT JOINT The **pivot joint** is a freely movable joint in which a bone moves around a central axis, creating rotational movement (Figure 14–5). An example is the joint between the radius and ulna of the lower arm.

GLIDING JOINT A **gliding joint** allows bones to make a sliding motion, either back and forth or side to side. Gliding joints are found in the carpals of the wrist and the tarsals of the ankle, and also between the vertebrae in the spine (Figure 14–6).

HINGE JOINT The **hinge joint** allows only extension and flexion, the reason for this being that the

convex surface of one bone fits into the **concave** surface of the second bone. The knee, elbow (Figure 14–7), and phalanges of the fingers and toes are all hinge joints.

CONDYLOID OR ELLIPSOIDAL JOINT **Condyloid** or **ellipsoidal joints** are formed where bones can move about one another in many directions but cannot rotate. This joint is named for a condyle-containing bone. A *condyle* is a curved process that fits into a fossa (cavity) in another bone for its articulation. This type of joint can be found at the metacarpals (bones in the palm of the hand) and phalanges (fingers), and between the metatarsals (foot bones, excluding the heel) and phalanges (toes) (Figure 14–8).

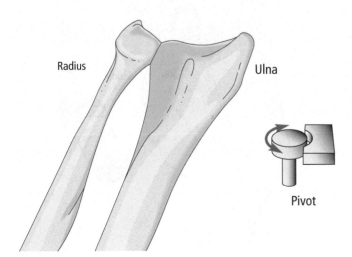

Figure 14–5 Pivot joint.

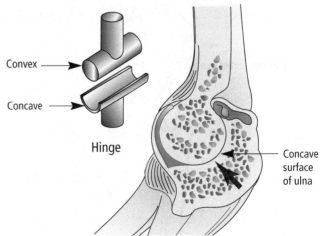

Figure 14–7 Hinge joint.

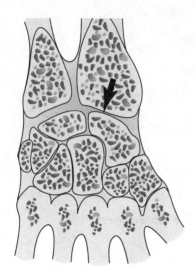

Figure 14–8 Condyloid joint.

BALL-AND-SOCKET JOINT In a **ball-and-socket joint**, one bone has a rounded end that fits into a concave cavity on another bone. This provides the widest range of movement possible in joints; for example, the hips (Figure 14–9) and shoulders can swing in almost any direction.

SADDLE JOINT In a **saddle joint**, the two bones have both concave and convex regions, with the shapes of both bones complementing one another. This joint also allows a wide range of movement. The only saddle joint in the body is in the thumb (Figure 14–10); it allows humans to turn and oppose their thumbs in cooperation with the fingers.

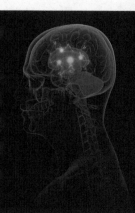

KEY CONCEPT

The six types of diarthroses are pivot joints, gliding joints, hinge joints, condyloid or ellipsoidal joints, ball-and-socket joints, and saddle joints. Each type allows a particular type of motion.

MOVEMENTS OF DIARTHROSES (SYNOVIAL JOINTS)

The range of motion in movable joints varies. Some joints are only slightly movable; others are capable of a wide range of motion. The ranges of motion of the movable joints determine the positions the human body can assume, and they play an important role in athletic activity.

The joints in the body that move most freely are the synovial joints. The greater the range of motion in a synovial joint, the more the joint relies on the attached muscles for stability.

The joints with the greatest amount of movement are the shoulders. The hips are a not-too-distant second: Some gymnasts have a range of motion in their hips nearly as great as that in their shoulders.

The stability of a joint is determined by three factors: the shape of the bones where they come together, the ligaments that join the bones, and

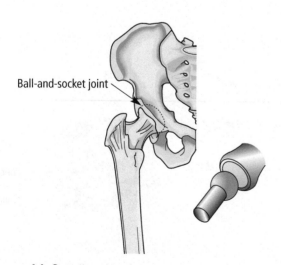

Ball-and-socket joint

Figure 14–9 Ball-and-socket joint.

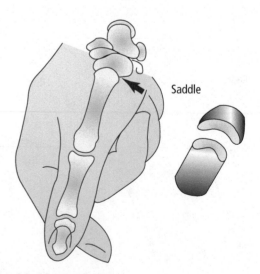

Saddle

Figure 14–10 Saddle joint.

muscle tone. In some joints, the shapes of the bones are well matched, resulting in a very stable joint (such as the hips); in others the opposite is true. The more ligaments a joint possesses, the stronger it is, but joints that rely on ligaments for bracing are not very stable. For most joints, however, muscle tone is the main stabilizing factor. The shoulder and knee joints, for example, are primarily stabilized in this way. Muscle tone keeps the tendons that attach the muscles to the bones taut, reinforcing the related joints.

Synovial joints allow 18 different types of movements:

- **Flexion** decreases the angle between two bones (Figure 14–11A).
- **Extension** increases the angle between two bones (Figure 14–11A).
- **Hyperextension** increases (extends) the angle between two bones beyond the normal range of motion (Figure 14–11B).
- **Abduction** describes movements of the limbs only; in abduction, the limb moves *away from* the midline of the body (Figure 14–11C).
- **Adduction** also describes movement of the limbs only; in adduction, the limb moves *toward* the midline of the body (Figure 14–11C).

- **Rotation** occurs when a bone turns on its axis toward or away from the midline of the body, in limbs, or between the atlas and axis (Figure 14–11D).
- **Circumduction** is the ability of a limb to move in a circular path around an axis. The proximal portion of the limb remains stationary, while the distal portion moves in a circle (Figure 14–11E).
- **Supination** refers to the act of turning the palm upward, performed by lateral rotation of the forearm. When applied to the foot, it generally implies movements resulting in raising of the medial margin of the foot (Figure 14–11F).
- **Pronation** refers to the act of turning the palm downward, performed by medial rotation of the forearm. When applied to the foot, it generally implies movements resulting in lowering of the medial margin of the foot (Figure 14–11F).
- **Plantar flexion** extends the foot, with the toes pointing down (Figure 14–11G).
- **Dorsiflexion** flexes the foot, bringing the toes up toward the lower leg (Figure 14–11G).
- **Inversion** turns the sole of the foot inward (medially) (Figure 14–11H).

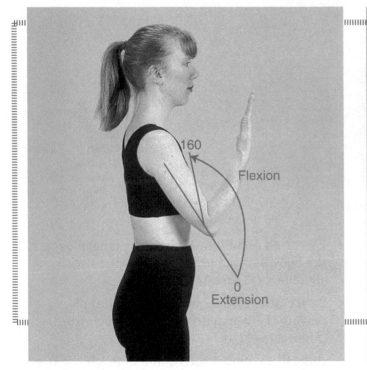

Figure 14–11A Flexion and extension.

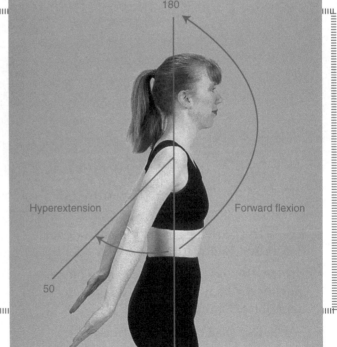

Figure 14–11B Hyperextension.

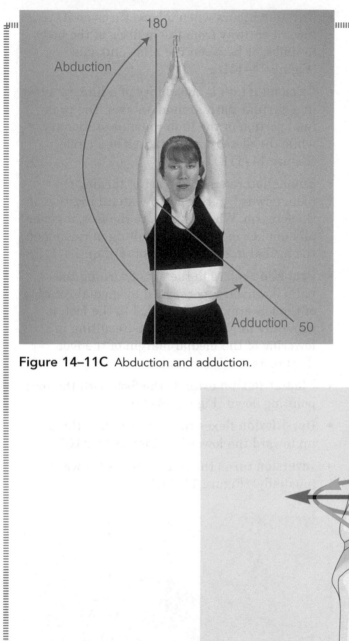

Figure 14–11C Abduction and adduction.

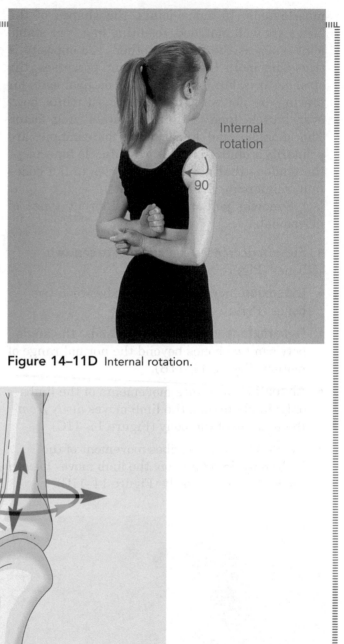

Figure 14–11D Internal rotation.

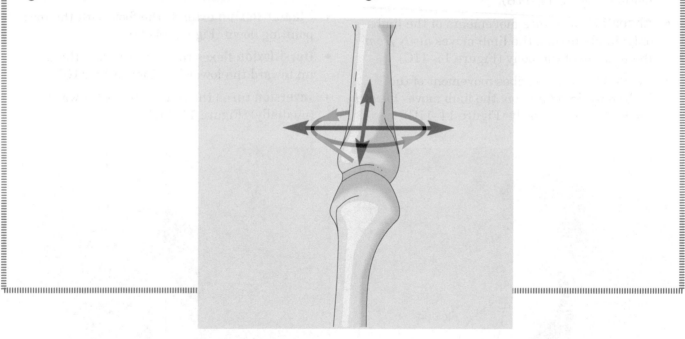

Figure 14–11E Circumduction.

- **Eversion** turns the sole of the foot outward (laterally) (Figure 14–11H).

- **Protraction** occurs in a transverse plane, moving the body part forward (shoulders, mandible) (Figure 14–11I).

- **Retraction** also occurs in a transverse plane, moving the body part backward (Figure 14–11J).

- **Elevation** occurs in the frontal plane, lifting the body part superiorly (upward), as with the shoulders (Figure 14–11K).

- **Depression** also occurs in the frontal plane, moving the body part inferiorly (downward) (Figure 14–11L).

- **Opposition** moves the thumb to touch the tips of the other fingers (Figure 14–11M).

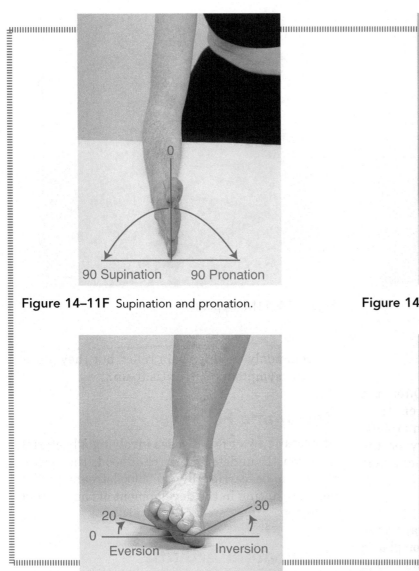

Figure 14–11F Supination and pronation.

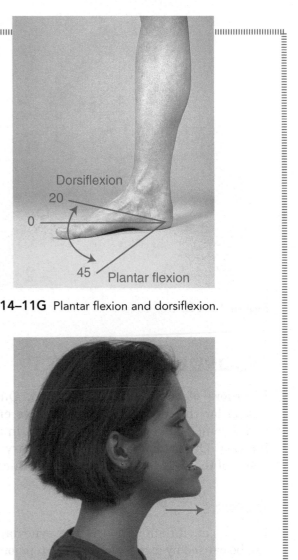

Figure 14–11G Plantar flexion and dorsiflexion.

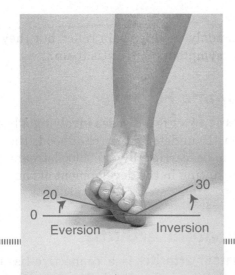

Figure 14–11H Eversion and inversion.

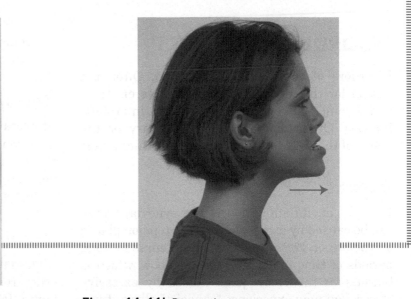

Figure 14–11I Protraction.

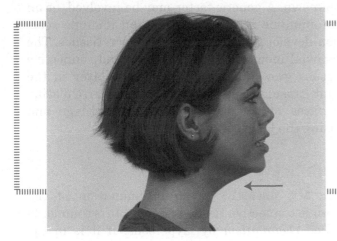

Figure 14–11J Retraction.

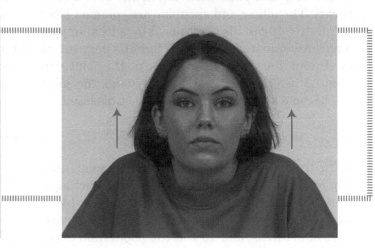

Figure 14–11K Elevation.

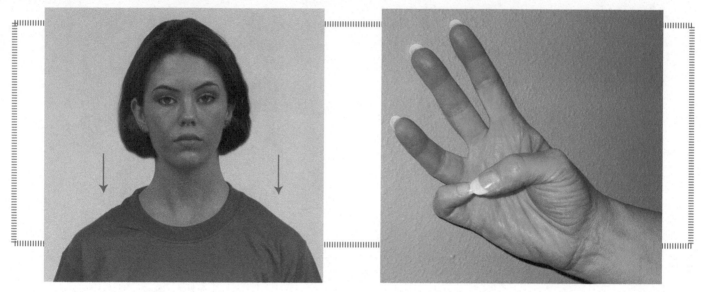

Figure 14–11L Depression.

Figure 14–11M Opposition.

DISORDERS OF JOINTS

Disorders of the joints are common. Often the reason for the disorder is excessive use or stress on the joint. This is commonly the case in athletic injuries. Other disorders are hereditary or the result of the deterioration that accompanies aging.

Bursitis

Bursitis, an inflammation of the synovial bursa, can be caused by excessive stress or tension placed on the bursa. For example, playing tennis for long periods of time may cause tennis elbow, which is bursitis in the elbow joint caused by excessive stress. You may experience "canoeist" elbow if you go canoeing and paddle for long hours. This is temporary. The elbow and shoulder are common sites of bursitis. It can also be caused by a local or systemic inflammatory process. If bursitis persists, as in chronic bursitis, the muscles in the joint can eventually degenerate or atrophy, and the joint can become stiff even though it is not diseased.

Arthritis

Arthritis, an inflammation of the entire joint, usually involves all the tissues of the joint: cartilage, bone, muscles, tendons, ligaments, nerves, blood supply, and so on. There are more than 100 varieties of arthritis, and 10% of the population experiences this disorder, which has no cure. Analgesics are commonly used for pain relief, but they affect only the symptom of arthritis (pain).

Rheumatic Fever

Rheumatic fever is a disease involving a bacterial infection. If undetected in childhood, the bacterium can be carried by the bloodstream to the joints, resulting in the development of rheumatoid arthritis.

Rheumatoid Arthritis

Rheumatoid arthritis is a connective-tissue disorder resulting in severe inflammation of small joints. It is severely debilitating and can destroy the joints of the hands and feet. The cause is unknown. A genetic factor may be involved, or an autoimmune reaction in which an immune reaction develops against a person's own tissues. The synovial membranes of the joints and connective tissues grow abnormally to form a layer in the joint capsule. This layer invades the articulating surfaces of the bone, destroying cartilage and fusing the bones of the joint.

Primary Fibrositis

Primary fibrositis is an inflammation of the fibrous connective tissue in a joint. It is commonly called *rheumatism* by laypersons. If it is in the lower back, it is commonly called *lumbago.*

Osteoarthritis

Osteoarthritis, sometimes referred to as *degenerative joint disease,* occurs with advancing age, especially in people in their seventies. It is more common in overweight individuals and affects the weight-bearing joints. Mild exercise can prevent joint deterioration and increase the ability to maintain movement at joints.

Gout

Gout is an accumulation of uric acid crystals in the joint at the base of the large toe and other joints of the feet and legs. It may also present in other joints throughout the body. It is more common in men than in women. These waste-product crystals can also accumulate in the kidneys, causing kidney damage.

ANATOMICAL PLANES

Medical professionals refer to sections of the body in terms of anatomical planes or flat surfaces. These planes are imaginary lines, vertical or horizontal, drawn through an upright body (Figure 14–12). In the anatomical position, the human body stands

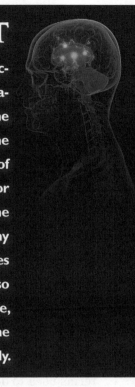

KEY CONCEPT

Medical professionals refer to sections of the body in terms of anatomical planes or flat surfaces. The coronal plane, also known as the frontal plane, allows discussion of anatomy related to the front or back of the body. The sagittal plane allows discussion of anatomy related to the right and left halves of the body. The axial plane, also known as the transverse plane, allows discussion related to the upper or lower portion of the body.

erect, eyes looking forward, arms at the sides, and the palms of the hands and the toes facing forward. The following terms are used to describe the specific planes of the body.

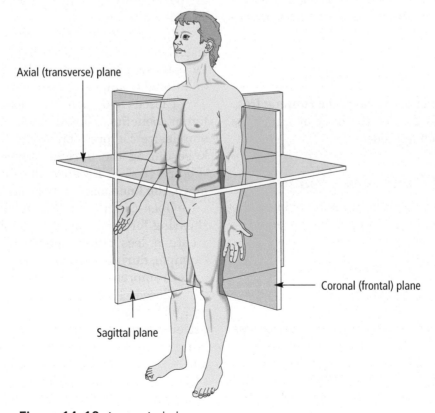

Axial (transverse) plane

Coronal (frontal) plane

Sagittal plane

Figure 14–12 Anatomical planes.

Table 14–1 Anatomical Terms Relating to Direction

ANATOMICAL TERM	DIRECTION
Medial	Toward the midline of the body
Lateral	Away from the midline of the body
Proximal	Nearest to a reference point
Distal	Farthest from a reference point
Inferior	Below
Superior	Above
Cephalad or Cranial	Toward the head
Caudal or Caudad	Toward the tailbone
Anterior	Toward the front
Posterior	Toward the back

It is important to understand how these terms and principles relate to movement about or within a specific surface or plane. Table 14–1 lists additional terms used to describe anatomical direction.

Coronal Plane (Frontal Plane)

The **coronal plane** is a vertical plane running from side to side. This divides the body or any of its parts into anterior (front) and posterior (back) portions.

Sagittal Plane (Lateral Plane)

The **sagittal plane** is a vertical plane running from front to back. This divides the body or any of its parts into right and left sides.

Axial Plane (Transverse Plane)

The **axial plane** is a horizontal plane dividing the body or any of its parts into upper and lower parts.

CLOSED AND OPEN KINEMATIC CHAINS

The concept of closed- and open-chain exercise was first discussed by Dr. Arthur Steindler in his book *Kinesiology of the Human Body: Under Normal and Pathological Conditions* (1955). Steindler defined *chains* as links of body parts, such as the foot, ankle, knee, and hip. Each link has an effect on the others. An example is walking, in which the foot, ankle, knee, and hip all play an important part in forward movement.

In a **closed kinematic chain** movement or exercise, the end of the chain farthest from the body is fixed; for example, in a squat the feet are fixed and the rest of the leg chain moves. Walking, or performing a pull-up or push-up, involves closed-chain motion.

In **open kinematic chain** movement or exercise, the end of the chain is free, such as in a seated leg extension. Waving a hand and kicking a ball are additional examples of open-chain movements.

Closed- and open-chain exercises provide different benefits. Closed-chain exercises tend to emphasize compression of joints; for example, the knee during the upright stance phase of squats (Figure 14–13). Because the distal end does not move, the knee joint is more stable.

Open-chain exercises tend to involve more shearing force parallel to the joint, and therefore create a less stable condition for exercise. For example, during a leg extension the knee is never under compression forces (Figure 14–14).

Closed chains tend to involve more muscles and joints than do open chains, and they lead to better coordination around each structure, which improves overall stability. Trunk movements are hard to categorize as closed- or open-chain because of the difficulty in assigning proximal and distal directions within the trunk.

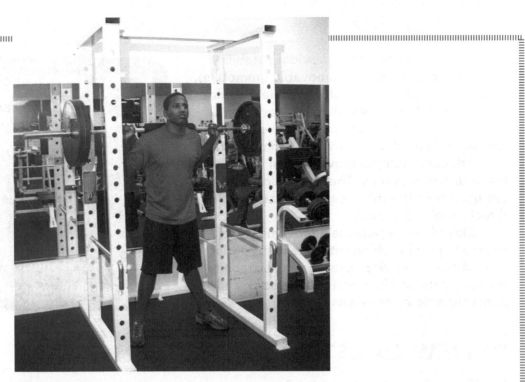

Figure 14–13 During this closed-chain exercise, the feet are fixed and do not move, creating compressive forces on the skeleton.

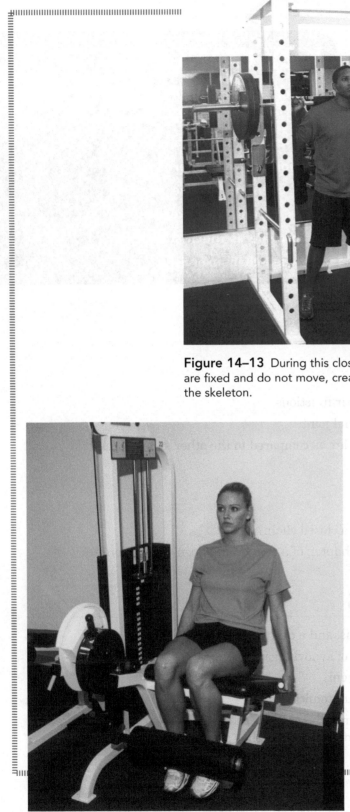

A

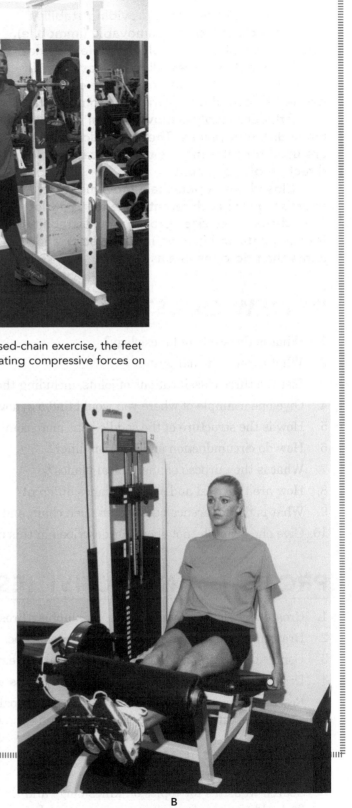

B

Figure 14–14A–B In this open-chain exercise, the feet move during the exercise, creating shear forces at the knee.

CONCLUSION

Joints allow motion while providing stability. Joints are classified as nonmovable (immobile), slightly movable, and freely movable. Besides providing stability, they allow at least 18 different movements. This creates the dexterity needed to complete a variety of complex tasks.

Athletics involves movement in and around many different planes. The anatomical planes are used for reference as to the location and direction of movement.

Closed- and open-chain movements and exercises provide different benefits to athletes. Closed-chain exercises provide more stability for the joints and involve more muscles and joints than do open chains.

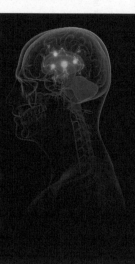

KEY CONCEPT

Closed- and open-chain exercises provide different benefits. Closed-chain exercises emphasize compression of joints, whereas open-chain exercises involve shearing forces. Open-chain exercises do not provide as much stability as do closed-chain exercises.

REVIEW QUESTIONS

1. What is the study of kinesiology?
2. What is the articular system?
3. List the three classifications of joints, including their functions.
4. Give one example of where you would find a synovial joint.
5. How is the structure of the saddle joint more complex as compared to the other synovial joints?
6. How do circumduction and rotation differ?
7. What is the purpose of anatomical planes?
8. How are the axial and sagittal planes different?
9. What is the difference between an open chain and a closed chain?
10. Give one example, not shown or described in this chapter, of a closed- and open-chain exercise.

PROJECTS AND ACTIVITIES

1. Create a model of a synarthrosis, an amphiarthrosis, and a diarthrosis.
2. Draw an example of each of the six different types of synovial joints.
3. Using stick figures, illustrate each synovial movement.
4. Draw a model of the human body divided into its anatomical planes.
5. Research open- and closed-chain exercises for repair of the anterior cruciate ligament (ACL). In a report, explain the difference between the two chains and describe when they are used in rehabilitation.

LEARNING LINKS

*   Search websites for topics on kinesiology and the various joints discussed in this chapter. Can you find additional information on programs of study or the relationship of athletics to kinesiology?
*   Search websites for additional information on the disorders and diseases discussed in this chapter. Do athletes tend to suffer from some joint disorders more than others?

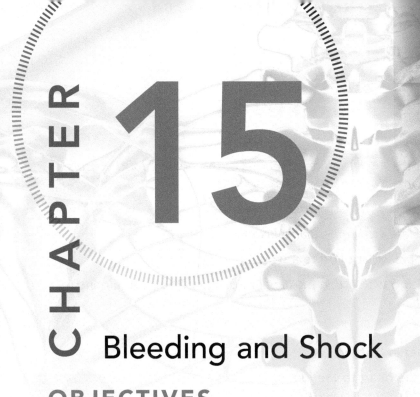

15

Bleeding and Shock

OBJECTIVES

Upon completion of this chapter, the reader should be able to:

- Describe the cardiorespiratory system
- List the components of the circulatory system
- Explain how blood circulates throughout the body
- Explain blood pressure and pulse
- Describe sudden cardiac death
- Describe equipment used to protect yourself and others from pathogens
- Explain what is meant by standard precautions
- Explain the guidelines for applying bandages
- Define the three basic types of bleeding
- Explain the signs of shock
- Explain the dangers associated with shock
- List and describe the eight types of shock
- Explain the care and treatment for shock

KEY TERMS

aorta *The heart's main artery, which carries nutrient-rich blood away from the heart to the body's cells.*

arterioles *The smallest of the arteries.*

atria *(singular: atrium) The upper chambers of the heart.*

capillaries *Tiny, microscopic blood vessels that connect arteries to veins.*

cardiac conduction system *The heart's electrical system, consisting of specialized cells within heart muscle that carry an electrical signal, which regulates the pumping of the heart.*

KEY TERMS CONTINUED

cardiac output *The output of blood by the heart per minute.*

cardiorespiratory system *The body system that includes the functions of the heart, blood vessels, circulation, and exchange of gases between the blood and the atmosphere.*

coronary arteries *The heart's own system of blood vessels.*

diastolic *The lowest pressure in the heart; relates to ventricular relaxation.*

gauze dressing *A woven, flexible, absorbent cloth applied to a wound.*

occlusive dressing *A petroleum-based dressing with a thin plastic film, designed to keep air and moisture from entering or escaping a wound.*

plasma *The yellowish, liquid part of blood.*

platelets *Tiny cell fragments in blood that aid in clotting.*

pulmonary artery *The artery that connects the heart to the lungs.*

pulse pressure *The difference between the diastolic and systolic pressures in the heart.*

pulse *The rhythmical beating of the heart.*

septum *The wall separating the left and right sides of the heart.*

shock *A potentially fatal physiological reaction usually characterized by significant drop in blood pressure, reduced blood circulation, and inadequate blood flow to the tissues; may occur in response to several conditions, including illness, injury, hemorrhage, and dehydration.*

standard precautions *Infection control guidelines designed to protect workers from exposure to disease spread by contact with blood or other bodily fluids.*

stroke volume *The amount of blood expelled through the ventricle with each beat.*

systolic *The highest pressure in the heart; correlates to ventricular contraction.*

target heart rate *The percentage of the maximum heart rate that is safe to reach during exercise.*

veins *Blood vessels that carry blood back to the heart.*

ventricles *The lower chambers of the heart.*

venules *The smallest of the veins.*

THE CARDIORESPIRATORY SYSTEM

The **cardiorespiratory system** includes the functions of the heart, blood vessels, circulation, and gas exchange between the blood and the atmosphere. The heart is responsible for pumping blood throughout the body through a complex system of pathways consisting of arteries, veins, and capillaries. Blood is enriched with oxygen when it passes through the lungs. As oxygen enters the bloodstream, carbon dioxide leaves it through the process called *respiration*.

THE CIRCULATORY SYSTEM

The circulatory system is the course taken by the blood through the arteries, capillaries, and veins, then back to the heart. The circulatory system uses blood to transport dissolved materials throughout the body. These include oxygen, carbon dioxide, nutrients, and waste. Oxygen from the lungs and nutrients from the digestive tract are transported to every cell in the body, allowing the continuation of cell metabolism. The circulatory system also picks up the waste products of cell metabolism and carries them to the lungs and

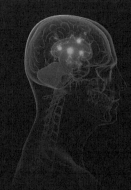

kidneys, where they can be expelled from the body. Without this important function, toxic substances would quickly build up in the body.

The Heart

The human circulatory system is organized into two major circulations. Each has its own pump, but both pumps are incorporated into a single organ, the heart. The two sides of the human heart are separated by partitions, the interatrial septum and the interventricular septum. Both septa are complete, so the two sides of the heart are anatomically and functionally separate pumping units. The right side of the heart pumps blood through the pulmonary circulation (the lungs). The left side of the heart pumps blood through the systemic circulation (the body).

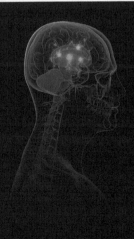

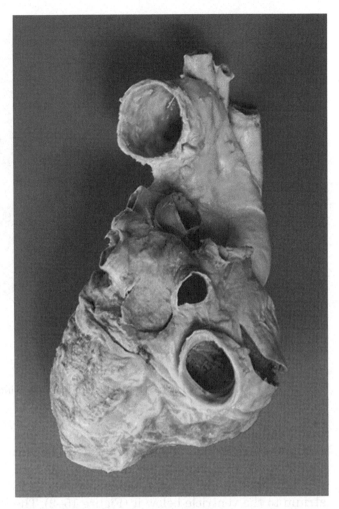

Figure 15–1 The human heart. Courtesy of Oak Ridge National Laboratory, Oak Ridge, TN.

The adult human heart is approximately the size of a closed fist. It is about 5 inches long and 3½ inches wide (Figure 15–1). It weighs just less than one pound and beats about 100,000 times each day. It pumps about 8,000 gallons of blood through 12,000 miles of vessels each day. Considering that the body is comprised of more than 100 trillion cells, all needing oxygen and nutrients, the heart is an amazing organ, and not to be taken for granted.

STRUCTURE OF THE HEART The human heart is primarily a shell with four chambers inside, each of which fills with blood. Two of these cavities are called **atria**. The other two are called **ventricles**. The two atria form the curved top of the heart. The ventricles meet at the bottom of the heart to form a pointed base that points toward the left side of the chest. The left ventricle contracts most forcefully, so the best place to feel the heart pumping is on the left side of the chest.

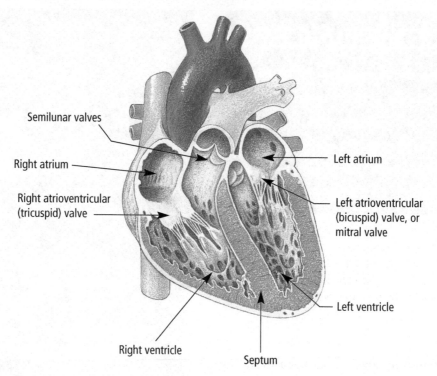

Semilunar valves

Right atrium

Right atrioventricular
(tricuspid) valve

Left atrium

Left atrioventricular
(bicuspid) valve, or
mitral valve

Left ventricle

Right ventricle

Septum

Figure 15–2 Human heart, showing valves and chambers.

The left side of the heart houses one atrium and one ventricle. The right side of the heart houses the others. A wall, the **septum**, separates the right and left sides of the heart. A valve connects each atrium to the ventricle below it (Figure 15–2). The mitral valve connects the left atrium with the left ventricle. The tricuspid valve connects the right atrium with the right ventricle.

The top of the heart connects to a few large blood vessels. The largest of these is the **aorta**, or main artery, which carries nutrient-rich blood away from the heart. Another important vessel, the **pulmonary artery**, connects the heart to the lungs as part of the pulmonary circulation system. The two largest veins that carry blood into the heart are the *superior vena cava* and the *inferior vena cava*. They are called "vena cava" because they are the "heart's veins." The superior is located near the top of the heart. The inferior is located beneath the superior.

On average, the heart muscle (also called the cardiac muscle) contracts and relaxes about 70 to 80 times per minute. As the cardiac muscle contracts, it pushes blood through the chambers and into the vessels. Nerves connected to the heart regulate the speed with which the muscle contracts. This is called **stroke volume**. The greater

the activity, the faster the heart will pump. The faster the heart pumps, the more oxygen and nutrients are carried throughout the body. This determines the **cardiac output**.

Located in the middle of the chest behind the breastbone, between the lungs, the heart rests in a moistened chamber called the pericardial cavity, which is contained within the ribcage. The diaphragm, a tough layer of muscle, lies below. As a result, the heart is well protected.

Blood

Blood is the only tissue that flows throughout the body. This liquid carries oxygen and nutrients to all parts of the body and transports waste products back to the lungs, kidneys, and liver for disposal. It is also an essential part of the immune system, crucial for fluid and temperature balance, a hydraulic fluid for certain functions, and a highway for hormonal messages.

Although blood appears to be red, it is actually composed of billions of cells in a yellowish liquid called **plasma** (Figure 15–3). The vast majority of these cells are red cells, which give the blood its red color. Besides the red cells, blood also contains several types of infection-fighting white

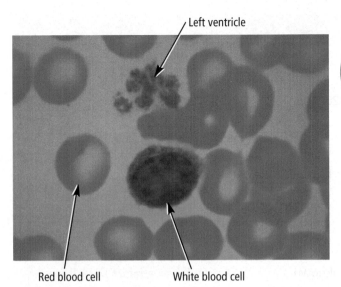

Left ventricle

Red blood cell   White blood cell

Figure 15–3 Photomicrograph of red blood cells with a white blood cell and a clump of platelets.

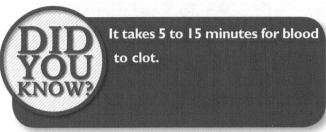

cells and tiny cell fragments, called **platelets**, that are essential for clotting.

All cells in the blood—red blood cells, all types of white blood cells, and platelets—are made in the bone marrow. This happens primarily in the flat bones of the body, such as the skull, the sternum, and the pelvis.

PLASMA Plasma is the river in which blood cells travel. It makes up 55% of blood's total volume. Plasma carries not only the blood cells but also nutrients (sugars, amino acids, fats, salts, minerals, etc.), waste products (CO_2, lactic acid, urea, etc.), antibodies, clotting proteins (called clotting factors), chemical messengers such as hormones, and proteins that help maintain the body's fluid balance.

RED BLOOD CELLS Most cells in the blood are red blood cells (erythrocytes), highly specialized cells that have been "stripped" of everything, including the nucleus, that might get in the way of doing their major job: transporting oxygen. The percentage of red blood cells in the total blood volume is called the *hematocrit*.

HEMOGLOBIN Red blood cells are filled with a special, red-colored molecule called hemoglobin. It picks up oxygen in areas where oxygen is abundant and releases it in tissues where the oxygen concentration is lowest.

WHITE BLOOD CELLS There are five distinct kinds of white blood cells: neutrophils, monocytes, lymphocytes, eosinophils, and basophils. Some of these specialized cells are able to change according to need and situations in the body. These cells can also leave the bloodstream, sliding out through the vessel walls to attack invaders at the site of an infection.

As an integral part of the immune system, white blood cells protect the body from numerous pathogens that can invade the body in many different ways. These pathways include ingestion, food, water, air, saliva, touch, bodily fluids, and sexual contact.

PLATELETS Platelets are fragments of a much larger cell, the megakaryocyte, which stays in the bone marrow after it differentiates and matures from the stem cell. Platelets leave the bone marrow and circulate throughout the body. When stimulated by substances from damaged tissue, the platelets release agents necessary to help initiate the clotting sequence and protect the integrity of the vasculature. Table 15–1 summarizes the types of blood cells found in the body, the life expectancy of each type of blood cell, and the function of each.

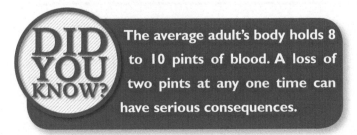

Table 15–1 The Life Spans and Functions of Blood Cells

BLOOD CELL	LIFE SPAN IN BLOOD	FUNCTION
Red blood cell (Erythrocyte)	120 days	O_2 and CO_2 transport
Neutrophil	7 hours	Immune defenses
Eosinophil	Unknown	Defense against parasites
Basophil	Unknown	Inflammatory response
Monocyte	3 days	Immune surveillance (precursor of tissue macrophage)
B Lymphocyte	Unknown	Antibody production (precursor of plasma cells)
T Lymphocyte	Unknown	Cellular immune response
Platelets	7–8 days	Blood clotting

Blood Vessels

Blood vessels are hollow tubes running throughout the body, through which the blood circulates. There are five types of blood vessels: arteries, arterioles, veins, venules, and capillaries. Besides circulating blood, the blood vessels provide two important means of measuring vital health statistics, pulse and blood pressure.

ARTERIES **Arteries** carry blood from the heart to all the organs and cells in the body (Figure 15–4). Arteries have muscular walls that allow them to grow larger (dilate) or smaller (constrict) as needed. The largest artery in the body is called the *aorta*. The aorta runs from the chest into the abdomen and receives blood directly from the powerful left ventricle of the heart.

Arteries decrease in size the closer they are to the cells they are nourishing. Very small arteries are known as **arterioles**. Table 15–2 lists the principal arteries and the areas of the body each serves.

VEINS **Veins** carry blood back to the heart. Veins have thinner walls than arteries and contain numerous one-way valves that help keep blood moving toward the heart (Figure 15–5). Deep veins in the lower limbs are surrounded by large muscle groups that compress the deep veins when the muscles contract. Compression of

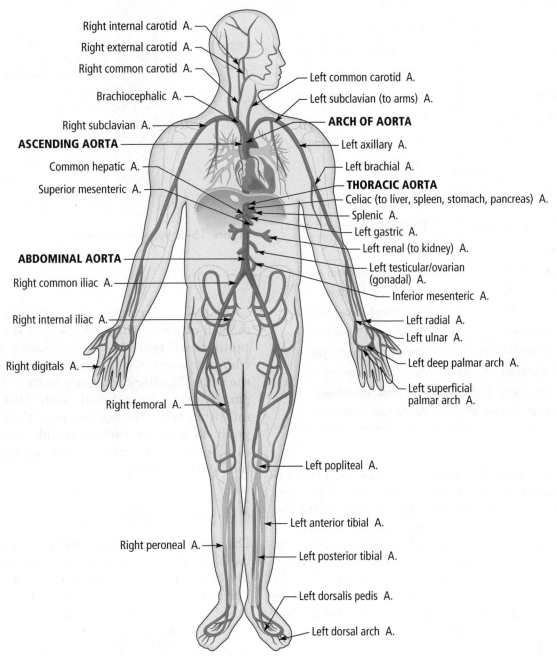

Right internal carotid A.
Right external carotid A.
Right common carotid A.
Brachiocephalic A.
Right subclavian A.
ASCENDING AORTA
Common hepatic A.
Superior mesenteric A.
ABDOMINAL AORTA
Right common iliac A.
Right internal iliac A.
Right digitals A.
Right femoral A.
Right peroneal A.

Left common carotid A.
Left subclavian (to arms) A.
ARCH OF AORTA
Left axillary A.
Left brachial A.
THORACIC AORTA
Celiac (to liver, spleen, stomach, pancreas) A.
Splenic A.
Left gastric A.
Left renal (to kidney) A.
Left testicular/ovarian (gonadal) A.
Inferior mesenteric A.
Left radial A.
Left ulnar A.
Left deep palmar arch A.
Left superficial palmar arch A.
Left popliteal A.
Left anterior tibial A.
Left posterior tibial A.
Left dorsalis pedis A.
Left dorsal arch A.

Figure 15–4 Arterial distribution.

Table 15–2 Principal Arteries

PRINCIPAL ARTERIES	AREA(S) SERVED
Common Carotid	Head and Face
Internal carotid	Brain
External *carotid*	Face (*pulse point*)
Vertebral	Spinal column and brain
Brachiocephalic	Right arm, head, and shoulder
Subclavian	Shoulder
Axillary	Axilla area
Brachial	Upper arm and elbow area (*pulse point*)
Radial	Arm, wrist (*pulse point*)
Thoracic aorta	Chest cavity
Celiac	Liver, spleen, stomach, and pancreas
Splenic	Spleen
Hepatic	Liver
Superior mesenteric	Small intestines and colon
Renal	Kidney
Common iliac	Lower abdominal area
Internal iliac	Pelvis and bladder
External iliac	Groin and lower leg
Femoral	Groin (*pulse point*)
Popliteal	Knee area (*pulse point*)
Anterior tibialis	Anterior lower leg
Posterior tibialis	Posterior lower leg
Dorsalis pedis	Ankle (*pulse point*)

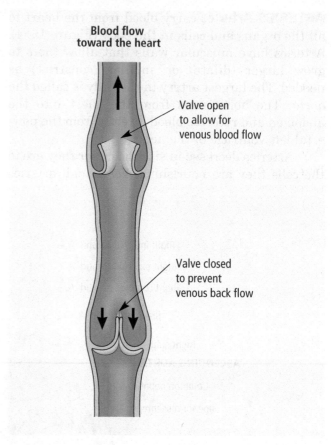

Blood flow toward the heart

Valve open to allow for venous blood flow

Valve closed to prevent venous back flow

Figure 15–5 Valves of the veins.

veins by muscular contractions in the extremities helps propel blood toward the heart and increases venous return. This action assists the heart in pumping blood throughout the body.

The largest veins are called the superior vena cava and inferior vena cava. These veins bring blood from the upper and lower body directly into the right atrium (Figure 15–6). The smallest veins are known as **venules**. Table 15–3 lists the principal veins and the areas of the body each serves.

CAPILLARIES Arteries and veins are connected to each other by tiny, microscopic vessels called capillaries (Figure 15–7). **Capillaries** are responsible for transferring oxygen and nutrients to the cells. Capillary walls are so thin that oxygen passes from the arterial blood through them into the cells in organs and tissues. Waste products such as carbon dioxide pass into the capillaries to be carried back by the veins to the heart and lungs.

Coronary Arteries

The heart requires large amounts of oxygen to do its job well, but it does not get that oxygen from the blood that is passing through its chambers. The heart has its own system of blood vessels, called **coronary arteries**, that are located around the heart muscle to provide blood and oxygen to all parts of the heart (Figure 15–8).

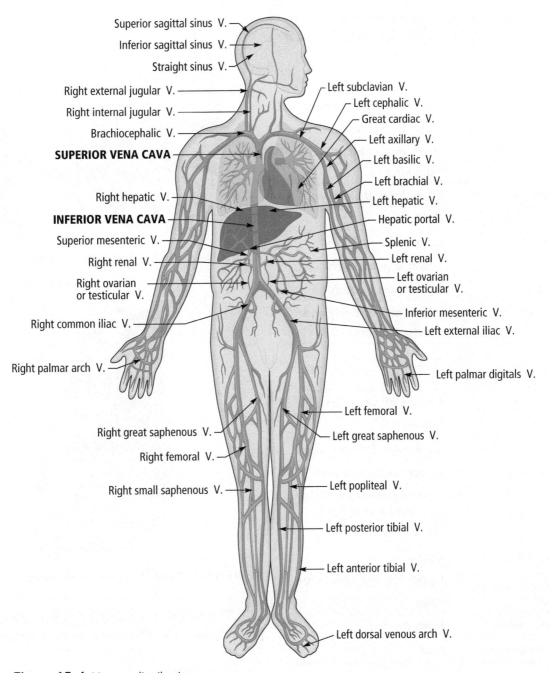

Figure 15–6 Venous distribution.

There are two primary coronary arteries, which branch off into smaller vessels. The right coronary artery feeds the right atrium and ventricle and the bottom of the left ventricle. The left main coronary artery supplies blood to the rest of the heart. This artery has two main branches, the left anterior descending and the circumflex. These quickly branch into smaller vessels.

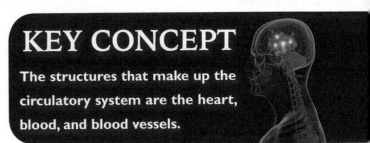

KEY CONCEPT

The structures that make up the circulatory system are the heart, blood, and blood vessels.

Table 15–3   Principal Veins

PRINCIPAL VEINS	AREA(S) SERVED
External jugular	Face
Vertebral	Spinal column and brain
Subclavian	Shoulder and upper limbs
Brachiocephalic	Right side of head and shoulder
Left cephalic	Shoulder and axillary
Axillary	*Axilla area*
Brachial	*Upper arm*
Radial	Lower arm and wrist
Superior vena cava	Upper part of body
Inferior vena cava	Lower part of body and abdominal area
Hepatic	Liver
Renal	Kidney
Hepatic portal	Organs of digestion
Splenic	Spleen
Superior mesenteric	Small intestine and colon
Common iliac 　Internal iliac 　External iliac	Lower abdominal and pelvis, bladder, and reproductive organs, Lower limbs
Great saphenous	Upper leg
Femoral	Upper leg and groin area
Popliteal	Knee
Posterior tibialis	Posterior leg
Dorsal venous arch	Foot

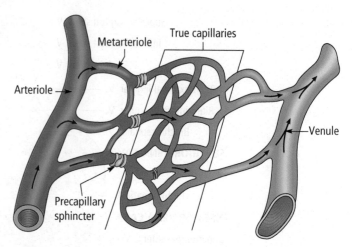

Figure 15–7 Capillary bed connecting an arteriole with a venule.

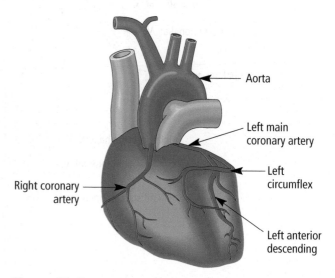

Figure 15–8 Coronary arteries of the heart.

THE HEART'S CONDUCTION SYSTEM

The heart is an electromechanical pump. The **cardiac conduction system**, made up of specialized cells within the heart muscle tissue, carries electrical signals, in a properly timed sequence, to muscle cells throughout the heart. These signals trigger the muscles to contract and thereby pump blood throughout the body. The signals must reach each chamber in an organized, controlled manner in order to maintain rhythmic contractions.

The heart's conduction system must function properly to make the heart pump effectively.

Blood Pressure

When the heart pumps blood into the arteries, the surge of blood filling the vessels creates pressure against the vessel walls. This pressure is measured in two aspects, **systolic** and **diastolic**. The systolic is the highest pressure and corresponds to ventricle contraction. The diastolic is the lowest pressure and represents ventricle relaxation.

The average systolic pressure in an adult is 120 mm/Hg (millimeters of mercury). The average diastolic pressure in an adult is 80 mm/Hg. The blood pressure would be recorded as 120/80. **Pulse pressure**, a figure derived from blood pressure, is the difference between the systolic and diastolic pressures. If blood pressure is 120/80, the pulse pressure would be 40.

Athletes, especially those who do prolonged aerobic activity, may have blood pressure readings considerably lower than the average because their hearts are stronger than normal and more efficient, using less effort to circulate the blood throughout the body.

Pulse

Pulse, the rhythmical beating of the heart, can be felt at different points on the body. The pulse is created by the alternating expansion and contraction of an artery as blood flows through it. The pulse can be felt in seven areas (Figure 15–9):

- Brachial artery—located at the crook of the elbow, along the inner border of the biceps muscle
- Common carotid artery—found in the neck, along the front margin of the sternocleidomastoid muscle, near the lower edge of the thyroid cartilage

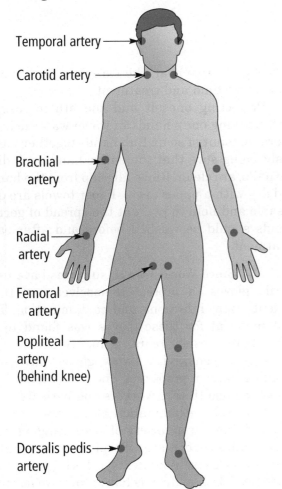

Figure 15–9 Points on the body where a pulse can be felt.

- Femoral artery—in the groin (inguinal) area
- Dorsalis pedis artery—on the anterior surface of the foot, below the ankle joint
- Popliteal artery—behind the knee
- Radial artery—at the wrist, on the same side as the thumb
- Temporal artery—slightly above the outer edge of the eye

The pulse rate of an athlete may be significantly slower than the average. As explained earlier, as the heart becomes stronger with aerobic activity, it becomes more efficient and thus does not have to pump as often.

TARGET HEART RATE **Target heart rate** is expressed as a range of percentages of the maximum heart rate that is safe to reach during exercise. For most healthy people, the American Heart Association recommends an exercise target heart rate ranging from 50 to 85% of the maximum heart rate, which is normally calculated as the number 220 minus one's age. Target heart rate is a sliding scale that decreases with age (Figure 15–10).

Target heart rate is a tool for measuring cardiovascular exercise, for athletes and nonathletes alike. Maintaining target heart rate for a period of 15 to 30 minutes each day will produce health benefits. It is important to note that some blood-pressure medications such as beta-blockers and diuretics helps to lower blood pressure and pulse rate. The maximum heart rate and therefore the target rate zone will therefore be affected. Individuals taking these medications should consult with their doctor prior to starting an exercise program.

Sudden Death in Competitive Athletes

An athlete who suddenly collapse during practice or competition may be the victim of a previously undiagnosed heart disease. In most competitive athletes under the age of 35, this is the result of *sudden cardiac disease (SCD)*. According to the American Heart Association, sudden death in athletes occur at a rate of 2.6 per 100,000 athletes.

SCD is a very real public health issue for both athletes and non-athletes. SCD in a young individual is devastating. Appropriate measures of

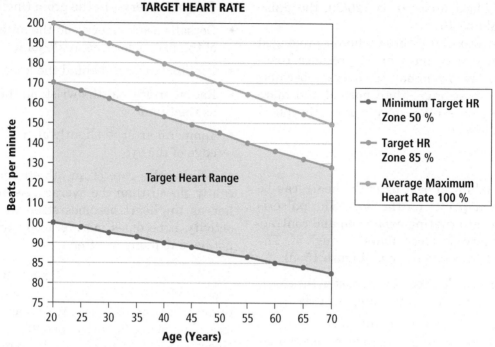

Figure 15–10 Target heart rate is calculated as follows:
Step 1: 220 − your age = your maximum heart rate (MHR)
Step 2: MHR × .50 = your lowest target heart rate
Step 3: MHR × .85 = your highest target heart rate.
Courtesy of the American Heart Association.

prevention and treatment are critical. However, based on the best available evidence, it is evident that measures conclusively effective in reducing athletic SCD remain unknown.

The best available data indicate that the total number of athletic deaths is relatively small. Proven strategies to prevent athletic sudden death are not currently available. Athletic trainers and their staff, along with the coaching staff, must be well trained in CPR and AED administration.

BODY SUBSTANCE ISOLATION

Open cuts and wounds are common in athletics. During care and treatment of these types of injuries, maintaining body substance isolation is critical to the health of both the athletic training staff and the athlete.

Protective equipment that the certified athletic trainer will use in the treatment of wounds and injuries includes sterile gloves, protective glasses, and a mask. The type of injury and wound care needed will dictate which of these barrier devices, if not all, will be used. Caregivers should always protect themselves first. After donning the proper protective gear, the caregiver can concentrate on first aid and treatment.

Protecting oneself and the athlete begins with washing one's hands in warm water using a liberal amount of soap. Rub hands together vigorously, being sure that the entire hand, including the nails, are clean. Rinse all soap from the hands and dry with a paper towel. Paper towels are disposable and help to prevent the spread of germs. Hands should be washed before and after each treatment.

GLOVES Since World War II, surgeons have used sterile gloves to protect themselves and their patients from infections and contamination. The best material for these gloves was found to be latex. Latex resists tears, is highly elastic, and offers good sensitivity. Latex gloves have outstanding barrier properties and are excellent for protecting health care workers and patients.

Disposable examination gloves are inexpensive and come in a variety of sizes, ranging from extra small to extra large. People with latex allergies can purchase nonlatex synthetic gloves as a substitute. Both materials have proven to be effective against bloodborne pathogens. Gloves *must* be worn when treating any injury involving bodily fluids, most notably blood.

Gloves must be discarded properly so that secondary exposure does not occur. Gloves should be taken off inside out, so as to trap any pathogens within the glove barrier. They should then be discarded in a garbage can lined with a red biohazard bag. Figures 15–11A through 15–11G show the proper procedure for application and removal of gloves.

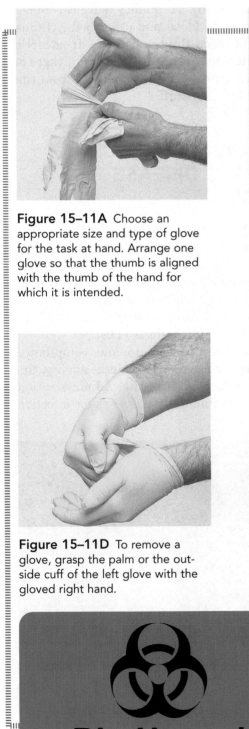

Figure 15–11A Choose an appropriate size and type of glove for the task at hand. Arrange one glove so that the thumb is aligned with the thumb of the hand for which it is intended.

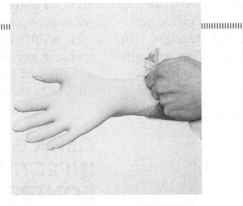

Figure 15–11B Grasp the front of the cuff with one hand, while inserting the other hand into the glove. Be sure to place each finger within its appropriate section. Pull at the cuff to ensure that the glove is completely applied to the hand.

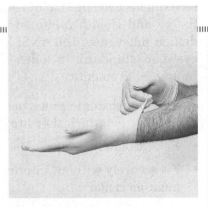

Figure 15–11C Repeat the process for the other hand.

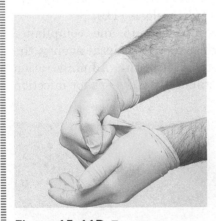

Figure 15–11D To remove a glove, grasp the palm or the outside cuff of the left glove with the gloved right hand.

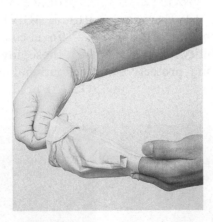

Figure 15–11E Pull the left glove toward the fingertips. The glove should turn inside out as it is removed.

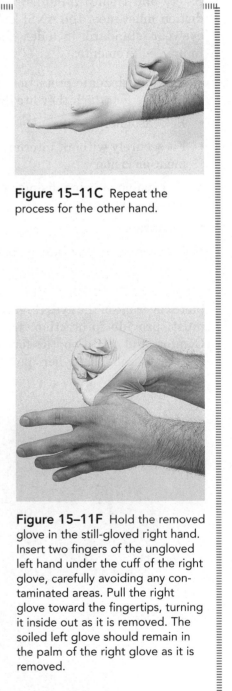

Figure 15–11F Hold the removed glove in the still-gloved right hand. Insert two fingers of the ungloved left hand under the cuff of the right glove, carefully avoiding any contaminated areas. Pull the right glove toward the fingertips, turning it inside out as it is removed. The soiled left glove should remain in the palm of the right glove as it is removed.

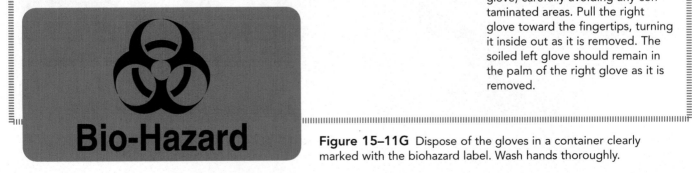

Bio-Hazard

Figure 15–11G Dispose of the gloves in a container clearly marked with the biohazard label. Wash hands thoroughly.

PROTECTIVE EYEWEAR In 1989, the American National Standards Institute (ANSI) developed standards for protective eyewear. The ANSI Z87.1 standard sets forth requirements for the design, construction, testing, and use of eye-protection devices, including standards for impact and penetration resistance. All safety glasses, goggles, and face shields used by employees under Occupational Safety and Health Administration (OSHA) jurisdiction must meet the ANSI Z87.1 standard. The eyewear standard includes the following minimum requirements:

- Provide adequate protection against the hazards for which they are designed
- Be reasonably comfortable
- Fit securely without interfering with movement or vision
- Be capable of being disinfected if necessary and be easy to clean
- Be durable
- Fit over, or incorporate, prescription eyewear

The primary purpose of using protective eyewear while treating injuries is to provide complete coverage of the eyes (Figure 15–12). Eyewear must provide protection from bodily fluids. Comfort and quality optics for visibility are other factors to consider when purchasing protective eyewear.

SURGICAL MASK The surgical mask, first used at the beginning of the twentieth century, was initially introduced to protect the patient. It was believed that the surgical mask would prevent harmful microorganisms from entering the patient's open wound. Surgical masks now are designed to protect both the patient and the caregiver (Figure 15–13). A quality surgical mask reduces exposure to blood and other bodily fluids with a 99% filtration fluid resistance. In athletic training, surgical masks should be worn if there is a danger of infectious disease spreading from the athlete to the training staff.

OSHA GUIDELINES FOR INFECTIOUS DISEASE CONTROL

The Centers for Disease Control and Prevention (CDC) is a federal organization that monitors outbreaks of infections and advises affected groups on how to handle the situation and control the spread of disease. The CDC has issued many advisories regarding common disease outbreaks such as hepatitis B (HBV) and tuberculosis (TB).

To encourage attention to and compliance with these advisories, another federal agency, the Occupational Safety and Health Administration (OSHA), produces standards and rules for infection

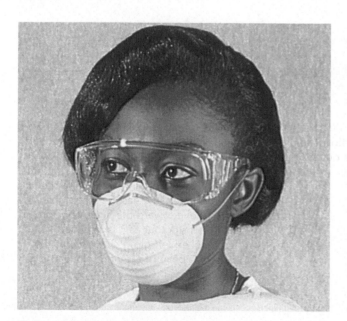

Figure 15–12 Protective glasses guard against splashes.

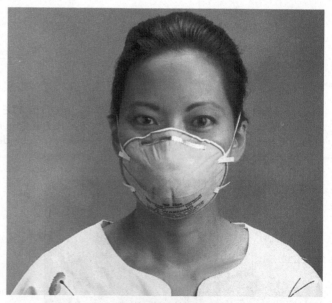

Figure 15–13 A mask provides protection from airborne diseases. Courtesy of 3M Health Care, St. Paul, MN.

Table 15–4 OSHA 1910.1030 (29 C.F.R. §1910.1030) Occupational Exposure to Bloodborne Pathogens

Intent: To eliminate or minimize occupational exposure to blood or other potentially infectious materials.

Applicable to: All employees with potential for occupational exposure to blood or other potentially infectious material.

Requirements:

- Exposure control plan
- Exposure determination
- Methods of compliance
  Universal precautions
  Engineering controls
  Work practice controls
  Personal protective equipment
  Housekeeping/waste disposal
  Hepatitis B vaccination
  Signs and labels on hazardous materials
  Training
- Postexposure follow-up

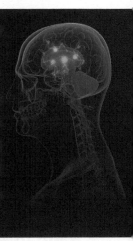

KEY CONCEPT

Standard precautions were developed to prevent contact with the blood of patients who may have infections that can be spread through bodily fluids and blood. All patients should be assumed to be infectious for bloodborne diseases.

control practice by medical care workers. One of the first published, in 1992, was the Bloodborne Pathogens rule (29 C.F.R. §1910.1030), which set out very clear provisions for employers regarding infection control practices. Table 15–4 outlines the rules and regulations of this standard.

Standard Precautions

Standard precautions are infection-control guidelines designed to protect workers from exposure to diseases spread by blood and certain bodily fluids. The Laboratory Centre for Disease Control, Health Canada, and the United States Centers for Disease Control have developed the strategy of standard precautions to prevent contact with patient blood and body fluids. Standard precautions stress that all patients should be assumed to be infectious for bloodborne diseases such as AIDS and hepatitis B, and require the following:

- Wash hands before and after all patient or specimen contact.
- Treat the blood of all patients as potentially infectious.

- Treat all linen soiled with blood or body secretions as potentially infectious.
- Wear gloves if contact with blood or bodily fluids is possible.
- Immediately place used syringes in a nearby impermeable container; do not recap or manipulate needles or sharps in any way.
- Wear protective eyewear and a mask if splatter with blood or body fluids is possible.
- Wear a mask if there is risk of infection by TB or other airborne organisms (HIV is not airborne).

WOUND CARE

The care of any wound requires proper treatment by the health care provider. Anyone giving aid to an injured athlete must first be protected from contamination and the risk of injury. The following principles should be followed when treating any wound.

Irrigate the wound with clean, cool water to wash away any foreign particles in the wound itself. Gentle washing with a mild soap (superficial cuts only) will help to control infection. All foreign particles must be removed, or infection will result. If this is not possible, the athlete must be referred to a doctor for additional treatment.

Minor cuts and abrasions should be washed, dried with a sterile gauze sponge, and treated with a first-aid cream to prevent infection. A dry, sterile bandage should then be applied to protect the wound and keep it clean. The bandage should be large enough to cover the entire injury. Be careful not to secure the bandage too tightly. A clean bandage should be applied daily. If the bandage gets wet or soaked through with drainage, replace it. The athlete should check for signs of infection regularly. These include redness, swelling, increased pain, oozing of pus and increase in body temperature. If a red streak is noticed going up the arm or leg, blood poisoning is possible. Immediate medical attention should be obtained.

The athlete should be instructed on how to clean and manage the wound. Proper care after the initial treatment is crucial. If the athlete allows the wound to become infected, healing time will be significantly longer and scarring worse.

Bandages and Dressings

Proper bandaging and dressing of a wound will ensure proper healing and infection control. The *dressing* is the material that is placed directly on the wound. It must be large enough to cover the injury, and sterile to prevent infection. The *bandage* is the material that holds the dressing in place.

The two primary types of dressing are gauze and occlusive. The **gauze dressing** comes in many different sizes and is made from cotton. It is woven into a flexible, absorbent cloth. The common sizes of gauze dressings are squares, 2 × 2 inches, 3 × 3 inches, and 4 × 4 inches (Figure 15–14). Special trauma dressings come in much larger sizes to accommodate injuries to the abdomen and chest.

An **occlusive dressing** is designed to prevent air and moisture from entering or escaping the wound. These dressings are often impregnated with petroleum gel or covered with a thin plastic film.

The bandage that holds the dressing in place should be large enough to conform to the wound. It

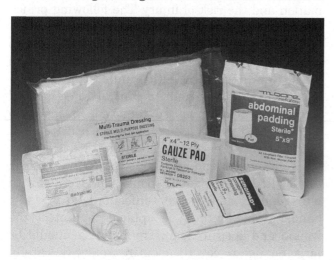

Figure 15–14 Dressings come in an assortment of sizes to accommodate different wounds.

must not be applied too tightly; just loose enough to allow any swelling that might occur. A bandage that is too tight may interfere with circulation.

There are many different types of bandages on the market today. Talk to your sports medicine representative about the best choices available for different applications. Follow these guidelines when applying bandages:

- Select the proper size and material for the injury.

- Remove anything that interferes with bandaging, such as rings, watches, earrings, and bracelets.

- Never reuse a dressing or bandage. Use only sterile material.

- Apply the bandage snugly, but not too tightly.

- Leave fingers and toes exposed (if possible) so that circulation can be checked.

BLEEDING

The three basic types of bleeding are arterial, venous, and capillary (Figure 15–15). All types of bleeding require immediate care and prompt control to prevent shock, infection, and possible loss of life. Bleeding may be from an artery, a major blood vessel that carries blood from the heart throughout the body. It may be from a vein, which carries blood back to the heart, or from a capillary, the smallest of the body's blood vessels. Chapter 22 addresses internal bleeding.

Arterial Bleeding

Arterial bleeding from a punctured or severed artery can be severe. A cut artery issues bright red blood from the wound in distinct spurts or pulses that correspond to the rhythm of the heartbeat. Because the blood in the arteries is under high pressure, an individual can lose a large volume of blood in a short period when damage to an artery occurs. Therefore, arterial bleeding is the most serious type. If not controlled promptly, it can be fatal. Follow these steps when arterial bleeding occurs:

- Treat the athlete for shock (described later in this chapter).

- Apply direct pressure; find and use pressure points as needed (Figure 15–9).

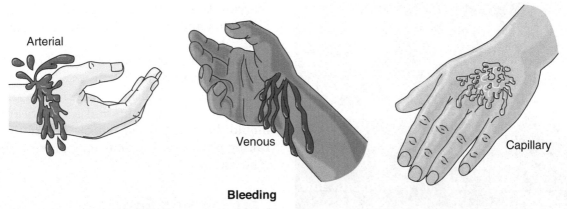

Bleeding

Figure 15–15 Arterial bleeding is bright red and spurts; venous bleeding is dark red and flows; capillary bleeding oozes.

- Activate the EMS system immediately.
- A tourniquet should be used only if bleeding cannot be controlled by direct pressure or the use of pressure points, or if death is imminent. Application of a tourniquet may result in loss of the limb. Write down the exact time the tourniquet was applied. Do not remove or loosen a tourniquet without a doctor's order.

Venous Bleeding

Venous bleeding is a result of the rupture of one or more veins. It is less severe than arterial bleeding, but can still be profuse. Blood flow will be steady, unlike the pulsating arterial flow. Because veins return oxygen-depleted blood to the lungs, the bleeding will appear bluish-red. Veins are closer to the surface than arteries, and therefore it is easier to control venous bleeding. The body's blood-clotting mechanism is also more effective during venous

than arterial bleeding. Direct pressure and compression bandaging are effective ways to manage venous bleeding. Additional layers of dressing may be needed on such a wound. The athlete will need to see a doctor immediately.

Capillary Bleeding

Bleeding from capillaries is slow and typically oozes. This type of bleeding occurs with scratches, minor cuts, and abrasions. Blood clotting normally occurs quickly. Because this type of bleeding is slow, the risk of infection is higher than with arterial or venous bleeding. Bandaging the wound with a sterile dressing will stop capillary bleeding and help prevent infection.

SHOCK

Shock is a precursor to death. Prompt recognition, treatment, and control are crucial for the survival of the victim. Shock occurs when the circulation system fails to send blood to all parts of the body. With shock, areas of the body are deprived of oxygen because blood flow or blood volume is too low to meet the body's needs. The result is damage to the limbs, lungs, heart, and brain. There are eight types of shock.

Hemorrhagic Shock

Hemorrhagic shock is loss of blood from an injury. The injury may be internal or external. Without enough blood in the system, blood pressure falls, and adequate oxygen is unavailable to the body. In athletics this can be caused by severe blunt

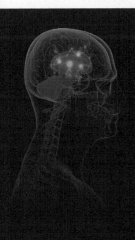

KEY CONCEPT

The three basic types of bleeding are arterial, venous, and capillary. Arterial bleeding can be severe. Venous bleeding is often less severe than arterial bleeding, but can often be profuse. Capillary bleeding is slow and can increase the risk of infection.

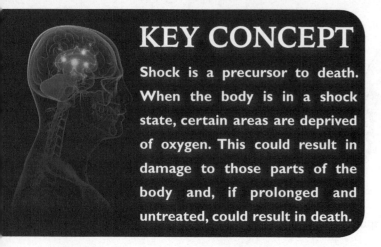

KEY CONCEPT

Shock is a precursor to death. When the body is in a shock state, certain areas are deprived of oxygen. This could result in damage to those parts of the body and, if prolonged and untreated, could result in death.

trauma, or internal injuries such as a ruptured spleen. It is uncommon to see severe external bleeding, resulting in hemorrhagic shock, in sports.

Respiratory Shock

Respiratory shock occurs when the lungs are unable to supply enough oxygen to the blood. It can be caused by disease, illness, or pulmonary contusion (bruising of the lungs). Injuries involving high velocity are more likely to cause pulmonary contusion, which occurs in response to passage of a shock wave through the tissue. Respiratory shock causes dyspnea (difficulty in breathing) and an elevated respiratory rate, leading to a collapse of the cardiorespiratory system. Without oxygen, major organs in the body can be damaged just minutes after symptoms appear. Hypoxemia (low oxygen in your blood) can cause hypoxia (low oxygen in the tissues) when the blood doesn't carry enough oxygen to your tissues to meet your body's needs. *Hypoxia* is sometimes used to describe both conditions.

Neurogenic Shock

Neurogenic shock is the loss of vascular control by the nervous system. This results from disruption of autonomic nervous system control over vasoconstriction. Under normal conditions, the autonomic nervous system keeps the muscles of the veins and arteries partially contracted. At the onset of most forms of shock, further constriction is signaled. The vascular muscles cannot maintain this contraction indefinitely. A number of factors, including increased fluid loss, central nervous system trauma, or emotional shock, can override the autonomic nervous system control. The veins and arteries immediately dilate, drastically expanding the volume of the circulatory system and thereby reducing blood pressure; this is called vasodilation.

Neurogenic shock can occur with any injury. An athlete who has suffered a significant injury should be treated for shock before it occurs. Taking proper precautions may prevent the onset of shock.

Cardiogenic Shock

Cardiogenic shock is caused by inadequate functioning of the heart. It can occur when the heart has sustained damage through disease, infection, or injury. It is extremely rare in athletics. However, athletes with previously undiagnosed heart defects or conditions may develop a sudden myocardial infarction, or heart attack.

Metabolic Shock

Metabolic shock occurs when there is a severe loss of bodily fluids, which may result from severe diarrhea, vomiting, or disease. In athletics, severe dehydration can cause metabolic shock. Chapter 25 discusses heat-related illnesses.

Anaphylactic Shock

Anaphylactic shock is caused by a severe *allergic reaction*. An allergic reaction is an exaggerated response by the body's immune system to what would otherwise be a harmless substance. Allergic or hypersensitivity reactions vary from annoying symptoms, such as itchy eyes and runny nose, to a life-threatening anaphylactic shock response, which may result in death from circulatory collapse or respiratory failure.

Some people are hypersensitive to insect stings, medications, and certain foods and food additives such as sulfites. Anyone who has had a serious allergic reaction should take the necessary precautions to avoid all future contact with the offending substance. All allergenic foods and medications should be avoided, as along with any drugs in the same class or with a similar chemical composition. A Medic Alert bracelet warning of the allergy should be worn.

Many persons who have a known sensitivity keep an *anaphylaxis kit* in their possession at all times. This kit usually contains epinephrine (adrenaline) and instructions on how to use this medication to combat allergic reactions.

A person suffering an extreme allergic reaction should be taken to the hospital as soon as possible, even if the symptoms seem to pass. Secondary reactions may occur up to several hours later.

Septic Shock

Septic shock is a life-threatening reaction to a severe infection. During septic shock, the body tissues and organs do not get enough blood and oxygen. Vital organs, such as the brain, heart, kidneys, and liver, may not function properly or may fail completely. In severe infections, germs make harmful toxins that can cause fluid to leak from blood vessels out into the tissues. These toxins may also prevent the heart from beating strongly enough. Together, these reactions lower blood pressure. If blood pressure falls too low, the body and its organs become deprived of oxygen.

In athletics, it is important to treat all wounds to prevent infection. An infection that does occur must be monitored closely so that it does not spread systemically. The symptoms of a systemic reaction may include fever, elevated breathing and heart rate, and dizziness. Septic shock is a medical emergency that requires treatment in the hospital.

Psychogenic Shock

Psychogenic shock is a physiological response to fear, stress, or emotional crisis that causes a person to faint. This type of shock is caused by a sudden temporary dilation of the blood vessels that reduces the normal volume of blood to the brain. This temporary condition will correct itself as soon as vascular control returns to normal and the individual regains consciousness.

Signs and Symptoms of Shock

The general signs and symptoms of shock are:

- Restlessness and anxiety
- Weak and rapid pulse
- Cold and clammy skin
- Profuse sweating
- Face that becomes pale and may eventually become cyanotic (blue) around the mouth
- Shallow respirations
- Dull, lusterless eyes with dilated pupils
- Thirst
- Nausea and vomiting
- Blood pressure that falls gradually and steadily
- Loss of consciousness

There are exceptions to this list—particularly anaphylactic shock, which has significantly different symptoms.

Shock may not cause all of these signs. If the person has been seriously injured, always be alert for the possibility or onset of shock. Treat for shock before it happens.

General Care and Treatment for Shock

The care for and treatment of shock are critical for the victim's well-being. The general guidelines for emergency handling of shock are:

- Activate the EMS system so help can arrive quickly. Call 911 immediately.
- Maintain a clear airway so breathing is not impaired.
- Control all bleeding.
- Elevate extremities 12 inches to help control swelling.
- Splint fractures, and elevate if well stabilized.
- Avoid rough and excessive handling that may cause additional injury.
- Prevent loss of body heat. If possible, a blanket should be placed under and upon the victim.
- In general, keep the victim in a supine position. A person complaining of chest pain may be more comfortable in a semi-reclining position.
- Do not give the victim anything to eat or drink. Any ingestion may result in choking or vomiting, which can cause additional problems.
- If you suspect that the person is having an allergic reaction, and you have access to an

epinephrine autoinjector and use it according to instructions.

- Record vital signs, such as pulse, blood pressure, and respiration rate, every five minutes. This will give the EMS personnel important data that can be used in the care of the patient.

- Constantly reassure the victim. Keeping the victim calm and reassured will help minimize the effects of shock until help arrives.

The goal in treating shock is to keep the victim from getting worse. Proper care, and reassuring the victim, will help meet this objective.

CONCLUSION

The cardiorespiratory system is responsible for the function of the heart, blood vessels, circulation, and breathing. The heart pumps oxygen-rich blood through the body to the capillaries by way of the arteries. Blood is returned to the heart from the capillaries through veins. When the heart pumps blood into the arteries, the surge of blood filling the vessels creates pressure against the vessel walls. This pressure is called the systolic and diastolic pressure. The rhythmic beating of the heart felt at different points on the body, called the pulse, is created by the alternating expansion and contraction of an artery as blood flows through it.

Anyone who works with athletes must always take preventive measures for protection against bloodborne pathogens and other diseases. Standard precautions are infection-control guidelines designed to protect workers from exposure to diseases spread by blood and certain bodily fluids. These precautions include the use of appropriate protective equipment such as gloves, protective eyewear, and masks or respirators. Different injuries and wound care will dictate which of these barrier devices, if not all, should be used. Caregivers should always protect themselves first.

There are three basic types of bleeding: arterial, venous, and capillary. All types of bleeding require immediate care to prevent shock and infection. Prompt control of bleeding is essential in avoiding shock and loss of life. Shock is a precursor to death; prompt recognition, treatment, and control are crucial for the victim's survival.

REVIEW QUESTIONS

1. Describe the importance of the cardiorespiratory system.
2. What is the difference between blood pressure and pulse?
3. How does blood circulate throughout the body?
4. What is the difference between a vein and an artery?
5. What is SCD?
6. What is the immediate treatment for SCD?
7. Describe the personal protective equipment a certified athletic trainer should use.
8. What two types of disposable examination gloves are available?
9. What is the ANSI standard for protective eyewear?
10. What are standard precautions?
11. What guidelines should be followed when treating any wound?
12. What guidelines should be followed when applying bandages?
13. Explain the differences between capillary, venous, and arterial bleeding.
14. Why is shock a precursor to death?
15. Name and describe the eight types of shock.
16. List the signs of shock.
17. How does one care for and treat shock?

PROJECTS AND ACTIVITIES

1. Create a matching exercise using the words in the Key Terms list. Include an answer key.
2. Take your blood pressure. Is it in the normal range? What is your pulse pressure?
3. Draw a picture of the human body indicating the various pressure points.
4. Visit your local EMS center. Ask them to show you the different types of dressings and bandages they use in the field. Write a summary of what you learned.
5. Create a quiz for the section on shock. Ask your teacher if you may give the quiz to the class.

LEARNING LINKS

- For more facts, interesting information, and a review of the circulatory system, visit http://www.innerbody.com.
- There are many websites related to the circulatory system. Do a search and share your favorite sites with your classmates.
- Visit the website of the Centers for Disease Control and Prevention and learn more about standard precautions and personal protection: http://www.cdc.gov

16

The Bones and Soft Tissues

Courtesy of Photdisc

OBJECTIVES

Upon completion of this chapter, the reader should be able to:

- Explain the difference between the axial and appendicular skeleton
- Define the functions of the skeletal system
- Describe the difference between long, short, and flat bones
- Define the six types of fractures
- Explain the difference between skeletal, smooth, and cardiac muscle
- Explain how muscle strains occur
- Explain how to treat muscle strains
- Describe the function of a nerve cell
- Explain the function of the nervous system
- Explain nerve injuries and their treatment
- List the different types of soft tissue injuries
- Explain how the body responds to injuries

KEY TERMS

abrasion *An injury that occurs when several layers of skin are torn loose or totally removed.*

acetylcholine *The chemical released when a nerve impulse is transmitted.*

action potential *The electric change occurring across the membrane of a nerve or muscle cell during transmission of a nerve impulse.*

afferent neuron *A nerve that carries nerve impulses from the periphery to the central nervous system; also known as a sensory neuron.*

angiogenesis *The formation of new blood vessels.*

KEY TERMS CONTINUED

antagonist *A muscle whose action opposes the action of another muscle.*

appendicular skeleton *The bones of the pelvis and shoulder girdles, and limbs.*

avulsion *An injury in which layers of the skin are torn off completely or only a flap of skin remains.*

axial skeleton *The bones of the head and trunk (skull, spine, sternum, and ribs).*

belly *The central part of a muscle.*

bursitis *Inflammation of the bursa (a padded cavity around a joint that decreases the friction between two surfaces).*

cardiac muscle *The type of muscle that makes up the heart.*

cellular dedifferentiation *A form of wound healing in which mature cells produce new cells with the same function.*

collagen fibers *A protein substance found in bone and cartilage.*

comminuted fracture *A break in which the bone is shattered into many pieces.*

compound fracture *A complete break in the bone where the bone ends separate and break through the skin; also known as an open fracture.*

concentric contraction *A contraction resulting in shortening of the muscle.*

connective tissue *Cells whose secretions support and connect organs and tissues in the body.*

contractibility *The ability to shorten or reduce the distance between parts.*

contusion *An injury resulting from a direct blow or force that does not interrupt the skin; typically bruising is seen at the injury site.*

delayed onset muscle soreness (DOMS) *The presence of soreness in the muscles a day or two after overuse of the muscles or a traumatic injury.*

diaphysis *The shaft of a long bone.*

eccentric contraction *A contraction of muscle resulting in lengthening of the opposing muscle.*

ecchymosis *Bruising.*

efferent neuron *A nerve that carries messages from the brain and spinal cord to muscles and glands; also known as a motor neuron.*

elasticity *The ability to return to original form after being compressed or stretched.*

epiphyseal plate fracture *A break in the bone at the growth plate (typically at the wrist or ankle).*

epiphysis *The end of a long bone.*

excitability *The ability to respond to stimuli; also known as irritability.*

extensibility *The ability to lengthen and increase the distance between two parts.*

external fixation *The use of a cast to maintain proper alignment of bones for the purpose of reduction.*

extracellular matrix (ECM) *Noncellular material that separates connective tissue cells.*

greenstick fracture *An incomplete break in the shaft of the bone; occurs in children.*

hematoma *The formation caused by pooling of blood and fluid within a tissue space.*

inflammation *Process that occurs when tissues are subjected to chemical or physical trauma; pain,*

KEY TERMS CONTINUED

heat, redness, and swelling occur.

insertion *The part of the skeletal muscle that is attached to the movable part of a bone.*

internal fixation *Surgical alignment of bones for the purpose of reduction.*

interneuron *A nerve that carries messages from a sensory neuron to a motor neuron; also known as an associative neuron.*

laceration *An injury that results from a tear in the skin; also known as a cut.*

leukocytes *White blood cells.*

lymphocytes *A group of white blood cells of crucial importance to the body's immune system.*

medullary canal *The center of the shaft of the long bone.*

membrane excitability *The ability of nerves to carry impulses by creating electrical charges.*

monocyte *Large, circulating white blood cells.*

mononuclear phagocytes *White blood cells that engulf and destroy waste material and foreign bodies in the bloodstream.*

motor unit *A motor nerve plus all of the muscle fibers it stimulates.*

muscle fatigue *The result of accumulation of lactic acid in the muscle.*

muscle tone *The state of partial contraction in which muscles are maintained.*

myelin sheath *The layers of cell membrane that wrap around nerve fibers; provides electrical insulation and increases the velocity of impulse transmission.*

myositis ossificans *A calcification that forms within the muscle; results from an improperly managed contusion.*

nerve fascicle *A small bundle of axons (nerve fibers) that transmits messages between the brain and other parts of the body.*

neuroma *A ball-like growth of nerve fibers that creates a nerve scar.*

neuromuscular junction *The point between the motor nerve axon and the muscle cell membrane.*

neutrophils *White blood cells that engulf and kill bacteria.*

origin *The part of the skeletal muscle that is attached to the fixed part of a bone.*

ossification *The process of bone formation.*

osteoblast *Type of bone cell involved in the formation of bony tissue.*

osteoclast *Type of bone cell involved in the resorption of bony tissue.*

osteocyte *A bone cell.*

periosteum *The fibrous tissue that covers the bone.*

prime mover *Muscle that provides movement in a single direction.*

puncture wound *An injury caused by a sharp object that penetrates the skin.*

reduction *The process of putting broken bones back into proper alignment.*

regeneration *The act of wound healing (tissue rebuilding).*

KEY TERMS CONTINUED

remodeling *The process of absorbing and replacing bone in the skeletal system.*

sarcolemma *The muscle cell membrane.*

sarcoplasm *The material within the muscle cell, excluding the nucleus.*

scar tissue *Fibrous connective tissue that binds damaged tissue.*

simple fracture *A break in the bone that may be complete or incomplete, but does not break through the skin; also known as a closed fracture.*

skeletal muscle *The type of muscle, attached to a bone or bones of the skeleton, that aids in body movements; also known as voluntary or striated muscle.*

smooth muscle *The type of muscle that is not attached to bone, and is nonstriated and involuntary; also known as visceral muscle.*

sphincter muscle *A type of circular muscle.*

spongy bone *Results from the breakdown of hard bone.*

sprain *An injury resulting from a fall, sudden twist, or blow to the body that forces a joint out of its normal position.*

strain *A muscle injury caused by the twisting or pulling of a muscle or tendon.*

stress fracture *A small, incomplete break in the bone that results from overuse, weakness, or biomechanical problems.*

synapse *The space between adjacent neurons through which an impulse is transmitted.*

synergists *Muscles that help steady a joint.*

tendonitis *Inflammation of the tendon (fibrous tissue connecting muscle to bone).*

transdifferentiation *A form of wound healing in which mature cells dedifferentiate and produce new cells that are then able to mature into cell types with a completely different function from the originating cells.*

THE SKELETAL SYSTEM

The average human adult skeleton has 206 bones that are joined to ligaments and tendons. These bones form a protective and supportive framework for the attached muscles and the soft tissues that underlie the skeleton (Figure 16–1).

The skeleton has two main parts: the **axial skeleton** and the **appendicular skeleton**. The axial skeleton consists of the skull, the spine, the ribs, and the sternum, and includes 80 bones. The appendicular skeleton includes two limb girdles (the shoulders and pelvis) and the attached limb bones. This part of the skeletal system contains 126 bones: 64 in the shoulders

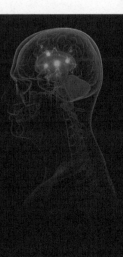

KEY CONCEPT

The skeleton has two main parts: the axial skeleton and the appendicular skeleton. The axial skeleton consists of the skull, spine, ribs, and sternum. The appendicular skeleton consists of the shoulder and pelvic girdles and the attached limb bones.

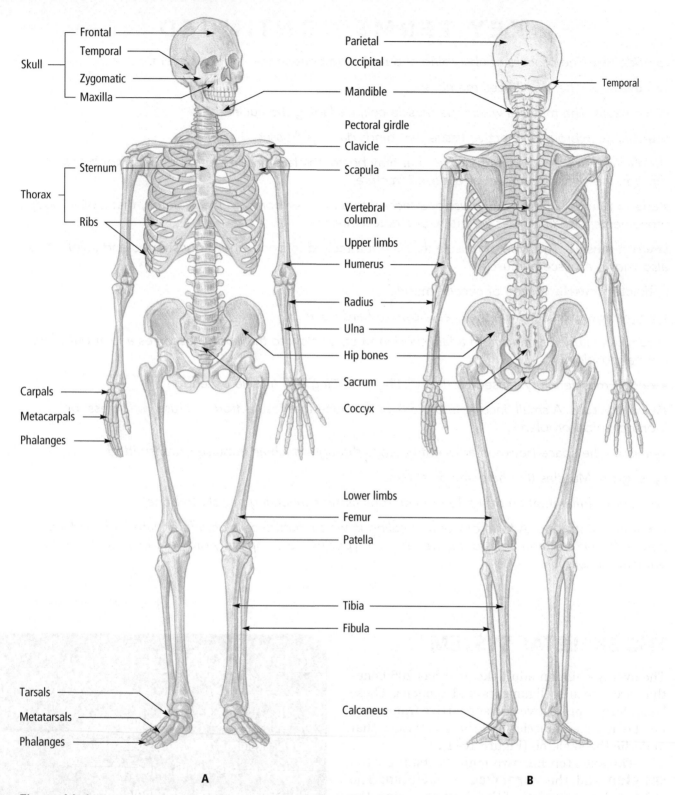

Figure 16–1 The human skeleton: (A) Anterior view. (B) Posterior view.

and upper limbs, and 62 in the pelvis and lower limbs. Babies are born with 270 soft bones—about 64 more than an adult; by adulthood, these 64 bones will have fused together into the 206 hard, permanent bones.

There are only minor differences between male and female skeletons. Men's bones tend to be larger and heavier than the corresponding women's bones, and a woman's pelvic cavity is wider to accommodate childbirth.

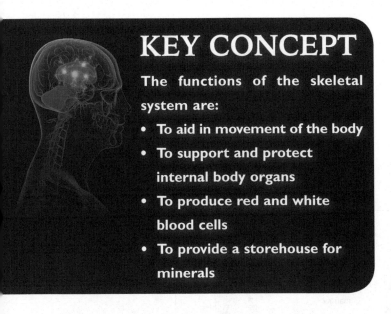

KEY CONCEPT

The functions of the skeletal system are:

- To aid in movement of the body
- To support and protect internal body organs
- To produce red and white blood cells
- To provide a storehouse for minerals

Functions of the Skeletal System

The skeleton plays an important part in movement because it acts as a series of independently movable levers, which the muscles can pull to move different parts of the body. It also supports and protects the internal body organs. The skeleton is not just a movable frame, but also an efficient factory that produces red and white blood cells from the bone marrow of certain bones. On average, 2.6 million red blood cells are produced each second by the bone marrow; these cells are used to replace those worn out and destroyed by the liver. The bones also store minerals, such as calcium and phosphorus, which can be supplied to other parts of the body. When minerals are present in excess in the blood, buildup will occur within the bones. When the supply of minerals within the blood is low, they will be withdrawn from the bones to replenish the supply.

BONES

Bones consist of microscopic cells called osteocytes (from the Greek word *osteon,* meaning "bone"). An **osteocyte** is a mature bone cell. Bone is made up of 35% organic material and 65% inorganic mineral salts, and water.

The organic matter derives from a protein called *bone collagen,* a fibrous material. Between these collagenous fibers is jellylike material. The organic substances of bone give it a certain degree of flexibility. The inorganic portion of bone is made from mineral salts such as calcium phosphate, calcium carbonate, calcium fluoride, magnesium phosphate, sodium oxide, and sodium chloride. These minerals give bone its hardness and durability.

A bony skeleton can be compared with steel-reinforced concrete. The collagenous fibers may be compared with flexible steel supports, and mineral salts with concrete. When pressure is applied to a bone, the flexible, organic material prevents bone damage, while the mineral elements resist crushing under pressure.

Bone Formation

The embryonic skeleton initially consists of collagenous protein fibers secreted by the osteoblasts (primitive embryonic cells). Later, during embryonic development, cartilage is deposited between the fibers. At this stage, the embryo's skeleton consists of collagenous protein fibers called hyaline cartilage (a clear, tough, smooth, slippery material). During the eighth week of embryonic development, **ossification** begins. That is, mineral matter starts to replace previously formed cartilage, creating bone. Infant bones are very soft and pliable at birth, because of incomplete ossification. A familiar example is the soft spot on a baby's head, the fontanel. The bone has not yet formed there, although it will harden later. Ossification by mineral deposit continues throughout childhood. As bones ossify, they become hard and more capable of bearing weight.

Structure of the Long Bone

A typical long bone contains a shaft, or **diaphysis**. This hollow cylinder of hard, compact bone is what makes a long bone strong and hard, yet light enough for movement. At each end (extreme) of the diaphysis is an **epiphysis** (Figure 16–2A).

In the center of the shaft is the broad **medullary canal** or cavity. This is filled with yellow bone marrow, mostly made of fat cells. The marrow also contains many blood vessels and some cells that form white blood cells, called *leukocytes.* The yellow marrow functions as a fat storage center. The *endosteum* is the lining of the marrow canal that keeps the cavity intact.

The medullary canal is surrounded by compact or hard bone. Haversian canals branch into the compact bone (Figure 16–2B). They carry blood vessels that nourish the osteocytes, or bone

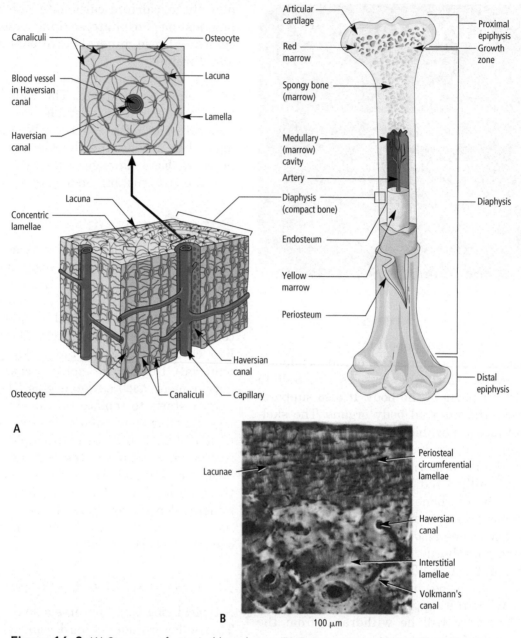

Figure 16–2 (A) Structure of a typical long bone. (B) Cross-section of bone. Photo from Bergman, R., Afifi, A., and Heidger, P., 1999, *Atlas of Microscopic Anatomy: A Functional Approach: Companion to Histology and Neuroanatomy 2e.* Reprinted with permission. http://www.vh.org/Providers/Textbooks/MicroscopicAnatomy/MicroscopicAnatomy.html.

cells. Where less strength is needed in the bone, some of the hard bone is dissolved away, leaving **spongy bone**.

The ends of the long bones contain the red marrow where some red blood cells, called *erythrocytes,* and some white blood cells are made. The outside of the bone is covered with the **periosteum**, a tough, fibrous tissue containing blood vessels, lymph vessels, and nerves. The periosteum is necessary for bone growth, repair, and nutrition.

Covering the epiphysis is a thin layer of cartilage, known as the *articular cartilage,* which acts as a shock absorber between two bones that meet to form a joint.

Growth

Bones grow in length and ossify from the center of the diaphysis toward the epiphyseal extremities. Using a long bone by way of example, it will grow lengthwise in an area called the *growth zone* (see Figure 16–2A). Ossification occurs here, causing the bone to lengthen; this causes the epiphyses to grow away from the middle of the diaphysis. It is a sensible growth process, because it does not interfere with the articulation between two bones.

A bone increases its circumference by the addition of more bone to the outer surface of the diaphysis by **osteoblasts**, bone cells that deposit the new bone. As girth increases, bone material is dissolved from the central part of the diaphysis. This forms an internal cavity called the *marrow cavity* or *medullary canal*. The medullary canal gets larger as the diameter of the bone increases.

The dissolution of bone from the medullary canal results from the action of cells called **osteoclasts**, immense bone cells that secrete enzymes. These enzymes digest the bony material, splitting off the bone minerals calcium and phosphorus and enabling them to be absorbed by the surrounding fluid. The medullary canal eventually fills with yellow marrow.

The length of a bone shaft continues to grow until all the epiphyseal cartilage is ossified. At this point, bone growth stops. This fact is helpful in determining further growth in a child. First, an x-ray of the child's wrists is taken. If some epiphyseal cartilage remains, there will be further growth. If there is no epiphyseal cartilage left, the child has reached his or her full stature (height).

The average growth in females continues for about 18 years; males grow for approximately 20 or 21 years. However, new bone growth can occur in a broken bone at any time. Bone cells near the site of a fracture become active, secreting large amounts of new bone within a relatively short time. Bone healing proceeds efficiently depending on the age and health of the individual.

German anatomist and surgeon Julius Wolff (1836–1902) stated, in 1892 that bone in a healthy person or animal will adapt to the loads under which it is placed. If loading on a particular bone increases, the bone will remodel itself over time to become stronger to resist that sort of loading. This concept is known as Wolff's Law.

Bone Types

Bones are classified into four types on the basis of their shape (Figure 16–3). *Long bones* are found in both upper and lower arms and legs. The bones of the skull are examples of *flat bones,* as are the ribs.

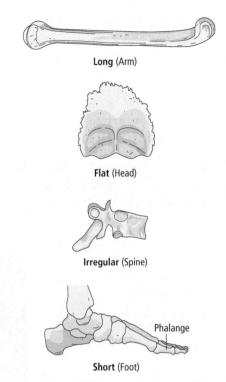

Figure 16–3 Bone shapes.

Irregular bones are represented by bones of the spinal column. The wrist and ankle bones are examples of *short bones,* which appear cubelike in shape.

The bones in the hand are short, making flexible movement possible. The same is true of the irregular bones of the spinal column. The thigh bone is a long bone needed to support the strong leg muscles and the weight of the body. The degree of movement at a joint is determined by bone shape and joint structure.

INJURIES TO BONES

Athletes push their bodies to the limit in practice and competition. Often, pushing to the limit can cause bone injuries. Contact sports result in thousands of fractures each year, in all age groups. Noncontact sports, such as cross country, cause fractures from falling and overuse.

Fractures

Bones are rigid, but they do give somewhat when an outside force is applied to them. When this force stops, bone returns to its original shape. For example, if someone falls forward and lands on an outstretched hand, there is an impact on the bones and connective tissue of the wrist as it hits the ground. The bones of the hand, wrist, and arm can usually absorb this shock by giving slightly and then returning to their original shape and position. If the force is too great, however, bones will break.

TYPES OF FRACTURES Fractures can be classified by the degree of injury to the bone. There are six major classifications of fractures:

- **Simple fracture**—occurs when the forces on the bone exceed the bone's ability to withstand them. Simple or closed fractures can be incomplete

or complete breaks in the bone, but the broken ends do not pierce the skin (Figure 16–4A–B). Also known as a closed fracture.

- **Compound fracture**—results in the fractured end penetrating the skin. This creates a danger of infection of the wound and the bone itself (Figure 16–5A–B). Also known as an open fracture.

- **Greenstick fracture**—named after the analogy of a child's bone and a young shoot of a plant, as compared to the bone of an adult,

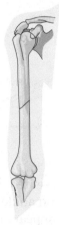

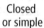

Closed
or simple

A

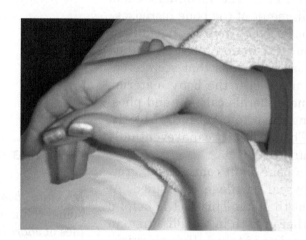

B

Figure 16–4A–B A simple, or closed, fracture often exhibits as a painful, swollen deformity. Photo B Courtesy of Dr. Deborah Funk, Alnaby Medical Center, Albany, NY.

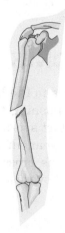

Open
or compound

A

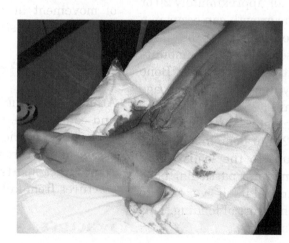

B

Figure 16–5A–B In a compound, or open, fracture, bone ends protrude through the skin. Photo B Courtesy of Dr. Deborah Funk, Alnaby Medical Center, Albany, NY.

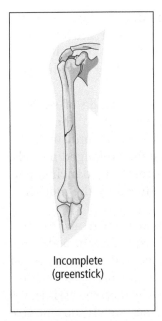

Incomplete
(greenstick)

Figure 16–6 Greenstick
or incomplete fracture.

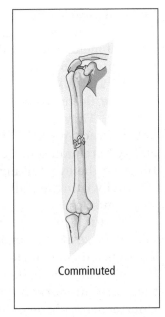

Comminuted

Figure 16–7 Comminuted
fracture.

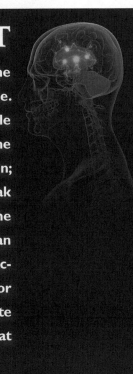

KEY CONCEPT

Fractures can be classified by the degree of injury to the bone. There are six types. The simple fracture is a break in the bone that does not penetrate the skin; the compound fracture is a break in the bone that penetrates the skin; the greenstick fracture is an incomplete break; the stress fracture is the result of overuse or weakness; and the epiphyseal plate fracture is a break that occurs at or near the growth plate.

analogized to a tree's older branch. Children's bones are more pliable than an adult's bones, and they can bend further. The force that created the break usually breaks only the outer part of the bend. In an adult, a corresponding amount of force would have broken the same bone completely (Figure 16–6).

- **Comminuted fracture**—occurs when forces on the bone are so great that the bone shatters into three or more pieces (Figure 16–7).

- **Stress fracture**—occurs when bone is stressed by overuse, poor muscle balance, lack of flexibility, weakness in soft tissues caused by previous injuries, or biomechanical problems. The stresses on the bone are greater than the body's ability to compensate, so a gradual deterioration of the bone occurs. Bones of the lower leg and foot are particularly prone to this condition.

- **Epiphyseal plate fracture**—the epiphyseal (growth plate) complex is very susceptible to injury in children. One reason for this type of injury is that the ligamentous and capsular structures around a joint are two to five times stronger than the most vulnerable part of the growth plate. Approximately 10% of all fractures in children involve the epiphyseal complex; the wrist and ankle are the most commonly affected areas. Seventy-five percent

of epiphyseal fractures occur in children between the ages of 10 and 16, usually as a result of sport participation.

- **Spiral fracture** is caused when force is applied to a bone in a twisting motion. Injuries where the end of an extremity is fixed while the rest of the limb remains in motion often result in this type of fracture. **Longitudinal fractures** occur along (or nearly along) the axis of the bone. This is most often used in the context of a long-bone fracture.

Signs and Symptoms

The general signs and symptoms that indicate a possible fracture are swelling, deformity, pain, tenderness, and discoloration. If the bone ends protrude through the skin, bleeding will occur. A nerve injury may also be present if sensation is lost below the site of the fracture.

Treatment

Bone is living tissue and is constantly in a state of turnover. Bones continually absorb and replace cells, a process known as **remodeling**. Because of this, the process of healing bone often occurs naturally. For a fracture to heal as quickly as possible, and without any deformity, the bones must sometimes be put back in proper position. This process, called **reduction**, involves the doctor manipulating the broken bone into proper alignment, then putting it in a cast. The use of a cast is called **external fixation**. For some breaks, immobilization through use of a cast may be enough to facilitate healing. Occasionally, surgery is required for more complicated breaks, such as comminuted fractures. Surgery for this purpose is known as **internal fixation**.

Healing depends on many factors, including the specific bone that was broken and the age of the individual. Some broken bones, especially in children, heal within a couple of weeks. Others may take months, even years.

MUSCLES

Body movements are determined by one or more of the three principal types of muscles: skeletal, smooth, and cardiac. These muscles are also described as striated, spindle shaped, and nonstriated because of the way their cells look under a microscope.

Skeletal Muscle

Skeletal muscles are attached to the bones of the skeleton. They are called striped or striated because they have cross-bandings (striations) of alternating light and dark bands running perpendicular to the length of the muscle (Figure 16–8). Skeletal muscle is also called *voluntary muscle,* because it contains nerves under voluntary control.

Skeletal muscle consists of bundles of muscle cells. Each muscle cell is known as a muscle fiber. The cell membrane is called the **sarcolemma**, and the contents of the cell, excluding the nucleus, are the **sarcoplasm**.

The fleshy body parts are made of skeletal muscles. They provide movement to the limbs, but contract quickly, fatigue easily, and lack the ability to remain contracted for prolonged periods. Blinking the eye, talking, breathing, dancing, eating, and writing are all produced by the motion of these muscles.

Smooth muscles (also known as visceral muscles) contain small, spindle-shaped cells There is only one nucleus, located at the center of the cell. They are called smooth muscles because they are unmarked by distinctive striations. Unattached to bones, they act slowly, do not tire easily, and can remain contracted for a long time (Figure 16–9).

Smooth muscles are not under conscious control; for this reason they are also called *involuntary muscles*. Their actions are controlled by the autonomic (automatic) nervous system. Smooth muscles are found in the walls of the internal organs, including the stomach, intestines, uterus, and blood vessels. They help push food along the length of the alimentary canal, contract the uterus during labor and childbirth, and control the diameter of blood vessels as blood circulates throughout the body.

Cardiac Muscle

Cardiac muscle is found only in the heart. Cardiac muscle cells are striated and branched, and they

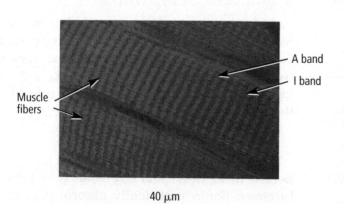
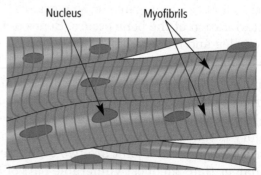

40 μm

Figure 16–8 Skeletal muscle cells. Photo from Bergman, R., Afifi, A., and Heidger, P., 1999, *Atlas of Microscopic Anatomy: A Functional Approach: Companion to Histology and Neuroanatomy* 2e. Reprinted with permission. http://www.vh.org/Providers/Textbooks/MicroscopicAnatomy/MicroscopicAnatomy.html.

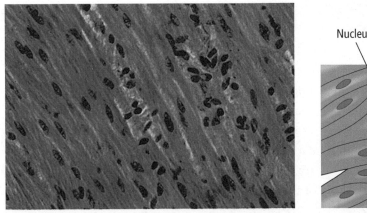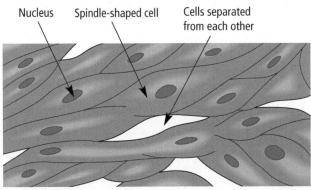

Nucleus   Spindle-shaped cell   Cells separated from each other

20 μm

Figure 16–9 Skeletal muscle cells. Photo from Bergman, R., Afifi, A., and Heidger, P., 1999, *Atlas of Microscopic Anatomy: A Functional Approach: Companion to Histology and Neuroanatomy* 2e. Reprinted with permission. http://www.vh.org/Providers/Textbooks/MicroscopicAnatomy/MicroscopicAnatomy.html.

are involuntary (Figure 16–10). Cardiac cells are joined in a continuous network without a sheath separation. The membranes of adjacent cells are fused at areas called *intercalated discs*. A communication system at the fused area will not permit independent cell contraction. When one cell receives a signal to contract, all neighboring cells are stimulated, and they contract together to produce the heartbeat. When the heart beats normally, it holds a rhythm of about 72 beats per minute; however, the activity of various nerves leading to the heart can increase or decrease its rate. Cardiac muscle requires a continuous supply of oxygen to function. If the oxygen supply is cut off for as little as 30 seconds, the cardiac muscle cells start to die.

KEY CONCEPT

The three main types of muscle are skeletal muscle, which is under voluntary control and aids in movement; smooth muscle, which is not under voluntary control but is controlled by the central nervous system; and cardiac muscle, which is involuntary and makes up the heart.

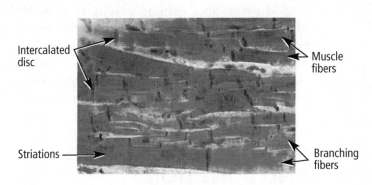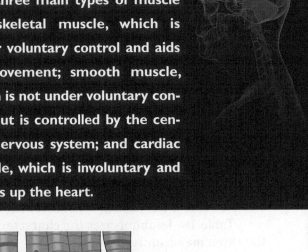

Intercalated disc — Muscle fibers
Striations — Branching fibers

Centrally located nucleus
Striations
Branching of cell
Intercalated disc

100 μm

Figure 16–10 Cardiac muscle cells. Photo from Bergman, R., Afifi, A., and Heidger, P., 1999, *Atlas of Microscopic Anatomy: A Functional Approach: Companion to Histology and Neuroanatomy* 2e. Reprinted with permission. http://www.vh.org/Providers/Textbooks/MicroscopicAnatomy/MicroscopicAnatomy.html.

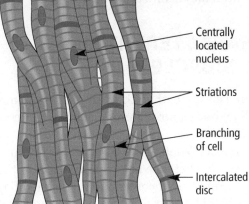

Table 16–1 Characteristics of Major Muscle Types

MUSCLE TYPE	LOCATION	STRUCTURE	FUNCTION
Skeletal muscle (striated, voluntary)	Attached to the skeleton and also located in the wall of the pharynx and esophagus.	A skeletal muscle fiber is long, cylindrical, multi-nucleated, and contains alternating light and dark striations. Nuclei are located at the edges of the fibers.	Contractions occur voluntarily and may be rapid and forceful. Contractions stabilize the joints.
Smooth muscle (nonstriated, involuntary)	Located in the walls of tubular structures and hollow organs such as in the digestive tract, urinary bladder, and blood vessels.	A smooth muscle fiber is long and spindle shaped, with no striations.	Contractions occur involuntarily and are rhythmic and slow.
Cardiac (heart) muscle	Located in the heart.	Short, branching fibers with a centrally located nucleus; striations are not distinct.	Contractions occur involuntarily and are rhythmic and automatic.

Sphincter Muscles

Sphincter muscles (or dilator muscles) are circular muscles in the openings between the esophagus and stomach, and the stomach and small intestine. They are also found in the walls of the anus, the urethra, and the mouth. They open and close to control the passage of substances.

Table 16–1 summarizes the characteristics of the three major muscle types.

CHARACTERISTICS OF MUSCLES

All muscles, whether they are skeletal, smooth, or cardiac, have four common characteristics. One is **contractibility**, a quality possessed by no other body tissue. When a muscle shortens or contracts, it reduces the distance between its parts or the space it surrounds. The contraction of skeletal muscles that connect a pair of bones brings the attachment points closer together, thus causing the bone to move. When cardiac muscles contract, they reduce the area in the heart chambers, pumping blood from the heart into the blood vessels. Likewise,

smooth muscles surround blood vessels and the intestines, causing the diameter of these tubes to decrease upon contraction.

Excitability or irritability is a characteristic of both muscle and nervous cells (neurons). It is the ability to respond to certain stimuli by producing electrical signals called **action potentials** (impulses).

Extensibility is the ability to be stretched. When the arm is bent, the muscles on the back of it are extended or stretched.

Muscles also exhibit **elasticity** (the ability to return to original length when relaxing). Collectively, these four characteristics of muscles—contractibility, excitability, extensibility, and elasticity—produce a veritable mechanical device capable of complex, intricate movements.

MUSCLE ATTACHMENTS AND FUNCTIONS

There are more than 650 different muscles in the body. For a given muscle to produce movement in any part of the body, it must be able to exert its force upon a movable object. Muscles must be attached to bones for leverage in order to have something to pull against. Muscles only pull, never push.

Muscles are attached to the bones of the skeleton by nonelastic cords called *tendons*. Bones are connected at joints. Skeletal muscles are attached to bones in such a way as to bridge these joints. When a skeletal muscle contracts, the bone to which it is attached will move.

Muscles are attached at both ends to bones, cartilage, ligaments, tendons, skin, or other muscles. The **origin** is the part of a skeletal muscle that is attached to a fixed structure or bone; it moves least during muscle contraction. The **insertion** is the other end, attached to a movable part; it is the part that moves most during a muscle contraction. The **belly** is the central body of the muscle.

The muscles of the body are arranged in pairs. One produces movement in a single direction and is called the **prime mover**; the other does so in the opposite direction and is called the **antagonist**. This arrangement of muscles with opposite actions is known as an antagonist pair.

By example, upper arm muscles are arranged in antagonist pairs (Figure 16–11). The muscle located on the front part of the upper arm is the biceps. One end of the biceps is attached to the scapula and humerus (its origin). When the biceps contract, these two bones remain stationary. The opposite end of the biceps is attached to the radius

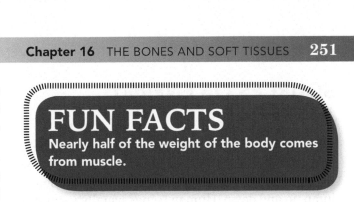

FUN FACTS
Nearly half of the weight of the body comes from muscle.

of the lower arm (its insertion); this bone moves upon contraction of the biceps.

The muscle on the back of the upper arm is the triceps. A simple demonstration will illustrate. Bend your elbow. With your other hand, feel the contraction of the belly of the biceps. At the same time, stretch your fingers out (around the arm) to touch the triceps; it will be in a relaxed state. Now extend your forearm; feel the simultaneous contraction of the triceps and relaxation of the biceps. Now bend your forearm halfway and contract the biceps and triceps. They cannot move, because both sets of muscles are contracting at the same time. In some muscle activity, the role of prime mover and antagonist may be reversed. When the arm is flexed, the biceps is the prime mover and triceps is the antagonist. When the arm is extended, the triceps is the prime mover, and the biceps is the antagonist.

Another group of muscles, called the **synergists**, help steady a movement or stabilize joint activity.

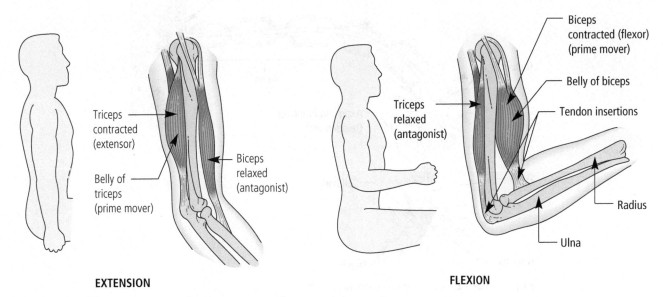

Triceps contracted (extensor)

Belly of triceps (prime mover)

Biceps relaxed (antagonist)

EXTENSION

Biceps contracted (flexor) (prime mover)

Belly of biceps

Tendon insertions

Triceps relaxed (antagonist)

Radius

Ulna

FLEXION

Figure 16–11 Coordination of prime mover and antagonistic muscles.

SOURCES OF ENERGY AND HEAT

When muscles work, they not only move the body but also produce the heat that bodies need. For instance, to get warm on a cold day, a person might jump up and down. Human beings usually maintain their body temperatures within a narrow range (98.6°F–99.8°F). Muscles need energy to contract and do their work. Their major source of energy is adenosine triphosphate (ATP), a compound found in the muscle cell. To make ATP, the cell requires oxygen, glucose, and other components, which are brought to the cell by the circulating blood. Extra glucose can be stored in the cell in the form of glycogen. When a muscle is stimulated, the ATP is broken down, producing the energy the muscle needs to contract. During this process, lactic acid, which is a by-product of cell metabolism, builds up.

CONTRACTION OF SKELETAL MUSCLE

Muscle movement occurs as a result of two major events: myoneural stimulation and contraction of muscle proteins. Skeletal muscles must be stimulated by nerve impulses to contract. A motor neuron (nerve cell) stimulates all of the skeletal muscles within a **motor unit**, which is a motor neuron plus all the muscle fibers it stimulates. The junction between the motor neuron's fiber (axon), which transmits the impulse, and the muscle cell's sarcolemma (muscle cell membrane) is the **neuromuscular junction** (see Figure 16–12). The gap between the axon and the muscle cell is known as the *synaptic cleft*.

When the nerve impulses reach the end of the axon, the chemical neurotransmitter **acetylcholine** is released. Acetylcholine diffuses across the synaptic cleft and attaches to receptors on the sarcolemma. The sarcolemma then becomes temporarily permeable to sodium ions (Na^+), which go rushing into the muscle cell. This gives the muscle cell excessive positive ions, which upset and change the electrical condition of the sarcolemma. This electrical upset causes an action potential (an electrical current).

Skeletal muscle contraction begins with the action potential, which travels along the muscle fiber length. The basic source of energy is glucose, and the energy derived is stored in the form of ATP and phosphocreatine. The latter serves as a trigger mechanism by allowing energy transfer

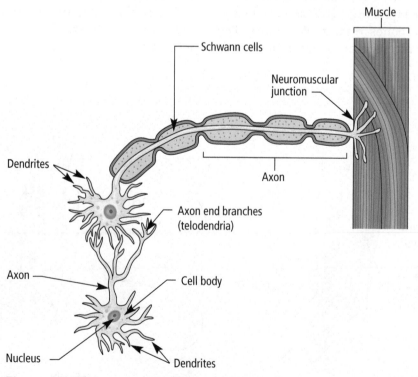

Figure 16–12 A neuron-stimulating muscle.

to the protein molecules, actin and myosin, within the muscle fibers. Once begun, the action potential travels over the entire surface of the sarcolemma, conducting the electrical impulse from one end of the cell to the other. This results in the contraction of the muscle cell. The movement of electrical current along the sarcolemma causes calcium ions (Ca^{++}) to be released from storage areas inside the muscle cell. When calcium ions attach to the action myofilaments (contractile elements of skeletal muscle), sliding of the myofilaments is triggered and the whole cell shortens. The sliding of the myofilaments is energized by ATP.

The events that return the cell to a resting phase include the diffusion of potassium and sodium ions back to their initial positions outside the cell. When the action potential ends, calcium ions are reabsorbed into their storage areas and the muscle cell relaxes and returns to its original length. Amazingly, this entire sequence takes place in just a few thousandths of a second.

While the action potential is occurring, acetylcholine (which began the process) is broken down by enzymes on the sarcolemma. For this reason, a single nerve impulse produces only one contraction at a time. The muscle cell relaxes until it is stimulated by the next release of acetylcholine (Figure 16–12).

MUSCLE FATIGUE

Muscle fatigue is caused by an accumulation of lactic acid in the muscles. During periods of vigorous exercise, the blood is unable to transport enough oxygen for the complete oxidation of glucose in the muscles. This causes the muscles to contract anaerobically (without oxygen).

Lactic acid normally leaves the muscle, passing into the bloodstream, but if vigorous exercise continues, the lactic acid level in the blood rises sharply. In such cases, lactic acid accumulates within the muscle. This impedes muscular contraction, causing muscle fatigue and cramps. After exercise, a person must stop, rest, and take in enough oxygen to convert the lactic acid back to glucose and other substances to be used by the muscle cells. The amount of oxygen needed is called the *oxygen debt*. When the debt is paid back, respirations resume a normal rate.

MUSCLE TONE

To function, muscles should always be slightly contracted and ready to pull. This is **muscle tone**. Muscle tone can be achieved through proper nutrition and regular exercise.

Muscle contractions may be isotonic or isometric. When muscles contract and shorten, it is called an *isotonic (concentric) contraction*. This occurs when we walk, talk, and so on. When the muscle lengthens, this is called eccentric contraction. An example is when the biceps contract (concentric) and the triceps lengthens (eccentric). When the tension in a muscle increases, but the muscle does not shorten, it is called an *isometric contraction*. This occurs with exercise, such as tensing the abdominal muscles. If they are not exercised, muscles become weak and flaccid. Muscles may also shrink from disuse. This is called atrophy. If they are over exercised, muscles will become enlarged. This is known as hypertrophy. In hypertrophy, the size of the muscle fiber (cell) enlarges.

Muscle Atrophy

Muscle atrophy is the wasting or loss of muscle tissue resulting from disease or lack of use. The majority of muscle atrophy in the general population results from disuse. Individuals whose jobs require little or no exercise are more likely to lose muscle tone and develop muscle atrophy. Children and young adults who lead sedentary lifestyles can also develop muscle atrophy, as well as other problems associated with a lack of regular exercise. Vigorous exercise will reverse this type of atrophy.

Muscle atrophy in athletics commonly occurs as a result of an injury. Injuries that require extended immobilization, or decrease in use, will cause the muscles associated with the injury to lose muscle tone.

Muscle Hypertrophy

Hypertrophy is an increase in the mass (size) of a muscle. The most common cause of muscle hypertrophy is exercise. Most athletes, regardless of their sport, have realized the value of resistance training to enhance athletic performance. When muscles are exposed to a progressive resistance weight-training program, they will gradually adapt to the new loads being placed on them. For muscles to be enlarged beyond their normal size, they must be exposed to a training stimulus that is sufficient to cause overcompensation in the muscle. High-volume, low-intensity training is typically used for this purpose.

INJURIES TO MUSCLES

Muscle injuries often occur as a result of a direct blow or from forces generated within the muscle itself. Damage within the muscle is typified by tearing of muscle fibers, connective tissue, and blood vessels.

Muscles have an ample blood supply and usually heal quickly. However, the injured area repairs itself by forming scar tissue, which is tight and inelastic in comparison to normal muscle tissue. Because of this inelasticity, previously injured muscles are prone to reinjury, formation of more scar tissue, and further tightness. Occasionally, adhesions may occur in which scar tissue binds together normally separate anatomical structures.

Strains

A **strain** is caused by twisting or pulling a muscle or tendon. Strains can be acute or chronic. An acute strain is caused by trauma or an injury such as a blow to the body; it can also be caused by improperly lifting heavy objects or over-stressing the muscles. Chronic strains are usually the result of overuse—prolonged, repetitive movement of the muscles and tendons. Interestingly, a strain from overuse might not be felt by the athlete initially. It could be a day or two before symptoms of mild overuse or traumatic injury appear. This is called **delayed-onset muscle soreness (DOMS)**.

Two common sites for strain are the back and the hamstring muscle (located in the back of the thigh). Contact sports such as soccer, football, hockey, boxing, and wrestling put participants at risk for strains. Gymnastics, tennis, rowing, golf, and other sports that require extensive gripping can increase the risk of hand and forearm strains. Elbow strains sometimes occur in people who participate in racquet, throwing, and contact sports (Figure 16–13).

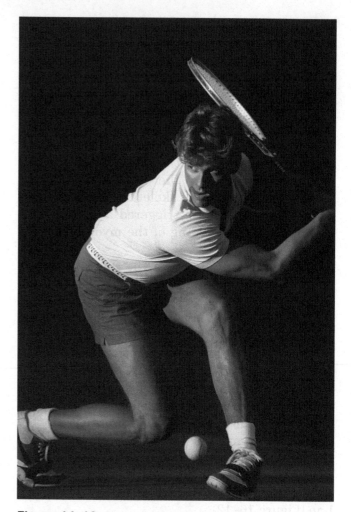

Figure 16–13 Strains to the elbow are common in individuals who participate in racquet sports such as tennis. Courtesy of Photodisc

SIGNS AND SYMPTOMS Athletes with a strain experience pain, muscle spasm, and muscle weakness. They can also have localized swelling, redness, heat, cramping, or inflammation and, with a minor or moderate strain, usually some loss of muscle function. Patients typically have pain in the injured area and general weakness of the muscle when they attempt to move it. Severe strains that partially or completely tear the muscle or tendon are often very painful and disabling.

TREATMENT Treatment for strains has two stages. The goal during the first stage is to reduce swelling and pain. At this stage, doctors usually advise patients to follow a formula of rest, ice, compression, and elevation (RICE) for the first 24 to 48 hours after the injury. The doctor may also recommend an over-the-counter or prescription nonsteroidal, anti-inflammatory drug, such as aspirin or ibuprofen, to help decrease pain and inflammation.

For people with a moderate or severe sprain, particularly of the ankle, a hard cast may be applied. Severe sprains and strains may require surgery to repair the torn ligaments, muscle, or tendons.

REHABILITATION The second stage of treating a strain is rehabilitation, the overall goal of which is to improve the condition of the injured part and restore its function. The health care provider will prescribe an exercise program designed to prevent stiffness, improve range of motion, and restore the joint's normal flexibility and strength. Some patients may need physical therapy during this stage.

When the acute pain and swelling have diminished, the health care provider or physical therapist will instruct the patient to do a series of exercises several times a day. These are very important because they help reduce swelling, prevent stiffness, and restore the normal, pain-free range of motion. The health care provider can recommend many different types of exercises, depending on the injury. For example, people with an ankle sprain may be told to rest the heel on the floor and write the alphabet in the air with the big toe. A patient with an injured knee or foot will work on weight-bearing and balancing exercises. The duration of the program depends on the extent of the injury, but the regimen commonly lasts for several weeks.

Another goal of rehabilitation is to increase strength and regain flexibility. Depending on the patient's rate of recovery, this process begins about the second week after the injury. The health care provider or physical therapist will instruct the patient to do a series of exercises designed to meet these goals. During this phase of rehabilitation, patients progress to more demanding exercises as pain decreases and function improves.

The final goal is return to full daily activities, including sports when appropriate. Patients must work closely with their health care provider or physical therapist to determine their readiness to return to full activity. Some people are tempted to resume full activity or play sports despite pain or muscle soreness. Returning to full activity before regaining normal range of motion, flexibility, and strength increases the chance of reinjury and may lead to a chronic problem.

The amount of rehabilitation and the time needed for full recovery after a strain depend on the severity of the injury and individual rates of healing. For example, a moderate quadricep strain may require one to three weeks of rehabilitation before a person can return to full activity. With a severe strain, it can take one to three months before the tissue damage is fully healed. Extra care should be taken to avoid reinjury.

There are many things people can do to help lower the risk of strains:

- Maintain a healthy, well-balanced diet to keep muscles strong.
- Maintain a healthy weight.
- Practice safety measures to help prevent falls (e.g., keep stairways, walkways, yards, and driveways free of clutter; salt or sand icy patches in the winter).
- Wear shoes that fit properly.
- Replace athletic shoes as soon as the tread wears out or the heel wears down on one side.
- Do stretching exercises daily.
- Be in proper physical condition to play a sport.
- Warm up and stretch before participating in any sports or exercise.
- Wear protective equipment when playing.

KEY CONCEPT

A strain is the result of twisting or pulling a muscle or tendon. It is characterized by pain, muscle spasm, and muscle weakness. Signs of a strain may include localized swelling, cramping, inflammation, and some loss of muscle function.

- Avoid exercising or playing sports when tired or in pain.
- Run on even surfaces.

Sprains

A **sprain** can result from a fall, a sudden twist, or a blow to the body that forces a joint out of its normal position. This results in overstretching or tearing of the ligament supporting that joint. Typically, sprains occur when the athlete falls and lands on an outstretched arm, slides into base, lands on the side of the foot, or twists a knee with the foot planted firmly on the ground (Figure 16–14). Although sprains can occur in both the upper and lower parts of the body, the most common site is the ankle.

SIGNS AND SYMPTOMS The usual signs and symptoms of a sprain include pain, swelling, bruising, and loss of the ability to move and use the joint. These signs and symptoms can vary in intensity, depending on the severity of the sprain. Sometimes people feel a pop or tear when the injury happens.

Doctors use many criteria to diagnose the severity of a sprain. In general, a grade I, or mild, sprain causes overstretching or slight tearing of

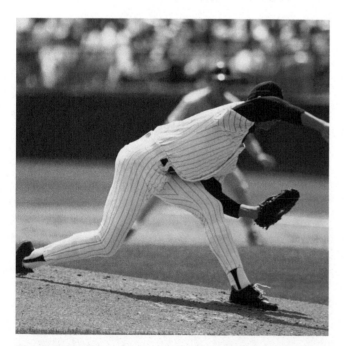

Figure 16–14 Overextending an arm while pitching can increase risk of a sprain. Courtesy of Photodisc

DID YOU KNOW? Ankle sprains are the most common injury in the United States, and often occur during sports or recreational activities. Approximately 1 million ankle injuries occur each year, and 85% of them are sprains.

the ligaments, but no joint instability. A person with a mild sprain usually experiences minimal pain, swelling, and little or no loss of functional ability. Bruising is absent or slight, and the person is usually able to put weight on the affected joint. People with mild sprains usually do not need an x-ray, but one is sometimes performed if the diagnosis is unclear.

A grade II, or moderate, sprain causes partial tearing of the ligament and is characterized by bruising, moderate pain, and swelling. A person with a moderate sprain usually has some difficulty putting weight on the affected joint and experiences some loss of function. An x-ray may be needed to help the doctor determine if a fracture is causing the pain and swelling. Magnetic resonance imaging (MRI) is occasionally used to help differentiate between a significant partial injury and a complete tear in a ligament.

Persons who sustain a grade III, or severe, sprain completely tear or rupture a ligament. Pain, swelling, and bruising are usually severe, and the patient is unable to put weight on the joint. An x-ray is usually taken to rule out a fractured bone.

TREATMENT AND REHABILITATION Treatment, rehabilitation, and prevention are similar to care for a strain.

Tendonitis

A *tendon* is a tough, flexible band of fibrous tissue that connects muscle to bone. When a muscle contracts, it pulls on a bone to cause movement. The structure that transmits the force of the muscle contraction to the bone is a tendon.

Tendons come in many shapes and sizes. Some are very small, like the ones that cause movements of the fingers; some are much larger, such as the Achilles tendon. When functioning normally, these tendons glide easily and smoothly as the muscle contracts.

When tendons become irritated, the action of pulling the muscle becomes difficult. If the normal smooth, gliding motion of the tendon is impaired, the tendon will become inflamed and movement will become painful. This is called **tendonitis**, or inflammation of the tendon.

The most common cause of tendonitis is overuse. People who begin an exercise program, or increase their level of exercise too quickly, can experience symptoms of tendonitis. The tendon is unaccustomed to the new level of demand, and this overuse may cause inflammation.

SIGNS AND SYMPTOMS The most common sign of tendonitis is pain and inflammation along a tendon, usually near a joint. Typically the pain is worse with movement and at night. The pain is usually dull initially, but becomes progressively worse as repeated overuse and movement aggravate the condition.

TREATMENT Treatment of tendonitis begins with avoidance of aggravating movements. This may mean stopping or reducing normal activities for a time to allow the inflamed tendon to heal. An alternative regimen may allow the athlete to keep active while healing.

Inflammation can also be treated with medications, including nonsteroidal anti-inflammatory drugs. Before beginning any medication program, consult a doctor. Other means of treatment include icing the injured tendon, ultrasound therapy, and physical therapy.

REHABILITATION To prevent and avoid tendonitis, athletes should slowly increase the intensity and type of exercise, and not try to achieve everything all at once.

Bursitis

Bursitis is inflammation of a bursa. There are hundreds of bursae scattered throughout the body. The function of a bursa is to decrease friction between two surfaces, such as where muscles, ligaments, and tendons glide over bones. The most common sites for bursitis are the hip, knee, elbow, and heel.

A bursa provides a slippery surface that has almost no friction. When a bursa becomes irritated or inflamed, though, it loses its gliding capabilities. Bursitis can result from a repetitive movement or prolonged or excessive pressure.

SIGNS AND SYMPTOMS Bursitis is usually characterized by joint pain and is often mistaken for arthritis. Symptoms are very similar to those of tendonitis; typically, pain in the joints upon movement, pain that is worse at night, and pain that is aggravated by continued movement and overuse.

TREATMENT The best treatment for bursitis is avoiding the activity that led to the inflammation. Nonsteroidal anti-inflammatory medications may also be beneficial. If conservative treatment fails, the physician may also try drainage of the bursa, injection of cortisone, and surgical excision. Surgical excision is rarely needed, but can be helpful in cases that will not resolve.

REHABILITATION To prevent bursitis from returning, the individual should strengthen the muscles around the joint, avoid repetitive stress, cushion joints, and take rest breaks.

Contusions

A **contusion** is a direct blow or blunt injury that does not interrupt (break) the skin. Typically, there is a bruise at the site of a contusion from injury to the blood vessels. Most contusions are mild and respond well to rest, ice, compression, and elevation (RICE). More serious contusions may need to be checked by a physician.

SIGNS AND SYMPTOMS Symptoms of a contusion include swelling, pain to the touch, redness, and **ecchymosis** (Figure 16–15). Ecchymosis is an accumulation of blood in the skin and subcutaneous tissues more than one centimeter in diameter. The general term for ecchymosis is *bruising*. Ecchymosis is often the result of injury; however, clotting and bleeding disorders can also cause ecchymosis. Ecchymosis presents as a bluish lesion at the earliest stages of onset. As the red blood cells in the lesion undergo progressive degeneration, the bruise progressively changes color from blue through green through purple to, finally, a brownish-yellowish discoloration.

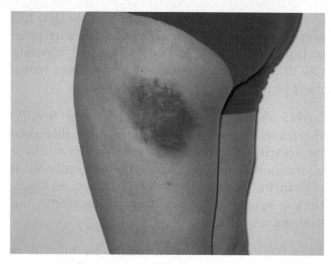

Figure 16–15 Bruising that results in a dark bluish-red patch is called ecchymosis.

Treatment

Treatment may include careful monitoring, for a minor contusion, or use of anti-inflammatory oral medications, compressive dressings, and ice to control swelling and pain. Treatment includes applying ice immediately after receiving the trauma. Ice should be applied with the body part in a stretched position, if possible; this keeps the muscle from tightening up in response to the injury. Physical therapy may be prescribed to aid in the healing of the contused tissues. Certain manual therapy techniques and modalities can be used to help decrease ecchymosis, decrease swelling, and increase range of motion.

If a contusion is not managed properly, certain side effects may occur. The most dangerous is **myositis ossificans**, a calcification that forms within the muscle. This condition usually requires surgical intervention.

REHABILITATION An athlete may return to participation when he or she has full range of motion, is at full strength, and is able to compete fully. When an athlete returns to participation after a contusion, the injured area should be protected with padding to prevent it from being struck again.

NERVES

Nerve tissue consists of two major types of nerve cells: neuroglia and neurons. Neuroglia, the cells that insulate, support, and protect the neurons, are sometimes referred to as "nerve glue."

All neurons possess the characteristics of being able to react when stimulated, and being able to pass the nerve impulse generated on to other neurons. These characteristics are *irritability* (the ability to react when stimulated) and *conductivity* (the ability to transmit a disturbance to distant points). Dendrites receive the impulse and transmit it to the cell body and then to the axon, where it is passed on to another neuron or to a muscle or gland. A **nerve fascicle**, or fasciculus, is a small bundle of axons (nerve fibers) that transmits messages between the brain and other parts of the body.

There are three types of neurons:

1. Sensory neurons, or **afferent neurons**, which emerge from the skin or sense organs and carry messages or impulses toward the spinal cord and brain.

2. Motor neurons, or **efferent neurons**, which carry messages from the brain and spinal cord to the muscles and glands.

3. Associative neurons, or **interneurons**, which carry impulses from the sensory neurons to motor neurons.

Function of the Nerves

Nerves carry impulses by creating electric charges in a process known as **membrane excitability**. Neurons have a membrane that separates the cytoplasm inside from the extracellular fluids outside the cell, thereby creating two chemically different areas. Each area has differing amounts of potassium and sodium ions, and other charged substances, with the inside part of the cell being more negatively charged than the outside. When a neuron is stimulated, ions move across the membrane, creating a current that, if large enough, briefly causes the inside of the neuron to be more positive than the outside area. This state is known as *action potential*. Neurons and other cells that produce action potentials are said to have membrane excitability.

To understand how impulses are carried along nerves, or throughout a muscle when it contracts, one needs to know more about membrane excitability. Ions cross a membrane through channels, some of which are open and allow ions to "leak" (diffuse) continuously. Other channels are called "gated" and open only during action potential. Another membrane opening is called a sodium-potassium pump, which, by active transport, maintains the flow of ions from higher to lower concentration levels across the membrane and restores the cytoplasm and extracellular fluid to their original electrical state after an action potential occurs. This action is in response to the imbalance between the cytoplasm and the extracellular fluid. When diffusion takes place, ions move from an area of greater concentration to an area of lesser concentration.

The following simplified description explains how this process works.

1. A neuron membrane is "at rest." There are large amounts of potassium (K^+) ions inside the cells, but not very many sodium (Na^+) ions. The reverse is true outside the cell in the extracellular fluid. Most of the open channels are for potassium to pass through, so it leaks out of the cell.

2. As the K^+ ions leave, the inside of the cell becomes relatively more negative until some K^+ ions are attracted back in, the electrical force balances the diffusion force, and movement stops. The inside is still more negative, and the amount of energy between the two differently charged areas is ready to carry an impulse. This state is called resting membrane potential (Figure 16–16A). The membrane is now polarized. The sodium ions are not able to move "in" because their channels are closed during the resting state; however, if a few do leak in, the membrane pump sends out an equal number.

3. Now suppose a sensory neuron receptor is stimulated by something (e.g., a sound) that causes a change in the membrane potential. The stimulus energy is converted to an electrical signal; if it is strong enough, it will depolarize a portion of the membrane and allow the gated Na^+ ion channels to open, initiating an action potential (Figure 16–16B).

4. The Na^+ ions move through the gated channels into the cytoplasm. The inside becomes more positive, until the membrane potential is reversed and the gates close to Na^+ ions.

5. Next, the K^+ gates open and large amounts of potassium leave the cytoplasm,

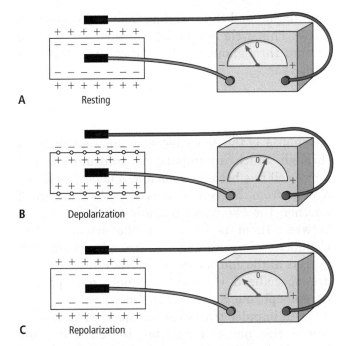

Figure 16–16 Sequence of events in membrane potential and relative positive and negative states. (A) normal resting potential (negative inside/positive outside). (B) Depolarization (positive inside/negative outside). (C) Repolarization (negative inside/positive outside).

resulting in repolarization of the membrane (Figure 16–16C). After repolarization, the sodium-potassium pump restores the initial concentrations of Na^+ and K^+ ions inside and outside the neuron.

This entire process occurs in a few milliseconds. When this action occurs in one part of the cell membrane, it spreads to adjacent membrane regions, continuing away from the original site of

KEY CONCEPT

The function of nerve cells is to carry impulses by creating electrical charges. This is done by moving electrically charged ions across a membrane. Ions move from an area of higher concentration to an area of lower concentration.

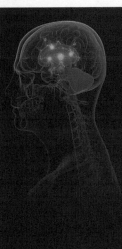

stimulation and thus sending "messages" over the nerve. This cycle is completed millions of times a minute throughout the body, day after day, year after year.

Synapse

A **synapse** is the space between adjacent neurons through which an impulse is transmitted. The nerve cell has both an axon and a dendrite. Messages go from the axon of one cell to the dendrite of another; the two never actually touch. The space between them is known as the *synaptic cleft*. Conduction is accomplished through neurotransmitters at the end of each axon. Neurotransmitters are specialized chemicals, namely epinephrine, norepinephrine, and acetylcholine.

An impulse travels along the axon to its end, where the neurotransmitter is released. This helps the impulse to "jump" the space between and reach the dendrite of the next nerve cell. The neurotransmitter between muscle cells and the nervous system is acetylcholine.

INJURY TO NERVES

With the growth of athletic participation has come a corresponding increase in sports-related neurological disorders. Peripheral nerve injuries in sports are caused by trauma, compression, and traction. Prompt evaluation and treatment of the athlete will enable an earlier return to competition. Spinal cord injuries and concussions are two of the most dangerous injuries that can be sustained in athletics. Both of these topics, as well as nerve injuries to the shoulder and elbow, are addressed in later chapters. Other sports-related nerve injuries are discussed here.

Nerves are fragile and can be damaged by pressure, stretching, or cutting. Injury to a nerve can stop signals to and from the brain, causing muscles to become unresponsive, along with a loss of feeling in the injured area. When a nerve is cut, both the nerve and the insulation are affected. Pressure or stretching injuries can cause the fibers that carry information to break and thus stop the nerve from working, without damaging its cover.

When nerve fibers are cut or broken, the end of the fiber farthest from the brain dies, although the insulation (**myelin sheath**) stays healthy. The end closest to the brain does not die, and after some time it may begin to heal. If the insulation was not cut, new fibers may grow down the empty cover of the tissue until they reach a muscle or sensory receptor. If both the nerve and insulation have been cut, and the nerve is not repaired, new nerve fibers may grow into a ball at the end of the cut, forming a nerve scar or **neuroma**. A neuroma can be painful and cause an electrical feeling when the person is touched.

The treatment for a cut nerve is to sew together the myelin sheath surrounding both ends of the nerve. The goal in repairing the nerve is to save the cover so that new fibers may heal and function be regained.

Once the nerve cover is mended, the nerve generally begins to heal three or four weeks after the injury. Nerves usually grow one inch every month, depending on the patient's age and other factors. This means that recovering from an injury to a nerve in the arm above the fingertips may require up to a year before feeling returns to the fingertips. The feeling of "pins and needles" in the fingertips is common during the recovery process. Though this can be uncomfortable, it usually passes and is a sign of recovery.

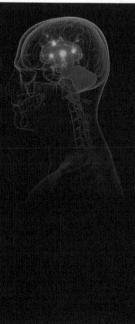

KEY CONCEPT

A nerve injury occurs because of pressure, stretching, or cutting of the nerve. Damage to a nerve interrupts its signals to the brain and can impair motor function and sensation as a result. Treatment for a cut nerve is to suture the myelin sheath around both ends of the nerve. The goal is to save the sheath so that new nerve fibers can grow.

SOFT-TISSUE INJURIES

Of the more than 10 million sports injuries that occur each year, most are due to either traumatic injury or overuse of muscles or joints. Many sports injuries can be prevented by proper conditioning and training, wearing appropriate protective gear, and using proper equipment. In athletics, there is always an inherent risk of injury.

Injuries due to minor trauma involving the soft tissue affect the skin, muscles, ligaments, and tendons. The recognition and prompt treatment of a soft-tissue injury often determines how quickly an athlete recovers from the injury.

Soft-tissue injuries are classified as open or closed. Open injuries include abrasions, lacerations, avulsions, and puncture wounds. Closed injuries include contusions, hematomas, and ecchymoses. Also in the closed category are sprains, strains, tendonitis, bursitis, and stress-related injuries, including stress fractures. Proper recognition and care of these injuries will help reduce the risk of infection and allow the body to heal faster.

Abrasions and Scrapes

Abrasions and scrapes occur when several layers of skin are torn loose or totally removed (Figure 16–17). Abrasions are painful, usually more painful than a deeper cut because the scraping of skin exposes millions of nerve endings.

TREATMENT Treatment includes washing the wound to remove all dirt and debris. Hydrogen peroxide may be used, but soap and water are as effective. If particles of dirt, rocks, or tar are embedded, it might be necessary to scrub the wound. This can be very painful and might require local anesthetic or oral pain medication before the wound is cleaned. Applying an antibiotic ointment to the wound will help keep the dressing from sticking to the wound and inhibit infection.

Abrasions usually are left open to the air, unless oozing fluid or blood is present. A nonstick adhesive dressing may be used for a couple of days, after which the wound may be left open to air. Generally, scrapes scab over quickly.

Loose skin flaps, if they are not dirty, may be left in place to help form a natural dressing for tender tissue. If the skin flap is dirty, it may be removed carefully with a clean nail clipper.

Pain may be mild to moderate, depending on the severity of the abrasion. Ice packs or cool towels might be helpful in relieving pain.

Check the date of the athlete's last tetanus immunization. One should be given every 10 years. Watch for signs of infection. Infection will not be obvious in the first 24 hours. Seek medical attention for the abrasion if any of the following symptoms occur:

- Pain increases after several days following the initial injury
- Redness or red streaks appear beyond the expected redness at the edges of the wound
- Swelling at the injured area, proximal or distal to the wound
- Purulent drainage (yellow, green, or bloody, foul-smelling pus)

Lacerations

A **laceration**, or cut, is a tear in the skin that results from an injury. Most minor lacerations have minimal bleeding, minimal pain, and no numbness or tingling at the site. Cuts that are less than 0.25 inches (6 mm) deep and 0.5 inches (1.3 cm) long, and have smooth edges, can usually be treated at home without stitches. Deeper lacerations should be treated by a physician (Figure 16–18).

TREATMENT Lacerations must be cleaned out with soap and water and well irrigated with clean water to remove any debris. The use of alcohol, iodine, mercurochrome, or peroxide on such a

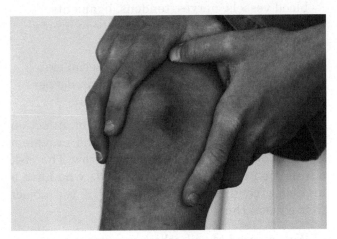

Figure 16–17 Abrasions can occur from contact with the ground, another player, or equipment. Courtesy of Photodisc

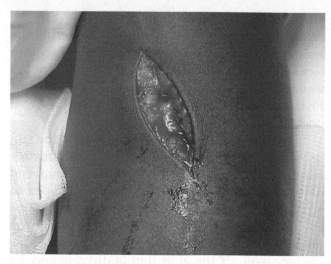

Figure 16–18 Deep lacerations may require professional medical care. Courtesy of Dr. Deborah Funk, Alnaby Medical center, Albany, NY.

wound may cause further damage and slow the healing process. Debris and bacteria can be drained from the wound by allowing some controlled bleeding for a brief time.

To stop bleeding, cover the wound with sterile gauze and apply direct, constant pressure to the wound site for 15 minutes or more. Once the wound has been cleaned, apply an antibiotic ointment to help to prevent infection and aid healing. Change the sterile dressing daily as needed.

For uncontrolled bleeding, or cuts that spurt blood in sync with the pulse (arterial bleeding), seek immediate professional medical attention.

Bruising, caused by blood clotting under the skin surface, may be seen around the laceration site. Some swelling may also be noted at the site. If bruising and swelling occur, apply ice to the site and elevate the area above the level of the heart. If bruising and swelling do not improve within 24 hours, contact a physician.

A physician should also be contacted if:

- The laceration is more than 0.25 inches (6 mm) deep and 0.5 inches (1.3 cm) long.

- The wound is in an area where it could be opened by simple movement of that body part.

- The wound is on the face, eyelids, or lips. The aesthetic outcome may be profoundly affected by scarring.

- There are deep cuts on the palm, finger, elbow, or knee.

- There is any loss of sensation or normal range of motion of a body part as a result of the cut.

Avulsions

An **avulsion** is an injury in which layers of skin are either torn off completely or a flap of skin only remains. This type of wound may cause considerable bleeding.

TREATMENT After cleaning the wound, if a skin flap remains connected, carefully replace it in its original position. Skin in the affected area often will survive. An injured party with a deep avulsion should see a doctor for possible stitches. If a large piece of skin has been torn off completely, place it in a plastic bag and put it on ice. The skin should not be frozen or soaked in water. Take the patient and the bag containing the skin to the patient's doctor, who may be able to save and replace the severed skin.

Puncture Wounds

Puncture wounds are caused by sharp, pointed objects that penetrate the skin. Nails, tacks, ice picks, knives, teeth, and needles can cause puncture wounds.

TREATMENT To treat a puncture wound:

- Find out whether any part of the object that caused the wound—such as lead (graphite) from a pencil—is still in the wound.

- Determine whether other tissues (such as blood vessels, nerves, tendons, ligaments, bones, or internal organs) have been injured by the object.

- Prevent infections, including bacterial skin infections, tetanus, and infections in deeper structures (such as bones and joints).

Puncture wounds are at risk of infection because they are difficult to clean and provide a warm, moist place for bacteria to grow. The risk of infection is greater in individuals who have a high-risk condition or disease, or if the object that caused the wound:

- Was exposed to soil, which may contain tetanus or other bacteria

- Went through the sole of a shoe (this increases the risk of a bacterial infection that is difficult to treat)
- Was injected into the skin under high pressure, such as paint from a high-pressure paint sprayer or a nail from a nail gun

A physician should be consulted if the object penetrated deeply, and for advice on the need for a tetanus shot. Seek medical attention if signs of infection appear.

Contusions

See discussion on Contusions earlier in the chapter.

Hematomas

A **hematoma** consists of blood and fluid that pool within a tissue space, compartment, or organ. They may form at any depth at almost any site in the body. Hematomas are usually the result of a contusion.

TREATMENT Treatment for typical hematomas is compression, cold pack, elevation, and rest (RICE). Local compression and padding may be needed for one or two weeks to assure complete resolution.

Ecchymosis

See discussion on Ecchymosis earlier in the chapter.

THE BODY'S RESPONSE TO INJURY

Inflammation is the body's reaction to invasion by an infectious agent or physical, chemical, or traumatic damage. The mechanism that triggers the body's response to injury is extremely sensitive. The body has the capacity to respond to minor injuries such as bruising, scratching, cuts, and abrasions, as well as to major injuries such as fractures, severe burns, and amputation of limbs.

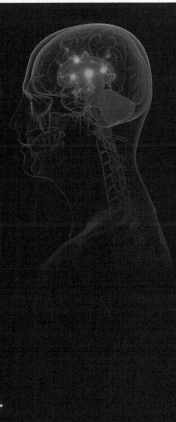

KEY CONCEPT

Treatment for soft-tissue injuries varies by injury:
- Abrasions are treated by washing with soap and water, applying antibiotic ointment, and leaving them open to air if not bleeding or oozing.
- Lacerations are treated by cleaning them with soap and water and applying a bandage with pressure to stop the bleeding.
- Avulsions must be cleaned. Any remaining skin flap should be replaced in its original position (completely detached skin can be placed on ice). This type of injury often requires treatment by a physician.
- Puncture wounds should be examined to determine if an object is still in the wound; if any underlying structures or organs were damaged; and if the object was contaminated and could increase the risk of infection. Puncture wounds should be checked by a physician.
- Contusions can be treated with ice, compressive dressings, and anti-inflammatory medications.
- Hematomas are treated with compression, cold packs, elevation, and rest.
- Ecchymosis usually does not require treatment unless severe.

Depending on the severity of the tissue damage from an injury, the integrity of the skin or internal surfaces may be breached. Damage to the underlying connective tissue and muscle, as well as blood vessels, can also occur. In this situation, infection can and frequently does result because the normal barrier to the entry of harmful organisms has been broken. It is important that the body respond to injury by healing and repairing damaged tissue, in addition to eliminating infectious agents (and their toxins) that have entered the wound.

The inflammatory response is humankind's oldest defense mechanism. The cells of the immune system are widely distributed throughout the body. When infection or tissue damage occurs, it is necessary to concentrate immune-system cells and their products at the site of damage. Three major events occur during this response:

1. Blood supply to the damaged tissue increases. This is performed by dilatation of the vessels.

2. Capillary permeability increases. This permits larger-than-usual molecules to escape from the capillaries, and thus allows specialized cells to reach the site of the injury.

3. **Leukocytes** (white blood cells) migrate out of the capillaries into the surrounding tissues. In the earliest stages of inflammation, **neutrophils** (an abundant type of granular white blood cells that are highly destructive to microorganisms) are particularly prevalent, but later **monocytes** (large, circulating white blood cells) and **lymphocytes** (nearly 25% of white blood cells, including B-cells and T-cells) also migrate toward the site of injury or infection.

Inflammatory responses must be well ordered and controlled. The body must be able to act quickly to reduce or stop the loss of blood, whereas tissue repair and reconstruction can begin a little later. A wide variety of interconnected cellular and body fluid mechanisms are activated when tissue damage and infection occur. Once leukocytes arrive at a site of inflammation, they release mediators that control the later accumulation and activation of other cells.

Inflammation can become chronic. In certain settings, the acute process gives way to a predominance of **mononuclear phagocytes** (white blood cells that engulf and absorb waste material, harmful microorganisms, and other foreign bodies in the bloodstream and tissues) and lymphocytes. This probably occurs to some degree with the normal healing process, but becomes exaggerated and chronic when there is ineffective elimination of damaged tissues.

Cell Regeneration

Regeneration is the act of wound healing. During the mechanism of regeneration, cells around the area of injury work to close and heal the wound. Once the damaged tissue is degraded by the leukocytes, generation of new tissue can begin. However, if the damage is severe enough, the wound may not be reparable to its pre-injury status. In such a case, the damaged tissue is replaced by fibrous or **scar tissue**.

Cellular Dedifferentiation

In a complex mechanism of regeneration known as **cellular dedifferentiation** cells revert to an earlier stage of development, becoming dedifferentiated from their mature functions, and reenter the cell cycle so they can proliferate to produce more cells with the same function. This form of regeneration may be useful in replacing cells that have become worn out, damaged, or are just in short supply.

Transdifferentiation

Regenerative complexity is seen in both cellular dedifferentiation and **transdifferentiation**. In this form of regeneration, cells once again are dedifferentiated from their mature function so that they can reenter the cell cycle and proliferate. However, once cellular proliferation has occurred, the new cells go one step further and become—that is, transdifferentiate into—cells with completely different functions than those from which they originated. This is extremely useful when a tissue or organ becomes impaired and loses some of its function. Through transdifferentiation, damaged cells can be replaced by neighboring cells, even though they are not of the same cell type. An example occurs in the pancreas, where duct cells dedifferentiate and then transdifferentiate into insulin-expressing beta cells.

Tissue Remodeling

Tissue remodeling is the process by which cells and molecules of the tissue are modified and reassembled to yield a new composition of cell types and an **extracellular matrix (ECM)**. There are four components to this process:

1. Formation of new blood vessels (**angiogenesis**), spanning the wound.
2. Migration and proliferation of fibroblasts (cells that give rise to connective tissue) to fill and bridge the wound.
3. Deposition of ECM.
4. Tissue remodeling (maturation and reorganization of the fibrous tissue into a scar).

The remodeling phase of an injury can last for over a year. During this phase, the **collagen fibers** thickened and strengthen. Collagen is a protein substance found in bone and cartilage. The fibers are mostly aligned with the axis of the wound, oriented by myofibroblast deposition and contraction. The tensile strength of the wound is increases as collagen molecules are modified and cross-linked by enzymes. Additionally, collagen fibers are modified to approach the ratio found in

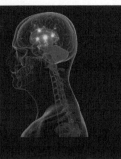

KEY CONCEPT

Inflammation is the body's reaction to invasion by an infectious agent or physical, chemical, or traumatic damage.

healthy tissue. As the amount of collagen within the matrix increases, the density of blood vessels diminishes. This remodeling tissue is *scar tissue,* which at its maximum tensile strength is only 70 to 80% as strong as normal tissue.

Repair cannot be accomplished solely by regeneration. It also involves replacement of lost cells and tissues by **connective tissue**. Connective tissue is the material between the cells of the body that gives tissues form and strength. In time, this produces fibrosis and scarring.

CONCLUSION

The skeleton provides support and protection to the internal organs of the body. It also is the foundation for muscle attachment and an efficient factory that produces red blood cells.

Many injuries associated with athletics are fractures—breaks in the bones resulting from excessive force or overtraining. Other injuries associated with athletics involve muscles, their attachments, and the various tissues surrounding them. These injuries can range from simple bruises to severe soft-tissue damage. The certified athletic trainer and sports medicine team must always be vigilant in recognizing, assessing, and managing these injuries.

REVIEW QUESTIONS

1. How many bones are in the adult skeleton? The infant skeleton?
2. List the differences between the axial and appendicular skeleton.
3. What are the distinct functions of compact and spongy bone?
4. Give one example each of a long, short, and flat bone.
5. What is bone marrow, and why is it important?
6. What are the six major classifications of fractures?
7. Explain the difference between skeletal, smooth, and cardiac muscle.
8. Explain how muscle strains occur.
9. How can muscle strains be prevented?
10. Explain nerve injuries and their treatment.
11. List and describe the different types of soft-tissue injuries.
12. How are different soft tissue injuries treated?

13. What is inflammation?
14. What is the function of a nerve cell?
15. How does the body repair injured tissue?
16. What is scar tissue?

PROJECTS AND ACTIVITIES

1. The nervous system sends electrical impulses up at to 250 miles per hour. How long would it take for an impulse from the brain to reach the foot of a person who is six feet tall?
2. Draw a nerve cell, including all major components.
3. Create a flowchart explaining membrane excitability.
4. Name some disorders of the nervous system? (Use the Internet as a resource to answer this question.)
5. Create a list of fun facts about the nervous system.
6. Create a matching exercise using the Key Terms. Include an answer key.
7. Rewrite the opening section on soft-tissue injuries using your own words.
8. Ask a radiologist or orthopedic surgeon from a local hospital or clinic to bring in x-rays used to examine bones. Lead a class discussion with your guest speaker.

LEARNING LINKS

• Review the skeletal, muscular, and nervous systems at http://www.innerbody.com.
• Visit http://www.teenshealth.org and click on the link for "Your Body." View the content on bones, muscles, and joints.
• Search for various other resources and activities related to the skeletal, muscular, and nervous systems. See if you can find additional websites that relate to athletic injuries to these systems.

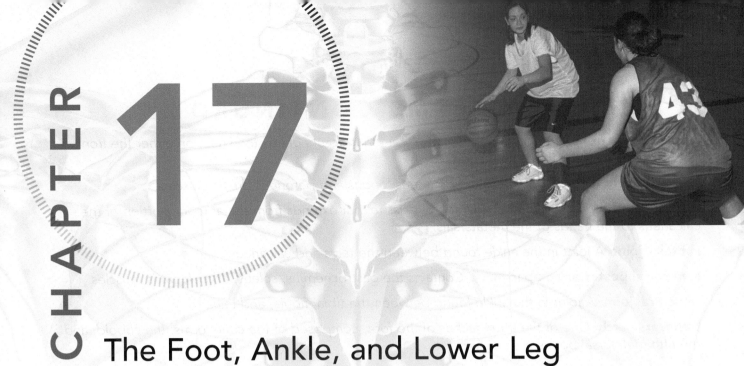

CHAPTER 17

The Foot, Ankle, and Lower Leg

OBJECTIVES

Upon completion of this chapter, the reader should be able to:

- Describe the anatomy of the foot and ankle
- Identify common injuries and conditions affecting the foot, ankle, and lower leg
- Explain what additional tests are described for the foot, ankle, and lower leg

KEY TERMS

Achilles tendon *A tendon in the back of the ankle and foot that attaches the gastrocnemius and soleus muscles to the calcaneus.*

anterior compartment *Contains the tibialis anterior, extensor digitorum longus, peroneus tertius, and extensor hallucis muscles.*

compartment syndrome *A serious condition that may develop when swelling exists in one or more of the four compartments of the leg or arm.*

cramp *A sudden, involuntary contraction of a muscle.*

deep posterior compartment *Contains the popliteus, flexor digitorum longus, flexor hallucis longus, and tibialis posterior muscles.*

extrinsic muscle *Muscle that is outside a body part, organ, or bone.*

intrinsic muscle *Muscle that relates to a specific body part or bone.*

lateral longitudinal arch *One of the three arches of the foot; composed of the calcaneus, talus, cuboid, and the fourth and fifth metatarsals; lower and flatter than the medial longitudinal arch.*

malleoli *Large, bony prominences located on either side of the ankle.*

medial longitudinal arch *The highest of the three arches of the foot; composed of the calcaneus, talus, navicular, cuneiforms, and the first three metatarsals.*

KEY TERMS CONTINUED

medial tibial stress syndrome (shin splints) *Pain that occurs below the knee, on either the front outside portion or the inside of the leg.*

peroneal compartment *Contains the peroneus longus and peroneus brevis muscles.*

plantar fascia *Wide, nonelastic, ligamentous tissue that extends from the anterior portion of the calcaneus to the heads of the metatarsals.*

subtalar joint *A joint in the ankle found between the talus and calcaneus.*

superficial posterior compartment *Contains the gastrocnemius, soleus, and plantaris muscles.*

talocrural joint *A joint in the ankle found between the tibia, fibula, and talus.*

transverse arch *One of the three arches of the foot; composed of the cuneiforms, the cuboid, and the fifth metatarsal bones.*

THE LOWER LEG

The lower leg, including the ankle and foot, is exposed to numerous types of trauma's during athletic practices and events. Even with protective equipment, such as the shin pads used in soccer, the lower leg is still susceptible to injury. Common injuries to the lower leg include contusions, strains, tendonitis, tendon ruptures, medial tibial stress syndrome (shin splints), stress fractures, compartment syndrome, and fractures.

THE FOOT AND ANKLE

It has been estimated that 15% of all sports injuries involve the ligaments, bones, and tendons of the ankle. Because the ankle absorbs three times the force of the body during running and jumping, it is not surprising that there are more than 20,000 ankle sprains in the United States every day (Figure 17–1).

Acting as shock absorbers, the feet cushion up to one million pounds of pressure during a single hour of strenuous exercise. Taking all this into consideration, the feet log approximately 1,000 miles per year.

The foot is responsible for some of the most minor, yet potentially debilitating, conditions suffered by athletes. These conditions include athlete's foot, turf toe, calluses, ingrown toenails, and blisters. If these conditions are not treated, they can be just as disabling for an athlete, as more serious foot problems.

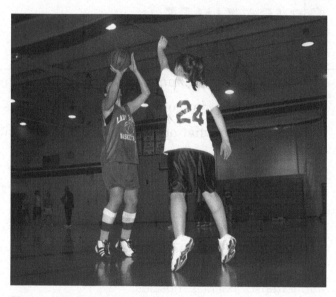

Figure 17–1 The foot, ankle, and lower leg must be fit and strong in those who participate in athletics.

Basic Anatomy of the Foot and Ankle

The foot stabilizes and supports the rest of the body during standing, walking, running, or jumping. Individually, the parts of the foot (bones, muscles, ligaments) are relatively weak. As a whole, the foot is strong enough to withstand most athletic demands. The key to the foot's function is a set of three arches, which help in absorbing the impact of walking, running, and jumping. These are the **transverse arch**, the **medial longitudinal arch**, and the **lateral longitudinal arch**. The medial longitudinal arch is the highest and most important of

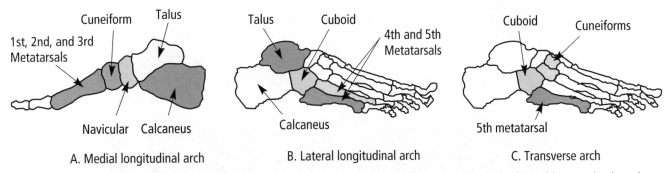

Cuneiform   Talus

1st, 2nd, and 3rd Metatarsals

Navicular   Calcaneus

A. Medial longitudinal arch

Talus   Cuboid

4th and 5th Metatarsals

Calcaneus

B. Lateral longitudinal arch

Cuboid   Cuneiforms

5th metatarsal

C. Transverse arch

Figure 17–2 The foot comprises three naturally occurring arches: the medial longitudinal, the lateral longitudinal, and the transverse arch.

the three arches. It is composed of the calcaneus, talus, navicular, cuneiforms, and the first three metatarsals. The lateral longitudinal arch is lower and flatter than the medial arch. It is composed of the calcaneus, talus, cuboid, and the fourth and fifth metatarsals. The transverse arch is composed of the cuneiforms, the cuboid, and the five metatarsal bases. The arches of the foot are maintained by the shapes of the bones as well as by ligaments. In addition, muscles and tendons play an important role in supporting the arches. Figure 17–2 illustrates the arches of the foot.

The feet contain about one-fourth of the total number of bones in the body. Each foot has 26 bones (7 tarsals, 5 metatarsals, and 14 phalanges), along with 38 joints. The tarsal bones consist of the talus, calcaneus, navicular, cuboid, and the medial, intermediate, and lateral cuneiform bones. The mid-foot region is made up of the five metatarsal bones. The toes have 14 bones known as the phalanges. Figure 17–3 illustrates the complicated bone structure of the foot and ankle.

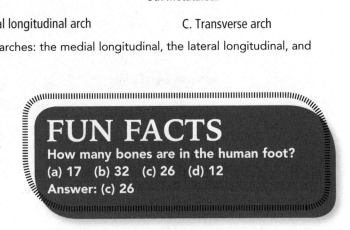

FUN FACTS
How many bones are in the human foot?
(a) 17   (b) 32   (c) 26   (d) 12
Answer: (c) 26

The ankle joint—the joint most commonly injured in athletics—is formed by a combination of two joints: the **talocrural joint**, made up of the tibia, fibula, and talus, and the **subtalar joint**, made up of the talus and calcaneus. The talus and calcaneus are the two largest bones of the foot. Large, bony prominences called **malleoli** are located

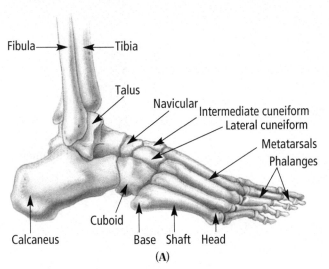

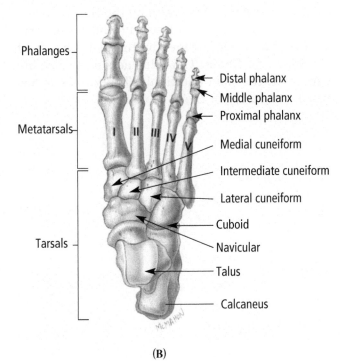

Figure 17–3 (A) Right ankle and foot lateral view. (B) Right ankle and foot superior view.

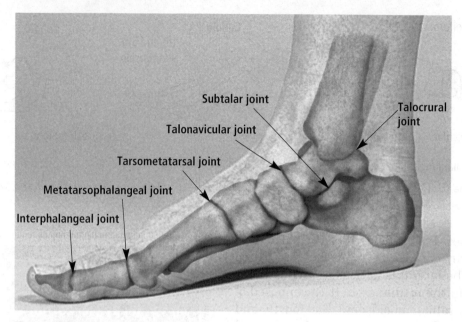

Figure 17–4 The joints of the ankle.

on either side of the ankle. They are the distal ends of the tibia (medially) and the fibula (laterally). The ankle joints are illustrated in Figure 17–4.

The tibia transmits the weight of the body to the talus. The fibula extends from the distal lateral side of the tibia, forming the lateral malleolus, which acts as a lateral stabilizer of the ankle joint. The talocrural is a hinge joint with most of its movement in dorsiflexion and plantar flexion. The subtalar joint has movement around the oblique axis.

The talus moves anteriorly and posteriorly in a cuplike cavity formed by the distal heads of the tibia and fibula. The talus acts as a movable saddle for the tibia and fibula. The talus sits forward and on top of the calcaneus.

Ligaments of the Foot and Ankle

Ligaments are tough bands of tissue that connect bones to each other. They provide strength and support to joints. Ligaments are named for the bones they connect. The ligaments most commonly injured on the lateral aspect of the ankle are the anterior talofibular, anterior tibiofibular, calcaneofibular, and posterior talofibular. On the medial aspect of the ankle the deltoid ligament is commonly injured. The triangular-shaped deltoid ligament consists of a superficial and deep layer that connects the talus to the medial malleolus. Figure 17–5 shows the ligament structure of the ankle.

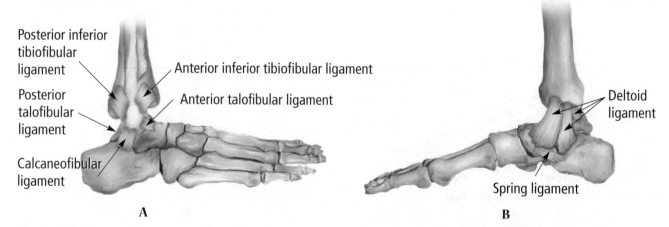

Figure 17–5 (A) Ligaments of the lateral aspect of the ankle. (B) Ligaments of the medial aspect of the ankle.

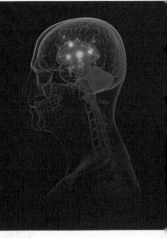

KEY CONCEPT

- The foot has three arches: transverse, medial longitudinal, and lateral longitudinal.
- The foot has 26 bones (7 tarsals, 5 metatarsals, and 14 phalanges).
- The foot has 38 joints.
- The ankle joint is made up of the talocrural and subtalar joints.
- There are five main ligaments in the ankle: anterior talofibular, anterior tibiofibular, calcaneofibular, posterior talofibular, and deltoid.

In the ankle, injuries to the ligaments, called *sprains*, are usually caused by unexpected twists of the joint. A sprain can be a stretch, tear, or complete rupture of one or more of the ankle ligaments.

BASIC ANATOMY OF THE LOWER LEG

The lower leg consists of two bones, the tibia and the fibula (Figure 17–6). The tibia, the largest of the two lower leg bones, is also known as the shin. In proportion to its length, the fibula is the slenderest bone in the body. It lies parallel with and on the lateral side of the tibia.

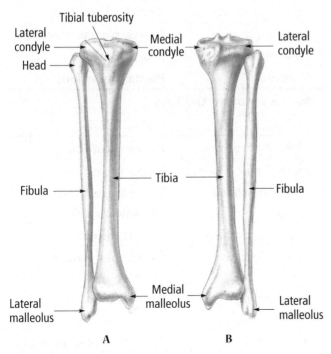

Figure 17–6 The tibia and fibula. (A) Anterior view. (B) Posterior view.

Muscles of the Lower Leg and Foot

The muscles of the foot are classified as either intrinsic or extrinsic. The **intrinsic muscles** are located within the foot and cause movement of the toes. These muscles are plantar flexors, dorsiflexors, abductors, and adductors of the toes. Several intrinsic muscles also help support the arches of the foot (Figure 17–7).

The **extrinsic muscles** are located outside the foot, in the lower leg (Figure 17–8). The powerful gastrocnemius muscle is among them. These muscles have long tendons that cross the ankle and attach on the bones of the foot to assist in movement. The talus, however, has no tendon attachments.

COMMON INJURIES OF THE FOOT AND ANKLE

Foot and ankle problems are among the most common health concerns in the United States. Studies show that at least three-quarters of the American population experiences foot problems of some degree of seriousness at some time in their lives.

Healthy feet are critical to a successful fitness program. The importance of foot care in exercise is stressed by the American Podiatric Medical Association (APMA). According to the American Academy of Podiatric Sports Medicine, an APMA affiliate, people do not realize the tremendous pressure that is put on their feet during exercise. For example, when a 150-pound jogger runs 3 miles, the cumulative impact on each foot is more than 150 tons.

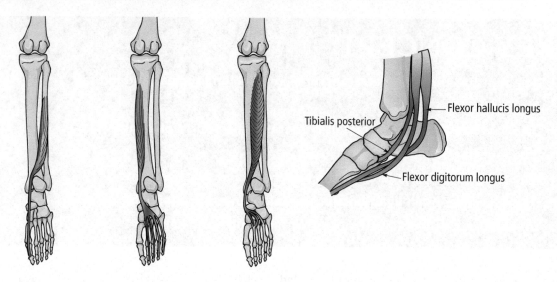

Flexor hallucis longus   Flexor digitorum longus   Tibialis posterior

Figure 17–7 Major intrinsic muscles of the lower leg and foot.

KEY CONCEPT

The intrinsic muscles cause movement of the toes and help support the arches of the foot. The extrinsic muscles aid in movement of the ankle and foot. Table 17–1 lists the names and functions of each muscle in the lower leg and foot.

Even without exercise-induced stress, foot problems contribute to pain in the knees, hips, and lower back, and also diminish work efficiency and leisure enjoyment.

Ankle Sprains

The ankle is susceptible to a variety of injuries, ranging from muscle strains and ligament sprains to dislocations and fractures. The most common injury is the ankle sprain. Dr. Carol Frey, associate professor at the University of Southern California, noted that sprains are the most common presentation in an orthopedic practice, and also the most common reason for emergency room visits (Frey, 1998) (Figure 17–9). There are about 27,000 sprains per day in the United States, accounting

Table 17–1 Muscles Moving the Foot and Toes	
Muscles Moving the Foot	
MUSCLE	FUNCTION
Gastrocnemius	Plantar flexes foot, flexes leg, supinates foot
Soleus	Plantar flexes foot
Tibialis posterior	Plantar flexes foot
Tibialis anterior	Dorsally flexes foot
Peroneus tertius	Dorsally flexes foot
Peroneus longus	Everts, plantar flexes foot
Peroneus brevus	Everts foot
Plantaris	Plantar flexes foot
Muscles Moving the Toes	
MUSCLE	FUNCTION
Flexor hallucis brevis	Flexes great toe
Flexor hallucis longus	Flexes great toe
Extensor hallucis longus	Extends great toe, dorsiflexes ankle
Interossei dorsalis	Abduct, flex toes
Flexor digitorum longus	Flexes toes, extends foot
Extensor digitorum longus	Extends toes
Abductor hallucis	Abducts, flexes great toe
Abductor digiti minimi	Abducts little toe

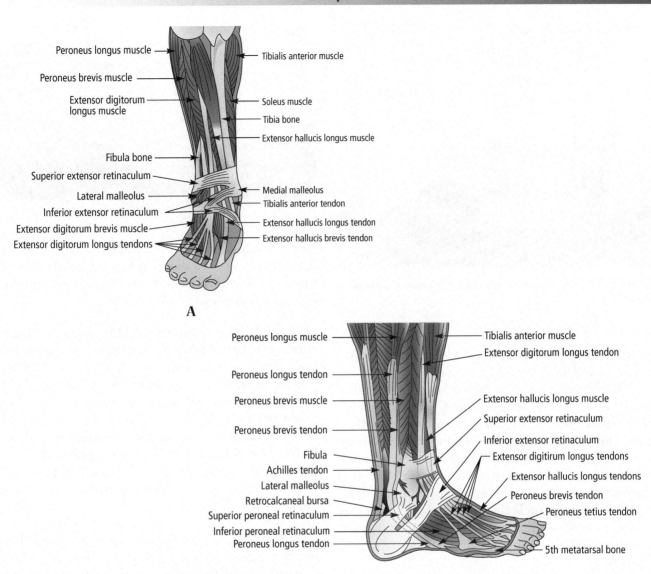

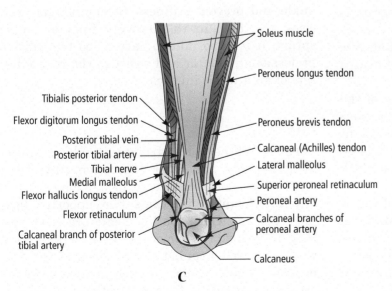

Figure 17–8 (A) Front view of the muscles of the foot. (B) Side view of the muscles of the foot. (C) Back view of the muscles of the foot.

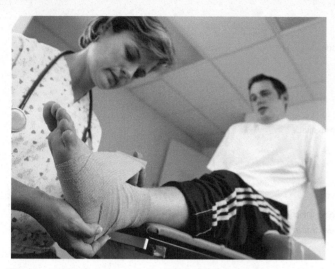

Figure 17–9 Ankle sprains are painful injuries. Courtesy of Photodisc

DID YOU KNOW? The most commonly sprained ligament of the ankle is the anterior talofibular ligament. Because it is the first lateral ligament that is stressed during inversion of the foot, it is most susceptible to damage.

for 45% of basketball injuries, 31% of soccer injuries, and 24% of volleyball injuries.

The mechanism of injury is usually a combination of excessive inversion and plantar flexion. More than 80% of all ankle sprains are of this type. The ligament most often injured is the anterior talofibular ligament. Other ligaments commonly involved in an inversion sprain are the calcaneofibular and posterior talofibular ligaments. Less common is the eversion sprain. On the medial side of the ankle, the tough, thick deltoid ligament helps prevent excessive eversion (turning outward of the heel).

SIGNS AND SYMPTOMS Whether the sprain is of the inversion or eversion type, it is usually placed into one of three categories: first degree (mild), second degree (moderate), or third degree (severe).

In a *first-degree sprain,* one or more of the supporting ligaments and surrounding tissues are stretched. There is minor discomfort, point tenderness, and little or no swelling. There is no abnormal movement in the joint to indicate lack of stability.

In a *second-degree sprain*, a portion of one or more ligaments is torn. There is pain, swelling, point tenderness, disability, and loss of function. There is slightly abnormal movement in the joint. The athlete may not be able to walk normally and will favor the injured leg.

In a *third-degree sprain,* one or more ligaments have been completely torn, resulting in

joint instability. There is either extreme pain or little pain (if nerve damage has occurred), loss of function, point tenderness, and rapid swelling. An accompanying fracture is possible.

TREATMENT Immediate treatment of an ankle sprain consists of protection, rest, ice, compression, and elevation (an approach known as PRICE). Splinting, taping, or bracing the ankle can help protect it from further injury. All activities that cause pain should be eliminated. For the first 24 hours, ice should be applied for 15 minutes, with an hour and a half allowed between applications. Use a compressive wrap around the ankle and the calf until the swelling subsides. Elevate the ankle above heart level.

REHABILITATION To restore function to the ankle, begin range-of-motion exercises. Stretching exercises also help to loosen the muscles around the ankle and prevent stiffness. Strengthening exercises, too, help in the recovery from an ankle sprain. It is important to have a sports medicine professional monitor and assist in the rehabilitation of all athletic injuries.

Arch Sprains

Each arch of the foot contributes to balance, movement, support, and shock absorption. Any of the arches of the foot (transverse, medial longitudinal, or lateral longitudinal) can suffer supportive ligament sprains. Once the ligaments are stretched, they fail to hold the bones of the foot in position. A weakened arch it cannot absorb shock as well as it normally would. Causes of arch problems include overuse, overweight, fatigue, training on hard surfaces, and wearing shoes that are not supportive or are in poor condition.

TREATMENT Treatment, as with other ligament sprains, includes cold, compression, and elevation. Most arch sprains are to the lateral arch or inner longitudinal arch.

Blisters

Blisters can occur on any part of the body where friction occurs. In athletics, blisters are most often found on the feet. As the layers of the skin rub together, friction causes separation. The body responds with fluid formation in this separation. This fluid creates pressure on nerve endings, which is perceived as pain. Once formed, blisters cannot be ignored. A neglected blister may break, creating an open wound. Proper treatment of a blister is mandatory to ensure maximum comfort of the athlete and to reduce the possibility of infection. Blisters can be very painful, and even debilitating, if not properly treated.

TREATMENT The goal of blister treatment is to relieve the pain, keep the blister from enlarging, and avoid infection. Signs of infection include red or warm skin around the blister, and pus coming from the blistered area. Small, intact blisters that do not cause discomfort usually need no treatment. The best protection against infection is a blister's own skin. Skin should not be removed from the blister unless it is flapping and causing additional discomfort. Finally, the blister should be covered with a bandage that is changed daily.

To prevent blisters, friction must be eliminated. Methods include the use of appropriate shoes and socks. Shoes should be the right size and type for the sport.

Great Toe Sprain (Turf Toe)

The great toe is very important in balance, movement, and speed. Occasionally, the ligaments supporting the toe will become sprained, resulting in *turf toe* and severely limiting the performance. Often, the mechanism of the injury is the foot sliding backward on a slippery surface, which forcefully hyperextends the big toe. Figure 17–10 illustrates the mechanism of a turf-toe injury.

TREATMENT As with any acute sprain, immediate care of turf toe is PRICE. The physician

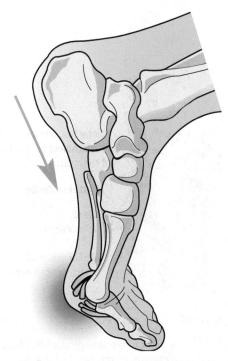

Figure 17–10 Hyperextension of the first metatarsophalangeal joint of the big toe is the mechanism of injury that causes turf toe.

may take x-rays to rule out a more severe injury. Most sprains of the great toe are minor. Once normal function returns, the certified athletic trainer will encourage constant foot/toe support to limit movement.

Plantar Fasciitis

The **plantar fascia** is a wide, nonelastic ligamentous tissue that extends from the anterior portion of the calcaneus to the heads of the metatarsals, supplying support to the longitudinal arch of the foot. This tissue can become strained from overuse, unsupportive footwear, a tight Achilles tendon, or running on hard surfaces. Figure 17–11 illustrates the plantar fascia region of the foot.

Most often, the cause of plantar fasciitis is chronic irritation. Cross-country and track athletes are prone to overuse injuries in which the plantar fascia is continually strained from running and jumping. Basketball and volleyball players are also susceptible to plantar fasciitis from repeated jumping and landing. An athlete with plantar fasciitis will experience pain and tenderness on the bottom of the foot near the heel. Untreated, this condition causes bone imbalance,

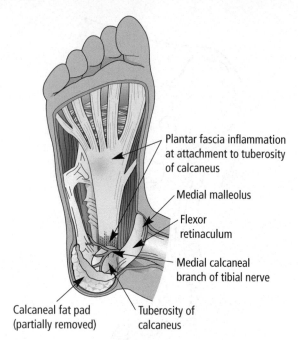

Figure 17–11 The plantar fascia region of the foot extends from the calcaneus to the base of the toes.

Labels in figure:
- Plantar fascia inflammation at attachment to tuberosity of calcaneus
- Medial malleolus
- Flexor retinaculum
- Medial calcaneal branch of tibial nerve
- Calcaneal fat pad (partially removed)
- Tuberosity of calcaneus

which can lead to heel spurs, muscle strains, shin splints, and other problems.

TREATMENT Basic treatment includes correcting training errors, icing, and massage. The athlete's shoes and activity level should be evaluated. Wearing shoes with more arch support may help decrease stress on the plantar fascia area. The use of a heel cup or cushion will help reduce the amount of shock and shear forces during activity.

Heel Bruise

The heel receives, absorbs, and transfers much of the impact from sports activities, especially running and jumping. Therefore, the ligaments, tendons, and the fat pad of the heel are all subject to stress and injury. A heel bruise is among the most disabling contusions in athletics. The heel must be protected during physical activity.

Treatment

Cold application before activity, and cold and elevation afterward, can help reduce swelling and pain. The certified athletic trainer can also supply the athlete with heel cups to help absorb the force of impact with the ground or floor; or a pad can be constructed to protect the bruised area.

Heel Spur

A *heel spur* is a bony growth on the calcaneus that causes painful inflammation of the accompanying soft tissue. This condition is aggravated by exercise. As the foot flattens, the plantar fascia is stretched and pulled at the point where it attaches to the calcaneus. Over time, the calcaneus reacts to this irritation by forming a spur of bony material.

TREATMENT The certified athletic trainer can locate a heel spur by pressing on the heel. The team physician may recommend taping the arch or using shoe inserts to help reduce the plantar fascia's pull on the calcaneus.

Fractures

Fractures of the foot and ankle immediately impair an athlete's ability to perform competitively in virtually any sporting activity. Athletes who suffer an ankle fracture usually cannot bear weight and have more swelling and pain than those with just a ligament sprain.

SIGNS AND SYMPTOMS Often, a site of point tenderness is present, and an obvious deformity may be seen. Fractures of the ankle and foot usually occur acutely in a traumatic episode.

An ankle fracture often presents with symptoms similar to those of an ankle sprain. It is important to complete a thorough examination of the involved extremity to avoid misassessing the injury. (Review Chapter 11 on assessment and evaluation of sports injuries.)

REHABILITATION OF FOOT AND ANKLE INJURIES

Returning an athlete to competition before healing is complete leaves the player susceptible to further injury. The best way to determine when healing is complete is by the absence of pain during stressful activity and the return of full range of motion, strength, power, and endurance to the affected muscle group. Before the beginning of any rehabilitation exercise program, the certified athletic trainer should consult with the sports medicine team to establish a program tailored for the individual athlete and the specific injury to be rehabilitated. The following list of exercises can be used as rehabilitative or preventive exercises (Figures 17–12 through 17–15). All exercises should begin with a few repetitions and sets, then gradually increase in intensity as the muscle groups get stronger.

COMMON INJURIES TO THE LOWER LEG

Injuries to the lower leg are common in athletics. These include contusions, sprains, strains, fractures, and inflammation of tendons and compartments of the lower leg. Prompt recognition and treatment will allow the athlete to continue activity.

Contusions

Contusions occur most often over the shin. The tibia lies just below the skin (subcutaneously) and is very sensitive to direct trauma. Trauma to this area of the leg can be very painful and disabling.

Contusions can also involve the muscular areas of the leg. A possible complication of a severe contusion to any of the leg muscles is significant swelling within the various compartments. In these closed spaces, swelling is not only uncomfortable but may also lead to compartment syndrome (discussed in greater detail later in this section). Another possible complication of a direct blow to the leg is damage to the peroneal nerve. This nerve is particularly vulnerable because it passes around the head of the fibula. A severe blow to this area may cause peroneal nerve injury, with pain radiating throughout the distribution of the nerve. Transient tingling and numbness to the lateral surface of the leg or dorsal surface of the foot may remain for a period of time. Occasionally, peroneal nerve damage will result in loss of function to the dorsiflexors and evertors of the foot, resulting in a condition known as *foot drop*. These symptoms are often temporary and recovery is usually complete.

Strains

The lower leg is the site of origin for the primary muscles responsible for transmitting power to the foot and ankle. The explosive and repetitive nature of various athletic activities subjects these muscles to extreme dynamic forces. Frequent and powerful use of leg muscles commonly results in injuries. Strains can occur anywhere along the muscles and normally result from a violent contraction, overstretching, or continued overuse. Symptoms may be present in the leg, about the ankle, or in the foot.

The most common leg strains occur to the calf muscles. Forcible contraction of these muscles during most athletic activities puts these muscles at risk.

Strains frequently occur in the area of the musculotendonous junction or at the insertion of the Achilles tendon into the calcaneus. These injuries may result from repetitive overuse or a single, violent contraction. Acute strains to the Achilles tendon have a tendency to become chronic and an area frequently complicated by tendonitis.

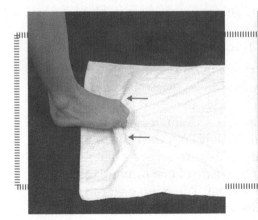

Figure 17–12 Using a towel spread out on the floor, the athlete curls the toes, bunching the towel underneath. This exercise strengthens the muscles in the foot.

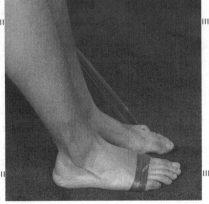
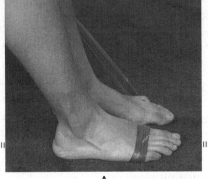
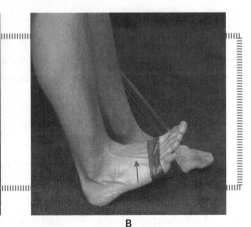

A   B

Figure 17–13A–B This exercise is for strengthening the tibialis anterior muscle of the lower leg. Using an elastic band, the athlete steps on one end while pulling up with the end wrapped around the foot.

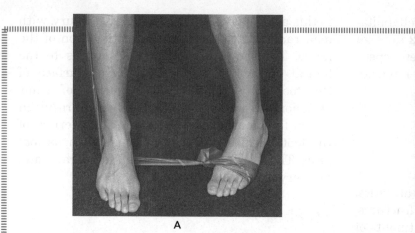

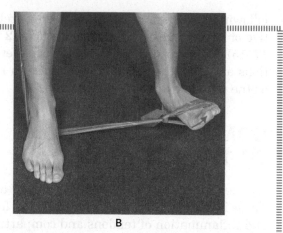

Figure 17–14A–B Strengthening exercises for the peroneus brevis muscle. The athlete steps inside a loop created in an elastic band. The opposite foot steps on the band to give resistance. The closer to the other foot, the more resistance; the further away, the less resistance. The athlete then everts the foot, working the peroneus brevis muscle.

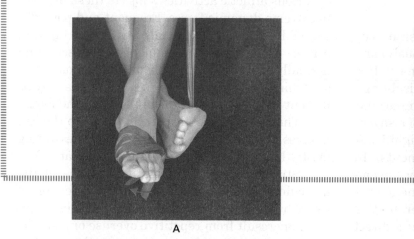

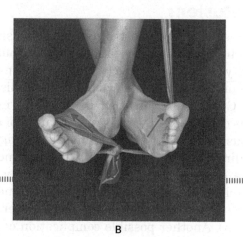

Figure 17–15A–B This exercise will strengthen the tibialis posterior muscle. Using elastic band material, the athlete loops one end around the foot. This is the side that will be worked. The athlete then crosses the other foot behind and inside the elastic band material. As illustrated by the arrows, the feet move in opposite directions.

Muscle Cramps

A **cramp** is a sudden, involuntary contraction of a muscle. Although the cause is unknown, several factors may contribute to the occurrence of a cramp:

- *Fatigue:* Working a muscle beyond its limits may cause the muscle to cramp.

- *Fractures:* After a fracture has healed, muscles usually atrophy. If the muscles involved are not strengthened to pre-injury status, cramps may occur.

- *Dehydration:* Lack of fluids can cause muscle cramps. An athlete who is exercising vigorously may lose 3.5 mL of water per hour. This rate of loss over a three- to four-hour period may account for loss of 4 to 6% of the athlete's total body weight. This causes a drop in blood volume and lessens the ability of the body to cool itself. Muscle cramping may result.

- *Lack of nutrients in diet:* A lack of fluids in the system may lead to an electrolyte imbalance that causes muscles to cramp. Electrolytes are minerals, such as sodium, magnesium, calcium, and potassium, that help the cells to function normally. An imbalance occurs when there is too much or too little of one or more electrolytes in the system. The main electrolytes affecting muscle cramping are potassium, sodium, and calcium.

- *Poor flexibility:* Good flexibility allows muscles to work through their full range of movement. Poor flexibility does the opposite, creating a situation in which the muscles may be worked beyond their limits. This may cause muscle strains or cramping.

- *Improperly fitted equipment:* Poorly fitted equipment may cause excessive strain. Excessive strain on any part of the body can result in a breakdown, which may be in the form of cramping or other injuries.

TREATMENT Treatment for muscle cramps includes passive stretching, fluid replacement, massage, rest, and ice. Water, sports drinks, or juice will help to rehydrate and restore the athlete's electrolyte balance. Most of the time, water is sufficient.

Passive stretching will help keep the muscle from forcefully shortening (Figure 17–16). Massage, along with passive stretching, will relax the muscle involved.

Achilles Tendonitis

The **Achilles tendon** derives its name from Achilles, the mighty warrior of Greek mythology. His mother dipped him into the magical waters of the river Styx at birth to give him physical invulnerability. According to legend, she held him by the heel, which was not touched by the mystic waters and therefore remained his only

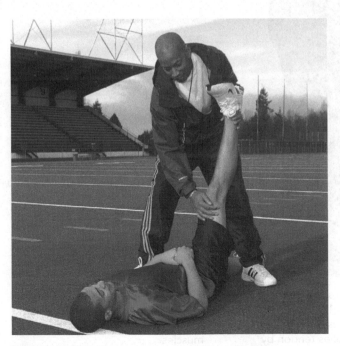

Figure 17–16 Slow, passive stretching will relax a cramped muscle.

vulnerable spot. Many years later, he was killed when an arrow struck him in the heel.

Achilles tendonitis is a painful condition caused by inflammation of the Achilles tendon. The Achilles tendon connects the gastrocnemius and soleus muscles of the posterior lower leg to the calcaneus. The gastrocnemius and soleus are strong leg muscles that attach to the foot and give us the ability to rise up on the toes, facilitating the act of walking. The Achilles tendon is vital to the ability to walk upright, so Achilles tendonitis can make walking almost impossible.

The inflammation that characterizes tendonitis reflects tearing of the tendon tissues caused by excessive stress. The problem may be caused by a single incident of overstressing the Achilles tendon, or it may result from an accumulation of lesser stresses that produce numerous small tears over time. The injury often occurs at the point where the tendon attaches to the heel, but it may occur at any point along the length of the tendon.

Sometimes overpronation causes the arch of the foot to flatten too much and the leg to twist more than normal. This, in turn, causes the gastrocnemius and soleus muscles to stretch more than normal. The force sustained by the Achilles tendon and the calcaneus increases, resulting in inflammation and pain.

SIGNS AND SYMPTOMS In most cases, symptoms develop gradually. Discomfort may be relatively minor at first and worsen if the patient tries to "work through" the pain. The initial discomfort is often attributed to the aches and pains that accompany fatigue. Repeated or continued overstress increases the inflammation; in severe cases, a rupture of the tendon can occur. This results in traumatic damage and severe pain that make walking virtually impossible. Other signs and symptoms of this condition include pain and crepitus (noise) upon palpation of the Achilles tendon and redness at the site of discomfort.

TREATMENT The best treatment for Achilles tendonitis is prevention. Stretching the Achilles tendon before exercise, even at the start of the day, will help maintain flexibility. The stretching exercises shown in Figures 17–17 through 17–21 will help the athlete maintain flexibility of the Achilles tendon.

It is important to find the cause of the problem, not just treat its symptoms. Chronic Achilles tendonitis should be assessed by a sports medicine physician or podiatrist. Solving a biomechanical

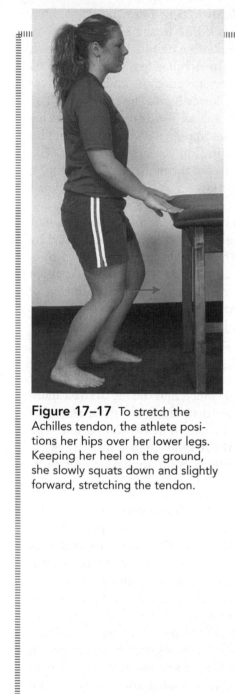

Figure 17–17 To stretch the Achilles tendon, the athlete positions her hips over her lower legs. Keeping her heel on the ground, she slowly squats down and slightly forward, stretching the tendon.

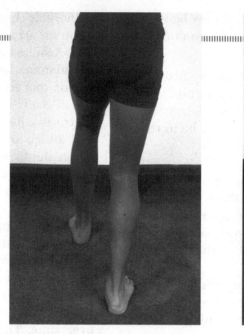

Figure 17–18 The athlete places the foot not to be stretched forward of the other. Both feet should be pointing straight ahead. As in Figure 17–17, the athlete slowly squats, stretching the Achilles tendon of the back leg.

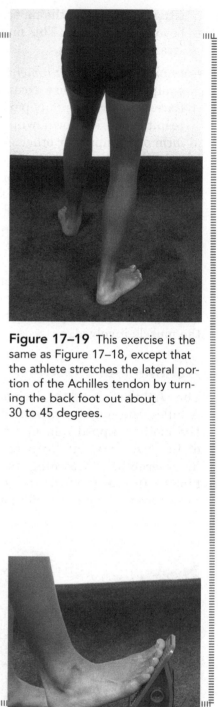

Figure 17–19 This exercise is the same as Figure 17–18, except that the athlete stretches the lateral portion of the Achilles tendon by turning the back foot out about 30 to 45 degrees.

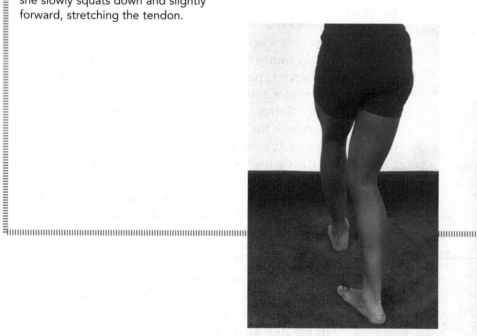

Figure 17–20 This exercise is the same as Figure 17–18, except that the athlete stretches the medial portion of the Achilles tendon by turning the foot in about 30 to 45 degrees.

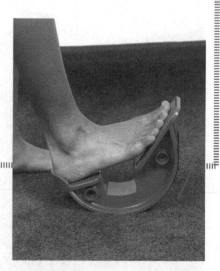

Figure 17–21 Commercial devices are available to assist in stretching the Achilles tendon and calf muscles.

problem with the foot or lower leg should allow resolution of this condition.

Conservative measures used to treat Achilles tendonitis include icing the injury, anti-inflammatory medication, and physical therapy. Resting the painful Achilles tendon will minimize aggravation of the inflammation and allow healing. A slow and careful return to activity should be monitored by the certified athletic trainer and physical therapist.

Achilles Tendon Rupture

Achilles tendon ruptures occur within the tendon substance itself, approximately one to two inches proximal to the insertion of the tendon into the calcaneus. Causes of Achilles tendon rupture include poor conditioning and overexertion. Ruptures usually occur when a sudden, eccentric force is applied to a dorsiflexed foot. Ruptures of the Achilles tendon may also occur as the result of direct trauma. Ruptured Achilles tendons must be surgically repaired. Rehabilitation may take up

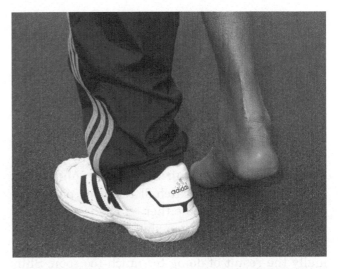

Figure 17–22 This athlete received surgery to repair a ruptured Achilles tendon. Notice the scar along the Achilles tendon.

to a year before the athlete is ready to return. Figure 17–22 shows a repaired Achilles tendon.

SPECIAL TESTS Certified athletic trainers use the Thompson test to see if the Achilles tendon is

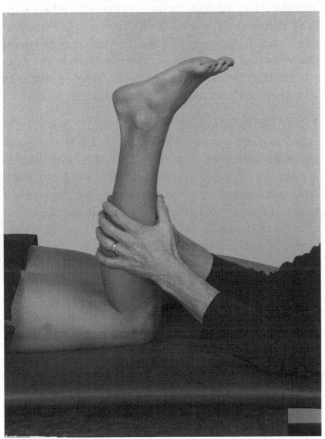

Figure 17–23 With the athlete prone and the knee bent to 90 degrees, the certified athletic trainer places the hands and fingers around the lower leg as shown.

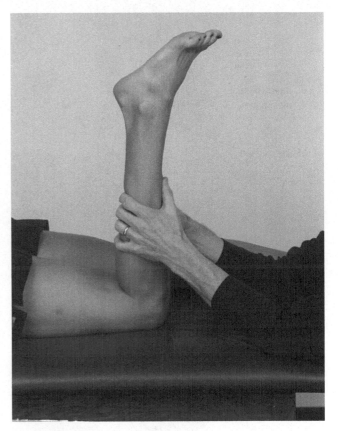

Figure 17–24 The certified athletic trainer squeezes the lower leg muscles. With an intact Achilles tendon, the foot will plantar flex, as is demonstrated here. The foot will not move if the tendon is ruptured.

intact. As shown in Figures 17–23 and 17–24, the resting calf muscles are gently squeezed. If the foot plantar flexes (points down), the Achilles tendon is intact. If the foot does not react, the Achilles tendon may be completely torn.

Medial Tibial Stress Syndrome (Shin Splints)

Medial tibial stress syndrome, or **shin splints** as it is often known, is a catchall term for pain that occurs below the knee either on the front outside part of the leg (anterior shin splints) or on the inside of the leg (medial shin splints). It is normally the result of doing too much too soon. Shin splints most often occur early in a training program or after training has been discontinued for a period of time and then resumed. It appears to be associated with repetitive activity on hard surfaces or forcible excessive use of the leg muscles,

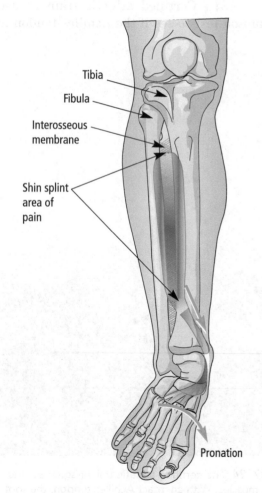

Tibia
Fibula
Interosseous membrane
Shin splint area of pain
Pronation

Figure 17–25 The area of pain and discomfort related to medial tibial stress syndrome (shin splints).

especially with running and jumping activities. Figure 17–25 illustrates the area of discomfort and pain with shin splints.

Among the causes of medial tibial stress syndrome is tightness of the gastrocnemius and soleus muscles. These muscles propel the body forward, placing additional strain on the tibialis anterior muscle in the front part of the lower leg. The tibialis anterior works to lift the foot upward and also prepares the foot to strike the running surface. Running on hard or uneven surfaces places greater forces on the lower leg complex. Varying the training schedule to include running on cushioned surfaces helps to ease the stresses placed on the leg.

Worn or ill-fitting shoes increase stress on leg muscles. Softer surfaces and shoe-cushioning materials absorb more shock, thereby transferring less force to the lower legs. How the athlete runs contributes to the overall health of the lower extremities. Athletes who run primarily on their toes put a tremendous amount of stress on the anterior portion of the leg, which may cause shin splints. Also, athletes who overpronate when running cause the muscles of the foot and leg to overwork in an attempt to stabilize the pronated foot; the repeated stress can cause the muscles to tear where they attach to the tibia. Finally, athletes who do too much too soon are also at risk.

TREATMENT Immediate treatment of shin splints consists of icing immediately after practice or competition, reducing the activity level, and gentle stretching of the posterior leg muscles. Long-term treatment should include a biomechanical assessment of the lower extremities to rule out any conditions that would expose the athlete to excessive stresses on the lower leg. Physical therapy, orthotic devices, anti-inflammatory medications, and a strengthening and flexibility program to help correct muscle imbalance may be helpful in alleviating and eliminating this condition. Athletes who are out of shape, beginning a new activity, or recovering from an injury are at much greater risk and must follow a graduated conditioning schedule to avoid overuse injuries.

Stress Fractures

Pain in the lower leg diagnosed as shin splints can actually be caused by a stress fracture. A *stress fracture* is an incomplete crack in the bone—a far more serious injury than shin splints. If the repeated stress placed on a bone is greater than the body's ability to heal it, stress fractures occur. These microscopic fractures (deteriorations) in the bone will eventually lead to a full fracture if left untreated. A bone scan is the definitive tool for diagnosing a stress fracture. However, there are clues that will signal whether the athlete should get a bone scan.

SIGNS AND SYMPTOMS If the examiner presses the fingertips along the shin and finds a definite "hot spot" of sharp, intense pain, it is a sign of a stress fracture. Shin-splint pain is more generalized. Usually, stress fractures feel better in the morning, because the bone was rested all night, whereas shin splints are worse in the morning, because the soft tissue tightens overnight.

Compartment Syndrome

Compartment syndrome may develop whenever there is swelling within one or more of the four compartments of the lower leg: the **anterior compartment, peroneal compartment, deep posterior compartment,** and **superficial posterior compartment.** Swelling may be caused by contusions, fractures, crush injuries, localized infection, excessive exercise, or overstretching. Anything that can cause an inflammatory response or uncontrolled swelling may result in increased pressure within these compartments. Figure 17–26 shows a cross-sectional view of the lower leg, with the four compartments identified.

SIGNS AND SYMPTOMS Depending on the cause of the condition, there may be sudden or gradual onset of symptoms in the afflicted leg. Swelling will be accompanied by point tenderness and pain in the affected muscle group. In later stages, numbness, weakness, and inability to use the affected muscle may develop. Compartment syndrome must be diagnosed immediately, or irreversible neurological, muscular, and vascular damage will occur. Any delay in treatment could result in permanent disability.

An athlete who has chronic compartment syndrome typically complains of lower leg pain

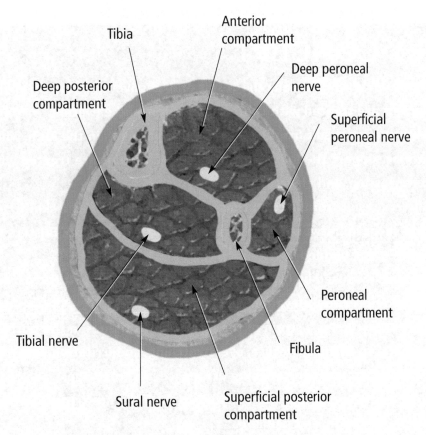

Figure 17–26 Compartments of the lower leg.

and tightness that occurs only with physical activity. A physical examination may reveal weakness and mild tenderness in the muscles of the respective compartments. The most common and consistent sign of compartment syndrome is a diffuse, intense pain that is exacerbated by movement, touch, pressure, and stretching. There is palpable tenseness in the affected compartment.

TREATMENT Treatment of compartment syndrome is immediate transportation to the nearest medical facility. Surgery usually will be needed.

Fractures

The tibia and fibula (the lower leg bones) are susceptible to fractures associated with athletic activity. Both bones are vulnerable because they are close to the surface, and force directly impacts them; there is little protective soft tissue around them.

Ten to fifteen percent of all lower-leg fractures are open fractures of the tibia, in which the bone protrudes through the skin. The tibia can be fractured by a direct blow, a twisting force, or occasionally from repetitive overuse, which produces a stress fracture. Acute tibial fractures are usually readily recognized because this is the weight-bearing bone in the lower leg, and symptoms are normally severe enough to require radiographic studies.

The fibula is normally fractured by a direct blow to the outside of the leg. The fibula is not a weight-bearing bone, but it acts as a lateral stabilizer of the leg. Fractures of the fibula present tenderness at the site of the injury, local swelling, and increased pain on any manipulation of the bone. The tenderness and swelling might be mistaken for a contusion because the athlete is often able to walk.

ADDITIONAL TESTS FOR THE FOOT, ANKLE, AND LOWER LEG

The following are standard methods of testing the various structures of the lower extremity.

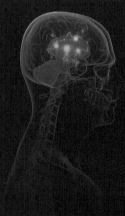

KEY CONCEPT

- Ankle sprains are usually the result of excessive inversion or plantar flexion. Sprains are treated with cold, compression, and elevation.

- Arch sprains result from overstretched ligaments in the arch, which then cannot support the foot or absorb shocks. Sprains are treated with cold, compression, and elevation.

- Blisters result from friction that causes the layers of the skin to separate; fluid seeps in between the layers and creates the blister. Blisters should be covered and padded.

- Turf toe is caused by hyperextension of the great toe. It is treated with ice, rest, compression, elevation, and support.

- Plantar fasciitis is a strain of the ligamentous tissues in the bottom of the foot due to chronic overuse, overstretching, and irritation. Treatment is targeted at correcting training errors, ice, and massage.

- Heel bruises occur due to repeated stress. They are treated with cold application, elevation, and padding.

- **Heel spurs** are a bony growth on the calcaneus that causes painful inflammation of the soft tissues. Management includes taping the arch and using shoe inserts.
- **Fractures** are breaks in bones. Treatment must be sought from a physician and will depend on the severity of the break.
- **Contusions** are injuries to the soft tissues.
- The exact cause of **muscle cramps** is unknown. Cramps can be relieved by passive stretching, fluid replacement, massage, rest, and ice.
- **Achilles tendonitis** is an inflammation of the Achilles tendon. The best treatment is prevention by stretching before beginning exercise.
- An **Achilles tendon rupture** is a complete tear of the tendon. This injury usually requires surgical treatment.
- **Medial tibial stress syndrome** (shin splints) is pain that occurs in the lower portion of the leg. Treatment consists of icing, reducing activity levels, and gentle stretching.
- **Stress fractures** are microscopic breaks in the bone due to repeated stress and overuse. Treatment from a physician should be sought.
- **Compartment syndrome** is damage to tissues resulting from swelling of one or more leg compartments. Immediate emergency treatment should be sought.

Anterior Drawer Test

This procedure tests the integrity of the anterior talofibular ligament. Figure 17–27 explains this procedure.

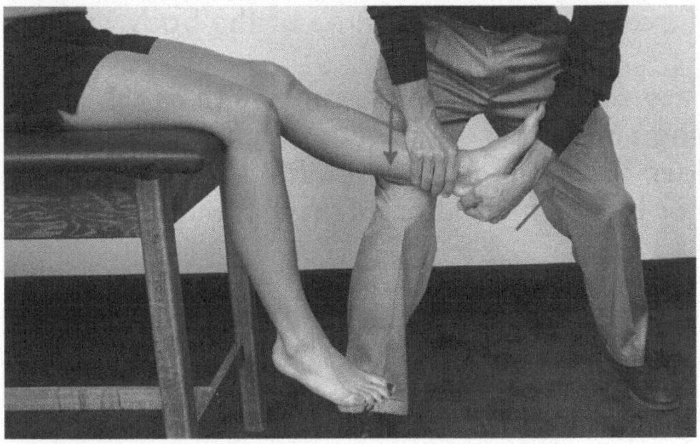

Plantar Fascia Test

The certified athletic trainer presses under the foot to locate plantar fascia pain. Figure 17–28 shows this test.

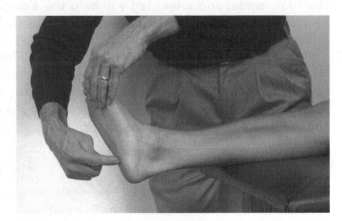

Figure 17–27 The certified athletic trainer stabilizes the top of the ankle with one hand and pulls up from the heel with the other hand. If there is forward movement of the foot, the anterior talofibular ligament may be torn.

Figure 17–28 The certified athletic trainer tries to locate plantar fascia pain at the medial calcaneus. Pressing in the area of the injury will help determine how much of the plantar fascia is affected.

Talar Tilt Test

This procedure tests the integrity of the calcaneofibular ligament. Figure 17–29 shows this test.

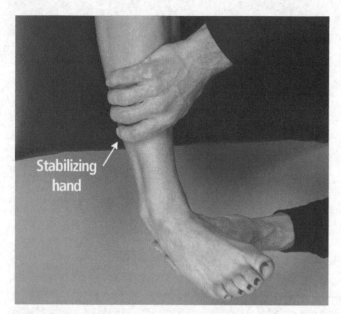

Figure 17–29 The calcaneofibular ligament is located laterally and stabilizes the ankle against direct inversion. With the patient sitting in a comfortable position, place the ankle in a neutral position (90 degrees, directly between dorsiflexion and plantar flexion). Grasp the calcaneus with one hand and the tibia-fibula with the other and apply a direct inversion stress. The test is positive if the talus tilts out from the lateral malleolus. Compare to the opposite ankle.

Tinel's Sign

Tarsal tunnel syndrome is an entrapment of the tibial nerve as it runs through the inside aspect of the foot and ankle. Pain, numbness, burning, and electric-shock sensations may be felt along the course of the tibial nerve, which includes the inside of the ankle, the heel, the arch, and the bottom of foot. Symptoms usually worsen with increased activity such as walking or exercise. Prolonged standing in one place may also be an aggravating factor. Figure 17–30 illustrates the Tinel's sign method of testing the tibial nerve.

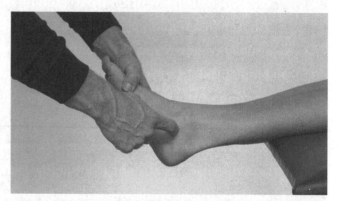

Figure 17–30 Tinel's sign is radiating pain caused by tapping the tibial nerve just below the lateral malleolus. Radiating pain is an indicator that the tibial nerve may be inflamed.

CONCLUSION

Injuries to the lower extremity are common in athletics. A solid understanding of the anatomy of the foot, ankle, and lower leg will help the examiner assess any injuries that occur. The examiner must also understand the different biomechanical forces applied to this area of the body during athletic participation.

Proper conditioning, equipment, and training are essential to the overall health of the athlete. The body generates great forces during running and jumping activities, all of which are translated to the foot and ankle. When an injury does occur, the informed athlete takes the necessary steps to heal the injury and correct any use or biomechanical problem that might have contributed to the injury in the first place.

REVIEW QUESTIONS

1. Describe the basic anatomy of the foot and ankle.
2. How many bones make up the foot and ankle?
3. What demands are placed on the lower extremity during athletic participation?
4. What type of ankle sprain is most common? Why?

5. List and explain the common injuries to the foot and ankle.
6. Why do athletes get muscle cramps? What can be done to prevent them?
7. Describe the signs, symptoms, and treatment for medial tibial stress syndrome.
8. What is the pathology of a stress fracture?
9. Explain the different compartments of the lower leg.
10. Describe three commonly used tests for lower leg injuries.
11. Look closely at Figure 17–26. This diagram is which leg—right or left? Why?

PROJECTS AND ACTIVITIES

1. Write a research paper on one aspect of the lower extremity.
2. Research how different athletic shoes change the biomechanics of the foot.
3. Visit your local sporting-goods store. Report on how many different types of athletic shoes are available for different foot conditions.
4. Make a chart listing injuries of the various structures of the lower extremity, injury causes, and treatments.

LEARNING LINKS

• Visit the website of the American Podiatric Medical Association at http://www.apma.org. What additional information can you find on the injuries discussed in this chapter?
• Visit http://www.sportsinjuryclinic.net and look for information on the injuries discussed in this chapter. Are any of them common in a particular sport?

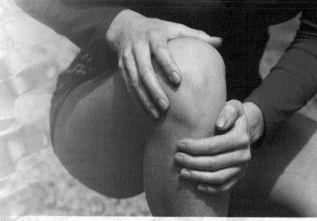

©Aleksandr Korobkov/Shutterstock.com

CHAPTER 18

The Knee

OBJECTIVES

Upon completion of this chapter, the reader should be able to:

- Describe the functions of the knee
- Describe the various physical demands associated with the lower extremities
- Describe the ligament structure of the knee
- Explain the purpose and function of the patellofemoral joint
- Understand the composition of the quadriceps muscle group
- Define various sports-related injuries of the knee
- Understand why females are more susceptible to ACL injures
- Describe special tests used to assess knee injuries

KEY TERMS

anterior cruciate ligament (ACL) *A ligament in the knee that attaches to the anterior aspect of the tibial plateau, restricting anterior movement of the tibia on the femur.*

articular cartilage *The thin layer of connective tissue over the ends of long bones.*

condyle *The rounded prominence found at the point of articulation with another bone.*

crepitus *A grinding noise or sensation within a joint.*

effusion *Swelling within the joint cavity.*

epiphyseal plate *The growth plate on the end of a bone.*

lateral collateral ligament (LCL) *A ligament that attaches to the femur and the fibula; maintains stability of the lateral aspect of the knee joint.*

lateral meniscus *Cartilage in the knee between the lateral femoral condyle and the lateral tibial plateau.*

KEY TERMS CONTINUED

medial collateral ligament (MCL) *A flat, longitudinal band found on the medial side of the knee joint.*

medial meniscus *Cartilage in the knee between the femoral condyle and the medial tibial plateau.*

patellar tendon *The tendon that encompasses the patella and extends distally across the front of the knee.*

patella *The kneecap.*

patellofemoral joint *The point where the kneecap and femur are connected in the trochlear groove.*

pes ansurine *The area where the sartorius, gracillus, and semitendinosus muscles attach to the anteriomedial tibia.*

posterior cruciate ligament (PCL) *A ligament in the knee that attaches to the posterior aspect of the tibial plateau, restricting posterior movement of the tibia on the femur.*

quadricep *A large group of four muscles in the front of the thigh.*

sesamoid *A small bone formed in a tendon where it passes over a joint.*

synovial fluid *A lubricating substance, produced by the synovial membrane, found in joints.*

synovial membrane *A layer of tissue that lines joint cavities and produces synovial fluid.*

tibial plateau *The top, flat portion of the tibia.*

tibiofemoral joint *The point where the tibia meets with the femur.*

valgus *Outward bending or twisting force.*

varus *Inward bending or twisting force.*

THE KNEE

The knee joint is one of the most complex joints in the body. Most movements and activities depend on the knee for support and mobility. Because the knee supports the majority of the body weight, it is at risk of overuse and traumatic injury in both contact and noncontact sports.

The knee is composed of three major bones and muscle groups. On top of the knee is the longest bone in the body, the femur. The end of the femur flares at its distal end into a pair of rounded prominences called **condyles**. One is medial, the other lateral. The shape of the condyles allows the femur to roll and spin on the flattened top portion of the tibia, the **tibial plateau**.

On the bottom of the knee is the tibia, which meets with the femur to form the **tibiofemoral joint**. The tibiofemoral joint is a weight-bearing, modified hinged joint held together with a joint capsule and several important ligaments

(Figure 18–1). The motions at this joint are limited to flexion, extension, and a few degrees of rotation of the tibia on the femur.

Understanding the anatomy of the knee joint and common mechanisms of injury will enable the certified athletic trainer to assess and manage injuries appropriately.

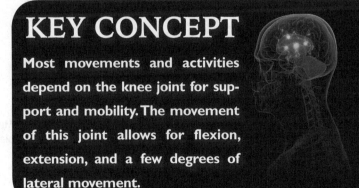

KEY CONCEPT

Most movements and activities depend on the knee joint for support and mobility. The movement of this joint allows for flexion, extension, and a few degrees of lateral movement.

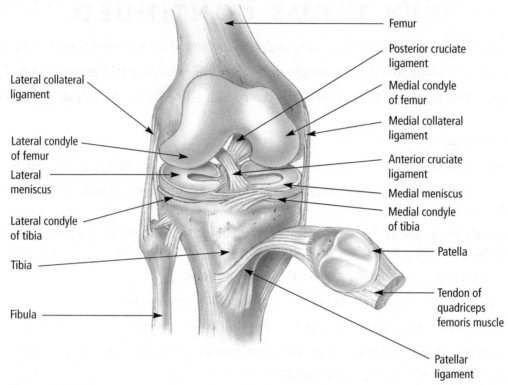

Figure 18–1 Major structures of the knee.

Cartilage

Two types of cartilage are found within the knee joint. The ends of both the tibia and femur are coated with a protective layer of **articular cartilage**, which provides a smooth surface for gliding of the joint. Interspersed between the tibia and femur are two crescent-shaped wedges of cartilage called *menisci* (Figure 18–2). The **medial meniscus** lies between the medial femoral condyle and the medial tibial plateau. The **lateral meniscus** lies between the lateral femoral condyle and the lateral tibial plateau.

The menisci play several very important roles in the health and function of the tibiofemoral joint. They aid in shock absorption, distribute forces, and improve stability of the femur as it

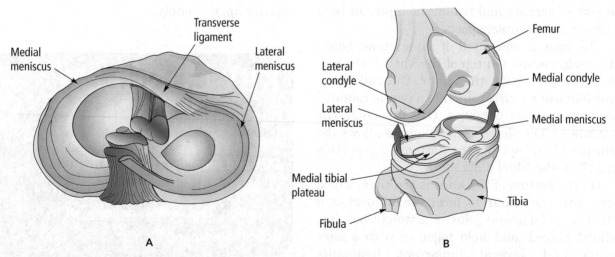

Figure 18–2 (A) The medial and lateral menisci of the knee (B) The menisci help make a more concave surface for the condyles to glide on, thereby making the knee joint more stable.

rides on the tibia. The menisci are bathed by the synovial fluid of the knee. The **synovial membrane** coats the inner surface of the fibrous joint capsule, but is only about four cells deep. It has many blood vessels, lymph vessels, and nerves. **Synovial fluid**, which is produced by the synovial membrane, lubricates the articulating surfaces of the joint and supplies nutrients to the articular cartilage. Synovial fluid is composed of nutrients needed by the joint structure.

Ligaments of the Knee

Four major ligaments connect the tibia and femur, controlling and guiding the movement of the tibia and femur in relation to each other. The four ligaments work together as a team, each assisting the others in their functions. Two ligaments on the outside of the joint capsule run roughly parallel to each other on the sides of the joint, vertically (see Figure 18–1). These are the *medial* and *lateral collateral ligaments*.

The **medial collateral ligament (MCL)** attaches to the femur above and the tibia below. The **lateral collateral ligament (LCL)** also attaches to the femur, but, unlike the MCL, it attaches to the head of the fibula instead of the tibia. These two ligaments provide medial and lateral stability of the knee joint.

Within the knee joint are two additional ligaments: the **anterior cruciate ligament (ACL)** and the **posterior cruciate ligament (PCL)**. *Cruciate* is derived from a Latin word meaning "cross." It is used to describe these two ligaments because they cross each other as they lie in the joint cavity (see Figure 18–1). The ACL attaches to the anterior aspect of the tibial plateau, whereas the PCL attaches to the posterior tibial plateau. It is easy to remember the direction these ligaments run, from their tibial attachments toward their femoral attachments, by remembering the following acronyms:

Anterior cruciate ligament:

APEX = **A**nterior-to-**P**osterior-**Ex**ternally

Posterior cruciate ligament:

PAIN = **P**osterior-to-**A**nterior-**In**ternally

Each cruciate ligament has a primary function. The ACL restricts anterior translation (movement) of the tibia on the femur; the PCL resists

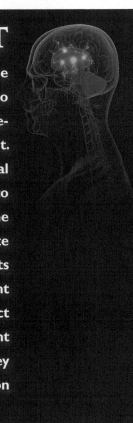

posterior translation of the tibia on the femur. Both cruciates have secondary functions of controlling rotation, medial stability, and lateral stability of the joint.

The Patellofemoral Joint

The **patella**, or kneecap, rides in the trochlear groove on the distal end of the femur. This is called the **patellofemoral joint**. The patella is a **sesamoid** (plate-shaped) bone that is enveloped within the quadriceps tendon on the front of the knee, and is part of the extensor mechanism. The quadriceps muscles, quadriceps tendon, patella, and patellar tendon constitute the structures of the extensor mechanism, which operate to actively straighten, or extend, the knee (Figure 18–3).

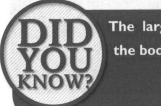

DID YOU KNOW?   The largest sesamoid bone in the body is the patella.

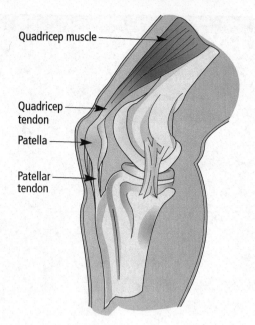

Figure 18–3 Lateral view of the knee, showing the patellofemoral joint.

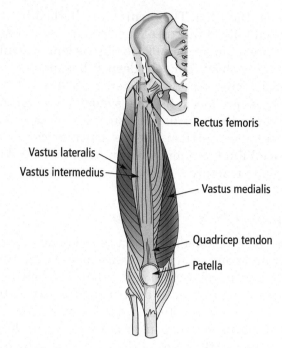

Figure 18–4 Front view of the quadricep muscles.

The primary role of the patella is to provide greater mechanical advantage in extension of the knee. Simply put, the presence of the patella allows knee flexion and extension to occur with a lesser amount of quadriceps force. It is estimated that the patella increases quadricep force by 33 to 50%. The back side of the patella, which articulates with the femur, is called the **retropatellar surface** and is covered with a thick layer of articular cartilage.

Muscles

The muscles that move the lower extremity are the strongest in the body. The large group of four

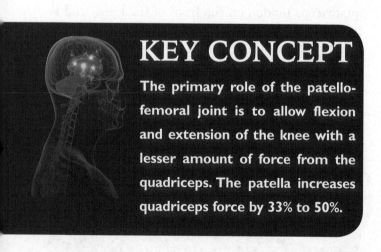

KEY CONCEPT

The primary role of the patello-femoral joint is to allow flexion and extension of the knee with a lesser amount of force from the quadriceps. The patella increases quadriceps force by 33% to 50%.

muscles in the front of the thigh are collectively called the **quadricep** muscles. These muscles are the vastus medialis, vastus intermedius, vastus lateralis, and the rectus femoris. They join together in the distal anterior thigh and attach to the patella through the quadriceps tendon (Figure 18–4). The tendon then encompasses the patella and extends distally across the front of the knee as the **patellar tendon**. The patellar tendon inserts onto the tibial tubercle on the proximal tibia. The quadriceps are very powerful knee extensors.

Two additional, long, straplike muscles in the thigh are the *sartorius* and the *gracillis*. These muscles attach to the anteriomedial tibia near the attachment of the semitendinosus. The area of these three attachments in close approximation is called the **pes ansurine**. They assist with flexion of the knee.

The hamstrings on the posterior thigh are divided into two groups. The medial hamstrings include the semitendinosis and semimembranosis, and the biceps femoris constitutes the lateral hamstrings (Figure 18–5). The hamstring muscles attach to the pelvis and femur proximally, and insert onto the posterior tibia. Because they cross the hip joint, they are also hip extenders.

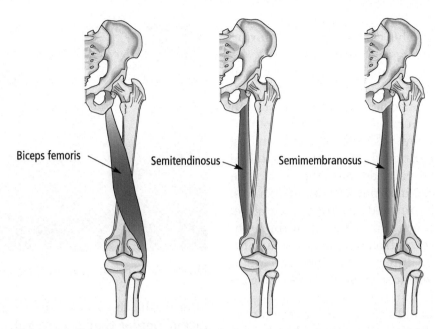

Figure 18-5 Hamstring muscles.

KNEE INJURIES

The knee can suffer either traumatic or overuse injuries. Recognizing which mechanism of injury is at fault will assist the certified athletic trainer in making correct assessments and directing appropriate interventions. The pathologies (conditions) listed here may be isolated, or may occur in combination with other injuries.

Patellofemoral Problems

Knee pain and dysfunction arising from the patellofemoral joint can be one of the most challenging injuries for both athlete and trainer. It is not always easy to identify this region as the source of an athlete's complaints, or to isolate the causative factors from the many possible causes. Understanding the biomechanics of the knee and entire lower extremity is essential for successful management of patellofemoral problems.

The patellofemoral joint is composed of the articulation of the patella with the femur. The patella is shaped like a triangle, with its apex directed inferiorly. Superiorly, it articulates with the trochlear groove found between the condyles on the distal articulating surface of the femur (Figure 18-6).

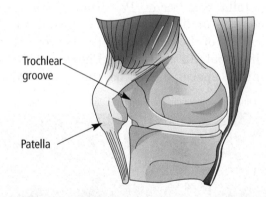

Figure 18-6 Trochlear groove.

SIGNS AND SYMPTOMS The classic complaint with a patellofemoral problem is aching pain in the front of the knee. More often than not, it is of gradual onset. The athlete may indicate that the site of pain is behind the kneecap. The athlete may also complain of the knee giving way. This is thought to be a protective response to pain caused by an aggravating factor, such as stair climbing. Some athletes may complain of a grinding noise, known as **crepitus**. This may concern the athlete, but is generally a benign condition.

The patella is subjected to increased forces during bent-knee weight-bearing activities, such as walking up and down stairs, squatting, and running. These activities tend to elicit pain in the patellofemoral joint. Pain can increase after prolonged knee flexion. This commonly occurs during long car rides or sitting in class or a theater.

Swelling is not common, but may occur in some instances. If present, it should be mild. Occasionally, a biomechanical assessment will reveal that the femurs of the legs are rotated inward. A frontal view with the athlete standing can reveal this condition. Instead of the patellae facing forward, the patellae may appear to face inward, indicating internally rotated femurs. This condition is termed *squinting patellae*. Excessive foot pronation, or lowering of the arch, can allow the lower extremity to rotate inward. Similarly, tight hip internal rotators and weak hip external rotator muscles may cause this condition as well.

The patella should slide or track in the center of the trochlear groove as the knee bends and extends (Figure 18–6). When the structures around the patella are out of balance, lateral tracking of the patella can occur. Palpation of the space between the undersurface of the medial and lateral borders of the patella and the femur can indicate if a patella is tilting (Figure 18–7). The amount of space should be the same. With a

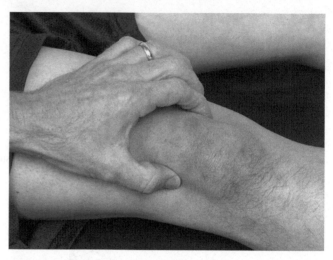

Figure 18–7 Palpating the patellar orientation on the femur.

lateral tilt, the space will be greater under the medial border than the lateral.

Provocation tests, such as a forward lunge or step-down test, can reproduce patellofemoral pain. These tests often are marked by a relative lack of control, and so comparison to the uninvolved side is always recommended.

TREATMENT Treatment of patellofemoral problems consists of correcting suspected causes. An athlete who pronates may need a shoe insert to support the arch, or low-dye taping. Weak external rotators of the hip and vastus medialis should be strengthened, and tight hip internal rotators should be stretched. Specialized taping of the patella can be effective (Figures 18–8A–C). The athlete with a lateral-tracking patella may

FUN FACTS
Pain that increases after prolonged knee flexion is often called *movie goer's sign*.

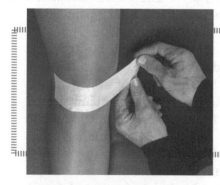

Figure 18–8A Patellar medial glide tape was developed by Jenny McConnell, PT. This figure shows application of cover roll skin tape across the patella and around the medial leg.

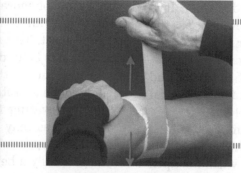

Figure 18–8B Application of short-stretch tape. After tape is secured to the patella, one hand lifts the medial leg muscles while a medially directed pull on the tape glides the patella medially.

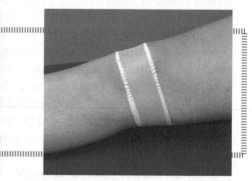

Figure 18–8C Finished knee taping.

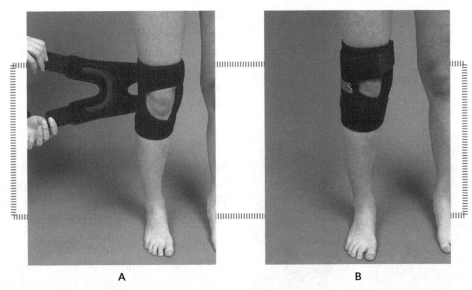

A   B

Figure 18–9A–B Commercial braces offer support and compression, as well as helping to discourage lateral tracking of the patella.

also benefit from a brace designed to resist this condition (Figure 18–9).

Bracing and taping should not be the sole treatment, however. They are used to make the patient comfortable for the rehabilitation process. Athletes must be fully rehabilitated before returning to athletics. It is very important to select strengthening exercises that do not cause pain, as pain may result in muscular inhibition and be counterproductive.

Patellar Tendonitis

Inflammation of the patellar tendon is often seen in sports that involve jumping. In fact, this condition is often referred to as *jumper's knee*. Sports that require fast running and abrupt changes of direction also place high forces on the patellar tendon. This high-force, repetitive strain frequently causes tendonitis of the patellar tendon.

Signs and Symptoms

Athletes with patellar tendonitis complain of anterior knee pain. The location of the pain is below the patella, over the site of the patellar tendon. Local tenderness on the tendon is a cardinal sign of patellar tendonitis. In some cases a small amount of local swelling occurs.

Treatment

Patellar tendonitis is usually the result of repetitive stress on the patellar tendon. Activity

modification should be considered to allow the tendon time to heal. Nonimpact activities such as cycling and swimming will allow the patellar tendon to heal. If the athlete has tight quadriceps, stretching them may help take strain off the patellar tendon. Ice application soon after exercise helps to keep inflammation from activity in check. Specialized braces and taping techniques may help control symptoms of patellar tendonitis.

SPECIAL TESTS The test demonstrated in Figure 18–10 can help detect patellar tendonitis. Figure 18–11 demonstrates the patellar dislocation apprehension test.

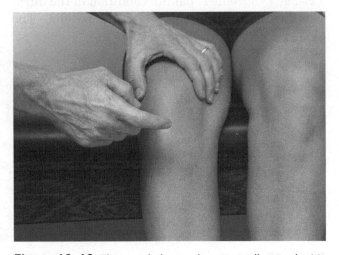

Figure 18–10 This test helps to detect patellar tendonitis and irritation. The athlete sits on the edge of a table with the knee in 90 degrees of flexion. The examiner taps the patellar tendon one to three times in rapid succession. A positive sign is sharp pain elicited on the patellar tendon.

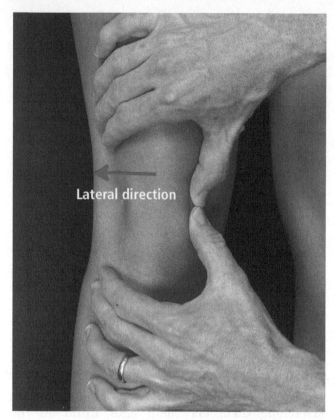

Figure 18–11 The patellar dislocation apprehension test is used to see if the athlete resists lateral positioning of the patella. If the athlete guards (flexes the quadriceps) and does not allow lateral movement of the patella, the examiner knows that an injury exists. This test uses both thumbs, positioned medially on the patella, applying gentle pressure across the patellofemoral joint.

Fat-Pad Syndrome

Fat-pad syndrome is painful condition in the infrapatellar region (area just below the patella). The *infrapatellar fat pad* (also known as Hoffa's fat pad) is a region of fatty tissue lying deep under the patellar tendon. This structure can become inflamed and painful. Because the infrapatellar fat pad lies underneath the patellar tendon, it is often confused with patellar tendonitis.

SIGNS AND SYMPTOMS Pain just below the patella is a characteristic sign of fat-pad syndrome. Movement of the knee often aggravates the symptoms, and often the knee is tender to palpation. Tenderness and swelling may be demonstrated in the anterior portion of the knee.

TREATMENT Strengthening exercises that avoid full knee extension, or leg presses that avoid full knee extension, may be tolerated well. The athlete may have to avoid activities that require rapidly kicking the knee into full extension. Specialized taping (Figures 18–12A–C), icing, and anti-inflammatory medications may help the athlete through the acute phase of this injury.

SPECIAL TESTS Figures 18–13A and B demonstrate a test to identify fat-pad syndrome.

Medial Collateral Ligament (MCL) Sprain

A blow to the outside of the knee (as in a football tackle), or a high-energy, twisting maneuver, are common causes of MCL injuries. These forces result in stretching and a **valgus** (outward) force on the medial tibiofemoral joint, which can damage this ligament. Pain and tenderness are felt on

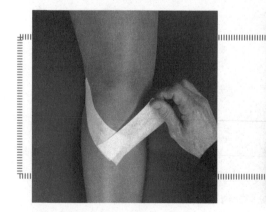

Figure 18–12A The fat-pad unloading tape application was developed by Jenny McConnell, PT. Cover roll skin tape is placed in a "v" along the inferior borders of the fat pad.

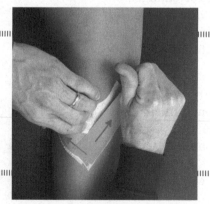

Figure 18–12B Application of short-stretch tape. The fat pad is lifted upward (parallel to the tape) while tension is applied to the two pieces of the short-stretch tape.

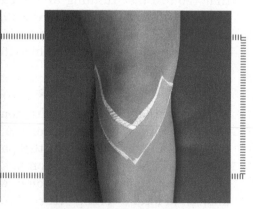

Figure 18–12C Finished knee taping.

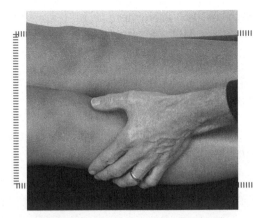

Figure 18–13A Fat-pad compression test: Pressure is applied to the proximal patellar tendon with quadriceps contracted, stressing only the tendon and not the fat pad.

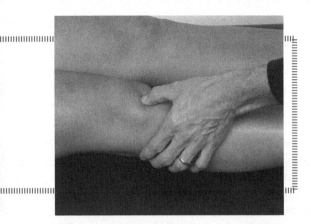

Figure 18–13B Pressure is applied over the proximal patellar tendon with a relaxed tendon, allowing compression of the fat pad.

the medial aspect of the knee. Extracapsular ligament sprains (the medial collateral and lateral collateral ligaments) are classified by their severity, on the grade I to grade III scale (Table 18–1). The injured athlete may have difficulty bearing weight on a leg with an acute grade II or III sprain.

SIGNS AND SYMPTOMS Examination may reveal limited motion in full flexion and extension, as well as swelling of the medial knee. Tenderness may be located on the MCL at the joint line, or on either of its bony attachment sites onto the tibia or femur. Varying degrees of pain

Table 18–1 Ligament Sprain Classification for the Medial Collateral and Lateral Collateral Ligaments

GRADE I SYMPTOMS

- Mild tenderness on the inside of the knee over the medial collateral ligament (lateral side of the knee for the lateral collateral ligament).
- Usually no swelling.
- When the knee is bent to 30 degrees and force is applied to the outside of the knee (stressing the medial collateral ligament), pain is felt, but there is no joint laxity (looseness). When force is applied to the inside of the knee, the test is for the lateral collateral ligament.

GRADE II SYMPTOMS

- Significant tenderness on the inside of the knee for the medial collateral ligament and the outside of the knee for the lateral collateral ligament.
- Some swelling seen over the ligament.
- When the knee is stressed as for grade I symptoms, there are pain and laxity in the joint, although there is a definite end point (the knee cannot be bent sideways completely).

GRADE III SYMPTOMS

- There is a complete tear of the ligament.
- Pain can vary and is sometimes not as bad as that of a grade II sprain.
- When the knee is stressed, there is significant joint laxity.
- The athlete may complain that the knee is very wobbly or unstable.

and laxity may be present with valgus stress testing for MCL injury.

TREATMENT Acute injuries should be treated with PRICE (protection, rest, ice, compression, and elevation). Protection may require a protective wrap, brace, or crutches. Once the acute phase passes, rehabilitation may proceed. Gentle active and passive range of motion, such as bending and extending the knee, can be performed in pain-free ranges. Care should be taken to avoid valgus and twisting forces. Once the knee obtains 110 to 115 degrees of flexion, cycling may be initiated. Submaximal effort strengthening can commence in the subacute stage, but only if tolerated without pain. Once the knee has full range of motion and normal strength, a functional progression should begin. All knee ligament injuries should be evaluated by the athlete's physician.

SPECIAL TEST The valgus stress test checks for MCL stability (Figure 18–14).

Lateral Collateral Ligament (LCL) Sprain

The LCL is on the lateral side of the knee and is not frequently involved in sports injuries. It can be injured by a blow to the medial side of the knee, resulting in a **varus** (inside) stress to the knee joint.

TREATMENT Treatment of LCL sprains is similar to that for MCL sprains (see preceding sections).

SIGNS AND SYMPTOMS Injury is confirmed with tenderness to palpation. Pain and laxity will be present with a varus stress test.

SPECIAL TEST The varus stress test checks for stability in the LCL (Figure 18–15).

Torn Anterior Cruciate Ligament

Before the passage of Title IX, which greatly expanded female sports participation, anterior cruciate ligament (ACL) injuries were seen primarily in male athletes. The incident of ACL injuries has since shifted, so that now more ACL tears are diagnosed in female than male athletes. Research has shown that females who participate in basketball and soccer are four to six times more likely to sustain an injury to the ACL than males who play the same sport. Seventy percent of ACL injuries in females come from noncontact situations. Each year, 1 in 10 female collegiate athletes and 1 in 100 female high school athletes will sustain a serious knee injury.

Orthopedic researchers reported that the following factors help to explain the increase in ACL injuries among the female athletic population

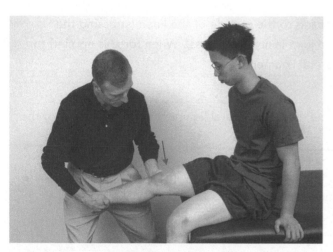

Figure 18–14 With the athlete's leg at full extension, the examiner presses laterally at the knee, while holding the leg at the ankle. Increased movement (compared to the uninjured knee) may be an indication of MCL damage.

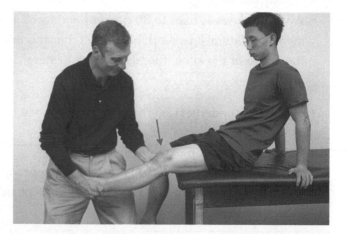

Figure 18–15 The varus stress test checks for LCL stability. With the athlete's leg at full extension, the examiner presses medially at the knee, while holding the leg at the ankle. Increased movement (compared to the uninjured knee) may be an indication of LCL damage.

(American Academy of Orthopaedic Surgeons, 1999):

- *Biomechanical factors.* Experts reported that females tend to use their quadriceps muscles more than male athletes, putting them at significantly increased risk of ACL injuries. The panel agreed that female athletes should learn to use their hamstring muscles more. The experts also concluded that females tend to land on a flat foot, rather than the toes, which can contribute to the increased injury rate.

- *Hormonal influences.* There need be no modification of activity or restriction from a sport at any time during the menstrual cycle, experts said. They also stated that a woman's hormones do not increase the chances of sustaining an ACL injury, but suggested that further investigation is warranted.

- *Environmental factors.* Functional knee braces do not prevent ACL injury, experts reported. They agreed that although the surface of an athletic shoe may improve performance, because it provides good traction on certain surfaces, it may also increase the risk of injury.

- *Anatomic risk factors.* The experts found insufficient data to support the theory that ACL size is related to injury risk. They also reported that no consensus could be reached on the role of the size of the femoral notch (the area within the knee that contains the cruciate ligaments) in injury occurrence.

Injury to the ACL can occur from contact or noncontact causes. As with the medial collateral ligament, a blow to the lateral knee can be a contact cause. Situations that place a loaded knee joint in a combined position of flexion, valgus, and rotation of the tibia on the femur can rupture the ACL in a noncontact manner. An example is a basketball player making a rapid change of direction (Figure 18–16). A falling skier could suffer this type of injury. Once an ACL is stretched or ruptured, it will not heal (Figure 18–17). ACL injuries are sometimes accompanied by meniscus tears and MCL sprains.

The anterior cruciate ligament (ACL) and the posterior cruciate ligament (PCL) do not follow the same grading scale as for MCL and LCL sprains.

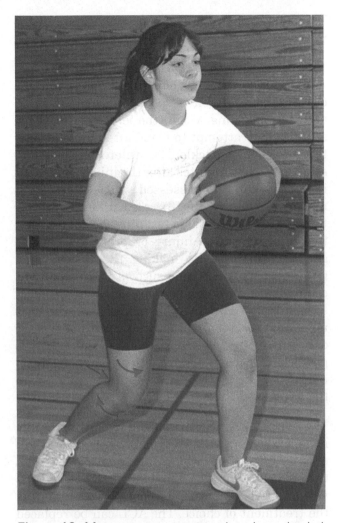

Figure 18–16 Noncontact situations that place a loaded knee joint in a combined position of flexion and interior rotation of the femur, valgus force, and external rotation of the tibia on the femur can rupture the ACL.

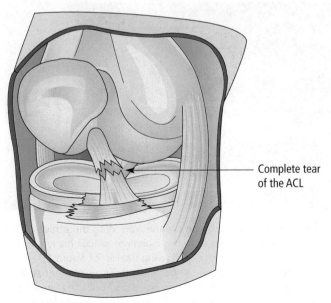

Complete tear of the ACL

Figure 18–17 An ACL tear.

They are either damaged or not. There is no middle ground.

SIGNS AND SYMPTOMS A classic sign of an ACL injury is the athlete complaining that he or she heard or felt a "pop," followed by rapid **effusion** (swelling within the joint cavity). Some athletes may attempt to stand after rupture, only to have the knee buckle. The athlete may feel nauseated for a few minutes after the injury. Ligament integrity can be assessed with Lachman's maneuver (Figure 18–18) or an anterior drawer test (Figure 18–19). This test must be done within five minutes of the injury or protective muscle guarding will set in, making the test invalid. Other injuries to the knee, such as a torn meniscus, could also prevent valid testing of this ligament. If special tests for ACL laxity are positive, the ligament may be torn; special tests are not always definitive, however. Diagnosis by the athlete's physician, in conjunction with a magnetic resonance imaging (MRI) examination, will confirm the diagnosis.

TREATMENT Acute care should include splinting, icing, and compressive wrapping. The athlete will need crutches. All athletes with suspected ACL tears should be referred to their family physicians for definitive diagnosis. Reconstructive surgery is the treatment of choice. The ACL can be replaced with a graft harvested from the athlete's patellar

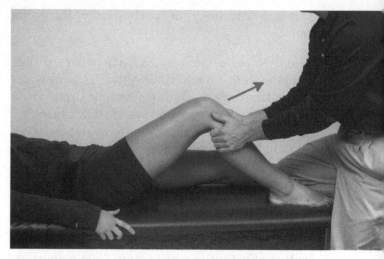

Figure 18–19 Anterior drawer test: The athlete is in a supine position with the knee bent approximately 90 degrees. The examiner applies anterior force to the proximal tibia. Excessive movement may indicate ACL damage.

tendon or hamstring, or from a cadaver. Surgery, followed by a comprehensive rehabilitation program under the direction of a physical therapist, should return the athlete to full participation within 6 to 12 months.

SPECIAL TESTS Figures 18–18 and 18–19 show tests for injury to the ACL.

Posterior Cruciate Ligament Tear

Posterior cruciate ligament injuries account for 3 to 20% of all knee ligament injuries (Figure 18–20). Little research has been done on the PCL, because it is injured far less often than the ACL.

The most common causes of PCL injuries are athletic, motor vehicle, or industrial accidents. Most athletic PCL injuries occur during a fall on the flexed (bent) knee with the foot plantar flexed (the toes pointing down with the top of the foot in line with the front of the leg). The tibia strikes the ground first and is pushed backward.

Hyperflexion (bending too far) of the knee without a direct blow to the tibia can cause an isolated PCL injury in which no other ligaments are damaged. The PCL can be injured in other ways, but these usually involve other ligaments as well, such as the ACL, medial and lateral collateral ligaments, and the posterolateral corner (back outer side) of the knee.

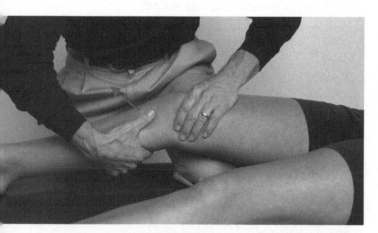

Figure 18–18 Lachman's maneuver: With the athlete lying in a supine position, the examiner places his knee under the athlete's knee, allowing flexion of about 20 degrees. The athlete must be relaxed. The examiner stabilizes the distal femur with one hand and pulls the proximal tibia forward with the other. Excessive movement (compared to the uninjured leg) may indicate ACL damage.

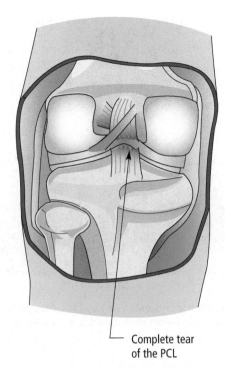

└─ Complete tear
of the PCL

Figure 18–20 Posterior cruciate ligament tear.

SIGNS AND SYMPTOMS A positive "sag test" is diagnostic of a PCL tear. The sag test is conducted with the athlete lying in the supine position, with the knee bent at 90 degrees. The knee should not have the appearance of bending (sagging) backwards. MRI imaging will reveal tears within this ligament.

TREATMENT Immediate care uses the PRICE approach. Suspected PCL tears should be assessed by the athlete's physician.

Physical therapy and a strong rehabilitation program aimed at strength restoration and proprioception enhancement are important for PCL injuries. Specific quadriceps strength and endurance training will compensate for the torn PCL, although there may be a small decline in the athlete's ability to participate in high-level activities. Rehabilitation may take several months. Some athletes choose to wear a knee brace for athletic participation. Surgery can be avoided in most cases.

Meniscus Tears

Each knee contains two menisci, one medial and one lateral. These fibrocartilaginous disks act as cushions between the ends of the femur and the tibia and fibula. The top of the tibia is flat, and the ends, or condyles, of the femur are rounded. The menisci help make a more concave surface for the condyles to rest and glide on, and thus make the knee joint more stable (refer to Figure 18–2).

The medial meniscus is attached to the ligaments on the back and medial side of the knee. Because it is attached so securely, it does not move freely. This causes it to be torn more often than the lateral meniscus, which is on the outside half of the joint. The lateral meniscus is attached only at the back of the knee and moves more freely as the knee is bent and straightened.

The menisci can be torn when the knee is twisted suddenly and one or both menisci become trapped between the femur and tibia. They can also be torn when the ligaments in and around the knee are torn. As one ages, the menisci can lose their rubbery consistency, soften, and fray. These weakened structures can be torn easily, with just a misstep around the house.

SIGNS AND SYMPTOMS Unlike ACL injury, which causes rapid swelling, isolated meniscal tears develop mild knee swelling slowly over several hours or more. Symptoms of a torn meniscus may include pain, popping, locking, or giving way of the knee. The tibiofemoral joint spaces may be tender.

TREATMENT Immediate care should include ice and compressive wrap. If the athlete cannot walk steadily, crutches may be needed. Knee supports, such as a neoprene sleeve, may make the athlete feel more comfortable. Knees showing indications of meniscal tears should be evaluated by a sports physician. Depending on the type and location of the tear and the severity of the symptoms, nonsurgical management may suffice. For meniscal injuries, this includes physical therapy to maintain or increase muscle strength and range of motion, activity modification, anti-inflammatory medications, support sleeves, and time. Generally, one to three months is a reasonable timeline for significant improvement. The physician can use magnetic resonance imaging (MRI) to confirm the existence of a meniscal tear, if necessary.

SPECIAL TESTS Figures 18–21A and B show a test for meniscal tears.

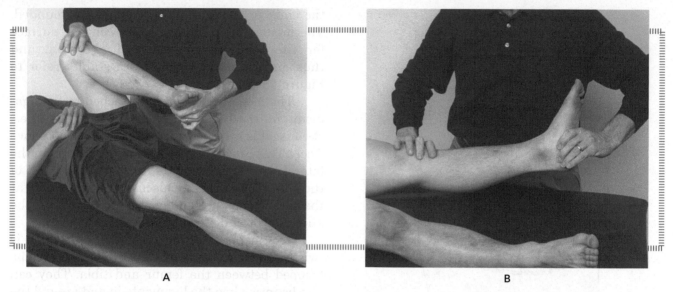

Figure 18–21A–B With the athlete lying supine, the examiner applies an internal and external tibial rotation while moving the knee from flexion to extension. A click that is felt while manipulation is being performed is a positive sign.

Epiphyseal (Growth-Plate) Injuries

The knee is subject to sports-induced trauma at the centers of bone growth in skeletally immature athletes. The growth plates at the end of long bones, the **epiphyseal plates**, are at risk from direct trauma. The growth plate is a zone of cartilage cells from which new bone is formed. The joint capsule and ligaments near these growth plates are two to five times stronger than the growth plate itself. Because the epiphysis is responsible for bone growth, injuries involving the epiphyseal growth plate may alter the length of the affected bone. Therefore, forces that would result in ligamentous injuries in adults have the potential to cause growth-plate injuries in children and younger athletes.

Because this type of injury can be quite serious in a growing athlete, return to play should be permitted only with a physician's approval.

Osgood-Schlatter Condition

Osgood-Schlatter condition is a group of symptoms involving the tibial tubercle epiphysis. The tibial tubercle is a small bump on the tibia where the patellar tendon of the quadriceps muscle attaches. This condition is a result of traction. The tibial tubercle is a growth center (apophysis or epiphysis) located just below the knee joint on the front of the tibia (Figure 18–22). This condition will most likely affect males of 12 to 16 and females of 10 to 14 years of age.

The layer under the hard bone of the tibial tubercle is fibrocartilage and is different from any of the body's other physes (growth cartilage areas). The tibial tubercle physis looks like a layered pastry. During the active growth years, these layers are loosely held together. Traction of the quadriceps

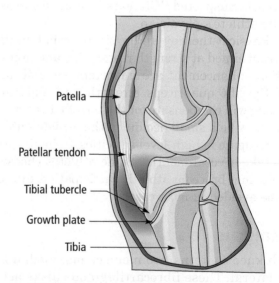

Patella

Patellar tendon

Tibial tubercle

Growth plate

Tibia

Figure 18–22 Osgood-Schlatter condition.

muscle may cause disruption and inflammation in the layers of the tubercle. In other words, if the femur is growing faster than the quadriceps muscle, the quadriceps will exert undue pressure on the growth center of the tibia (where the patellar tendon attaches), causing pain.

SIGNS AND SYMPTOMS Signs and symptoms of Osgood-Schlatter condition include:

- Pain over the tibial tubercle
- Swelling over the tibial tubercle (Figure 18–23)
- Weakness in the quadriceps muscle group
- Increased pain and swelling with activity
- Visible lump
- Pain to the touch over the affected area

Athletes who suffer from this growth-related problem are susceptible to, although not likely to develop, an avulsion fracture of the tibial tubercle. If the growth center has too much traction on it for too long a period of time, the bone fails and a fracture results. The quadriceps muscle is elastic—much like an extended spring—so if a fracture occurs, the bone fragment will be displaced.

TREATMENT Preventing this problem from progressing to a season-ending injury is fairly easy. If the three symptoms of pain, swelling, and flexibility

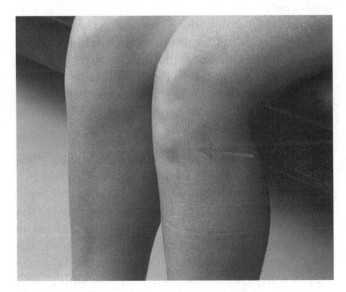

Figure 18–23 Notice the enlarged tibial tubercle on the left knee. This is a permanent result of Osgood-Schlatter condition.

are managed, the athlete should be able to participate at a competitive level.

During competition, the athlete should wear a protective pad. The most effective is a standard volleyball knee pad, which will protect the sensitive tibial tuberosity from impact. Impact to the swollen tuberosity is the most common cause of increased pain.

Some athletes feel pain reduction or relief when a neoprene sleeve is combined with the knee pad. The neoprene sleeve places subtle pressure on the swollen area and retains heat. The light pressure seems to relieve pain by compressing the separating physis. Combined with the protection afforded by the pad, it will help to alleviate the most common symptoms during competition.

After activity, ice should be applied to control inflammation. This should be done daily, even for those without pain, to control the swelling associated with activity and control pain. Nonsteroidal anti-inflammatory medications also help to control these symptoms. All medications should be taken in accordance with instructions from the athlete's personal physician.

Improving flexibility is one of the most important treatments for controlling symptoms for the duration of the growth spurt. At first glance, one might expect that stretching the quadriceps muscles would be beneficial. In reality, stretching the hamstrings is more important. Increased hamstring tightness causes the quadriceps to pull harder during athletic activities. This places more traction force on the tibial tubercle. Increasing hamstring flexibility will help to alleviate the pain. Quadricep stretching will only increase the traction forces on the quadricep attachment, possibly increasing pain and swelling. Quadricep stretching should be performed with caution, so as not to exacerbate any pain, but gentle stretching is appropriate and useful.

Stretching should be done at least four times daily. Ideally, the suffering athlete should stretch six times a day. At the minimum, every athlete should stretch after waking, before athletic activities, after athletic activities, and before bedtime. These stretching sessions should address all major muscle groups, with added time emphasizing tight spots. Each stretch should be held for 10 to 30 seconds and repeated 3 to 5 times.

An athlete who feels intensifying pain and cannot participate on a daily basis should return to a physician for further consultation. Removal from athletics for a short time may help relieve the pain enough to allow the athlete to return to competition. If the athlete has to be removed from competition, rehabilitation exercises that not exacerbate the symptoms should be performed to maintain aerobic fitness and strength. Exercises to avoid include knee extensions, heavy squats, power cleans, and plyometrics. Any exercise that involves explosive use of the quadricep mechanism may aggravate symptoms. Appropriate exercises for improving aerobic fitness are cycling (with a high seat post), slide board, and swimming. Stair-climbing activities may or may not aggravate symptoms, so do them only if appropriate. For maintaining muscular strength, exercises such as straight leg raises, body-weight squats, hamstring curls, and calf raises should be performed to minimize strength loss rather than to increase strength.

Allowing an athlete with Osgood-Schlatter condition to continue to lift weights and compete at a high level is appropriate if participation in these activities does not increase pain. Decreasing the intensity of training may be all the adjustment needed to control the pain and swelling associated with this condition.

Iliotibial Band Syndrome

Iliotibial band syndrome occurs when there is inflammation of the iliotibial band (a thick band of fibrous tissue that runs down the outside of the leg). This band begins at the hip and extends to the outer side of the tibia just below the knee joint (Figure 18–24). It functions in coordination with several thigh muscles to provide stability to the outside of the knee joint.

The irritation usually occurs over the outside of the knee joint, at the lateral epicondyle (lateral end of the femur). The iliotibial band crosses bone and muscle at this point. Between these structures is a bursa that should facilitate a smooth, gliding motion. However, when inflamed, the iliotibial band does not glide easily, and pain associated with movement

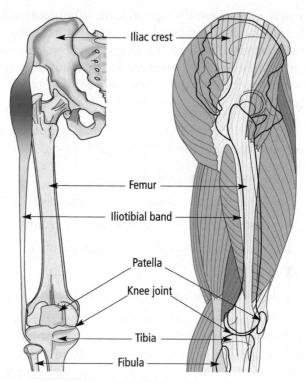

Figure 18–24 Iliotibial band.

results. As noted, the function of the iliotibial band is to provide stability and assist in flexion of the knee joint. When irritated, movement of the knee joint becomes painful. Usually the pain worsens with continued movement and resolves with rest.

People who suddenly intensify their level of activity, such as runners who increase their mileage, often develop iliotibial band syndrome. Others who are prone to iliotibial band syndrome include individuals with mechanical problems—people who overpronate, have leg-length discrepancies, or are bowlegged.

TREATMENT Treatment of iliotibial band syndrome begins with an analysis of the athlete's gait and training program to rule out mechanical problems or training errors that may predispose the athlete to the condition. Proper footwear, icing the area of pain, and stretching will help treat iliotibial band syndrome. Modifying the athlete's training program, along with cross-training, will

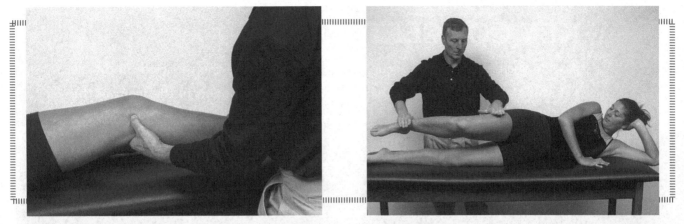

Figure 18–25 With the athlete in a supine position, the examiner passively flexes and extends the knee. This is done while applying pressure with the thumb on the distal iliotibial (IT) band (overlying the lateral femoral epicondyle). If the athlete has pain under the examiner's thumb when the knee is at approximately 20 to 30 degrees of flexion, IT band friction syndrome is indicated.

Figure 18–26 The athlete lies on the unaffected side. While the athlete lifts and keeps the affected leg up, and moves it in a bicycle-pedaling pattern, the examiner places downward pressure on the leg. If the athlete feels pain over the distal IT band during this test, IT band friction syndrome is indicated.

be helpful. The athlete will need to reduce his or her activity level until symptoms subside.

SPECIAL TESTS Testing for iliotibial band syndrome is demonstrated in Figures 18–25 and 18–26.

Fractures

Fractures in the area of the knee are the result of high-energy trauma. Fortunately, they are not seen frequently in athletes, especially in younger athletes. Fractures vary in location and severity.

A fracture of the patella is usually the result of direct impact to the anterior knee. This can occur when the knee strikes the ground or some other hard sport surface. A football player with a poorly fit knee pad may be vulnerable if he falls onto the knee. Another example is a tennis player who lands on her knee on concrete or asphalt.

Distal femoral and proximal tibial fractures may occur from violent twisting injuries such as falls from heights (Figure 18–27). A pole vaulter who misses the landing pit may sustain such an injury.

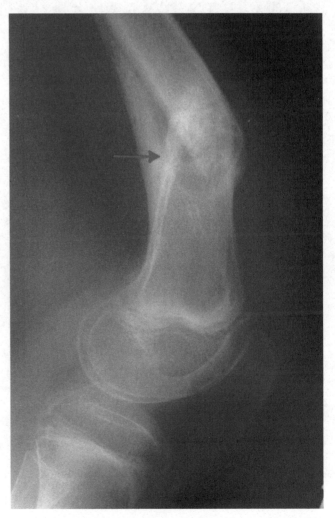

Figure 18–27 Fracture of the distal femur near the knee.

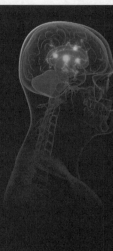

KEY CONCEPT

A wide variety of injuries occur to the knee. Some of the most common are:

- Patellofemoral problems, characterized by aching pains in the front of the knee. Treatment must focus on correcting the suspected causes.

- Patellar tendonitis, inflammation of the patellar tendon, often seen in sports that involve jumping. Activities must be modified to allow the tendon time to heal.

- Fat-pad syndrome, a painful condition affecting the infrapatellar region. Specialized taping, icing, and anti-inflammatory medications may help relieve the pain. Activities that involve full extension of the knee should be avoided.

- Medial collateral ligament sprains, which are caused by application of a force to the outside of the knee that stretches and damages the ligament. Treat with PRICE.

- Lateral collateral ligament sprains, which result from force applied to the medial side of the knee. Treat with PRICE.

- Tearing of the anterior cruciate ligament, which usually results from the knee joint being placed in a position of flexion, valgus, and rotation. The athlete usually feels or hears a pop. Treatment includes splinting, icing, and compressive wrapping. Surgery is often indicated.

- Posterior cruciate ligament tears, which result from falling on a flexed knee with the foot pointing downward. Treat with PRICE.

- Meniscus tears, which are caused by sudden twisting of the knee. Immediate treatment should be application of ice and a compressive wrap.

- Epiphyseal injuries, which may result in alteration in the length of the bones involved.

- Osgood-Schlatter condition, a group of symptoms involving the tibial tubercle epiphysis. To prevent the condition from worsening, address the pain, swelling, and flexibility.

- Iliotibial band syndrome, an inflammation of the iliotibial band that usually occurs over the knee joint. Treatment for this syndrome involves assessing and correcting problems of gait and training.

- Fractures of the knee, which are the result of high-energy trauma.

CONCLUSION

The knee is the largest joint in the body, and one of the most prone to injury. It is made up of the femur, tibia, and patella. The knee also contains large ligaments that help in controlling motion. These ligaments connect bones and brace the joint against abnormal types of motion. Other parts of the knee, like cartilage, cushion the joint and help it absorb shock during motion.

REVIEW QUESTIONS

1. Describe the function of the knee. What is the difference between articular cartilage and the meniscus?
2. List the four major ligaments of the knee and their functions.
3. Explain the function of the patellofemoral joint.
4. What makes up the quadricep muscle group?
5. Explain the various injuries of the knee associated with athletics.
6. What are some possible reasons why female athletes have a greater incidence of ACL injuries?
7. Why is an epiphyseal injury significant in children?
8. Why is Osgood-Schlatter condition painful?
9. Describe three of the special tests for the knee discussed in this chapter.
10. Describe three commonly used tests for lower leg injuries.

PROJECTS AND ACTIVITIES

1. Create a model of the knee. Include all major structures.
2. Interview someone who has or has had Osgood-Schlatter condition. Write a paper on your findings.
3. Make an appointment with an athletic trainer in your school or area. Ask her or him what knee injuries were addressed this school year, and their outcomes.

LEARNING LINKS

- Visit http://www.sportsknee.com; click on the "Education" tab at the bottom of the screen; then view the tutorials and animations of the knee.
- Learn more about the anterior cruciate ligament by visiting http://www.aclsolutions.com.
- Browse the website http://www.kneeguru.co.uk for more information on knee anatomy and knee injuries.

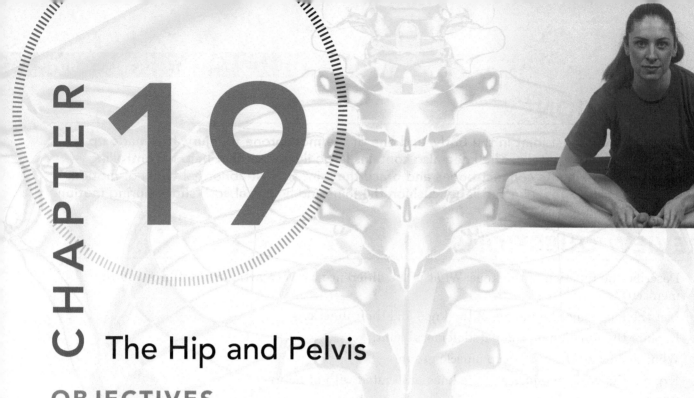

CHAPTER 19

The Hip and Pelvis

OBJECTIVES

Upon completion of this chapter, the reader should be able to:

- Explain the importance of the hip and pelvis as a support structure for the human body
- Describe the skeletal structure of the hip and pelvis
- List the primary muscles of the hip and pelvis
- Describe common injuries associated with the hip and pelvis
- Explain what overuse injuries are and how they can be managed

KEY TERMS

adductor muscles *A muscle group that aids in adduction of the hip; consists of the adductor longus, adductor brevis, and adductor magnus muscles.*

coccyx *The tailbone.*

greater sciatic notch *A space in the pelvis through which the sciatic nerve travels to the legs.*

hamstring muscles *A muscle group that aids in hip movement; consists of the biceps femoris, semitendinosus, and semimembranosus muscles.*

hip flexors *A muscle group that aids in flexion of the hip; consists of the iliopsoas, sartorius, pectineus, and rectus femoris muscles.*

iliac crest contusion *A painful injury caused by a direct blow to the hip, resulting in ecchymosis, tenderness, and swelling; also known as a hip pointer.*

iliac crest *The upper ridge of the ilium.*

iliac fossa *The broad, slightly concave inner surface of the ilium.*

ilium *A broad, flared bone that makes up the upper and lateral sections of the pelvis.*

ischium *The portion of the pelvis attached to the pubis in front and the ilium laterally in the back; bears the weight of the body when sitting.*

KEY TERMS CONTINUED

obturator foramina *The large openings in the ischium through which blood vessels and nerves pass to the legs.*

pubis *The bone in the pelvis to the front and below the bladder.*

sacrum *The portion of the vertebral column between the lumbar vertebrae and the coccyx; composed of five fused vertebrae.*

symphysis *The center of the pubis where the two sides of the pubis are fused together.*

THE HIP AND PELVIS

The hip is one of the most stable joints in the body, although it allows a great deal of motion. It is well protected and surrounded by muscle on all sides. The hip is a freely movable, ball-and-socket joint that lies between the head of the femur and the acetabulum of the pelvis (Figure 19–1).

The hip is where the muscles of the back, abdomen, hamstrings, quadriceps, abductors, adductors, and gluteals attach. These muscles are shorter than the leg muscles, allow rotation, and help stabilize the joint. Most hip injuries result from these small muscles being overused or pushed too hard. This arrangement of bones, ligaments, muscles, and tendons makes the hip the strongest joint in the body.

The pelvis is made up of several flattened bones that form a ring and function as a support structure for the human skeleton. The function of the pelvis is to transmit weight from the axial skeleton to the lower limbs when standing, or to the ischial tuberosities when sitting. The pelvis:

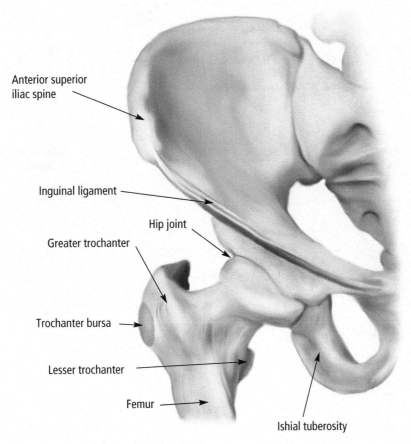

Anterior superior iliac spine

Inguinal ligament

Hip joint

Greater trochanter

Trochanter bursa

Lesser trochanter

Femur

Ishial tuberosity

Figure 19–1 Anatomy of the hip joint.

- Provides attachments for various muscles that attach onto and control the lower limbs
- Houses parts of the digestive and urinary tracts
- Houses reproductive systems

Important differences exist in the size and structure of the hip and pelvis in men and women (Figure 19–2). A woman's bone structure is slightly less dense than a man's, and the pelvis is smaller, shorter, and wider. Additionally, the bony protrusions for muscle attachment are not as sharply defined.

Skeletal Structure

The ilium, sacrum, ischium, pubis, and coccyx are the structures of the pelvis.

The **ilium** is a broad, flared bone that constitutes the upper and lateral sections of the pelvis. The primary features of the ilium are:

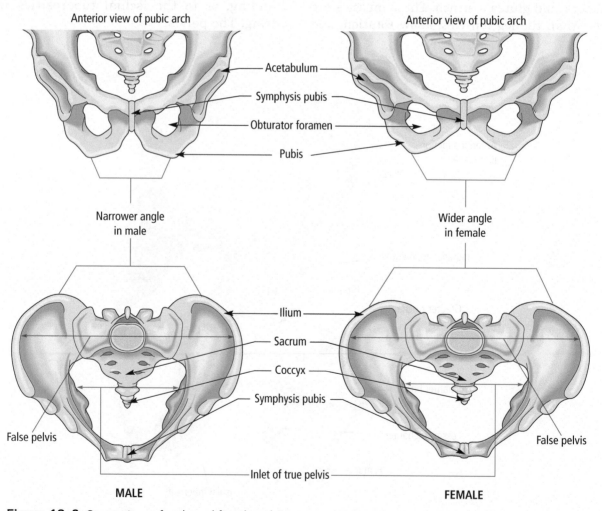

Figure 19–2 Comparison of male and female pelvises.

- The **iliac crest**, which marks the upper ridge of the ilium
- The **greater sciatic notch**, which allows the sciatic nerve to pass to the legs below
- The **iliac fossa**, the broad, slightly concave inner surface of the ilium

The fossa, pubis, and ischium create a basin in which the lower abdominal organs rest. The **sacrum**, the portion of the vertebral column between the lumbar vertebrae and the structures of the coccyx, is composed of five vertebrae fused together to form a single bone structure.

The **ischium** bears the body weight when sitting, and is attached to the pubis in front and to the ilium laterally and to the back. The large openings in the ischium on either side of the pelvis, just below the pubis, are the **obturator foramina**. The obturator foramen is the large opening in each ischium. These openings admit blood vessels and nerves from the abdominal cavity to the inside of the upper legs.

The **pubis** is located just to the front and below the bladder. In the center of the pubis is the **symphysis**, which marks the line where the two sides of the pubis are fused.

The **coccyx** (tailbone) is composed of three to five rudimentary vertebrae. Often, the first of these coccygeal vertebrae is separate, while the remainder are fused together. The articulation between the coccygeal vertebrae and the sacrum allows some flexibility in the coccyx, which is particularly beneficial in taking the stresses of sitting and falling. The coccyx is extremely susceptible to shock fracture, as might be induced from a fall.

Furthermore, because a number of nerve pathways pass near this area, damage to the coccyx threatens damage to the nerves of the lower body. The juncture of the first coccygeal vertebra with the sacrum occurs at the lower facet of the sacrum.

Primary Muscles of the Pelvis, Hip, and Thigh

Strong capsular ligaments surround and support the hip joint. Muscles from the lower back, pelvis, and thigh contribute to strength and stability. The head of the femur is covered with a smooth layer of cartilage, which helps to absorb shock and reduce friction during movement, while synovial fluid further cushions the joint and transports essential nutrients to joint structures.

Attached to the pelvis are groin and torso muscles that are involved in supporting and moving the trunk, as well as the upper and lower extremities. The bones of the hip and pelvis are supported by these ligaments: ligamentum teres, transverse acetabular, iliofemoral, pubofemoral, and inguinal (Figure 19–3).

A number of important muscle groups are located in the hip and pelvic region. The largest muscle group includes the gluteal muscles. The gluteus medius, gluteus minimus, and gluteus maximus assist in hip extension, internal and external rotation, and abduction. Muscles that assist in hip flexion (**hip flexors**) are the iliopsoas, sartorius, pectineus, and rectus femoris. Hip adduction is performed by the group of muscles known as the **adductor muscles**. The hip adductor group is

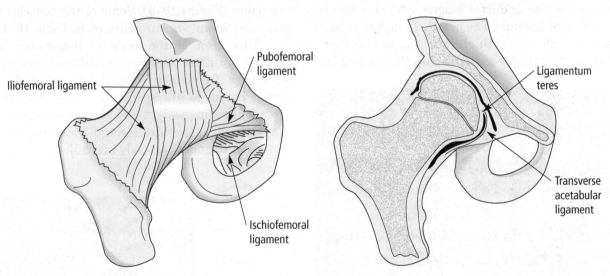

Figure 19–3 Ligaments of the hip.

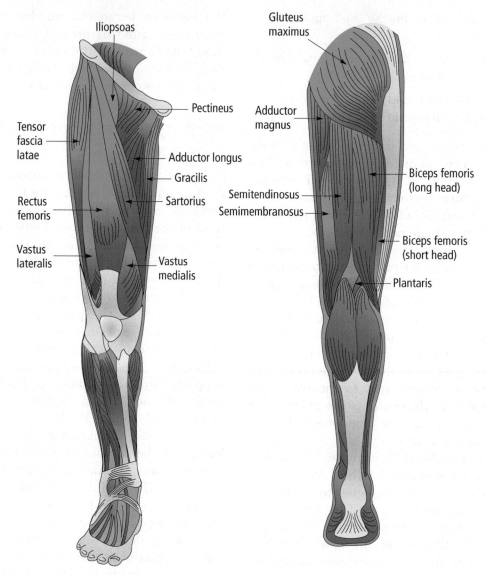

Figure 19–4 Primary muscles of the pelvis, hip, and thigh.

composed of the adductor longus, adductor brevis, and adductor magnus. The muscle groups that compose the bulk of the thigh (quadriceps and **hamstring muscles**) also assist in hip flexion and hip extension (Figure 19–4). Some of the muscles that move the femur are summarized in Table 19–1.

This area of the body is innervated by a number of different nerves. Additional anatomical structures frequently injured are fat pads and bursa. Fat pads are specialized soft-tissue structures for bearing weight and absorbing impact. The synovial sacs generally located over bony prominences throughout the body are called *bursae*.

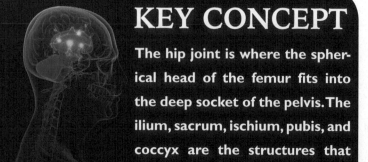

KEY CONCEPT

The hip joint is where the spherical head of the femur fits into the deep socket of the pelvis. The ilium, sacrum, ischium, pubis, and coccyx are the structures that constitute the pelvis.

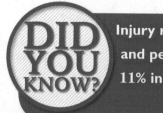

Injury rates involving the hip and pelvis range from 2% to 11% in runners.

Table 19-1 Muscles That Move the Femur

MUSCLE	ORIGIN	INSERTION	FUNCTION
Psoas major	Transverse process of lumbar vertebrae	Femur	Flexes, rotates thigh medially
Psoas minor	Last thoracic and lumbar vertebrae	Junction of ilium and pubis	Flexes trunk
Iliacus	Last thoracic and lumbar vertebrae	Junction of ilium and pubis	Flexes, rotates thigh medially
Gluteus maximus	Ilium, sacrum, and coccyx	Fascia lata, gluteal ridge	Extends, rotates thigh laterally
Gluteus medius	Ilium	Tendon on femur	Abducts, rotates thigh medially
Gluteus minimus	Ilium	Femur	Abducts, rotates thigh medially
Tensor fascia lata	Ilium	Femur	Tenses fascia lata
Abductor brevis	Pubis	Femur	Abducts, rotates thigh
Adductor magnus	Ischium, ischiopubic ramus	Femur	Adducts, extends thigh
Obturator externus	Ischium, ischiopubic ramus	Femur	Rotates thigh laterally
Pectineus	Junction ilium and pubis	Femur	Flexes, adducts thigh

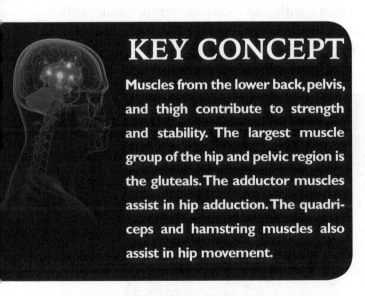

KEY CONCEPT

Muscles from the lower back, pelvis, and thigh contribute to strength and stability. The largest muscle group of the hip and pelvic region is the gluteals. The adductor muscles assist in hip adduction. The quadriceps and hamstring muscles also assist in hip movement.

COMMON INJURIES AND CONDITIONS OF THE HIP AND THIGH

Injuries to the hip and thigh are very common in athletics. The major injuries and conditions are discussed in the following subsections.

Bursitis

The most frequent location for bursitis is over the outside of the hip. This is called greater trochanteric bursitis (refer to Figure 19–1). This condition is commonly seen in athletes who do not sufficiently stretch and warm up this area.

SIGNS AND SYMPTOMS Tenderness over the outside of the hip, a symptom of bursitis, can frequently be made worse by walking, running, or twisting the hip in certain directions.

TREATMENT The initial treatment for bursitis is limiting activity, followed by stretching exercises and ice massage. Nonsteroidal, anti-inflammatory medicines are also quite helpful.

Fracture

A *hip fracture* refers to a break of the top part of the femur where it connects to the pelvis. Hip fractures are classified into many types, the most common being femoral neck fractures, intertrochanteric fractures, and subtrochanteric fractures (Figure 19–5).

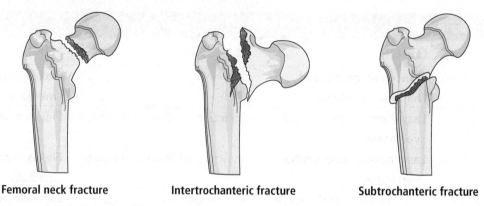

Femoral neck fracture   Intertrochanteric fracture   Subtrochanteric fracture

Figure 19–5 Common fractures of the proximal femur at the hip.

The most common cause of hip fractures is falling. The majority of these fractures occur in the elderly. Extreme trauma, such as motor vehicle accidents and impact injuries from athletics, may cause hip fractures in younger patients.

SIGNS AND SYMPTOMS Most hip fractures are diagnosed by a history of a fall or an accident followed by severe hip pain. The leg may appear abnormally rotated. Any attempt to move the hip will result in a significant increase in pain. X-rays are used to confirm the diagnosis. Occasionally, a bone scan or MRI is needed to prove that a fracture is present.

TREATMENT Hip fracture treatment is highly individualized. Treatment choices must be discussed with the surgeon and made according to the patient's fracture type and medical condition.

Quadriceps and Hip Flexor Strains

Strains of the quadriceps and hip flexors are common in sports requiring jumping, kicking, or repetitive sprinting. Most quadriceps strains involve the rectus femoris. Hip flexor strains may involve the rectus femoris and/or iliopsoas muscle. With grade I and II injuries, the major concern is preventing reinjury and complete disruption (grade III strain) (Figure 19–6).

TREATMENT Initial treatment includes icing, compression with an elastic wrap, and anti-inflammatory medications. As with all medications, a physician should be consulted.

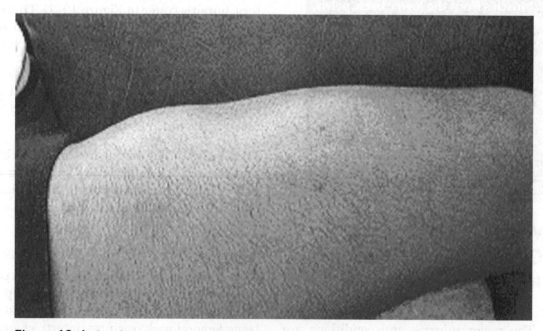

Figure 19–6 Quadricep rupture in an athlete.

REHABILITATION Rehabilitation should be progressive and sport specific. For example, for quadriceps strains caused by running, range-of-motion exercises and stretching should commence early and progress to strengthening exercises, walking, pool-running, jogging, limited speed running, and full-speed sprints as soon as the athlete is free of pain. Figures 19–7 and 19–8 demonstrate stretching that is useful for the hip flexors.

Hamstring Strains

The hamstring muscles bend and flex the knee. Strong hamstring muscles are especially important for power and balance when sprinting and jumping.

Counterparts to the quadriceps muscles in the front of the thigh, they are involved in almost every leg movement.

The hamstrings are composed of three separate muscles: the biceps femoris, semitendinosus, and semimembranosus (Figure 19–9). These muscles originate at the ischial tuberosity of the pelvis and attach behind the knee. They span two joints and are prone to strain during athletic activity. Any of the three hamstring muscles may be injured, but the long head of the biceps femoris is most frequently affected.

A hamstring strain is commonly called a "pulled hamstring." Pulling the hamstrings too far or too fast stretches the muscle fibers, which causes the strain. A hamstring strain can range from microtears in a small area of muscle to a complete tear in the muscle or the tendons that attach the muscle to bone.

In general, the term *hamstring strain* refers to mild or moderate damage in the muscle tissue. Completely tearing the muscles, or separating them from connective tendons, is usually a more serious injury, a *hamstring tear*.

Sudden, explosive starts and stops, and chronic overuse of the hamstring muscle-tendon unit, are the most common causes of pulled hamstrings. More severe hamstring pulls often result

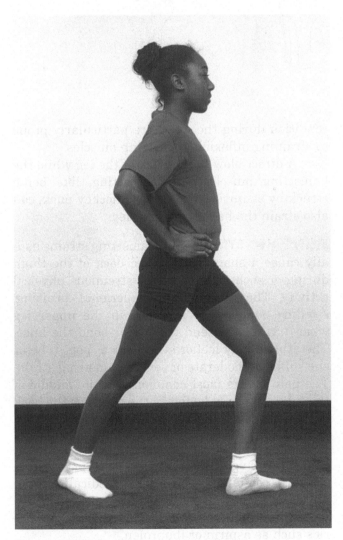

Figure 19–7 The athlete stands with the leg to be stretched behind the other leg and rotated slightly outward. She then shifts weight forward to the opposite leg, putting the hip flexor muscles in a stretch. Posture should be erect, with hips thrust forward.

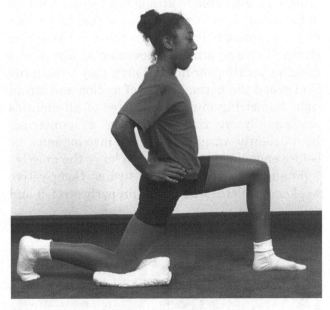

Figure 19–8 This stretch is similar to the one described in Figure 19–7, except that the athlete kneels on a towel (which serves as a cushion), then thrusts forward with the hips, still maintaining an erect posture. A stretch should be felt in the area of the hip flexors.

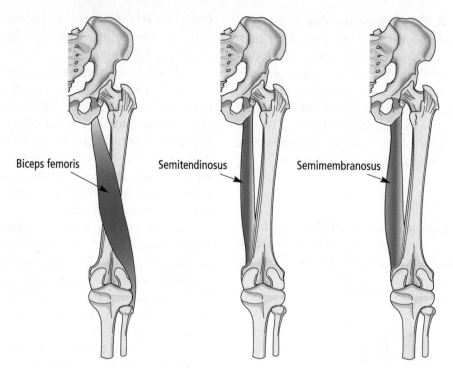

Biceps femoris   Semitendinosus   Semimembranosus

Figure 19–9 Hamstring muscles.

from sprinting or making a quick start or stop when the leg is extended. Chronic hamstring strains can also result from overtraining that puts stress on fatigued hamstring muscles.

When the quadriceps muscles are overdeveloped in relation to the hamstring muscles, the athlete may be able to straighten the leg with an imbalanced force that damages the hamstring muscles. Inflexibility also can cause a hamstring strain. Certain athletic movements, like ballet dancing, tackling, or martial arts, may stretch the leg beyond the normal range of motion and strain tight hamstring muscles. Athletes of all abilities are equally at risk of pulling a hamstring. Insufficiently warming up the hamstring muscles before engaging in athletics can leave the muscles tight and at risk for pulls and strains. Competitive weekend athletes who do not properly stretch and

condition during the week are particularly prone to straining inflexible hamstring muscles.

A direct blow to the back of the leg while the hamstring muscles are contracting, like being struck by a squash racquet or a hockey puck, can also strain the hamstring muscles.

SIGNS AND SYMPTOMS Hamstring strains usually cause a sharp pain in the back of the thigh during or soon after sports or strenuous physical activity. The athlete may experience bruising, swelling, and loss of strength in the upper leg when trying to extend the hip or bend the knee. The athlete may feel or even hear a "pop" if he or she suffers a moderate or severe hamstring strain. The pain occurs most commonly in the middle of the thigh, but may be felt in the pelvis or the back of the knee if the tendons are damaged.

TREATMENT Nonsurgical treatment usually can heal hamstring strains. Physicians typically prescribe a combination of RICE, medication, and physical therapy. Most patients receive adequate pain relief from nonprescription anti-inflammatories such as aspirin or ibuprofen.

Depending on the severity of the injury, the athlete's physician may prescribe crutches to keep weight off the injured leg for up to three weeks. Massage from a trained therapist can

FUN FACTS

After a butcher cleans a pig, he hangs up the ham—strings it up—by the muscle group at the back of the leg. It is this process that gave hamstrings their name.

help relax and tone the hamstring muscles after an injury.

REHABILITATION The athlete should begin a rehabilitation program as soon as possible after a hamstring strain. Rehabilitation progresses into a weight-training program focused on balancing strength between the hamstrings and quadriceps muscles. Rushing through the rehabilitation process and returning to sports before the athlete has completely recovered risks reinjury of the hamstring. Athletes can expect to return to sports at full strength, following most hamstring strains. Mild strains can usually be rehabilitated in 2 to 10 days. Moderate strains may take between 10 days and 6 weeks to heal. Severe strains may require 6 to 10 weeks of rehabilitation before the athlete can return to competition.

To prevent reinjury, it is important to keep leg muscles strong and flexible. The athlete should make the exercises learned in rehabilitation part of an everyday exercise routine. The athlete should also maintain cardiovascular fitness, so that the legs are prepared for quick starts and stops during physical activities. Figures 19–10 through 19–15 demonstrate stretching techniques for the hamstring.

Adductor (Groin) Strains

Adductor strains are common in sports requiring sudden, sideways changes in direction, such as skating, soccer, track and field, and tennis. Most involve the adductor longus. Typically, an adductor strain is a grade I or II strain (mild or moderate) and is characterized by groin pain when running or kicking. The adductors originate on the pelvic bone and attach at intervals along the length of

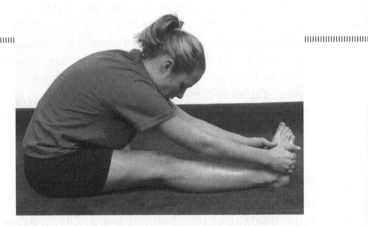

Figure 19–10 Seated, single-leg hamstring stretch.

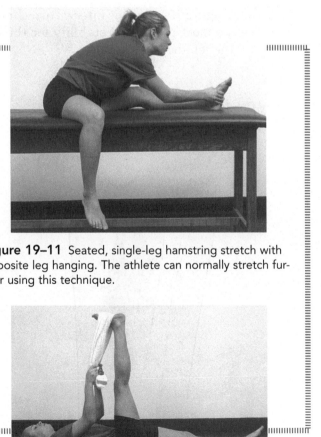

Figure 19–11 Seated, single-leg hamstring stretch with opposite leg hanging. The athlete can normally stretch further using this technique.

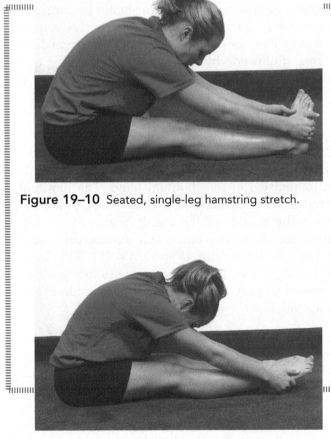

Figure 19–12 Double-leg hamstring stretch. Notice that the toes are pointed forward to isolate the hamstrings.

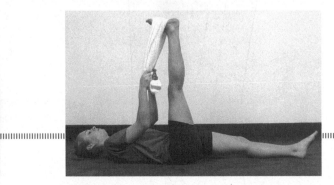

Figure 19–13 Supine, single-leg towel stretch. Using a towel, the athlete can slowly pull the leg back to stretch the hamstrings.

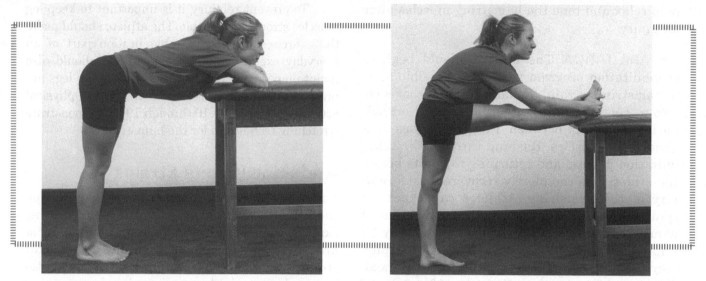

Figure 19–14 Standing bench stretch. This is a good beginning stretch for the hamstrings. It is important that the feet are flat, legs straight, and the back as flat as possible.

Figure 19–15 This exercise is similar to the one described in Figure 19–14, except that one leg is supported on a bench. This is an excellent stretch for athletes who want to gain additional mobility. It is not advised for athletes who have hamstring strains.

the femur (Figure 19–16). This interval attachment provides the most power and stability for the hip joint and the femur.

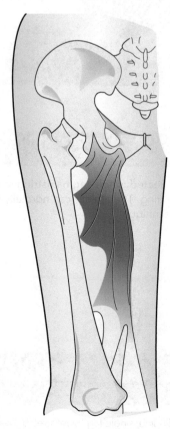

Figure 19–16 Adductor muscles of the hip.

TREATMENT Adductor strains are difficult to treat, and the risk of reinjury is high. As with hamstring strains, the athlete should be carefully monitored during rehabilitation. Treatment involves rest, ice, and anti-inflammatory medications, followed by adductor stretching and strengthening exercises. Figure 19–17 shows a stretching exercise for the adductor muscles.

Iliotibial Band Syndrome

Iliotibial band syndrome occurs when there is inflammation of the iliotibial band. The iliotibial band is a thick band of fibrous tissue that runs down the outside of the leg. It begins at the hip and extends to the outer side of the tibia, just below the knee joint (Figure 19–18). The band functions in coordination with several of the thigh muscles to provide stability to the outside of the knee joint.

SIGNS AND SYMPTOMS Irritation usually occurs over the outside of the knee joint, at the lateral epicondyle end of the femur. The iliotibial band crosses bone and muscle at this point.

Between these structures is a bursa that should facilitate a smooth, gliding motion. However, when inflamed, the iliotibial band does not glide easily, and pain associated with movement of the

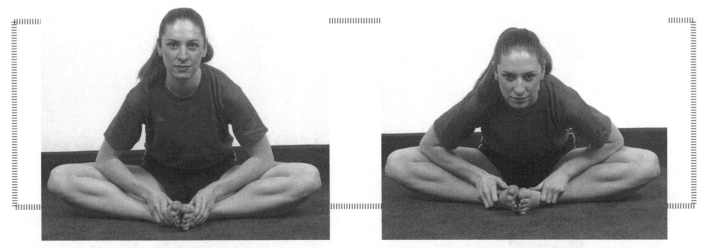

Figure 19–17A In a sitting position, the athlete pulls her heels in as far as possible.

Figure 19–17B In this position, the athlete leans forward, stretching the adductor muscles of the hip.

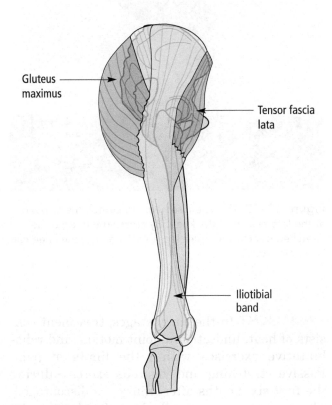

Gluteus maximus

Tensor fascia lata

Iliotibial band

Figure 19–18 Iliotibial band.

knee joint is the result. Usually the pain worsens with continued movement and resolves with rest.

People who suddenly increase their level of activity, such as runners who add mileage, often develop iliotibial band syndrome. Others who are prone to iliotibial band syndrome are individuals with mechanical problems, as well as people who overpronate, have leg-length discrepancies, or are bow-legged.

TREATMENT Treatment of iliotibial band syndrome begins with analysis of the athlete's gait and training program, to rule out mechanical problems or training errors that may predispose the athlete to this condition. Proper footwear, icing the area of pain, and stretching help to treat iliotibial band syndrome. The athlete will need to reduce activity level until symptoms subside. Figures 19–19 and 19–20 demonstrate stretches for the iliotibial band. (Iliotibial band syndrome is also discussed in Chapter 18.)

Quadriceps Contusions

Quadriceps contusions are common in football, rugby, soccer, and basketball. In these sports, contusions are usually caused by a direct blow to the thigh from a helmet or knee. The injury may limit motion and affect gait. The severity of the contusion is usually graded by the range of motion in the hip at the time of evaluation.

TREATMENT Treatment consists of immediate compression, ice (applied during the first 24–48 hours), and crutches to assist with weight bearing. Massage is contraindicated and may in fact cause further damage (bleeding and increased pain).

Complete recovery can be expected, but painless full range of motion should be achieved before the athlete returns to sports. Recovery time may range from two days to six months, depending on the severity of the injury and the development of complications such as myositis ossificans.

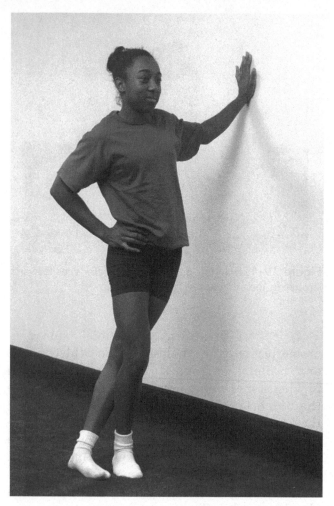

Figure 19–19 Stretching the iliotibial (IT) band is not easy, but this exercise will help. As shown, the athlete leans against a wall with the leg to be stretched crossed behind the other leg. It is important to cross the feet to put as much stretch on the IT band as possible.

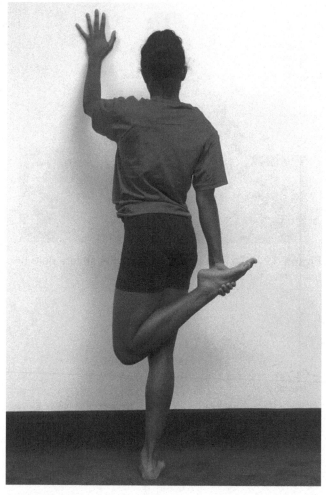

Figure 19–20 This exercise helps to stretch the IT band at the lateral side of the knee. By crossing the leg to be stretched behind the other leg, the IT band at the knee can be stretched.

Myositis Ossificans

Myositis ossificans is a very painful condition in which an ossifying mass (calcium deposit) forms within the muscle see figure 19-21 and 19-22. In many cases, myositis ossificans is the result of recurrent trauma to a quadricep muscle that was not properly protected after an initial injury. A history of injury should always be investigated to rule out other causes.

SIGNS AND SYMPTOMS A hard, painful mass in the soft tissue of the thigh and progressive loss of bending motion of the injured knee are indications of myositis ossificans. The definitive diagnosis of this condition is made by x-ray, but usually not until at least four weeks after the injury.

TREATMENT In the early stages, treatment consists of heat, limitation of joint motion, and rehabilitative exercises within the limits of pain. Passive stretching and vigorous exercise during the first six months after injury are discouraged. The calcium mass usually is reabsorbed by the body; however, resorption may take three to six months. Surgical excision may be necessary if pain and limited motion persist beyond one year.

Iliac Crest Contusions

The **iliac crest contusion**, or "hip pointer," is a very painful injury caused by a direct blow to the hip. Hip pointers are common in football players who wear improperly fitting hip pads.

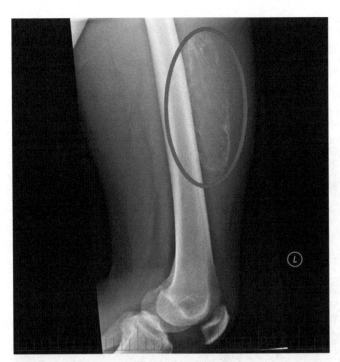

Figure 19-21 Myositis Ossificans present in the greater quadriceps area.

SIGNS AND SYMPTOMS Extreme tenderness, swelling, and ecchymosis over the iliac crest are classic signs and symptoms of a hip pointer (Figure 19–22).

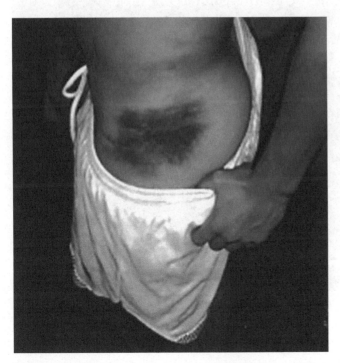

Figure 19–22 Iliac crest contusion (resulting from a fall on the hip during a slide tackle in a soccer game).

TREATMENT Treatment involves application of ice and compression.

REHABILITATION Return to sport should be dictated by the athlete's pain level. The injured area should be padded to protect it from further injury.

Overuse Injuries

Overuse injuries are common in athletes who focus their efforts on one sport. These injuries are caused by the cumulative effect of very low levels of stress, such as that caused by the repetitive action of running. Chronic muscle strains, stress fractures, tendonitis (overuse/overload fatigue within the tendon), snapping hip (iliopsoas tendon snapping over the head of the femur), and bursitis (inflammation and thickening of the bursal wall) are examples of overuse injuries.

An athlete with an overuse injury should rest from the sport that aggravated the injury, and use cross-training techniques. Exercises that work different parts of the body to maintain cardiovascular conditioning will help the athlete to return to the sport sooner.

Stress Fractures

Stress fractures of the pelvis occur most often in runners and dancers. Stress fractures of the femur usually occur in runners.

SIGNS AND SYMPTOMS The injured athlete may complain of chronic, ill-defined pain over the groin and thigh, and initially be diagnosed with a muscle strain. If there is no history of acute injury, a stress fracture should be considered. If the symptoms do not resolve with rest and rehabilitative exercise, the athlete should be examined by a sports medicine specialist. Diagnosis is performed by using x-rays and/or bone scans.

TREATMENT Treatment of stress fractures consists of rest and non-weight-bearing endurance exercises, such as running in water or swimming.

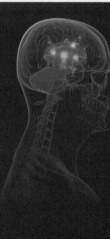

KEY CONCEPT

In athletics, there are several common injuries to the hip and pelvic region:

- Bursitis is inflammation of bursae toward the outside of the hip. Treatment is to rest and ice the affected area. Anti-inflammatory medication is also helpful.

- Fractures of the hip usually result from a fall and result in severe hip pain. Treatment will depend on the fracture type.

- Quadriceps and hip flexor strains usually occur in athletes whose sports require repetitive sprinting, jumping, and kicking. Treatment consists of ice, compression, and anti-inflammatory medications.

- Hamstring strains result when these muscles are pulled too far too fast. Treatment is usually a combination of RICE, medication, and physical therapy.

- Adductor strains usually result from sudden, sideways changes in direction. Typically, they are difficult to treat; rest, ice, anti-inflammatory medications, and stretching are recommended.

- Iliotibial band syndrome is an inflammation of the iliotibial band. Treatment includes analysis of gait and modification of the athlete's training regimen.

- Quadriceps contusions are the result of a direct blow to the thigh. Treatment consists of compression, ice, and protection from weight bearing.

- Myositis ossificans is a painful condition in which a calcium deposit forms within the muscle. Treatment involves heat, limitation of joint movement, and rehabilitative exercises.

- Iliac crest contusions are a result of a direct blow to the hip. Treatment involves ice and compression.

- Overuse injuries are the result of the cumulative effects of low-level stress on one particular area. Treatment may include developing a more well-rounded training routine.

- Stress fractures of the pelvis occur most often in runners and dancers. Treatment consists of rest and non-weight-bearing exercises.

CONCLUSION

The hip is a stable joint that is well protected and surrounded by muscle on all sides. It allows substantial range of motion. Because the hip is a freely movable, ball-and-socket joint, the muscles that protect it are prone to injuries. Injuries of the hip usually result from these muscles being overused or pushed too hard.

The pelvis is made up of several flattened bones that form a ring and function as a support structure for the human skeleton. The function of the pelvis is to transmit weight from the axial skeleton to the lower limbs, when standing, or to the ischial tuberosities, when sitting. The pelvis provides attachments for various muscles, which insert into and control the lower limbs; it also houses parts of the digestive and urinary tracts, and the reproductive system in both males and females.

Injuries to the hip and thigh are very common in athletics. They include muscle strains, ligament sprains, inflammation of bursae, contusions, and fractures. The iliotibial band, which provides stability to the knee and assists in flexion of the knee joint, can also become inflamed. When the IT band is irritated, movement of the knee joint becomes painful.

REVIEW QUESTIONS

1. Describe the differences of the hip and pelvis between men and women.
2. Explain the importance of the hip and pelvis as a support structure for the human body.
3. List the common injuries and conditions of the hip and thigh. Briefly describe each.
4. List the primary muscles of the hip and pelvis. The hamstrings are made up of three different muscles. What are they?
5. Describe the causes of hamstring strains.
6. Explain the causes of iliotibial band syndrome.
7. How does myositis ossificans develop?
8. What is a "hip pointer"?
9. What can be done to avoid overuse injuries?

PROJECTS AND ACTIVITIES

1. Using the library or the Internet, research "core muscle group." How does this pertain to the hip and pelvis? Explain.
2. Select one of the common injuries and conditions of the hip and thigh explained in this chapter. Research and write a paper on this topic.
3. Create a stretching chart using the stretching exercises explained in this chapter.

LEARNING LINKS

- Visit http://www.sportsknee.com; click on the patient education animation link to view the anatomy of the hip. (This site also has a nice animation of the knee and shoulder.)
- Visit https://www.hss.edu/condition-list_hip-pelvis.asp; excellent information and graphics on the hip and pelvis.

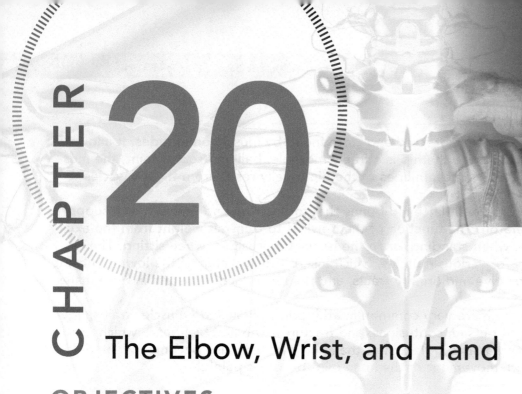

CHAPTER 20

The Elbow, Wrist, and Hand

OBJECTIVES

Upon completion of this chapter, the reader should be able to:

- Define the major components of the elbow
- Describe the major injuries and conditions of the elbow, wrist, and hand
- Explain the treatment for tendonitis of the elbow, wrist, and hand
- List the different bones of the hand
- Describe the location of the radial, median, and ulnar nerves

KEY TERMS

anatomical snuffbox *A depression on side/back of the hand, just beneath the thumb, that is formed by two tendons (the extensor pollicis brevis and the extensor pollicis longus).*

baseball (mallet) finger *An injury to the finger resulting from tearing of the finger tendon and damage to the cartilage.*

boutonnière deformity *A tear of the extensor tendon of the PIP joint, at the middle of the finger, and the DIP joint that controls the fingertip.*

boxer's fracture *A break in the fifth metacarpal leading to the little finger.*

carpal tunnel syndrome *An inflammatory disorder caused by irritation of the tissues and nerves around the median nerve.*

carpal tunnel *A passageway that runs from the forearm through the wrist.*

carpals *The eight bones that make up the wrist.*

Colles's fracture *An injury to the lower arm bone just above the wrist.*

cubital tunnel syndrome *Irritation, compression, and entrapment of the ulnar nerve.*

deQuervain's tenosynovitis *Tendonitis originating in the base of the thumb.*

dislocation *The displacement of any bone from its normal position.*

epicondylitis *A chronic strain of the medial or lateral epicondyle in the elbow.*

KEY TERMS CONTINUED

gamekeeper's thumb *Injury to the thumb that results in tearing or stretching of the MP joint or rupture of the ulnar collateral ligament.*

ganglion *A small, hard lump above a tendon or in the capsule that encloses a joint.*

humerus *The bone of the upper arm.*

ischemia *Decreased blood supply to an organ or tissue resulting from pressure, swelling, trauma, or a fracture.*

jersey finger *An injury to the finger resulting in tearing of the flexor tendon in the fingertip.*

lateral epicondyle *The bony end of the humerus that lies to the outside of the elbow joint.*

medial epicondyle *The bony end of the humerus that forms with the elbow joint.*

median nerve *Nerve within the brachial plexus that crosses the anterior elbow, passes between the heads of the pronator teres, and runs distal to the joint.*

metacarpals *The bones that form the structure of the hand.*

olecranon bursitis *Inflammation of the bursa located over the olecranon process of the elbow.*

phalanges *The finger bones.*

pronator teres syndrome *Entrapment or compression of the median nerve.*

radial nerve *Nerve within the brachial plexus that passes anteriorly to the lateral epicondyle and lies in a tunnel of several muscles and tendons.*

radial tunnel syndrome *Entrapment of the radial nerve.*

radius *The bone on the thumb side of the forearm.*

scaphoid fracture *A break in the scaphoid bone in the thumb.*

subluxation *The abnormal movement of one of the bones that constitute a joint.*

tendonitis *Inflammation of the tendons caused by overuse or repetitive motion.*

tennis elbow *A chronic strain of the lateral epicondyle in the elbow; another name for epicondylitis.*

ulnar nerve *Nerve within the brachial plexus that passes through the cubital tunnel in the posterior aspect of the medial epicondyle.*

ulna *The bone of the inner forearm.*

Volkmann's contracture *Condition in which the muscles in the palm side of the forearm shorten, causing the fingers to form a fist and the wrist to bend.*

THE ELBOW, WRIST AND HAND

Many human activities—from shooting an arrow, to playing the piano, to shooting a basketball—would be impossible without the healthy functioning of the elbow, wrist, and hand. This area of the body is one of the most intricate, yet most vulnerable to injury.

THE ELBOW

The elbow is composed of three bones: the **humerus, ulna,** and **radius**.

The humerus articulates with the radius and ulna, forming a hinge joint. Many structures, including ligaments, nerves, muscles, and bursa sacs, surround the elbow joint (Figure 20–1). These structures aid in moving and protecting the elbow.

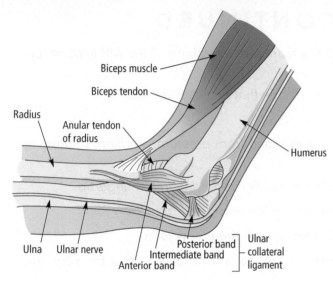

Figure 20–1 The elbow joint.

Muscles of the Elbow

Three muscles flex the forearm at the elbow: the brachialis, the biceps brachii, and the brachioradialis (Figure 20–2). Table 20–1 lists the muscles that move the elbow and the functions they perform. Two muscles extend the arm: the triceps brachii and the anconeus.

COMMON INJURIES OF THE ELBOW

Injuries involving the elbow and forearm are common in almost any athletic activity. Many different types of forces and stresses affect the elbow during the rigors of various sports. The elbow is prone to repetitive overuse injuries.

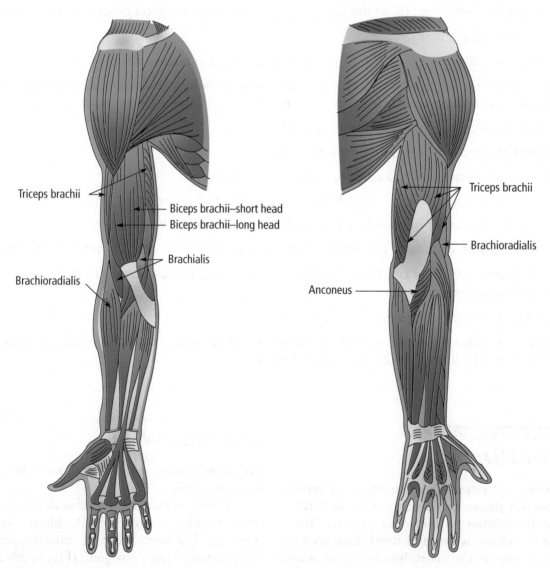

Figure 20–2 Muscles of the elbow.

Table 20–1 Muscles That Move the Elbow

MUSCLE	FUNCTION
Brachialis	Flexes forearm
Triceps brachii (3 heads)	Extends and adducts forearm
Biceps brachii (2 heads)	Flexes arm, flexes forearm, supinates hand
Anconeus	Extends forearm
Brachioradialis	Flexes forearm

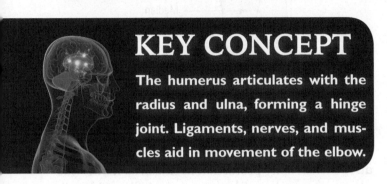

KEY CONCEPT

The humerus articulates with the radius and ulna, forming a hinge joint. Ligaments, nerves, and muscles aid in movement of the elbow.

Repetitive sports activities probably cause the most common of these injuries. Activities that place the arm in extension (a straight position)—throwing a baseball or football, or swinging a bat, club, or racquet—tend to cause most elbow injuries (Figure 20–3).

A variety of athletic injuries can result from direct trauma to the area; indirect trauma (such as falling on an outstretched hand); or acute and chronic stresses associated with throwing and swimming. These mechanisms of injury can result in contusions, sprains, strains, dislocations, fractures, and nerve involvement.

Contusions

Contusions are common to this area of the body, and may involve the muscles of the forearm and subcutaneous bony prominences of the elbow. An athlete's forearms absorb the brunt of many impacts during athletic activity, especially contact sports. Direct blows to these muscular areas can result in bruising and subsequent bleeding, producing stiffness during function and active range of motion. The direct blow that causes the contusion may also be responsible for additional trauma such as a fracture. Proper management during treatment of contusions includes ensuring that the area is protected from additional trauma and

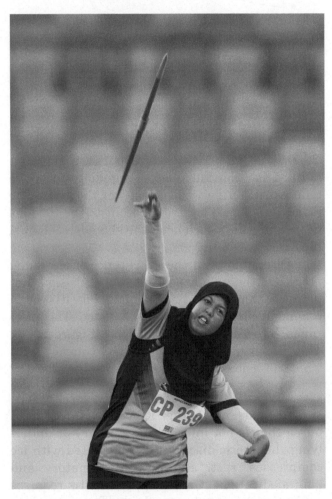

Figure 20–3 The elbow is subjected to tremendous stress during athletic competition. Shahjehan/Shutterstock.com

guarding against the possible development of a condition called myositis ossificans, in which bone grows in skeletal muscle. (See Chapter 19 for further discussion.)

TREATMENT Treatment is the same as for any contusion: rest, ice, compression, and elevation (RICE). Protective padding will help ensure that the injured area does not sustain another impact.

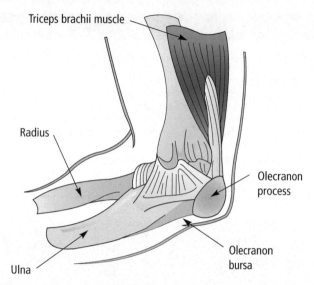

Figure 20–4 Olecranon bursa of the elbow.

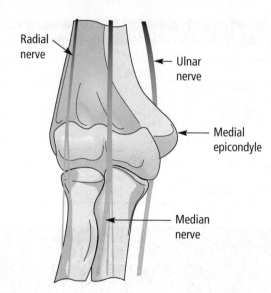

Figure 20–5 The three major nerves of the elbow.

Olecranon Bursitis

Bursitis is inflammation of a bursa, a tiny, fluid-filled sac that functions as a gliding surface to reduce friction between tissues of the body. The major bursae are located adjacent to the tendons near large joints such as in the shoulders, elbows, hips, and knees.

Direct blows to the subcutaneous olecranon process of the ulna can result in a contusion that produces an acute hemorrhagic bursitis or a common, chronic **olecranon bursitis**. The olecranon bursa can become infected (Figure 20–4). This is partially a result of the frequency with which abrasions occur over the tip of the elbow.

TREATMENT The treatment of any form of bursitis depends on whether it involves infection. A bursa that is not infected (from injury or underlying rheumatic disease) can be treated with ice compresses, rest, and anti-inflammatory and pain medications. Occasionally, bursitis requires aspiration of the bursa fluid. This procedure involves removal of the fluid with a needle and syringe under sterile conditions. It can be performed in the doctor's office, although the fluid is sometimes sent to the laboratory for further analysis.

Ulnar Nerve Contusion

Almost everyone has suffered an ulnar nerve contusion at one time or another. As the nerve passes behind the **medial epicondyle** of the humerus, it runs subcutaneously in a groove and passes through the cubital tunnel (Figure 20–5). The relative lack of bony protection in this area makes the ulnar nerve vulnerable to trauma. A direct blow to this area may cause immediate pain and burning sensations shooting down the ulnar side of the forearm to the ring and little fingers. This paresthesia, commonly referred to as "hitting the funny bone," is normally transient and disappears in a few minutes, depending on the severity of the blow. Pain and numbness may persist for some time.

Strains to the Elbow

Strains to the muscles and structures of the elbow are common athletic injuries, which normally occur as a result of the tremendous stresses placed on the elbow joint, especially in sports requiring throwing or swimming motions. Overuse can cause irritation of the muscle fibers, resulting in microscopic tears. Continued trauma to this area can develop into overuse syndromes and chronic degenerative processes.

Strains are divided into acute and chronic types. Acute strains occur when a sudden overload is applied to the elbow joint. The resulting injury is a strain to the muscles or tendons of the elbow. The most common areas of acute strains are the common flexor tendon around the medial epicondyle and the common extensor tendon over the **lateral epicondyle**. Chronic strains occur when a previous injury is not addressed properly. This can be caused by overuse, which increases inflammation or degeneration of the flexor tendon, causing pain and weakness.

SIGNS AND SYMPTOMS The symptoms of acute strain to the musculature supporting the elbow include history of an incident of sudden, excessive overload, followed by tenderness over the involved area and pain on function or resisted motion. If the injury results in a rupture of a tendon, there may also be a palpable gap, a bunching of the injured muscle, and a loss of efficient function of the involved muscle.

Epicondylitis

Chronic strains commonly occur in the region of the medial and lateral epicondyles of the humerus at the elbow. These overuse conditions are usually caused by repeated overload of the musculotendinous units attaching to one of the epicondyles. Additional factors that may predispose or aggravate **epicondylitis** include faulty techniques or mechanics, weak muscle groups, and inappropriate equipment.

An overuse condition is named according to the athletic activity being engaged in at the time it develops. **Tennis elbow** is a name commonly given to pain on the lateral side of the elbow, because it was first noted in tennis players (Figure 20–6). *Golfer's elbow* names the same condition, except on the other side of the elbow. However, tennis players can also develop pain on the medial epicondyle, depending on which muscle groups are irritated or overloaded. *Pitcher's elbow, bowler's elbow,* and *javelin thrower's elbow* are other names given to elbow epicondylitis that develops because of the sport in which the athlete is involved.

Little League elbow is a term used to describe elbow problems that result from repetitive throwing by immature athletes. This term may encompass a variety of conditions within the elbow, such as epicondylitis or an injury to the epiphysis (growth plate) of the medial epicondyle of the humerus. This epiphysis, normally the last epiphyseal center to close in the elbow area, is one of the weakest. Symptoms may be of acute or gradual onset. When onset is sudden, the injury is more likely to involve an avulsion of the epicondyle. Acute pain and tenderness over the epicondyle indicate that an immature athlete should be referred to a physician for further assessment. More commonly, Little League elbow is a chronic condition, and the symptoms usually include persistent discomfort and stiffness about the elbow. Symptoms are aggravated by use of the arm.

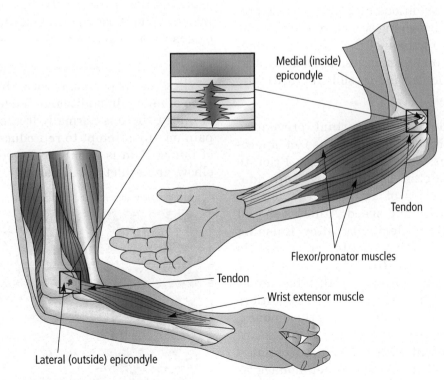

Figure 20–6 The lateral epicondyle is frequently injured in racquet sports.

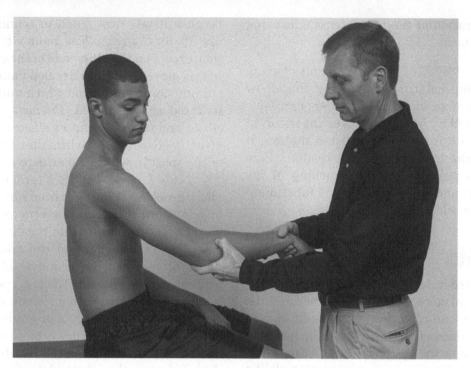

Figure 20–7 Location of tenderness found with lateral epicondylitis (tennis elbow) on the common extensor tendon.

SIGNS AND SYMPTOMS Initial symptoms of chronic strain are local tenderness over the involved epicondyle, pain on use of the involved muscles, and perhaps swelling (Figure 20–7). Resisted wrist motion often reproduces pain. Without proper treatment, these conditions may develop into prolonged, degenerative changes resulting in chronic epicondylitis, contractures of the elbow (a permanent shortening of the muscles, tendon, or scar tissue) reduced friction, and possible rupture of the muscle tendon unit.

TREATMENT The most important preventive measures are proper technique, use of appropriate equipment, and limited stress. Prior to competition, athletes should warm up adequately with a series of activities that slowly increase in intensity and speed. Athletes should stretch to maintain flexibility after finishing their sporting activity. Acute epicondylitis should be treated with RICE, the mainstay for treating soft-tissue injuries. Athletes must modify activities that aggravate the condition. This may be as simple as decreasing the amount, frequency, or intensity of activity. Athletes are often more compliant with a decreased regimen if they are allowed to increase other, nonaggravating activities.

Sprains of the Elbow

Sprains of the elbow joint are moderately common in athletics. Because of the configuration of the ulna in the trochlear notch, the elbow is a relatively stable joint. Injuries involving the ligamentous system of the elbow most commonly result from forced hyperextension or valgus/varus (side-to-side) forces.

SIGNS AND SYMPTOMS Athletes may describe a "click" or "pop," along with sharp pain, at the time of injury. In addition to tenderness at the site of injury, there is normally localized swelling and pain on any attempt to reproduce the mechanism of injury. Pain is usually relieved by bending the elbow, and athletes will normally hold the injured

FUN FACTS

If the elbow had been placed closer to the hand, the forearm would have been too short to bring the glass to the mouth; and if it had been closer to the shoulder, the forearm would have been so long that it would have carried the glass beyond the mouth.

—Benjamin Franklin (1706–1790)

extremity in some degree of flexion. Swelling and muscle spasms often limit complete extension. It may be difficult to determine significant instability of the elbow joint unless there has been a complete dislocation and rupture of ligaments. To prevent loss of motion and chronic disability, it is important to recognize significant ligamentous injuries to the elbow and initiate proper treatment procedures.

TREATMENT The treatment for elbow sprains is the same as for elbow strains. One of the many special braces marketed today may help athletes with elbow sprains and strains. However, wearing a brace has the potential to harm the injured area, because the brace changes the compression exerted and the biomechanics of motion from the compressive force. It is always important to consult a physician before using any brace or equipment designed to alleviate a condition.

SPECIAL TESTS Figures 20–8 and 20–9 show tests used to determine if the lateral collateral or medial collateral ligament of the elbow has been sprained.

Dislocations of the Elbow

The elbow is the second most frequently dislocated major joint, after the shoulder. Dislocations involving the elbow joint are not common, but can be serious. The most common type of elbow dislocation is posterior displacement of the ulna and

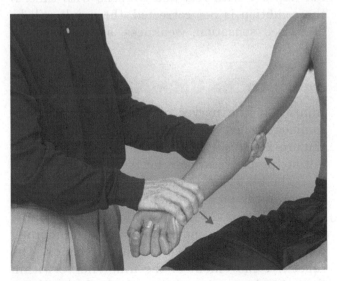

Figure 20–8 Varus stress testing for the elbow lateral collateral ligament.

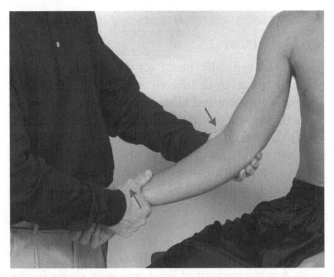

Figure 20–9 Valgus stress testing for the elbow medial collateral ligament.

radius in relationship to the humerus. This normally occurs as a result of a fall onto an outstretched hand with the elbow in extension. As the elbow is forced into hyperextension, the olecranon process is levered against the humerus, which can force the ulna backward (posteriorly). The collateral ligaments will be severely stretched or ruptured, but the annular ligament often remains intact, so that the head of the radius usually accompanies the ulna in its posterior displacement.

SIGNS AND SYMPTOMS Elbow dislocations that remain displaced should be easily recognized, as there will be obvious deformity, with the olecranon process abnormally prominent, loss of elbow function, and considerable pain.

The initial examination must include an evaluation of the circulation and nerve function to the distal portion of the extremity (hands and fingers). Determine the presence or absence of a radial pulse, as well as sensory and motor functions of the hand. All elbow dislocations should be properly immobilized and referred to a physician immediately.

TREATMENT Transportation to the athlete's physician or the nearest medical facility is critical. Because there is a possibility of vascular and neurological impairment, prompt reduction of the dislocation is important. Children who have elbow injuries should be evaluated with particular care because of multiple growth plates in that area. Although elbow dislocations occur in children, fractures are more common.

Fractures of the Elbow and Forearm

Fractures typically occur as the result of either direct trauma to the forearm or elbow, or indirect stresses transmitted through the upper extremity (usually as the result of falling on an outstretched arm). Excessive forces associated with throwing and swinging activities may also cause a fracture. Fractures in the elbow area are among the most frequent in children and skeletally immature athletes. Many involve the epiphysis, because the ligamentous structures in young athletes are much stronger than the bony and cartilaginous components of the growth plate.

A wide variety of fractures may occur in the elbow area and involve the distal humerus, proximal ulna, or radius. They can range from simple avulsions, in which a small piece of bone flakes off, to serious and complicated fractures.

SIGNS AND SYMPTOMS The signs and symptoms associated with fracture injuries are directly related to the degree of severity. There may or may not be visible or palpable deformity. Point tenderness is normally present at the site of injury, and varying amounts of hemorrhaging or swelling are common. The athlete may also demonstrate a limited range of motion, disability at the elbow or hand, and an increase in pain at the fracture site upon attempted movement.

TREATMENT Treatment involves immobilization, ice, elevation, and prompt referral to a physician or medical clinic. Serious elbow fractures and dislocations are of great concern and must be treated as a medical emergency.

Volkmann's Contracture

Volkmann's contracture is a serious condition that occurs in the absence of blood flow (**ischemia**) to the forearm. This can be caused by increased pressure in the arm from swelling, trauma, or fracture. The increased pressure compresses blood vessels and decreases blood flow to the arm. If left undiagnosed, the decreased blood flow will injure the muscle, causing it to shorten. When the muscle shortens, it pulls on the joint at the end of the muscle just as it would if it were normally contracted. This causes the joint to bend; it remains bent and cannot be straightened. This condition is

called a *contracture*. In Volkmann's contracture, the muscles involved are on the palm side of the forearm. Their contraction normally causes the fingers to form a fist and flex down the wrist.

There are three levels of severity in Volkmann's contracture:

• *Mild*—flexion contracture of two or three fingers only, with no or limited loss of sensation

• *Moderate*—all fingers are flexed and the thumb is stuck in the palm; the wrist may be stuck in flexion, and there is usually loss of some sensation in the hand

• *Severe*—all muscles in the forearm that flex or extend the wrist and fingers are involved; this is a severely disabling condition

The injury classically associated with this condition is an elbow fracture in children. Other conditions that can cause increased pressure in the forearm include any forearm fracture, burns, bleeding disorders, excessive exercise, injection of certain medications into the forearm, and animal bites.

SIGNS AND SYMPTOMS Signs and symptoms include severe pain when a muscle running through a compartment is passively moved. For example, when the doctor moves the fingers up and down, the patient who has Volkmann's contracture or a compartment syndrome in the forearm will experience severe pain. The forearm may be tensely swollen and shiny. There is also pain when the forearm is squeezed. The pain does not improve with rest and worsens with time. If the condition is not corrected, the result will be decreased sensation, weakness, and paleness of the skin.

Injury to the Ulnar Nerve

Injuries to the nerves of the elbow are not as common as musculoskeletal injuries to this area (Figure 20–10). It is important to recognize and initiate proper treatment for these conditions.

The **ulnar nerve** passes through the cubital tunnel in the posterior aspect of the medial epicondyle (Figure 20–11). The floor of this tunnel is the medial epicondyle groove; the remaining components are formed by fascial bands. The repetitive movement of the ulnar nerve within the cubital tunnel, and the relative lack of bony protection here, make this nerve vulnerable to paresthesia in the distribution of the ulnar nerve in the hand (the little finger and the and ring finger).

Injury to the Radial Nerve

The **radial nerve** passes anteriorly to the lateral epicondyle and lies in a tunnel formed by several muscles and tendons (see Figures 20–5 and 20–12). The radial nerve can become entrapped in the tunnel area, especially during activities requiring repetitive pronation and supination of the forearm. This radial nerve entrapment is called **radial tunnel syndrome**. Although this condition occurs infrequently, it should be considered in the assessment of lateral epicondylitis (tennis elbow), as the symptoms are very similar. It can also be difficult to differentiate between epicondylitis and nerve entrapment because the conditions may occur together.

SIGNS AND SYMPTOMS The athlete will exhibit pain over the lateral aspect of the elbow. However, with nerve entrapment, the tenderness may be present over the anterior radial head instead of the common extensor tendon. Symptoms may also be reproduced by resisting supination with the elbow flexed 90 degrees, or resisting extension of the middle finger with the elbow extended. Radial tunnel syndrome should be considered as a possible cause of lateral elbow pain when conservative treatment of lateral epicondylitis has failed and symptoms continue for an extended period of time.

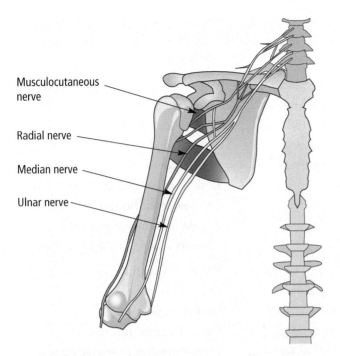

Figure 20–10 Brachial plexus of the shoulder showing the radial, median, and ulnar nerves. Notice how the three nerves pass down the arm and around the elbow joint.

compression forces and tension stresses at the elbow. The ulnar nerve can become irritated, compressed, or entrapped in this tunnel due to repetitive throwing or swinging activities. This is often referred to as **cubital tunnel syndrome**.

SIGNS AND SYMPTOMS Symptoms may include pain along the inner aspect of the elbow, tenderness over the medial epicondylar groove, and

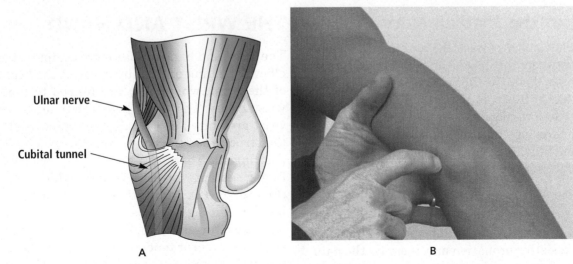

Figure 20–11 (A) Ulnar nerve passing through the cubital tunnel. (B) Location of the cubital tunnel. The ulnar nerve is superficial in the tunnel.

Table 20–2   Peripheral Nerve Injuries of the Elbow and Forearm

PERIPHERAL NERVE	ORIGIN	SENSATION	EFFECT OF INJURY
Ulnar nerve	C_7, C_8, T_1	Dorsal and palmar surfaces of the hand, including the little finger and ulnar half of the ring finger.	Weakness of wrist flexion and ulnar deviation; Flexion loss of distal interphalangeal (DIP) joints of the little and ring fingers; Loss of extension of fingers Loss of flexion of fingers; Inability to abduct or adduct fingers inability to adduct thumb
Median nerve	C_5, C_6, C_7, C_8, T_1	Radial half of the palm, including palmar surface of the thumb, index, middle, and radial half of the ring finger. Also the dorsal surfaces of the same fingers.	Weakness with flexion and radial deviation; Loss of pronation; Loss of thumb opposition; Loss of flexion at metacarpophalangeal (MCP) joints
Radial nerve	C_5, C_6, C_7, C_8, T_1	Back of the arm, forearm, wrist, thumb, index finger, and part of the middle finger, radial half of the back of the hand.	Loss of wrist extension, supination, extension at MCP joints, extension and abduction of the thumb; triceps reflex, weakness of elbow flexion, and ulnar and radial deviation

"C" denotes cervical vertebra.

Injury to the Median Nerve

The **median nerve** crosses the anterior elbow and passes between the heads of the pronator teres muscle, just distal to the joint (see Figures 20–5 and 20–10). At this point it is vulnerable to entrapment or compression due to hypertrophy of the pronator teres or activities that involve repetitive pronation of the forearm. This condition is referred to as **pronator teres syndrome**.

SIGNS AND SYMPTOMS Symptoms include pain radiating down the anterior forearm, with numbness and tingling in the thumb, index, and middle fingers. Resistive pronation may increase the pain. Table 20–2 summarizes nerve injuries in the elbow.

THE WRIST AND HAND

The wrist and hand are far more complex than the elbow. The ulna and radius meet at the beginning of the wrist, where they are hinged to the other wrist bones. The eight bones that make up the wrist are known as **carpals**; the **metacarpals** form the structure of the hand, and the **phalanges** form the fingers. There are three phalanges in each finger, except for the thumb which has two (Figure 20–12). In all, there are 27 bones in the hand, including the wrist.

Each finger is supplied with two types of tendons: an extensor tendon on top, which straightens the finger, and a flexor tendon on the bottom, which bends the finger. Three large nerves run the

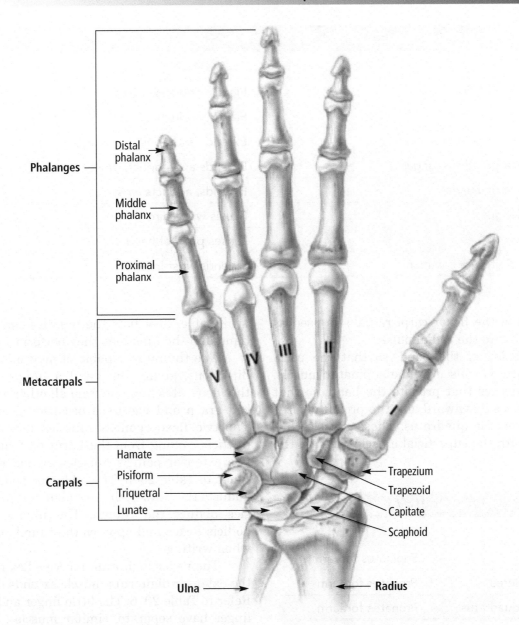

Phalanges
- Distal phalanx
- Middle phalanx
- Proximal phalanx

Metacarpals

Carpals
- Hamate
- Pisiform
- Triquetral
- Lunate
- Trapezium
- Trapezoid
- Capitate
- Scaphoid

Ulna

Radius

Figure 20–12 Bones of the wrist and hand.

length of the arm to send information to the brain and to create movement and sensation.

Muscles of the Hand and Wrist

Numerous muscles coordinate the movement of the hand and wrist bones. Two flexor carpi muscles flex the wrist. Three extensor carpi muscles extend the wrist with the assistance of the extensor digitorum communis. Table 20–3 lists the muscles that move the wrist and the functions they perform. These muscles are also involved in abducting and adducting the wrist. When the pulse is taken,

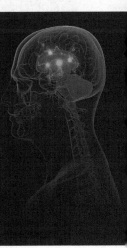

KEY CONCEPT

The hand, including the wrist, consists of 27 bones. The carpals are the 8 bones that make up the wrist. The 5 metacarpals form the structure of the hand. The 14 phalanges are the bone of the fingers.

Table 20-3 Muscles That Move the Wrist

MUSCLE	FUNCTION
Flexor carpi radialis	Flexes, abducts wrist
Flexor carpi ulnaris	Flexes, adducts wrist
Extensor carpi radialis brevis	Extends and abducts wrist joint
Extensor carpi radialis longus	Extends and abducts wrist
Extensor carpi ulnaris	Extends, adducts wrist
Palmaris longus	Flexes wrist joint
Palmaris brevis	Tenses palm of hand
Extensor digitorum communis	Extends wrist joint

the tendon of the flexor carpi radialis is used as the site to locate the radial pulse.

Supination of the hand, so that the palm faces upward, is caused by the supinator muscle. The two muscles that pronate the hand, so that the palm faces downward, are the pronator teres and the pronator quadratus. These muscles are found beneath the superficial muscles deep in the arm. Table 20-4 lists the muscles that move the hand and the functions they perform.

The thumb is capable of movement in many directions, giving the hand a unique capability that separates humans from all other animals. We can grasp and use tools because of our thumbs. The two flexor pollicis muscles flex the thumb (*pollicis* coming from the Latin for "thumb"). The two extensor pollicis muscles extend the thumb. Refer to Table 20-5. The adductor pollicis muscle adducts the thumb; the two abductor pollicis muscles abduct the thumb. The unique opponens pollicis flexes and opposes the thumb and is used when writing.

The flexor digitorum muscles flex the fingers; the extensor digitorum muscle extends the fingers. Refer to Table 20-6. The little finger and the index finger have separate, similar muscles. The inter-

Table 20-4 Muscles That Move the Hand

MUSCLE	FUNCTION
Supinator	Supinates forearm
Pronator teres	Pronates forearm
Pronator quadratus	Pronates forearm

Table 20-5 Muscles That Move the Thumb

MUSCLE	FUNCTION
Flexor pollicis longus	Flexes second phalanx of thumb
Flexor pollicis brevis	Flexes thumb
Extensor pollicis longus	Extends terminal phalanx
Extensor pollicis brevis	Extends thumb
Adductor pollicis	Adducts thumb
Abductor pollicis longus	Abducts, extends thumb
Abductor pollicis brevis	Abducts thumb
Opponens pollicis	Flexes and opposes thumb

Table 20–6 Muscles That Move the Fingers	
MUSCLE	FUNCTION
Flexor digitorum profundus	Flexes terminal phalanx
Flexor digiti minimi brevis	Flexes little finger
Interossei dorsalis	Abduct, flex proximal phalanges
Flexor digitorum superficialis	Flexes middle phalanges
Extensor indicis	Extends index finger
Interossei palmaris	Adduct, flex proximal phalanges
Abductor digiti minimi	Abducts little finger
Opponens digiti minimi	Rotates, abducts fifth metacarpal
Extensor digitorum communis	Extends the fingers

ossei muscles, found between the metacarpals, cause abduction of the proximal phalanges of the fingers. The tendons of the extensor digitorum are visible on the surface of the hand. Extend the fingers to view these tendons. Figure 20–13 summarizes some of the muscles in the wrist and hand.

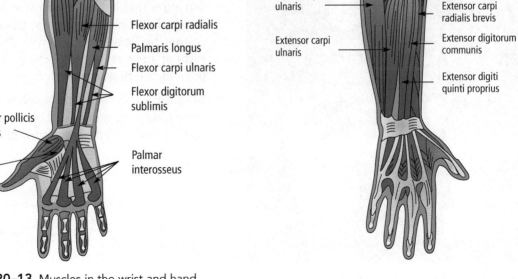
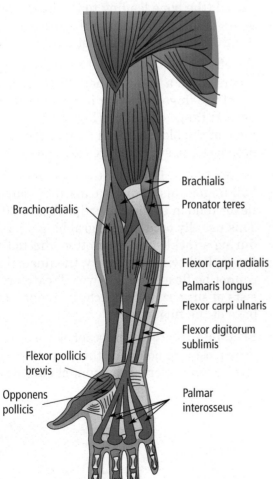

Figure 20–13 Muscles in the wrist and hand.

HAND AND WRIST INJURIES

Along with our highly developed brains, it is our hands that make our species unique. Our hands allow us to grasp and manipulate objects, enabling us to write, play sports, and perform countless other tasks. Our hands are also highly developed sensory organs, containing the many nerve endings that produce our sense of touch.

We use our hands to protect ourselves by deflecting potentially dangerous objects and breaking the force of falls. Because the bones of the hand and wrist are small and delicate, they are easily broken. Minor cuts, abrasions, and burns are common; however, these can result in damaged tendons, nerves, or arteries, or can lead to infection.

Athletes have a greater potential for injuries to the hands and wrist because these structures come into contact with other players, equipment, or the playing surface. The certified athletic trainer must understand the types of hand and wrist injuries and their proper treatment (Figure 20–14). Common injuries to the hand and wrist include fractures, dislocations, contusions, sprains, tendonitis, and nerve impingements.

Fractures of the Wrist and Hand

Many types of fractures to the hand and wrist are possible:

- **Finger fractures.** These can involve any of the three bones (phalanges) in each finger (two in

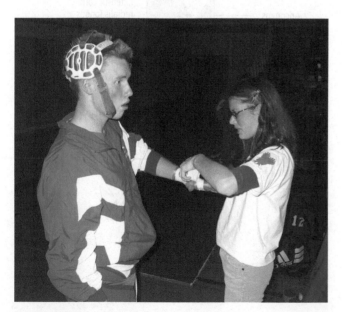

Figure 20–14 Athletic training student aide assisting a wrestler with wrist taping.

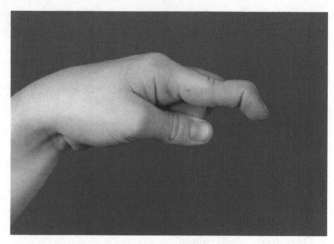

Figure 20–15 Baseball (mallet) finger.

the thumb). Most finger fractures can be treated with a finger splint, but if the fracture is severe it may be necessary to use pins, wires, or screws to repair the finger.

- **Boxer's fracture,** a fracture to the fifth metacarpal (the bone leading to the little finger) is, as its name implies, often the result of slamming a clenched fist against a solid object.

- **Baseball (mallet) finger.** This painful injury occurs when a ball or other object strikes the tip of the finger, bending it down beyond its normal range of motion (Figure 20–15). The force of the blow tears the finger tendon and damages the surrounding cartilage.

- **Jersey finger.** Basically the opposite of baseball finger, this injury is caused by tearing the flexor tendon to the fingertip (Figure 20–16). This usually occurs from grabbing a jersey during a tackle and most often affects the ring finger. Following the injury, the fingertip cannot be flexed (bent down). Treatment consists of surgery to reattach the tendon to the base of the fingertip.

- **Scaphoid fracture.** The scaphoid—perhaps the bone most commonly fractured in athletics—can receive a considerable amount of force when the

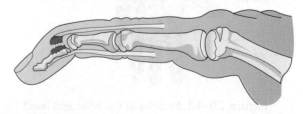

Figure 20–16 Jersey finger.

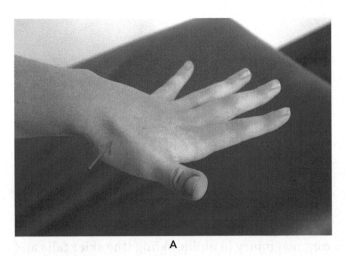

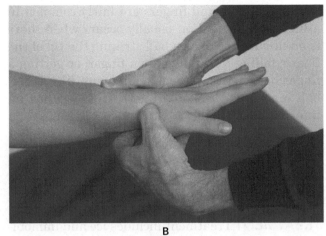

Figure 20–17 (A) Location of the anatomical snuffbox on the hand. (B) Pressure exerted over the scaphoid bone will trigger a pain response if a fracture is present.

wrist is placed into extension. An example is falling on an outstretched hand. Palpation at the **anatomical snuffbox** will cause pain, a positive sign that a fracture may be present (Figure 20–17). Careful evaluation will prevent misdiagnosing this as a wrist sprain.

- **Colles's fracture.** A very common fracture of the lower arm bone (radius), just above the wrist (Figure 20–18). It occurs when a person extends his or her hand in an attempt to break a fall, and the force of the impact is absorbed by the wrist.

TREATMENT As with all fractures, treatment includes rest, ice, compression, elevation, and support. Evaluation by a physician for proper care is advised.

Dislocations and Subluxations of the Hand and Wrist

A **dislocation** is the displacement of any bone from its normal position. A **subluxation** is the abnormal movement of one of the bones that constitute a joint. Dislocations and subluxations of the bones of

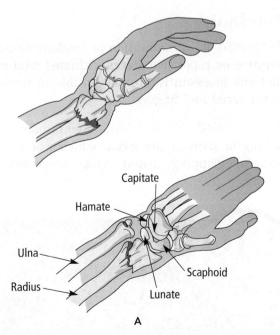

Capitate

Hamate

Ulna

Radius

Scaphoid

Lunate

A

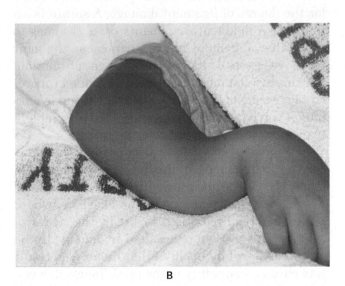

B

Figure 20–18 Colles's fracture. Courtesy of Dr. Deborah Funk, Albany Medical Center, Albany, NY.

the wrist, hand, and fingers are fairly common in athletics. A dislocation usually occurs when there is an accident such as a ball striking the tip of the finger; falling forcefully onto a finger; or getting a finger hooked in a piece of equipment (like a football mask or a basketball net). This is called an interphalangeal dislocation.

SIGNS AND SYMPTOMS A dislocation causes immediate pain and swelling. The finger looks swollen and crooked. The athlete will usually be unable to bend or straighten the dislocated joint.

TREATMENT Treatment includes ice and immobilization, as well as immediate consultation with a physician. Only physicians can reduce a dislocation, thereby making it a priority for immediate treatment.

Contusions

Contusions are caused by direct blows or falling onto a hard surface. Unique to the fingers and toes are contusions of the nails. When a nail becomes contused, blood pools under it. Pressure from this injury is painful and may require a physician to drain the blood from beneath the nail. Athletes should refrain from attempting this themselves, as the risk of infection is high. Chapter 16 describes treatments for soft-tissue injuries, including contusions.

Sprains of the Wrist and Hand

Sprains are discussed in detail in Chapter 16. However, certain tests can be performed to check for the degree of ligament damage. A *sprain* is an injury to a ligament. Ligaments connect bones to each other. Ligament injuries can cause the joint to move beyond its normal range of motion. Sprains are commonly classified as grade I (microscopic tearing of the ligament), grade II (up to one-half of the ligament torn), and grade III (complete tear or rupture of the ligament).

Gamekeeper's thumb is a sprain of the ulnar collateral ligament of the metacarpophalangeal joint (MPJ). The term originated in the 1950s to describe an injury unique to gamekeepers, whose profession required them to break the necks of rabbits. This procedure resulted in damage to the ulnar collateral ligament of the thumb. The result was chronic instability of the MPJ. Today, this is a

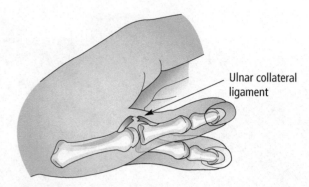

Figure 20–19 Gamekeeper's thumb.

common injury in alpine skiing (the skier falls and sprains the thumb). This type of injury occurs when force is applied to the medial side of the thumb, forcing the MPJ to hyperextend so that it stretches, tears, or even ruptures the ulnar collateral ligament (Figure 20–19). When this occurs, the thumb becomes very unstable.

TESTS Figure 20–20 demonstrates the test used to determine gamekeeper's thumb. Figure 20–21 demonstrates taping that can help stabilize the injury.

Ligament injury to the medial collateral and lateral collateral ligaments of the fingers can result in finger instability. Figures 20–22 and 20–23 show ligament stability testing of the phalanges by applying varus (medial) and valgus (lateral) stresses to the individual ligaments of the fingers.

Tendonitis

Tendonitis is inflammation of tendons caused by overuse or repetitive stress. Athletes who repeat motions incessantly are susceptible to tendonitis of the wrist and fingers.

SIGNS AND SYMPTOMS Symptoms include aching or pain at the wrist, which worsens with forceful gripping, rapid wrist movements, or

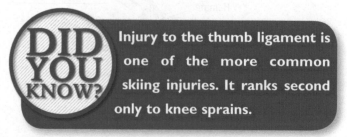

DID YOU KNOW? Injury to the thumb ligament is one of the more common skiing injuries. It ranks second only to knee sprains.

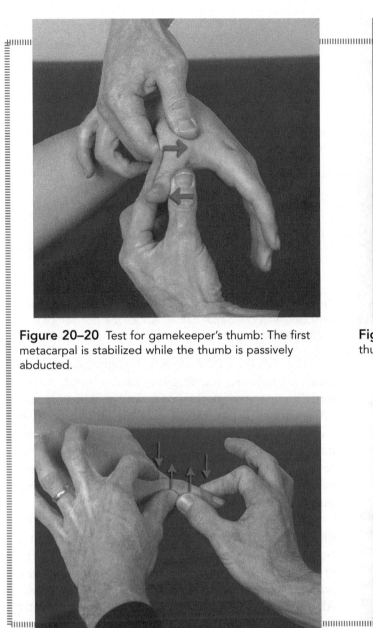

Figure 20–20 Test for gamekeeper's thumb: The first metacarpal is stabilized while the thumb is passively abducted.

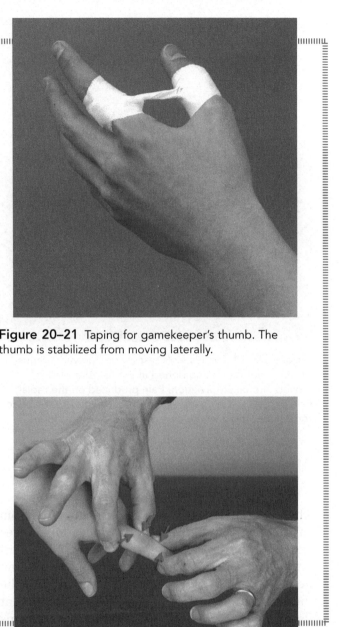

Figure 20–21 Taping for gamekeeper's thumb. The thumb is stabilized from moving laterally.

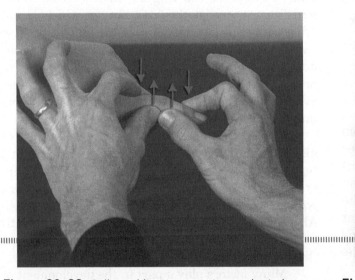

Figure 20–22 Collateral ligament testing to the index finger proximal interphalangeal (PIP) joint. The PIP joint is gently stressed in a varus direction (pressure applied inward). Pain or excessive laxity (movement) indicates injury to the collateral ligament.

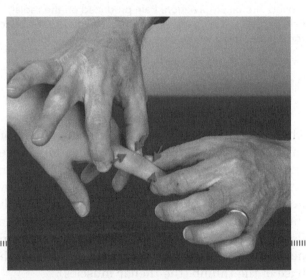

Figure 20–23 Collateral ligament testing to the index finger PIP joint. The PIP joint is gently stressed in a valgus direction (pressure applied outward). Pain or excessive laxity (movement) indicates injury to the collateral ligament.

moving the wrist and fingers to an extreme position. Tendons cross the wrist from the forearm to the hand on all sides of the wrist. The most common sites for tendonitis of the wrist are at the base of the thumb near the anatomical snuffbox (a condition known as **deQuervain's tenosynovitis**), on the back of the wrist, and on the palm side of the wrist.

TREATMENT Tendonitis of the hand and fingers is treated the same as any other tendonitis: with rest, ice, and anti-inflammatory medications.

SPECIAL TESTS Figure 20–24 demonstrates a test used to determine the existence of tendonitis in the wrist.

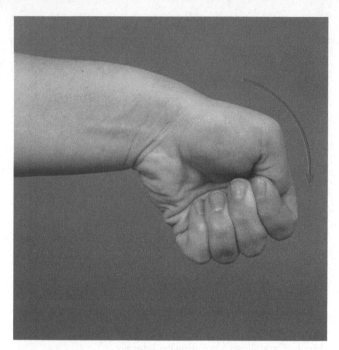

Figure 20–24 Finkelstein's test for deQuervain's tenosynovitis. With the thumb buried in the fist, the wrist is moved into ulnar deviation. Pain produced on the radial side of the wrist is an indication of tendonitis of the abductor pollicis longus and extensor pollicis brevis tendons.

Nerve Impingement and Carpal Tunnel Syndrome

The **carpal tunnel** is a passageway that runs from the forearm through the wrist. Bones form three walls of the tunnel, and a strong, broad ligament bridges over them, forming a tunnel. The median nerve, which supplies feeling to the thumb, the index and ring fingers, and the nine tendons that flex the fingers, pass through this tunnel. This nerve also provides function for the muscles at the base of the thumb (the thenar muscles).

Usually, **carpal tunnel syndrome (CTS)** is considered an inflammatory disorder caused by repetitive stress, physical injury, or other conditions that cause the tissues around the median nerve to become swollen. It occurs when the protective linings of the tendons within the carpal tunnel become inflamed and swell, or when the ligament that forms the roof becomes thicker and broader (Figure 20–25). Just as stepping on a hose slows the flow of water through the hose, so compression on the median nerve fibers by the swollen tendons and thickened ligament slows down the transmission of nerve signals through the carpal tunnel.

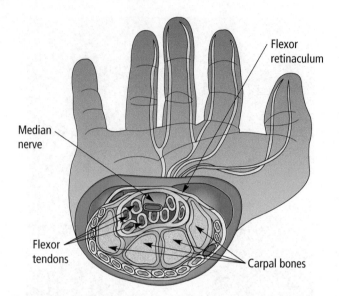

Figure 20–25 Cross-sectional view of the forearm at the wrist, showing the carpal tunnel. Notice the position of the median nerve.

SIGNS AND SYMPTOMS Symptoms include pain, numbness, and tingling in the wrist, hand, and fingers (except the little finger, which is not affected by the median nerve). Patients may also experience a sense of weakness and develop a tendency to drop things. They may lose the sense of heat and cold, or feel that their hands are swollen even though there is no visible swelling. Symptoms may occur when the hand is busy or at rest.

Carpal tunnel syndrome is one of a group of disorders categorized by several different terms: *repetitive stress injuries, cumulative trauma disorder, overuse syndromes, chronic upper limb pain syndrome,* and *repetitive motion disorders.* All these problems are generally associated with repetitive, forceful use of the hands that damages the muscles and bones of the upper extremities.

Many factors play a part in the development of carpal tunnel syndrome: repetition, high force, awkward joint posture, direct pressure, vibration, and prolonged constrained posture. Athletic injuries such as bone dislocations and fractures can narrow the carpal tunnel, thereby exerting pressure on the median nerve. Certain other medical conditions, such as rheumatoid arthritis, diabetes, and hypothyroidism, can also cause inflammation in the carpal tunnel, resulting in median nerve entrapment.

TREATMENT The affected hand and wrist should be rested for at least two weeks; this allows the swollen, inflamed tissues to shrink, and relieves pressure on the median nerve. Ice may provide relief.

Some people wear a wrist splint or brace at night or during the sports season to help keep the wrist from bending. The splint is used for several weeks or months, depending on the severity of the problem. Except for anecdotal reports, no evidence exists that such supports help over the long term. Some experts believe that wrist supports may exacerbate the problem by reducing circulation and restricting movement so that the shoulder muscles tense up. In severe cases, surgical decompression of the median nerve may be required.

SPECIAL TESTS Figures 20–26 through 20–28 demonstrate tests that can be used to investigate the possibility of carpal tunnel syndrome.

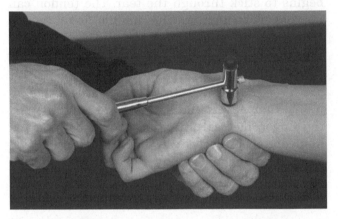

Figure 20–26 Tinel's sign at the carpal tunnel. A reflex hammer or fingertip is tapped on the carpal tunnel. Tingling or shooting pain into the palm, thumb, index finger, and frequently into the long finger indicates carpal tunnel syndrome.

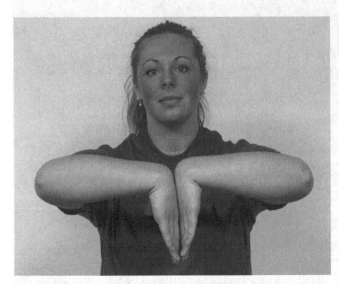

Figure 20–27 Phalan's test. If holding this position for 60 seconds or less produces tingling or shooting pain in the palm, thumb, index, and long finger, carpal tunnel syndrome is indicated.

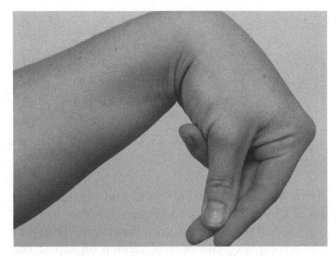

Figure 20–28 Modified Phalan's test. If holding the thumb, index, and long fingers in this position for 60 seconds or less produces tingling or shooting pain in the median-nerve distribution of the hand, carpal tunnel syndrome is suspected.

Ganglion Cyst of the Wrist

A **ganglion** is a small, usually hard lump above a tendon or in the capsule that encloses a joint (Figure 20–29). A ganglion is also called a *synovial hernia* or *synovial cyst.*

This condition is common in people who bowl or who play handball, racquetball, squash, or tennis. Runners and athletes who jump, ski, or play contact sports often develop foot ganglia. A ganglion usually appears on the back of the wrist, but can also occur on the palm side or at the base of the fingers. These fluid-filled cysts arise from the tissue that lines the joints or tendons. The size of ganglion cysts can increase during periods of irritation, but they often resolve spontaneously. Ganglion cysts are benign and noncancerous.

TREATMENT A small, painless cyst need not be treated. If the cyst enlarges rapidly, becomes painful, or interferes with use of the hand, the athlete should seek treatment.

Boutonnière Deformity

Boutonnière deformity is an extensor tendon injury affecting two joints of the finger, the proximal interphalangeal (PIP) joint at the middle of the finger and the distal interphalangeal (DIP) joint that controls the fingertip. These joints allow the finger to bend and flex. In boutonnière deformity, there is a tear in the central part of the tendon that extends the finger. The finger bends

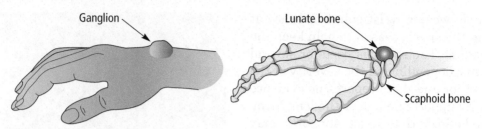

Figure 20–29 Ganglion cyst of the hand.

down at the middle (PIP) joint and is pulled back up at the end (DIP) joint (Figure 20–30).

When the finger is hit or bent forcibly in just the wrong way, the central tendon on top of the

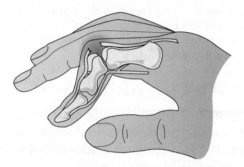

Figure 20–30 Boutonnière deformity is a tear of the extensor tendon of the PIP joint, at the middle of the finger, and the DIP joint that controls the fingertip.

finger tears away from its attachment to the top of the bone in the middle of the finger. A jammed finger can cause this injury. The tear in the tendon looks like a buttonhole (hence the French name *boutonnière*), and the end of the finger bone begins to stick through the tear. The tendon can no longer straighten the middle joint, which remains bent. The joint at the end of the finger flips upward.

SIGNS AND SYMPTOMS If the athlete has an injury that affects the ability to flex and extend the finger, medical attention should be obtained immediately. A doctor can diagnose the condition and limit damage. The finger joints will be painful and tender. The finger will appear misshapen, and the athlete will not be able to straighten it.

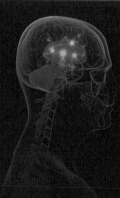

KEY CONCEPT

Common elbow injuries include:

- Contusions, the result of force applied to the bony prominences of the elbow. Treatment consists of RICE.
- Olecranon bursitis, which is inflammation of the bursa. Treatment depends on the presence of infection. If the bursa is not infected, bursitis can be treated with ice, rest, and anti-inflammatory pain medications.
- Ulnar nerve contusion, or "hitting the funny bone," results from a direct blow to the ulnar nerve. Treatment is usually unnecessary, as this condition generally subsides on its own.
- Elbow strains, which result from stress being placed on the elbow. Treatment is aimed at prevention through proper technique, use of appropriate equipment, and limitation of the stress on the joint.

- Elbow sprains, resulting from forced hyperextension by side-to-side forces on the joint. Treatment is similar to that for strains; commercial braces may help.
- Elbow dislocations, which result from the bones in the joint being displaced. The athlete must be transported to the nearest medical facility.
- Fractures of the elbow and forearm, resulting from forces that crack and break the bony structures. Treatment involves immobilization, ice, elevation, and prompt referral to a physician.
- Volkmann's contracture, a serious condition that results from a lack of blood flow to the forearm.
- Nerve injuries, which can occur to the ulnar, radial, or median nerve.

Common injuries to the wrist and hand include:

- Fractures resulting from excessive force on the bony structure of the hand and wrist. Treatment includes ice, immobilization, and immediate treatment by a physician.
- Contusions, which result from force or a fall onto a hard surface.
- Sprains, resulting from forces that place stress on the joints and cause ligament damage.
- Tendonitis, an inflammation of the tendons in the wrist and fingers.
- Nerve damage, which can occur to the nerves in the hand and fingers as a result of repetitive stresses on the hand and wrist. Treatment should include rest , and icing may provide some relief.
- Ganglion cysts, small, hard lumps above a tendon that encloses a joint.
- If the cyst is painless, treatment is not necessary.
- Boutonnière deformity, an injury to the extensor tendon that affects two joints of the finger. After this injury, there is a limited period of time only during which treatment can be effective.

TREATMENT There is a limited period during which treatment of any kind can be effective. Over time, the sensitive tissues of the hand and fingers lose their elasticity, increasing the difficulty of returning them to normal. Many people fail to seek early treatment for this condition, thinking they have only a "jammed finger." With prompt treatment, the probability of returning the finger to normal is much improved.

STRENGTHENING EXERCISES FOR THE WRIST

After an injured wrist or hand has healed, it will be necessary to strengthen this area before resuming athletic participation. Figures 20–31 and 20–32 illustrate simple exercises for the wrist.

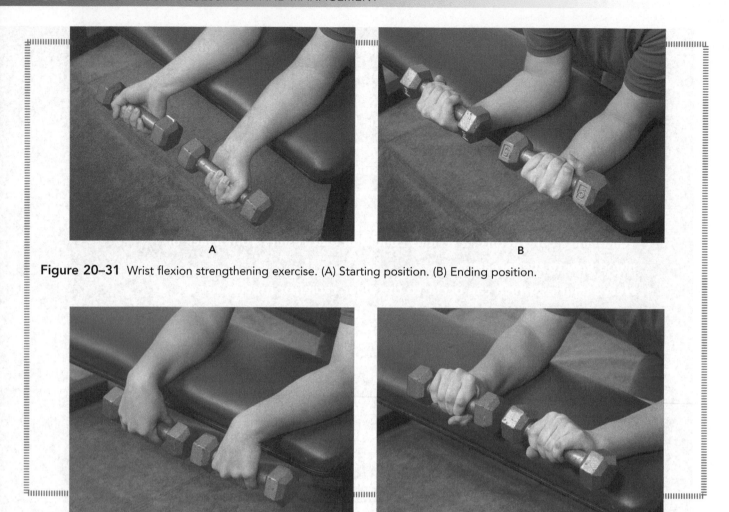

Figure 20–31 Wrist flexion strengthening exercise. (A) Starting position. (B) Ending position.

Figure 20–32 Wrist extension strengthening exercise. (A) Starting position. (B) Ending position.

CONCLUSION

The elbow, wrist, and hand contain some of the most intricate and complex joints in the body. Understanding the anatomy, biomechanics, and mechanisms of injury associated with this area of the body will enable the certified athletic trainer to assess and plan appropriate treatment for the athlete.

Injuries involving the elbow and forearm are common in almost any athletic activity. Many different types of forces and stress are applied in the elbow area during the various motions involved in different sports. The elbow is prone to overuse injuries, especially from sports or activities that require repetitive activity.

REVIEW QUESTIONS

1. Define the major components of the elbow, wrist, and hand.
2. Why is transitory paresthesia of the elbow called "hitting the funny bone"?
3. Describe the signs and symptoms for, tennis elbow.
4. Why is an elbow dislocation a medical emergency?

5. Describe the location of the radial, median, and ulnar nerves.
6. List all the bones in the hand.
7. List and describe the different types of fractures of the wrist and hand.
8. What is the treatment for tendonitis of the elbow, wrist, or hand?
9. What is the difference between a dislocation and a subluxation?
10. What is a ganglion cyst?

PROJECTS AND ACTIVITIES

1. Using the Internet, research carpal tunnel syndrome. What did you find?
2. Create an outline drawing of the elbow, wrist, and hand. Use these outline drawings to assemble a coloring book.
3. Research three current news articles on the elbow, wrist, and hand. These articles should be recent (within one month). Write a review of each article.
4. Create a mnemonic to help remember the bones of the hand.
5. Using several Key Terms in this chapter, create a crossword puzzle.

LEARNING LINKS

• Look for companies that sell support products for the wrist and hand. Compare and contrast the different products you find. Does the research exist supporting the use of these products?

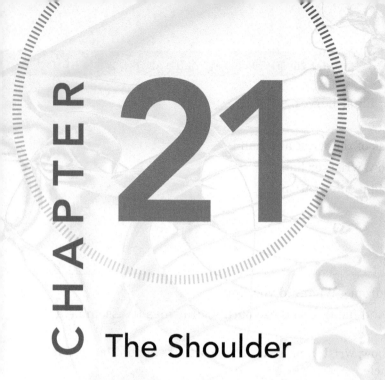

CHAPTER 21

The Shoulder

OBJECTIVES

Upon completion of this chapter, the reader should be able to:

- Name the three articulations that constitute the shoulder girdle complex
- Describe how stability of the shoulder is maintained
- Recite the names of the four muscles that come together to form the rotator cuff
- Explain the anatomy of the shoulder girdle complex
- Identify major injuries and conditions of the shoulder
- Describe special tests used in evaluating shoulder injuries

KEY TERMS

acromioclavicular joint *The joint formed by the acromion of the scapula and the clavicle.*

acromioclavicular separation *A traumatic sprain to the AC joint, usually caused by a direct blow to the shoulder.*

acromion process *The lateral triangular projection of the spine of the scapula that forms the point of the shoulder and articulates with the clavicle.*

anterior shoulder dislocation *of the humerus that occurs in the anterior inferior direction.*

biceps tendon *The tissue that connects the biceps muscle to the shoulder girdle.*

biceps tendonitis *Inflammation of the tendon that connects the biceps to the shoulder girdle.*

brachial plexus *A group of peripheral nerves that exit the spinal cord and extend from the vertebrae into the shoulder.*

dynamic stability *Mobility with steadiness of a joint.*

force couple *Two forces acting in opposite directions to rotate a part around an axis.*

glenohumeral joint *The synovial ball-and-socket joint of the shoulder.*

glenoid fossa *A slightly concave projection of the scapula.*

KEY TERMS CONTINUED

glenoid labrum *A ring of cartilage attached to the margin of the glenoid cavity of the scapula.*

head of the humerus *The upper portion of the humerus bone, where the bone attaches to the scapula.*

Hill-Sachs lesion *Indentation of the posterior humeral head (visible on X-ray), resulting from the humerus hitting the glenoid during dislocation.*

impingement syndrome *A condition that occurs when the space between the humeral head below and the acromion above becomes narrowed.*

referred pain *Pain that is felt in one body area (such as the shoulder), but that originates elsewhere in the body.*

rotator cuff *A collective set of four deep muscles of the glenohumeral joint.*

scapulothoracic joint *The area that provides movement of the scapula over the back side of the ribcage.*

sternoclavicular joint *The area where the clavicle and the sternum connect.*

stinger (burner) *An injury caused by stretching or compressing the brachial plexus.*

synergistically *Acting together; a group of muscles act together to enhance the movement of a joint or limb.*

THE SHOULDER GIRDLE COMPLEX

The shoulder joint, a complex and fascinating area of the human body, includes three primary articulations: the glenohumeral joint, the acromioclavicular joint, and the sternoclavicular joint. Movements are performed and guided with the aid of ligaments, cartilage, and layers of muscles. Together these structures make up the *shoulder girdle complex*.

The structure of this joint allows a wide degree of mobility—at the expense of stability. Any of the muscles and tendons that contribute to the movement and coordinated stability of these joints can become strained in a shoulder injury.

Structure and Function

Mobility with stability of a joint is termed **dynamic stability**. The shoulder joint is able to accomplish dynamic stability through the coordinated movements of the scapula, or shoulder blade, working in concert with the humerus, or upper arm bone. The upper end of the humerus has a hemisphere-formed portion called the **head of the humerus**. It attaches to a slightly concave projection of the scapula called the **glenoid fossa**. The anatomical name of this synovial ball-and-socket joint is the **glenohumeral joint** (Figure 21–1). The glenohumeral joint is like a golf ball on a tee: The golf ball is the head of the humerus, and the tee is the glenoid fossa. Without its numerous muscles, ligaments, and soft tissue, the arm would simply fall off. Ball-and-socket joints permit multiple directions of movement.

The hip is also a ball-and socket joint, but it differs from the shoulder. The hip, as compared to the glenohumeral joint, has a relatively deep socket and small head. The hip is inherently stable because of this joint geometry. The tradeoff for this stability is limited mobility. Contrast this with the glenohumeral joint: The glenoid fossa is shallow and small in surface area compared to the humeral head.

Superior to the glenohumeral joint is the upper lateral aspect of the scapula, or shoulder blade, called the **acromion process** (Figure 21–1). It is easily palpated as the hard spot on top of the shoulder. It is here that the clavicle, or collar bone, connects to form the **acromioclavicular joint**

FUN FACTS

The shoulder is the only joint of the body with 360 degrees of rotation.

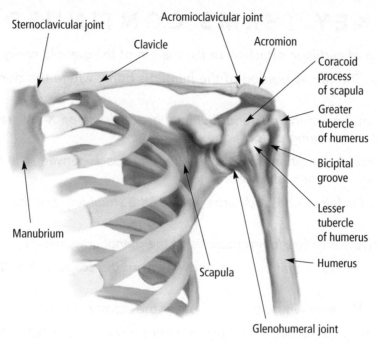

Figure 21–1 The shoulder girdle.

(or AC joint). This joint is especially exposed to injury in contact sports. The other end of the clavicle is attached to the sternum, or breastbone, named the **sternoclavicular joint**, or SC joint. Although injuries to the SC joint can be debilitating, they are rarely seen in sports and so are not addressed in this chapter. The clavicle and its movements via the joints at both ends allow the scapula to move up and down, protract, retract, and rotate.

The scapula is highly mobile, sliding over the back side of the thorax (ribcage) area (Figure 21–2). Even though it is not a true joint, it is referred to as the **scapulothoracic joint**. Stability of this joint is derived entirely from muscle action.

The shoulder complex is the most mobile of the upper extremity joints. Being able to position your hand into the proper location is one thing, but having it both strong and stable at the same time is an even more amazing feat. It is this ability that allows athletes to perform a wide array of activities like

throwing, swimming, or swinging on gymnastic uneven bars. Dynamic stability is essential for both normal and athletic function. Several muscle groups working together **synergistically** are responsible for dynamic stability of the shoulder. Both controlled and coordinated muscle action are the primary source of glenohumeral joint stability.

The Rotator Cuff

The **rotator cuff** is a collective set of four deep muscles of the glenohumeral joint. These muscles are critical for normal function and often are implicated in shoulder problems.

The four rotator-cuff muscles arise from the scapula and insert onto the superior aspect of the humerus, surrounding the head of the humerus (Figure 21–3). As the muscles merge near their insertion onto the humerus, the tendons fuse to form one continuous, broad structure.

The four muscles of the rotator cuff are:

- Subscapularis—inserts onto the humerus anteriorly
- Supraspinatus—inserts onto the humerus anteriosuperiorly
- Infraspinatus—inserts onto the humerus posterosuperiorly
- Teres minor—inserts onto the humerus posteriorly

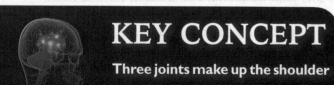

KEY CONCEPT

Three joints make up the shoulder girdle: the sternoclavicular joint, the acromioclavicular joint, and the glenohumeral joint.

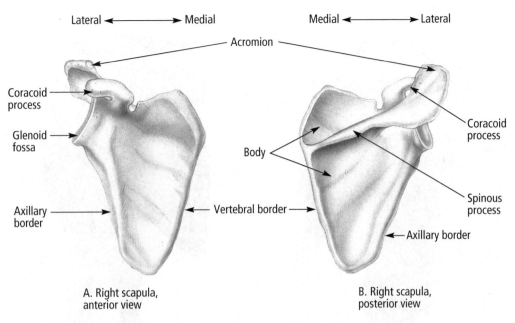

Figure 21–2 The scapula: (A) Anterior view (B) Posterior view.

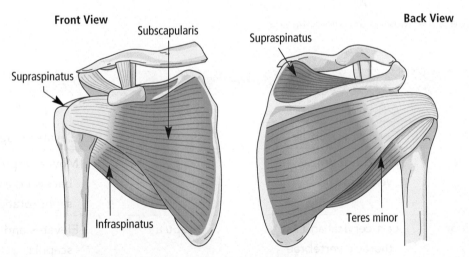

Figure 21–3 Muscles of the rotator cuff of the shoulder.

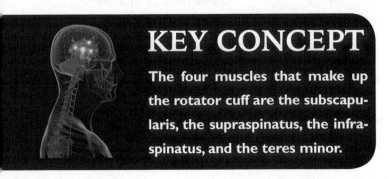

KEY CONCEPT

The four muscles that make up the rotator cuff are the subscapularis, the supraspinatus, the infraspinatus, and the teres minor.

The deep rotator-cuff muscles work in conjunction with the large, powerful, superficial muscles of the glenohumeral joint to move the arm (Figure 21–4). The most important superficial muscle used in abduction of the arm is the *deltoid*. Adequate strength and endurance of all shoulder muscles are equally essential. In fact, without adequate rotator-cuff function, many overhead activities are difficult or impossible. Table 21–1 summarizes the muscles of the shoulder girdle and their functions.

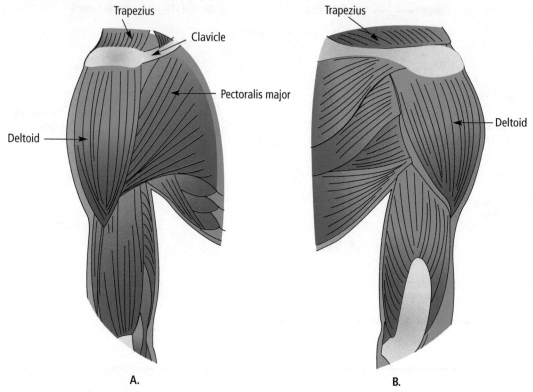

Trapezius
Clavicle
Pectoralis major
Deltoid

Trapezius
Deltoid

A.

B.

Figure 21–4 Muscles that move the arm.

Table 21–1	Muscles of the Shoulder Girdle		
MUSCLE	ORIGIN	INSERTION	FUNCTION
Levator scapulae	Cervical vertebrae	Scapula	Elevates scapula
Rhomboid major	2nd–5th thoracic vertebrae	Scapula	Moves scapula backward and upward; slight rotation
Rhomboid minor	Last cervical and 1st thoracic vertebrae	Scapula	Elevates and retracts scapula
Pectoralis minor	Ribs	Scapula	Depresses shoulder and rotates scapula downward
Trapezius	Occipital bone 7th cervical 12th thoracic	Clavicle	Draws head to one side; rotates scapula
Serratus anterior	8th, 9th rib	Scapula	Moves scapula forward away from spine and downward and inward toward chest wall
Coracobrachialis	Scapula	Humerus	Flexes, adducts arm

(*continues*)

Table 21–1 Muscles of the Shoulder Girdle (*continued*)

MUSCLE	ORIGIN	INSERTION	FUNCTION
Pectoralis major	Clavicle; sternum 6 upper ribs	Humerus	Flexes, adducts, rotates arm medially
Teres major	Scapula	Humerus	Adducts, extends, rotates arm medially
Teres minor	Scapula	Humerus	Rotates arm laterally and adducts
Deltoid	Clavicle, scapula	Humerus	Abducts arm
Supraspinatus	Scapula	Humerus	Abducts arm
Infraspinatus	Scapula	Humerus	Rotates humerus outward
Latissimus dorsi	Lower 6 thoracic; lumbar vertebrae; sacrum; ilium lower 4 ribs	Humerus	Extends, adducts, rotates arm medially, draws shoulder downward and backward

Muscle Force Couple

The actions of the deltoid and rotator-cuff muscles combine to produce what is called a **force couple**: two equal forces acting in opposite directions to rotate a part around its axis. With active arm movement, the rotator-cuff muscles compress and depress the humeral head and prevent it from sliding off the glenoid. While the deltoid is lifting the arm, it also produces an upward-directed force on the humerus. The action of the rotator cuff's pulling down and the deltoid's lifting up balance one another, allowing the humeral head to spin while remaining in place on the glenoid.

Rotator-cuff problems may throw off this coordinated interplay. The dynamic stability of the rotator cuff can be compared to a large man and a little boy teaming up to raise a very long, heavy ladder. The large man possesses most of the force to raise the ladder upward (create the primary motion), while the little boy holds (stabilizes) the bottom of the ladder to prevent it from sliding or lifting off the ground (Figure 21–5). The deltoid raises the arm, while the rotator cuff stabilizes the humeral head on the glenoid fossa.

KEY CONCEPT

The stability of the shoulder is maintained by the combined effort of the deltoid muscle and the rotator-cuff muscles. This is called a force couple: two equal forces acting in opposite directions to rotate the bones of the shoulder girdle around an axis.

Scapulothoracic Mechanics

The base of support of the shoulder complex comes from the scapula. This flat bone glides over the posterior thoracic wall, keeping this base of support in functional alignment with the upper extremity. Continual repositioning of the scapula beneath a moving humeral head ensures optimal muscle length and joint approximation (Figure 21–6).

Several muscles of the upper back work together to create movement of the scapula, which takes place in several different planes

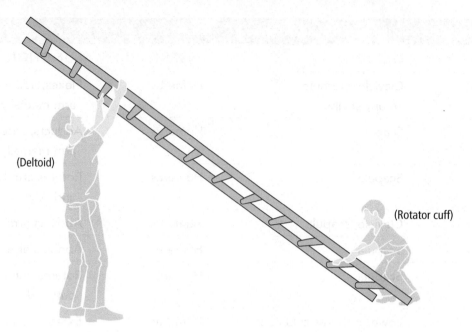

Figure 21–5 Illustration of dynamic stability of the rotator cuff. The large man possesses most of the force to raise the ladder upward (create the primary motion), while the little boy holds (stabilizes) the bottom of the ladder to prevent it from sliding or lifting off the ground. The deltoid raises the arm, while the rotator cuff stabilizes the humeral head on the glenoid fossa.

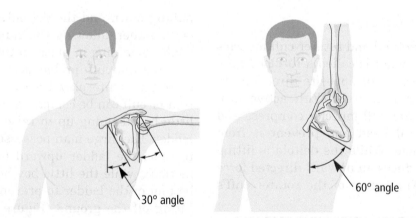

Figure 21–6 The scapula rotates as the arm is elevated.

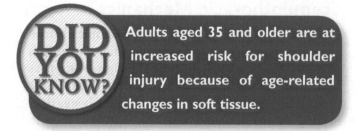

(Figures 21–7A–D). The scapular muscles are the upper, middle, and lower trapezius; the rhomboids; the serratus anterior; and the pectoralis minor. Disrupted function of any scapular muscle, from any cause, can result in limited or abnormal mobility of the entire upper extremity (Figure 21–8).

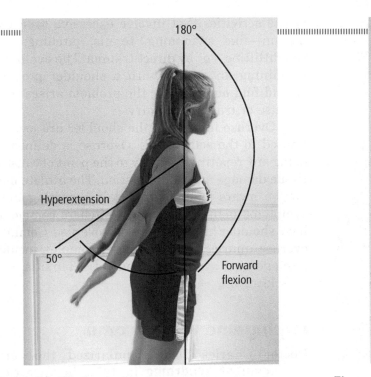

Figure 21–7A Forward flexion, hyperextension.

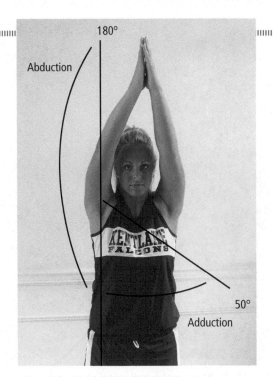

Figure 21–7B Abduction, adduction.

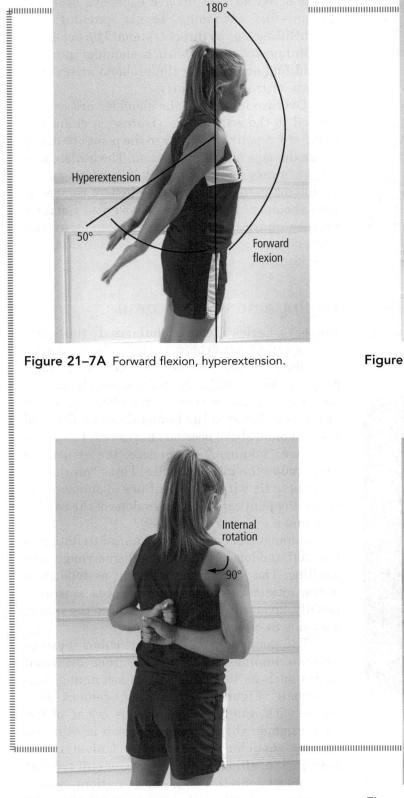

Figure 21–7C Internal rotation.

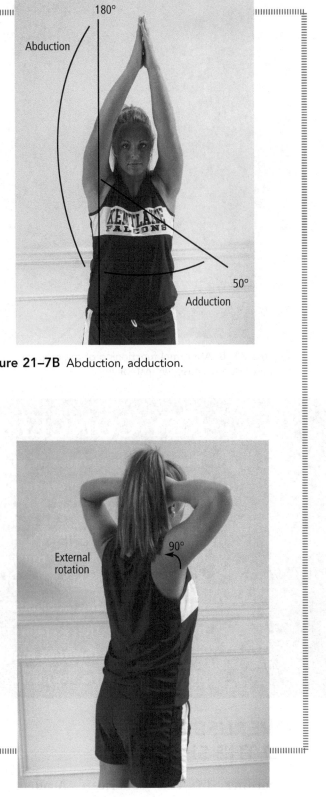

Figure 21–7D External rotation.

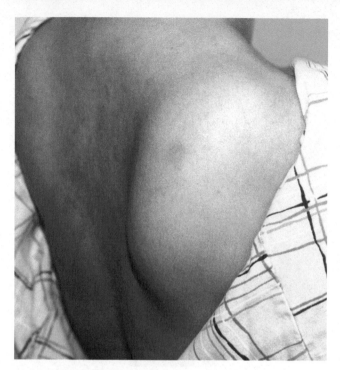

Figure 21–8 Abnormal functioning of the scapula (winged) due to muscular instability.

KEY CONCEPT

The shoulder complex is made up of three joints. Movement of the shoulder complex occurs with the aid of ligaments, cartilage, and layers of muscles. Stability of the shoulder complex results from the coordinated movements of the scapula and humerus. This is the most mobile of the upper extremity joints.

OVERUSE INJURIES TO THE SHOULDER

According to the American Academy of Orthopaedic Surgeons (2006), approximately 7.5 million people annually see a doctor about a sprain, strain, dislocation, or other shoulder problem. Shoulder injuries can be caused by sports activities that involve excessive overhead motion—like swimming, tennis, pitching, and weightlifting—or by direct trauma. The evaluator examining an athlete with a shoulder problem should find out whether the problem arises from overuse or traumatic injury.

Overuse injuries of the shoulder are usually limited to the soft tissues. Overuse is defined as doing any repetitive activity to the point of causing tissue damage and inflammation. The athlete may not be aware that an injury is occurring until symptoms manifest. Baseball pitchers commonly have shoulder injuries related to overuse. Common overuse injuries of the shoulder complex include impingement syndrome, tendonitis, bursitis, and muscle strain.

Impingement Syndrome

Doctor Charles Neer popularized the term **impingement syndrome** in 1972, in an article published in the *Journal of Bone and Joint Surgery* (Neer, 1972). The term is widely used to describe a situation that occurs when the space, or interval, between the humeral head below and the acromion above becomes narrowed. The bones can then "impinge," or squeeze, the structures that occupy the interval space. Three "pinchable" structures lie within the confines of subacromial space: the joint capsule, the tendons of the rotator cuff, and a bursa (Figure 21–9).

Impingement causes mechanical irritation of the cuff tendons, resulting in hemorrhage and swelling. This is commonly known as tendonitis of the rotator cuff. The supraspinatus muscle is usually involved. This can also affect the bursa, resulting in bursitis.

The shoulder complex is particularly susceptible to impingement injuries from overhead sports such as baseball, tennis, swimming, and volleyball (Figure 21–10). Impingement syndrome with rotator-cuff tendonitis is one of the most common shoulder injuries seen in athletes. At the shoulder clinic at the University of Washington, afflictions of the rotator cuff account for almost one-third of new patient visits. According to Marty Louzon, a physical therapist and certified athletic trainer, 95% of overuse injuries seen in swimmers are related to the shoulder (Louzon, 1998).

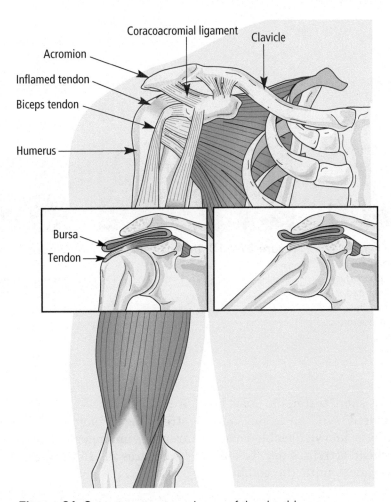

Figure 21–9 Impingement syndrome of the shoulder.

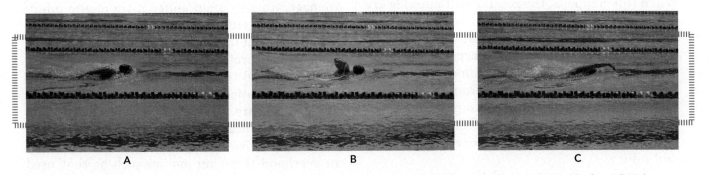

A   B   C

Figure 21–10A-B-C The shoulder is susceptible to overuse injuries in sports that make demanding use of overhead movements.

SIGNS AND SYMPTOMS The signs and symptoms of impingement syndrome include:

- Pain and tenderness in the glenohumeral area
- Pain or weakness with active abduction in midrange

- Limited internal rotation compared to noninvolved side
- Confirmation with special tests (Hawkins impingement test)
- Tenderness to palpation in the subacromial area

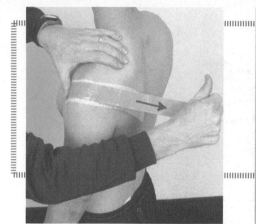

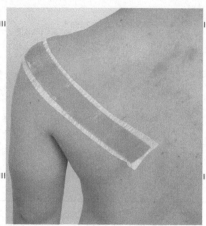

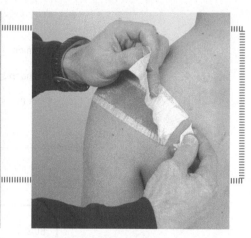

Figure 21–11A Humeral head relocation taping was developed by Jenny McConnell, PT. This procedure is used to help with humeral head stability of the shoulder. The clinician's left thumb provides a posterior glide to the humeral head as the short-stretch tape is applied.

Figure 21–11B The finished taping.

Figure 21–11C Carefully work tape off using adhesive remover. This tape adheres to the skin, so remove it carefully to prevent removing skin with it.

TREATMENT Improper sport technique may be the cause of impingement syndrome and may have to be addressed by a knowledgeable coach. Cross-training for overhead activities may be substituted for regular workouts until the condition resolves.

Muscle fatigue of the rotator cuff will disrupt the force couple of the glenohumeral joint. When this happens, the rotator-cuff muscles are no longer able to keep the head of the humerus positioned on the glenoid fossa. Because the deltoid is so strong, it may overpower fatigued cuff muscles and pull the humeral head up against the overhanging acromion process. Prevention includes attention to preseason conditioning. In baseball, counting and limiting the number of pitches can prevent excessive fatigue and injury.

Excessive movement of the humeral head results in narrowing of the subacromial space. Treatment includes preseason conditioning, cross-training, and exercise. Specialized taping techniques may aid in keeping the humeral head stable. One such technique is shown in Figures 21–11A–C.

SPECIAL TESTS Figures 21–12 through 21–14 demonstrate tests for the presence of impingement syndrome.

REHABILITATION AND PREVENTION Many stretching techniques and exercises are suitable for treating impingement syndrome as demonstrated by Figures 21–15 through 21–21.

Rotator-Cuff Tears

Rotator-cuff injuries occur in both young and old. Younger athletes often suffer a traumatic injury such as falling onto an outstretched hand. A young athlete may put unusual demands on the shoulder, as may older professional athletes. As people age, the muscle and tendon tissues of the rotator cuff lose some elasticity, become more susceptible to tearing, and are often injured while performing everyday activities.

In repetitive-use injury, an action (commonly an overhand throwing motion such as that used by baseball pitchers) leads to a chronic condition, and ultimately to a tear in the tendons that form the attachment of the rotator cuff. Rotator-cuff tears may be of partial or full thickness. Partial-thickness tears do not completely sever the tendon and may respond well to nonoperative treatments. Full-thickness tears require surgery for correction. Surgery may also be used to treat partial-thickness tears that do not respond to nonoperative treatment.

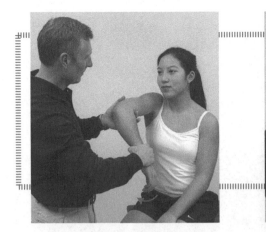

Figure 21–12 Hawkin's impingement test for rotator-cuff tendonitis. The athlete stands or sits with the arm and elbow each flexed to 90 degrees, and the arm internally rotated. The clinician applies overpressure to internal rotation. Produces symptoms of anterior shoulder pain.

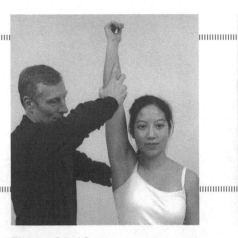

Figure 21–13 Neer's impingement test for rotator-cuff tendonitis. The athlete stands or sits. The clinician passively flexes the arm to end range and applies gentle overpressure. Produces symptoms of anterior shoulder pain.

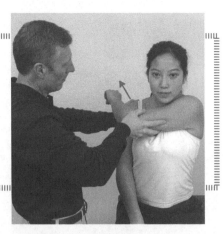

Figure 21–14 Crossover impingement test for rotator-cuff tendonitis. The athlete stands or sits. The clinician passively horizontally adducts the arm to end range (as far as possible). Pain produced in the AC joint is a positive sign for rotator-cuff tendonitis.

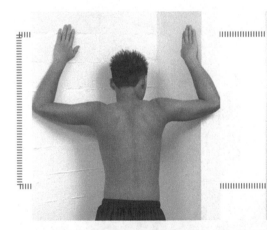

Figure 21–15 Corner stretching exercise for the pectoral muscles. The athlete stands in a corner with hands supporting against both wall surfaces. Leaning forward stretches the pectoral muscles.

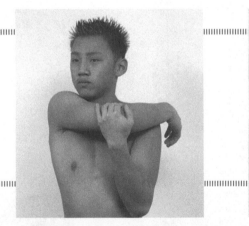

Figure 21–16 Horizontal stretching exercise for the posterior shoulder complex. This exercise will help to stretch the muscles on the back side of the shoulder.

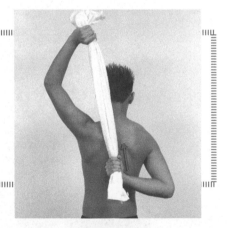

Figure 21–17 Using a towel, the athlete stretches the right shoulder into an internally rotated position.

SIGNS AND SYMPTOMS If the rotator cuff is partially torn, the athlete will feel pain but will still be able to move the arm in a normal range of motion. With a complete rupture of the tendon, the athlete will be unable to move the arm in a normal range of motion. Individuals with rotator-cuff tears are usually unable to actively lift the arm overhead; when they attempt it, the shoulder can be observed to shrug or hike.

Most rotator-cuff tears cause a vague pain in the shoulder area and may result in a "catching" sensation when the arm is moved. The larger the tear in the tendon, the more weakness the individual senses when trying to move the arm. Most

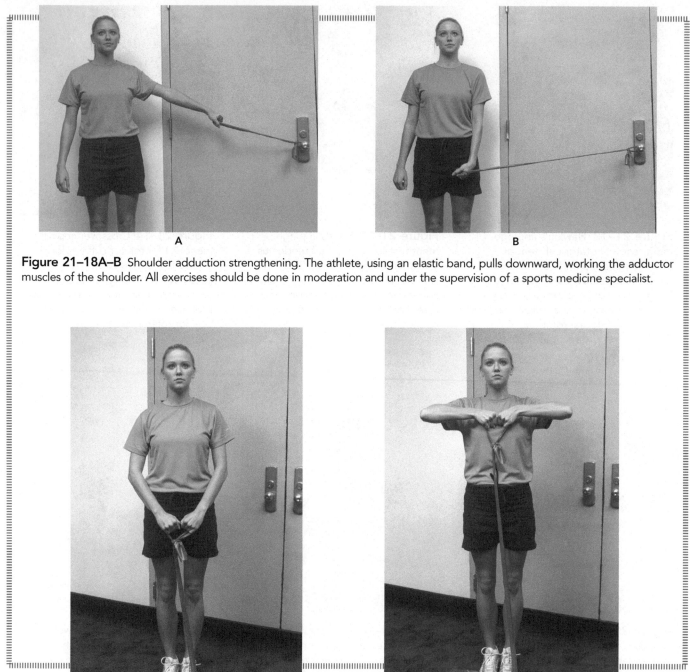

Figure 21–18A–B Shoulder adduction strengthening. The athlete, using an elastic band, pulls downward, working the adductor muscles of the shoulder. All exercises should be done in moderation and under the supervision of a sports medicine specialist.

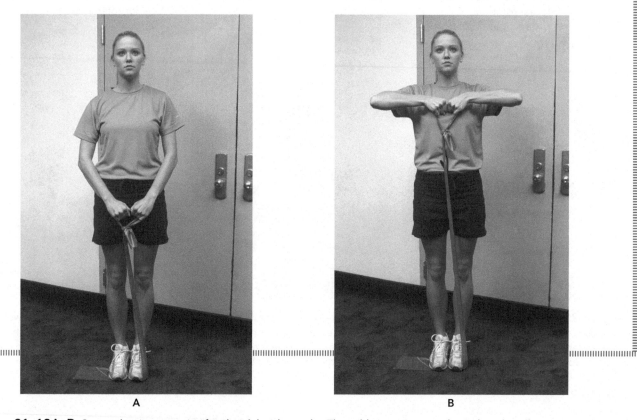

Figure 21–19A–B Strengthening exercise for the deltoid muscle. The athlete, using an elastic band, pulls upward, close to the body. This stretch should be held for 5 to 10 seconds.

people report an inability to sleep on the affected side, because of pain.

Varying degrees of disability accompany this injury. The tear can be small or large. In some cases, rotator-cuff tears are initially diagnosed as impingements until the actual tear is found. Because the rotator-cuff muscles are no longer able to depress the humeral head, X-rays may reveal that the humeral head is riding up and reducing the acromiohumeral

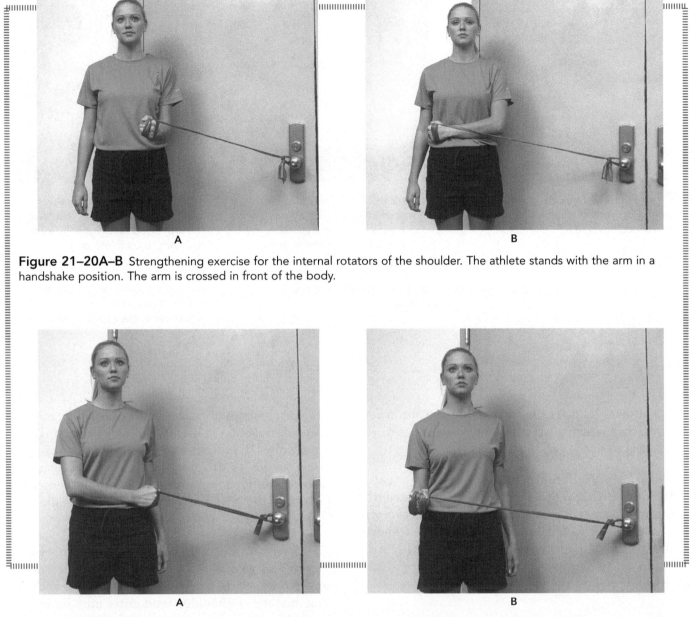

Figure 21–20A–B Strengthening exercise for the internal rotators of the shoulder. The athlete stands with the arm in a handshake position. The arm is crossed in front of the body.

Figure 21–21A–B Strengthening exercise for the external rotators of the shoulder. This exercise is the opposite of the exercise in Figure 21–20. Here the athlete stands with the arm across the body and pulls outward into a handshake position.

interval space. An MRI can detect tears in the rotator cuff.

Small and partial-thickness tears may respond to a shoulder rehabilitation program. Surgery, followed by a rehabilitation program, may be required for small and most moderate to large tears.

SPECIAL TESTS Figures 21–22 through 21–24 show tests that can determine the existence and extent of a rotator-cuff injury.

Muscle Strains

Strains can be caused by overuse or traumatic injuries. Overuse strains often occur at the start of a sports season or with an increase in activity level during the season.

SIGNS AND SYMPTOMS Muscle strains are characterized by pain and tenderness in the area of the muscle belly. Symptoms can be provoked by direct palpation, stretch, and contraction against

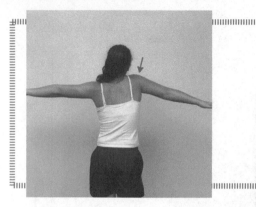

Figure 21–22 Shoulder hiking during active abduction indicates a rotator-cuff problem.

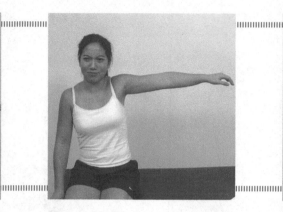

Figure 21–23 Drop-arm sign for rotator-cuff integrity. The athlete sits or stands with arm overhead, the slowly lowers the arm to the side. The clinician observes for pain and loss of control occurring in midrange when the arm is being lowered.

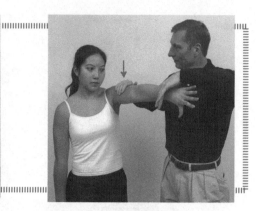

Figure 21–24 Supraspinatus manual muscle strength test. With the arm lifted up diagonally from the body, the athlete points the thumb toward the floor and resists a downward force to the arm. This test, as compared to the other side, will determine if there is a weakness in the supraspinatus muscle.

resistance. Mild strains can resolve within a few days, but severe strains may require several months to heal.

TREATMENT Treatment of muscle strains includes PRICE, gentle stretching, and a strengthening program. Cross-training during recovery is also helpful. A functional progression of sports drills prior to return will allow the athlete to ramp up to the level of intensity she or he had attained before the injury.

Biceps (Long-Head) Tendonitis

Discomfort in the front of the shoulder may be **biceps tendonitis**. Because the **biceps** (long head) **tendon** lies adjacent to the rotator cuff, the condition could be confused with rotator-cuff tendonitis. Both can be caused by impingement and are treated similarly.

Biceps Tendon Rupture

Biceps tendon ruptures are not common in athletics, but are dramatic when they do occur. Sudden onset of pain in the front of the shoulder, associated with a "pop" during vigorous activity, is

the typical symptom of this injury. Drooping of the biceps muscle at the distal arm will be seen. This is a grade III injury; a complete rupture of the biceps tendon to the long head. The short head of the biceps tendon remains attached to the corocoid process of the scapula. This deformity is called a "Popeye" muscle.

SIGNS AND SYMPTOMS The athlete may see an area of ecchymosis (bruising) in the upper anterior arm following the rupture. An athlete with a prior history of shoulder tendonitis may be more prone to this injury because of the weakened tendon. Even though the damage is usually restricted to the tendon, a visit to a doctor to rule out additional injury is warranted. Surgery is usually not needed.

TREATMENT The athlete can normally return to full activity after a period of conservative care, without surgery. Protection, rest, and ice in the acute phase, with a gradual return to strengthening and sports over the next few weeks, is usually the treatment of choice. There may be a small loss of shoulder flexion strength in the long term, but not enough to result in loss of high-level function.

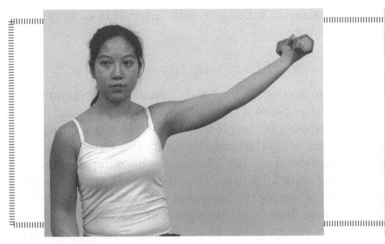

Figure 21–25 Gilchrist's sign for biceps long-head dislocation or subluxation. The athlete sits or stands with arm fully elevated, holding a 2-pound weight, then slowly lowers the arm sideways with the palm facing upward. The clinician observes for a painful click or snap in the shoulder at about 90 degrees.

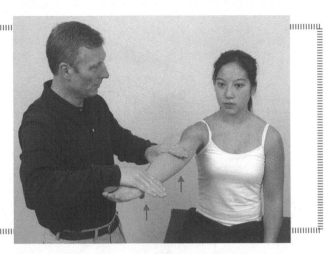

Figure 21–26 Speed's test for biceps long-head tendonitis. The athlete sits or stands, shoulder flexed to 90 degrees, with palm facing up. The clinician applies downward pressure to the arm. Produces symptoms of pain in the bicipital groove if positive.

SPECIAL TESTS Figures 21–25 and 21–26 demonstrate testing to identify biceps tendon injury.

TRAUMATIC SHOULDER INJURIES

Traumatic shoulder injuries have a sudden onset and are often the byproduct of a blow to the arm or shoulder, or of the shoulder joint being forced beyond its physiologic limits. Common traumatic injuries to the shoulder complex are glenohumeral dislocation, acromioclavicular separation, fractures, and tendon ruptures.

Anterior Shoulder Dislocation

The term *shoulder dislocation* is used in reference to the glenohumeral joint. With this a traumatic injury, the head of the humerus is dislocated completely off of the glenoid fossa. The direction in which it dislocates will depend on the nature of the injury. The head of the humerus can come out of the socket anteroinferiorly (front and down), inferiorly (down), or posteriorly (back). The most common direction is anteroinferiorly (simply referred to as anterior).

The mechanism of injury of an **anterior shoulder dislocation** occurs when the arm is abducted to the side, with the elbow bent, and a force applied to the arm causes external rotation (Figure 21–27). The anterior and posterior glenohumeral structures tear, allowing the head of the humerus to come out of the glenoid fossa and resulting in visible deformity (Figure 21–28). This dislocation is extremely painful at the time of the injury and requires immediate care by a physician. The athlete may need sedation before the humerus can be relocated. Also, the natural guarding of the muscles of the shoulder complex

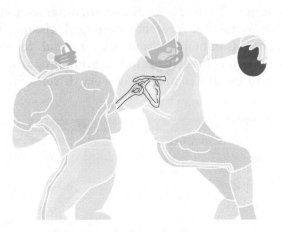

Figure 21–27 An anterior dislocation can occur when the arm is forced into abduction, extension, and external rotation.

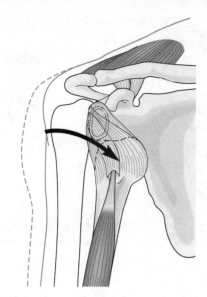

Figure 21–28 Anterior shoulder dislocation.

often prevents the physician from relocating the humerus.

With dislocations, a comprehensive medical examination is always necessary to evaluate for other possible injuries such as fractures, glenoid labial tears, or axillary nerve damage. If the posterior aspect of the head of the humerus hits the front of the glenoid hard enough at the time of dislocation, an indentation on the posterior humeral head can be observed on an X-ray. This is called a **Hill-Sachs lesion**.

It is critical that a first-time dislocation remain just that: the first and only dislocation event. Depending on age, if the initial injury is not properly managed and fully rehabilitated, the athlete may be at high risk for recurrent dislocations (Table 21–2). Immobilization in a sling after reduction protects damaged tissue. The length of immobilization may extend to eight weeks. An aggressive rehabilitation program will help to ensure complete recovery. If conservative

Table 21–2	Chance of Recurrent Dislocation
AGE	REINJURY RATE
Under 20	80–90%
20–30	60%
Over 40	40%

treatment fails, surgical intervention may be needed.

Glenoid Labrum Injuries

The deepest of the soft tissues in the shoulder is the **glenoid labrum**, positioned around the periphery of the glenoid fossa, which is a cartilaginous ring that acts to keep the humeral head positioned on the glenoid by blocking unwanted movement. Its action is similar to that of a wedge placed under the bottom of a door, which keeps the entire door from moving out of place.

Injury to the glenoid labrum can occur with trauma, such as an anterior shoulder dislocation. When the head of the humerus comes off the front of the glenoid, some structures tear (Figure 21–29). Another type of tear, called a *degenerated tear*, occurs with repeated traumas.

Baseball pitchers are susceptible to degenerative changes of the labrum. Certain activities may cause the anterior aspect of the joint to become lax (loose), thus permitting the humeral head to slip forward (translate). When battered by repeated slipping, the labral rim will degenerate over time and eventually fail.

SIGNS AND SYMPTOMS Signs and symptoms of injury to the glenoid labrum include pain and a catching or popping sensation. This injury results in limitation of use of the arm. There may be varying degrees of weakness. Special tests, as well as an MRI, will help with an accurate diagnosis.

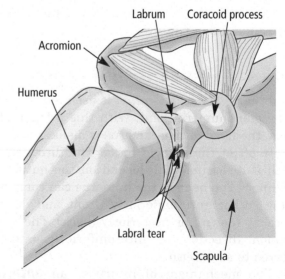

Figure 21–29 Example of a labral tear in the shoulder.

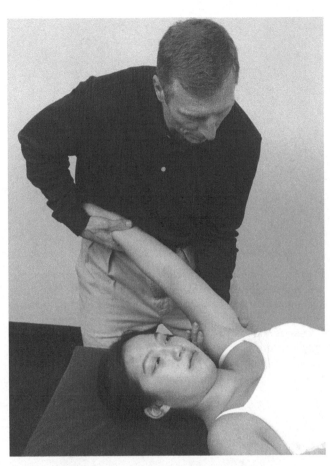

Figure 21–30 Clunk test for glenoid labrum tears. The athlete is supine on a treatment table. The clinician passively abducts the arm with one hand while "bouncing" the humeral head anteriorly with the other. A click or pop produced in the shoulder may be an indication of a labral tear.

TREATMENT Some degenerative labral tears, as well as mild tears, may respond well to a guided strengthening program, with special attention given to the rotator cuff. Athletes who may have labial tear must be referred to a physician for diagnosis. Surgery to trim off degenerate flaps or repair tears may be required. If surgery is performed, proper rehabilitation must follow.

SPECIAL TEST Figure 21–30 demonstrates a test that can be done to detect tears of the glenoid labrum.

Multidirectional Instabilities

Some athletes are able to voluntarily dislocate their shoulders. They discover that their shoulders slip out of joint with very little provocation and without an initial injury. This is usually a bilateral condition; that is, it may affect both shoulders. These individuals tend to be hyperelastic, or overly flexible.

They may have problems with sports requiring overhead movements. This condition can prove frustrating to both the athlete and the medical specialist if it does not improve with exercise. A thorough assessment of the shoulder will prevent this condition from being confused with repeat traumatic dislocations. The sulcus sign test will be positive (see Figure 21–31).

Weight-bearing exercises such as pushups, plyometrics, and weight training are often helpful. This condition is normally not improved by surgical intervention.

SPECIAL TESTS Figures 21–31 through 21–34 demonstrate tests that can identify shoulder instability.

Acromioclavicular Separation

Acromioclavicular separations are traumatic sprains of the acromioclavicular (AC) joint (Figure 21–35). The mechanism of injury is usually a direct blow to the tip of the shoulder. A football player's falling on the tip of his shoulder or on his outstretched arm commonly results in this type of injury.

SIGNS AND SYMPTOMS The athlete will complain of pain in the vicinity of the AC joint. Deformity of the joint, caused by the clavicle disassociating from the acromion, will be evident depending on the degree of sprain. Table 21–3 provides a rating scale for AC sprains.

TREATMENT A physician referral should be made for all shoulder separations. First-degree sprains may be treated conservatively with PRICE, with "E" meaning exercise in this instance. Exercises to restore range of motion and strength may be initiated as tolerated. Strengthening exercises that raise the arms over the head, such as military presses, are not recommended until the individual is fully healed.

Second-degree separations often require three to four weeks of immobilization (Figure 21–36). Third-degree separations will require six to eight

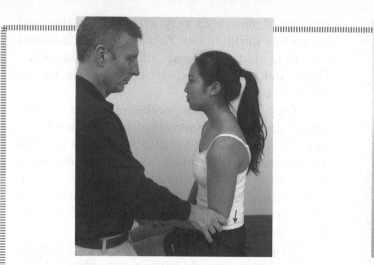

Figure 21–31 Sulcus sign test for inferior stability of the shoulder. The athlete sits or stands, with a relaxed shoulder. The clinician holds the elbow and distracts the arm inferiorly (pulls downward). A positive sign is gapping between the lateral acromion and humeral head.

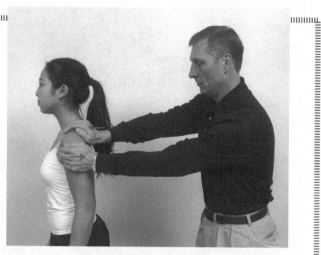

Figure 21–32 Posterior glide test for posterior glenohumeral instability. The athlete stands, arms at the side. The clinician, standing behind the athlete, braces the posterior shoulder while pulling the anterior superior humerus. Excessive movement (as compared to the uninjured side) may indicate posterior glenohumeral instability.

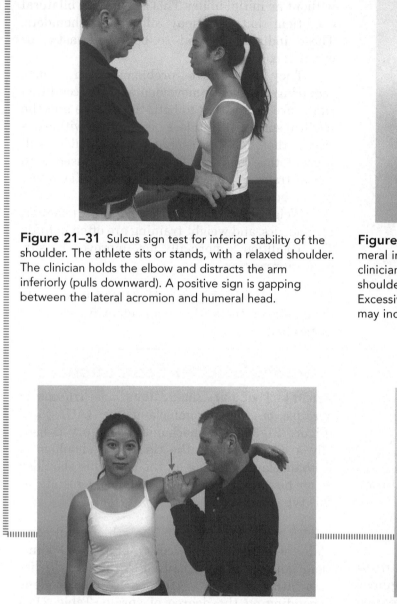

Figure 21–33 Feagin's test for inferior glenohumeral instability. The athlete stands, with arm resting on clinician's shoulder. The clinician, with athlete's arm resting on the shoulder, gently pulls down on the arm at the shoulder. Excessive movement (as compared to the uninjured side) may indicate inferior glenohumeral instability.

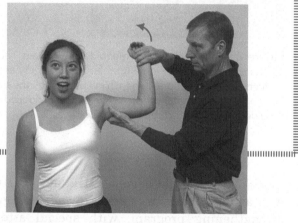

Figure 21–34 Anterior apprehension test for anterior shoulder instability. The athlete sits or stands, with the arm in 90 degrees of abduction and external rotation and elbow flexed 90 degrees. The clinician gently applies external rotation. This test is considered positive if the athlete has a reaction of apprehension and possibly a sense of instability.

weeks of immobilization. Of the three categories, second-degree sprains are most painful. Second- and third-degree sprains may leave some permanent cosmetic deformity of this joint, but should not impede adequate function in the long run.

Once healing has completed, gradual rehabilitation should be initiated, followed by functional testing prior to return to sports.

SPECIAL TESTS Figure 21–37 demonstrates a test for detection of an AC separation.

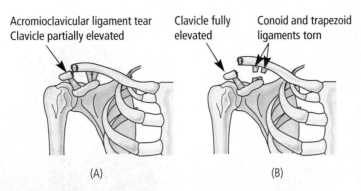

Acromioclavicular ligament tear
Clavicle partially elevated

Clavicle fully elevated

Conoid and trapezoid ligaments torn

(A) (B)

Figure 21–35 Acromioclavicular separation. (A) Second degree. (B) Third degree.

Table 21–3 Acromial Clavicular Sprain Rating Scale

CLASSIFICATION	DEGREE OF INJURY	PATHOLOGY
First-degree AC sprain	Mild sprain. AC joint ligaments remain intact.	Minimal pain. Mild tenderness. No deformity or swelling. Full, or almost full, ROM. Clavicle is stable.
Second-degree AC sprain	Moderate to severe sprain. Partial tearing of AC joint ligaments.	Severe pain at injury. Moderate to considerable tenderness. Some swelling/elevation of distal clavicle. Restriction of ROM.
Third-degree AC sprain	Severe sprain. Complete rupture of AC joint ligaments.	Moderate to considerable pain. Moderate to severe tenderness. Obvious swelling/elevation of the distal clavicle. Athlete may not want to move the arm.

Brachial Plexus Injury

An injury to the brachial plexus, often referred to as a **stinger** or **burner**, is a painful and disabling injury that occurs when the head and neck are forcibly pushed or hit to one side, stretching the brachial plexus on the opposite side. Sometimes, the nerves in the brachial plexus are compressed on that same side. The nerves become irritated as a result of being stretched or compressed.

The **brachial plexus** is a group of peripheral nerves that leave the spinal cord and extend from the vertebrae into the shoulder, giving the arm its ability to function (Figure 21–38). These nerves are injured when the athlete suffers a stinger.

SIGNS AND SYMPTOMS A stinger causes intense pain from the neck down to the arm. The athlete may feel like the arm is on fire or may have a pins-and-needles sensation. The arm or hand may be weak and numb, with intense pain in the area of the brachial plexus in the shoulder. These symptoms can last from several minutes to several hours or more. Weakness in the affected arm can last for several days, depending on the severity of the injury.

Injuries to the brachial plexus should always be referred to a sports medicine specialist. The family or team doctor may do neck X-rays to be sure there is no damage to the vertebrae. If the injury is serious, further testing may be ordered.

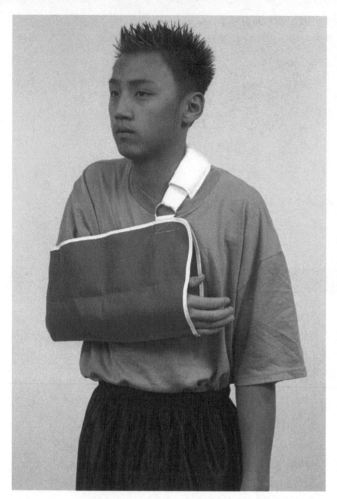

Figure 21–36 Shoulder injuries often require periods of immobility and support to heal.

TREATMENT Treatment includes medical referral and careful compliance with the treatment plan prescribed by sports medicine specialists. Treatment may include:

- Resting the neck and arms until the pain and symptoms cease
- Ice pack on the neck and shoulders for 20 minutes every 3 to 4 hours
- Taking an anti-inflammatory medication under the direction of the doctor
- Beginning exercises to strengthen the neck and shoulders

Return to activities will be determined by the sports medicine staff. Subsequent stingers will be the cause for further testing and perhaps neurological studies. Chronic stingers may eliminate the athlete from further competition in contact sports. Each injury creates a little more

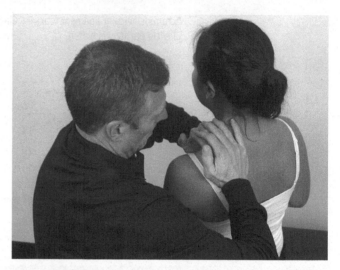

Figure 21–37 Acromioclavicular (AC) shear test. The athlete sits or stands, with arms at the side. The clinician, using both hands, squeezes between the anterior and posterior shoulder. If this test produces pain, the AC joint may be sprained.

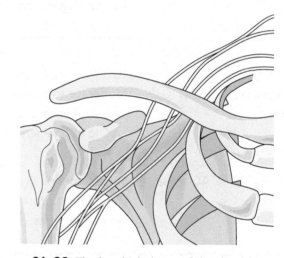

Figure 21–38 The brachial plexus of the shoulder.

scar tissue, which may develop around the nerves of the brachial plexus like an intricate spider web, entrapping the nerves. If the athlete receives another blow to this area, the brachial plexus may be unable to flex, and will shatter instead. This shattering of the brachial plexus can tear the major nerves of the arm, causing permanent neurological damage.

The only way to avoid stingers is to keep the muscles of the neck and shoulders as strong as possible. Proper equipment that fits well is important, to evenly distribute the impact of a collision. Proper tackling and blocking techniques will also lessen the chance that a stinger will occur.

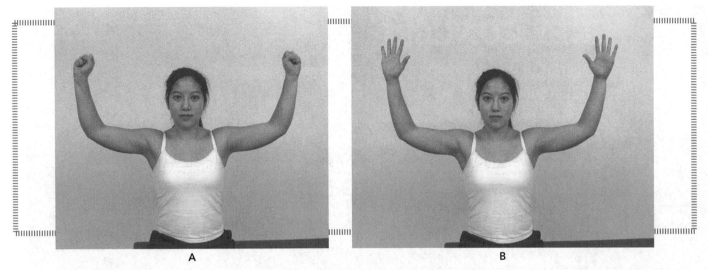

Figure 21–39A–B Roos test for thoracic outlet syndrome (TOS). This tests whether the brachial plexus has sustained a stretch injury. With arms abducted 90 degrees, externally rotated, and the elbows flexed 90 degrees, the athlete opens and closes the hands about once a second over the period of one minute. Reproduction of tingling in the arm(s) and hand(s) indicates TOS.

SPECIAL TESTS Figure 21–39 demonstrates a testing technique used to determine damage from a stinger.

Fractures of the Shoulder

Bone is seated within soft tissue. Therefore, an injury to a bone always results in injury to soft-tissue structures as well. When a fracture is either suspected or diagnosed, the evaluator must also consider possible injury to joints, muscles, ligaments, vessels, and nerves. As with other traumatic injuries, fractures to the shoulder complex are usually caused by an impact or blow to the shoulder (from another athlete, the ground, or equipment).

SIGNS AND SYMPTOMS Some fractures can be recognized if deformity or exposed bone is visible. Ecchymoses or bruising may also be present. Figure 21–40 shows the deformity associated with a fractured clavicle. Sagging of the shoulder downward and forward, along with inability to lift the arm, are additional signs of a fractured clavicle. Fractures of the clavicle account for approximately 5% of shoulder fractures. Falling onto the shoulder or an outstretched arm may put undue pressure on the clavicle to the point of breaking. Fractures can be partial or complete. The athlete's physician will determine the degree and method of treatment.

When a fracture is suspected, the certified athletic trainer should support the arm and shoulder using a sling.

Common areas for shoulder fractures include the clavicle and humerus. Sometimes the glenoid and scapula can sustain fractures. Scapular fractures may not be seen on standard X-rays, but will show up on bone scans.

TREATMENT Suspected fractures should be supported, and the athlete taken to the emergency room. Accurate diagnosis can be made from appropriate imaging studies ordered by a physician.

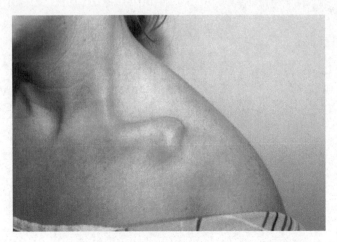

Figure 21–40 Deformity associated with a fractured clavicle.

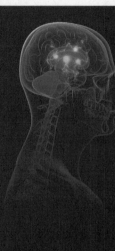

KEY CONCEPT

Injuries to the shoulder result from overuse or trauma. Common overuse injuries include:

- Impingement syndrome, resulting from narrowing of the space between the humeral head and the acromion. Treatment for this injury usually involves correction of improper technique, preseason conditioning, and specialized taping.

- Rotator-cuff tears, in which there is damage to the muscles that make up the rotator cuff. There can be varying degrees of tears; treatment depends on the severity of the tear.

- Muscle strains, which usually resolve within a few days. Immediate treatment is with PRICE.

- Biceps tendonitis, an inflammation of the tendon that lies adjacent to the rotator cuff.

- Biceps tendon rupture, the tearing away of the tendon from its point of attachment.

Traumatic injuries to the shoulder include:

- Anterior shoulder dislocation, in which the head of the humerus comes out of the socket. Immediate treatment by a physician should be sought.

- Glenoid labrum injuries, which can occur with a shoulder dislocation. Structures in the glenoid fossa are torn or damaged. Treatment for mild injuries includes strengthening the area. For more involved injuries, surgery may be required.

- Multidirectional instabilities, which are injuries that occur when the joint slips out of place with little or no force. Weight training to strengthen the area is often helpful.

- Acromioclavicular separations, which result from a direct blow to the tip of the shoulder. There are varying degrees of sprain with this injury. The athlete should see a physician.

- Injury to the brachial plexus, which results in pain and is caused by a blow to the head and neck that stretches the nerves on the opposite side. Treatment may include rest, ice packs, anti-inflammatory medication, and strengthening exercises.

- Shoulder fractures, which are breaks to the bones in the shoulder complex. Treatment should be sought from a physician.

IS IT A SHOULDER INJURY?

Pain in the shoulder region does not always indicate a shoulder problem. The astute clinician needs to maintain a sense of suspicion when the pieces of the puzzle do not seem to fit. **Referred pain** to the shoulder area can originate in other areas of the body. Cardiac problems can refer pain to the left shoulder, neck, and arm. Pinched or stretched nerves in the neck and brachial plexus areas, pulmonary pathology, and visceral pathology can all cause pain to be felt in the upper back and shoulder region. A spleen injury can cause a symptom called *Kehr's sign*, which refers pain to the left shoulder and down the upper portion of the left arm. Several in-depth textbooks on referred pain should be in every certified athletic trainer's personal library.

ADDITIONAL STRETCHING AND STRENGTHENING EXERCISES FOR THE SHOULDER

In addition to the exercises shown in the section on shoulder impingement, the exercises shown in Figures 21–41 through 21–44 will help to stretch and strengthen the shoulder girdle. Table 21–4 summarizes the special tests that can be done for shoulder problems and injuries.

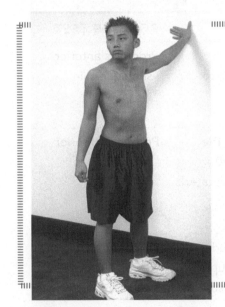

Figure 21–41 Wall stretch for the pectoralis major muscle. Athlete stands sideways with the arm extended and hand externally rotated against a wall. Gentle rotation of the body will put this muscle into a stretch.

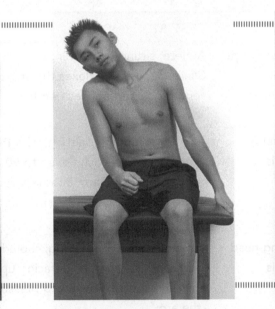

Figure 21–42 Upper trapezius stretch. Athlete, in a sitting position, holds onto the table with one hand as he stretches away from the support. This will stretch the upper trapezius muscle.

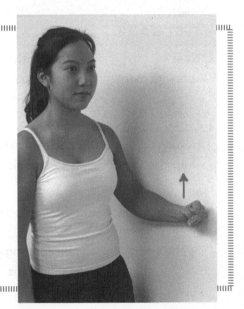

Figure 21–43 Isometric abduction of the deltoid muscle. Athlete, standing sideways against a wall, lifts upward against the wall with the forearm. Isometric contraction exercises should be held for 5 to 10 seconds.

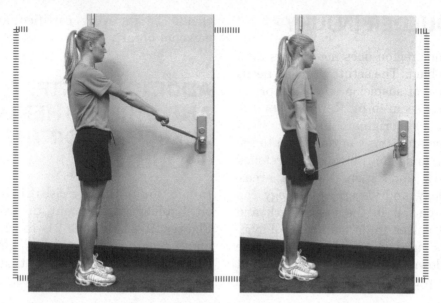

Figure 21–44A–B Elastic band shoulder extension strengthening exercise.

Table 21–4 Tests for Shoulder Problems

TEST NAME	INDICATES	TEST METHOD	POSITIVE TEST
Neer's impingement	Tendonitis; Biceps long head, supraspinatus	Athlete: sitting or standing. Clinician: passively flexes the arm to end range and applies gentle overpressure.	Produces anterior shoulder pain
Hawkin's impingement	Supraspinatus tendonitis	Athlete: standing or sitting, with the arm and elbow each flexed to 90 degrees and the arm internally rotated. Clinician: applies overpressure to internal rotation.	Produces anterior shoulder pain
Speed's test	Biceps long-head tendonitis	Athlete: sitting or standing; shoulder flexed to 90°, with palm facing up. Clinician: applies downward pressure to the arm.	Produces pain in the bicipital groove
Gilcrist's test	Subluxating biceps long head	Athlete: sitting or standing; with arm fully elevated and holding a two-pound weight, slowly lowers arm sideways with the palm facing upward. Clinician: observes.	A painful click or snap in the shoulder at about 90 degrees
Drop-arm sign	Rotator-cuff pathology, possible tear	Athlete: sitting or standing with arm overhead; slowly lowers the arm to the side. Clinician: observes.	Shoulder pain and loss of control when arm reaches midrange

(*continues*)

Table 21–4 Tests for Shoulder Problems (*continued*)

TEST NAME	INDICATES	TEST METHOD	POSITIVE TEST
Cross-arm adduction	AC joint pathology	Athlete: sitting or standing. Clinician: passively adducts the arm horizontally to end range.	Pain produced in the AC joint
Anterior apprehension test	Anterior shoulder instability	Athlete: sitting or standing, with the arm in 90 degrees of abduction and external rotation, and elbow flexed 90 degrees. Clinician: gently applies external rotation.	Athlete has reaction of apprehension and possibly a sense of instability; may be painful.
Sulcus sign	Inferior or global instability	Athlete: sitting or standing with shoulder relaxed. Clinician: holds the elbow and distracts the arm inferiorly (pulls downward).	Gapping between the lateral acromion and the humeral head
Clunk test	Glenoid labrum tear	Athlete: supine on a treatment table. Clinician: passively abducts the arm with one hand while "bouncing" the humeral head anteriorly with the other.	A click or pop is produced in the shoulder

CONCLUSION

The upper extremity is one of the most challenging areas of the body to treat. Understanding the mechanisms of injury associated with damage to the shoulder complex will enable the certified athletic trainer to assess and plan appropriate rehabilitation for the athlete. Certified athletic trainers must also understand the causes of common upper extremity conditions so that they can adequately assess and manage the many different injuries associated with this area of the body.

REVIEW QUESTIONS

1. Explain the anatomy of the shoulder girdle complex.
2. What are the four muscles of the rotator cuff?
3. What is muscle force couple?
4. Explain the three articulations that constitute the shoulder girdle complex.
5. Explain impingement syndrome and its effect on the upper extremity.
6. List the signs and symptoms of a rotator-cuff tear.
7. What happens when the shoulder becomes dislocated?
8. Describe an AC sprain and its treatment.
9. How can pain be referred to another part of the body?
10. Pick three of the special tests for the shoulder explained in this chapter. Describe the examinations and the conditions for which they test.

PROJECTS AND ACTIVITIES

1. Create a matching quiz out of the words listed in the Key Terms section. Include an answer key with your quiz.

2. Write a three-page report on rotator-cuff injuries in athletics.

3. Develop a teaching unit on the shoulder to be taught to sixth-graders. Include lesson plans, diagrams, handouts, quizzes, and tests. The unit should last one week, with each class being 30 minutes long.

4. Teach your shoulder unit from number 3 to a sixth-grade class.

5. Visit your local sporting-goods store. Make a list of the different braces and supports available for the shoulder.

6. Ask the baseball coach at your school what he or she does to minimize injuries to players' shoulders. Write a summary of what you learn.

LEARNING LINKS

- Visit http://www.omahashoulder.com/shoulder-animations/ to view animations of various shoulder conditions and repairs.

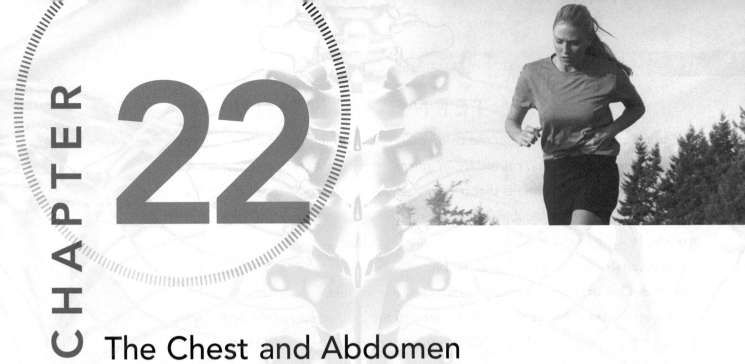

22

The Chest and Abdomen

OBJECTIVES

Upon completion of this chapter, the reader should be able to:

- Describe the anatomy of the thoracic cavity
- Explain what organs are housed within the abdominopelvic cavity and their location
- Explain the difference between the large and small intestine
- Explain where the liver and kidneys are located
- Describe the structures and functions of the organs of respiration
- Explain the chemical factors associated with respiration
- Explain the treatment for hyperventilation
- Explain how the treatment for a pneumothorax and a tension pneumothorax differ
- Explain the breathing and respiratory process
- Discuss the significance of chest and abdominal injuries
- Describe the various injuries and treatments associated with the thoracic cavity
- Describe the various injuries and treatments associated with the abdominal cavity

KEY TERMS

abdominal cavity *The area of the body that contains the stomach, liver, gallbladder, pancreas, spleen, small intestine, appendix, and part of the large intestine.*

abdominopelvic cavity *The area from below the diaphragm to the pubic floor; there is no separation between the abdomen and the pelvis.*

absorption *The passage of a substance into bodily fluids and tissues.*

afferent arteriole *Structure that takes blood from the renal artery to the Bowman's capsule.*

alveolar sacs (alveoli) *Air sacs found in the lung.*

KEY TERMS CONTINUED

ascending colon *The portion of the colon that travels up the right side of the abdominal cavity.*

asthma *Airway obstruction caused by an inflammatory reaction to a stimulus.*

bilirubin *One of two pigments that determines the color of bile; reddish in color.*

Bowman's capsule *The double-walled capsule around the glomerulus of a nephron.*

bronchiole *One of the small subdivisions of a bronchus.*

bronchoconstriction *Narrowing of the bronchioles.*

bronchus *One of the two primary branches of the trachea.*

cardiac sphincter *Circular muscle fibers around the cardiac end of the esophagus.*

cardiac tamponade *A buildup of fluid in the pericardium.*

cecum *A pouch at the proximal end of the large intestine.*

celiac plexus *A cluster of nerves located in the upper middle region of the abdomen; also known as the solar plexus.*

cellular respiration *The use of oxygen to release energy from the cell; also known as oxidation.*

chest contusion *Bruising over the central area of the chest as a result of a compressive blow to the chest.*

cilia *Tiny, lashlike processes of protoplasm.*

collecting tubule *The structure in the nephron that collects urine from the distal convoluted tubule.*

colon *The large intestine.*

common bile duct *The passage that brings bile to the duodenum.*

cortex *The outer portion of an organ.*

crepitus *A grating feeling produced by fractured bone ends rubbing together.*

cystic duct *The duct from the gallbladder to the common bile duct.*

descending colon *The portion of the colon that travels down the left side of the abdominopelvic cavity.*

distal convoluted tubule *The tubular structure that ascends to the cortex from the loop of Henle.*

duodenum *The first part of the small intestine.*

edema *Swelling.*

efferent arteriole *The structure that carries blood from the glomerulus.*

epigastric region *The upper region of the abdomen.*

epiglottis *Elastic cartilage that prevents food from entering the trachea.*

exercise-induced asthma *Airway narrowing as a result of increased physical activity.*

expiration *Exhalation; the process of breathing air out.*

external respiration *Breathing; the act of inspiration and expiration.*

false ribs *The five pairs of lower ribs that connect to the seventh rib rather than to the sternum, or make no anterior connection*

KEY TERMS CONTINUED

flail chest *A fracture of three or more consecutive ribs on the same side of the chest.*

gallbladder *A small, pear-shaped organ that stores and concentrates bile.*

glomerulus *Capillaries inside the Bowman's capsule.*

glottis *The space within the vocal cords of the larynx.*

glycogen *A polysaccharide formed and stored in the liver.*

hematuria *Blood in the urine.*

hemopneumothorax *An accumulation of blood in the pleural space.*

hemoptysis *Coughing up blood.*

hepatic duct *The structure that carries bile from the liver to the common bile duct.*

hernia *A protrusion of abdominal tissue through a portion of the abdominal wall.*

hilum *The indentation along the medial border of the kidney.*

hypertrophic cardiomyopathy *Thickening of the cardiac muscle.*

hyperventilation *Breathing faster than required for proper exchange of oxygen and carbon dioxide.*

hypogastric region *The lower region of the abdomen.*

ileum *The lower part of the small intestine, extending from the jejunum to the large intestine.*

inspiration *Inhalation; the process of breathing air in.*

internal respiration *The exchange of carbon dioxide and oxygen between the cells and the lymph surrounding them; the oxidative process of energy in the cells.*

jaundice *A buildup of bilirubin and bile in the bloodstream, which tints skin and eyes a yellowish color.*

jejunum *The section of small intestine between the duodenum and the ileum.*

Kehr's sign *Pain that radiates to the left shoulder and down the left arm; results from a spleen injury or rupture.*

kidney contusion *Bruising of the kidney.*

larynx *The voice box.*

loop of Henle *The proximal convoluted tubule that descends into the medulla.*

mediastinum *The intrapleural space separating the sternum in front and the vertebral column behind.*

medulla *The inner portion of an organ.*

myocardial contusion *Bruising of the heart muscle.*

nasal septum *The partition between the two nasal cavities.*

nephron *The functional unit of the kidney.*

olfactory nerve *Nerve that supplies the nasal mucosa and provides a sense of smell.*

oxidation *The use of oxygen to release energy from the cell.*

paradoxical *The opposite of what is expected.*

KEY TERMS CONTINUED

pelvic cavity *The area of the body containing the urinary bladder, reproductive organs, rectum, and the remainder of the large intestine.*

pharynx *The throat.*

pleural space *The space between the lung and the chest wall.*

pleura *Serous membrane protecting the lungs and lining the internal surface of the thoracic cavity.*

Pleurisy *Inflammation of the lining of the lungs.*

pneumothorax *Condition in which air enters the pleural space between the chest wall and lung.*

proximal convoluted tubule *The twisted tubular branch off the Bowman's capsule.*

pyloric sphincter *A valve that regulates the movement of food from the stomach to the duodenum.*

rales *A crackling sound heard when breathing.*

rectum *The portion of the colon that opens into the anus.*

renal fascia *The tough fibrous tissue covering the kidney.*

renal pelvis *The funnel-shaped structure at the beginning of the ureter.*

respiration *The physical and chemical process by which the body supplies the cells and tissues with oxygen and rids them of carbon dioxide.*

retroperitoneal *Located behind the peritoneum.*

rib contusion *Bruising of the intercostal muscles by a direct blow to the ribs.*

rib fracture *A break in the bony structure of the thorax.*

side stitches *Pain that occurs just under the ribcage during vigorous exercise.*

sigmoid colon *The S-shaped portion of the colon.*

sinus *A recessed cavity of hollow space, filled with air, around the nasal cavity.*

spirometer *A device that measures the volume and flow of air during inspiration and expiration.*

spleen *A large lymphatic organ that filters blood and helps activate the immune system.*

spontaneous pneumothorax *The rupture of a weakened area of the lung, which allows air to escape into the pleural space.*

stomach *A major organ of digestion located in the upper left quadrant of the abdominal cavity.*

sucking chest wound *An open wound in the chest that allows air to enter and become trapped in the pleural space.*

sudden death syndrome *The rapid collapse and death of an otherwise healthy person; usually the result of an unknown congenital disorder.*

tension pneumothorax *Condition in which air entrapped in the pleural space puts pressure on the lung and heart.*

thoracic cavity *The upper central area of the body, which is subdivided into two cavities, the left pleural cavity (containing the left lung) and the right pleural cavity (containing the right lung).*

tidal volume *The amount of air that moves in and out of the lungs with each breath.*

trachea *The windpipe.*

KEY TERMS CONTINUED

transverse colon *The portion of the colon that veers left across the abdomen to the spleen.*

true ribs *The first seven pairs of ribs, which connect directly to the sternum.*

umbilical area *The area located around the navel.*

ureters *The long, narrow tubes that convey urine from the kidney to the bladder.*

urethra *The tube that takes urine from the bladder to the outside of the body.*

urinary bladder *A muscular, membrane-lined sac that holds urine.*

urinary meatus *The outside opening of the urethra.*

vermiform appendix *A fingerlike projection, of unknown function, that protrudes into the abdominal cavity to the lower left of the cecum.*

villi *Hairlike projections.*

THE THORACIC CAVITY

The organs that constitute most of the body systems are located in four cavities: cranial, spinal, thoracic, and abdominopelvic (Figure 22–1). The cranial and spinal cavities are within a larger region known as the dorsal (posterior) cavity. The thoracic and abdominopelvic cavities are found in the ventral (anterior) cavity.

The diaphragm divides the ventral cavity into two parts: the upper thoracic and lower abdominopelvic cavities.

The central area of the **thoracic cavity** is called the *mediastinum*. It lies between the lungs and extends from the sternum (breastbone) to the

vertebrae of the back. The esophagus, bronchi, lungs, trachea, thymus gland, and heart are located in the thoracic cavity. The heart itself is contained within a smaller cavity, called the *pericardial cavity.*

The thoracic cavity is further subdivided into two pleural cavities: The left lung is in the left cavity, and the right lung is in the right cavity. Each lung is covered with a thin membrane called the **pleura**.

RIBS AND STERNUM

The thoracic area of the body is protected and supported by the thoracic vertebrae, ribs, and sternum.

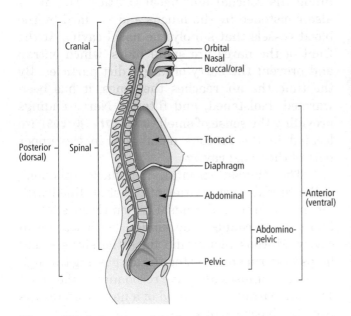

Figure 22–1 Cavities of the body.

KEY CONCEPT

The thoracic cavity contains the lungs and extends from the sternum to the vertebrae of the back. The major organs of the cardiac and respiratory system lie within the thoracic cavity. These vital organs are protected by the bony structures of the ribs. This bony structure also provides support for the torso.

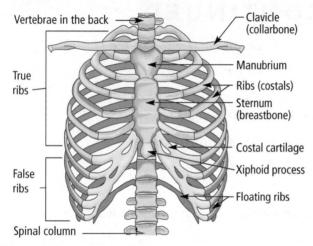

Figure 22–2 Ribs and sternum.

The sternum (breastbone) is divided into three parts: the upper region (manubrium), the body, and a lower cartilaginous part called the xiphoid process. Attached to each side of the upper region of the sternum, by means of ligaments, are the two clavicles (collarbones).

Seven pairs of costal cartilages join seven pairs of ribs directly to the sternum. These first seven pairs are known as **true ribs** (Figure 22–2). The human body contains 12 pairs of ribs. The next three pairs are **false ribs**, because their costal cartilages attach to the seventh rib instead of directly to the sternum. Finally, the last two pairs of ribs, connected neither to the costal cartilages nor to the sternum, are special false ribs called *floating ribs*.

THE RESPIRATORY SYSTEM

The respiratory system obtains oxygen for use by the millions of body cells and eliminates the carbon dioxide that is produced in cellular respiration. Oxygen and nutrients stored in the cells combine to produce heat and energy. Oxygen must be in constant supply for the body to survive.

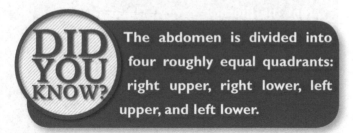

The abdomen is divided into four roughly equal quadrants: right upper, right lower, left upper, and left lower.

The respiratory system provides the structures for the exchange of oxygen and carbon dioxide in the body through respiration, further delineated into external respiration, internal respiration, and cellular respiration. This system is also responsible for the production of sound; the larynx contains the vocal cords. When air is expelled from the lungs, it passes over the vocal cords and produces sound.

Air moves into the lungs through several passageways: nasal cavity, pharynx, larynx, trachea, bronchi, bronchioles, and alveoli.

The Nasal Cavity

Air enters the respiratory system through two oval openings in the nose, the *nostrils*. From there, air enters the nasal cavity, which is divided into a right and left chamber, or smaller cavity, by a partition known as the **nasal septum**. Both cavities are lined with mucous membranes.

Protruding into the nasal cavity are three turbinate, or nasal conchae, bones. These three scroll-like bones (superior, middle, and inferior concha) divide the large nasal cavity into three narrow passageways. The turbinates increase the surface area of the nasal cavity and cause turbulence in the flowing air. This makes the air move in various directions before exiting the nasal cavity. As air moves through the nasal cavity, dust and dirt particles are filtered from it by the mucous membranes and swept away by **cilia** lining the conchal and nasal cavities. The air is also moistened by the mucus and warmed by the blood vessels that supply the nasal cavity. At the front of the nares are small hairs, which entrap and prevent the entry of larger dirt particles. By the time the air reaches the lungs, it has been warmed, moistened, and filtered. Nerve endings providing the sense of smell (**olfactory nerves**) are located in the mucous membrane in the upper part of the nasal cavity.

The **sinuses**—frontal, maxillary, sphenoid, and ethmoid—are cavities of the skull filled with air in and around the nasal region (Figure 22–3). Short ducts connect the sinuses with the nasal cavity. Mucous membrane lines the sinuses and helps to warm and moisten the air passing through them. The sinuses also give resonance to the voice. The unpleasant voice sound of a nasal cold results from the blockage of sinuses.

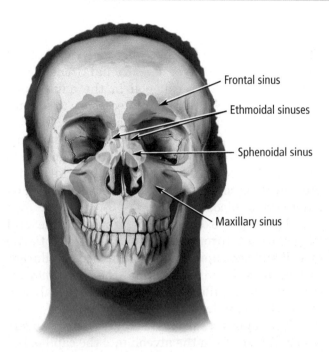

Figure 22–3 Paranasal sinuses.

The Pharynx

After air leaves the nasal cavity, it enters the **pharynx**, commonly known as the throat. The pharynx serves as a common passageway for air and food. It is about five inches long and can be subdivided into the nasopharynx, oropharynx, and laryngopharynx. The nasopharynx lies above and behind the soft palate. The left and right eustachian tubes open directly into the nasopharynx, connecting with each middle ear. Because of this connection, nasopharyngeal inflammation can lead to middle-ear infections. The oropharynx, also called the oral part of the mouth, extends from the soft palate, behind the mouth, to just above the hyoid bone. The laryngopharynx is located below the oropharynx and is superior to the larynx. Air travels down the pharynx on its way to the lungs; food travels this route on its way to the stomach.

The **epiglottis** is the flap of cartilage lying behind the tongue and in front of the entrance to the larynx. At rest, the epiglottis is upright and allows air to pass through the larynx and to the lungs. During swallowing, it folds back to cover the entrance to the larynx, preventing food and drink from entering the trachea. The larynx draws upward and forward to close the trachea. At the end of each swallow, the epiglottis moves up again, the larynx returns to rest, and the flow of air into the trachea continues. (See Figure 22–4.)

The Larynx

The **larynx**, or voice box, is a triangular chamber found below the pharynx. The laryngeal walls are composed of nine fibrocartilaginous plates. The largest of these is commonly called the Adam's apple. During puberty, the vocal cords become larger in the male; therefore, the Adam's apple is more prominent in men.

The larynx is lined with a mucous membrane, continuous from the pharyngeal lining above to

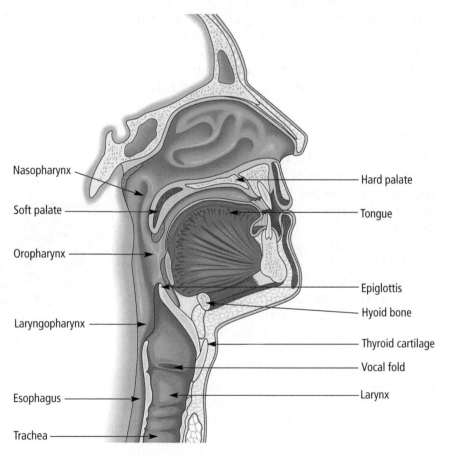

Figure 22–4 Sagittal section of the face and neck.

the tracheal lining below. Within the larynx are the vocal cords. There is a space between the vocal cords known as the **glottis**. When air is expelled from the lungs, it passes the vocal cords. This sets off a vibration, creating sound. The action of the lips and tongue on this sound produces speech.

The Trachea

The **trachea**, or windpipe, is a tubelike passageway some 11.2 centimeters (about 4.5 in.) in length. It extends from the larynx, passes in front of the esophagus, and continues to form the two bronchi (one for each lung). The walls of the trachea are composed of alternate bands of membrane and 15 to 20 C-shaped rings of hyaline cartilage. These C-shaped rings are virtually noncollapsible, keeping the trachea open for the passage of oxygen into the lungs. However, the trachea can be obstructed by large pieces of food, tumorous growths, or the swelling of inflamed lymph nodes in the neck.

The walls of the trachea are lined with both mucous membrane and ciliated epithelium. The function of mucus is to entrap inhaled dust particles; cilia then sweep the dust-laden mucus upward to the pharynx. Coughing and expectoration (spitting out) dislodges and eliminates the particle-laden mucus from the pharynx (Figure 22–4).

The Bronchi and the Bronchioles

The lower end of the trachea separates into the right and the left **bronchus**. There is a slight difference between the two bronchi; the right bronchus is somewhat shorter, wider, and more vertically positioned.

As the bronchi enter the lung, they subdivide into bronchial tubes and smaller **bronchioles**. The divisions are Y-shaped. The two bronchi are similar in structure to the trachea in that their walls are lined with ciliated epithelium and ringed with hyaline cartilage; however, the bronchial tubes and smaller bronchi are ringed with cartilaginous plates instead of incomplete C-shaped rings. The bronchioles have no cartilaginous plates or fibrous tissue. Their thinner walls are made from smooth muscle and elastic tissue lined with ciliated epithelium. At the end of each bronchiole is an alveolar duct that ends in a saclike cluster called **alveolar sacs (alveoli)** (see Figure 22–5).

The Alveoli

The alveolar sacs consist of many alveoli, each of which has a single layer of epithelial tissue. There are about 500 million alveoli in the adult lung, about three times the amount necessary to sustain life. Each alveolus forming a part of the alveolar sac possesses a globular shape. Their inner surfaces are covered with a lipid material known as *surfactant*, which helps to stabilize them and prevent their collapse. Each alveolus is encased by a network of blood capillaries.

The rapid exchange of carbon dioxide and oxygen occurs through the moist walls of both the alveoli and the capillaries. In the blood capillaries, carbon dioxide diffuses from the erythrocytes, through the capillary walls and into the alveoli, and is then exhaled through the mouth and nose.

The opposite process occurs with oxygen, which diffuses from the alveoli into the capillaries, and from there into the erythrocytes.

The Lungs

The lungs are fairly large, cone-shaped organs that fill the two lateral chambers of the thoracic

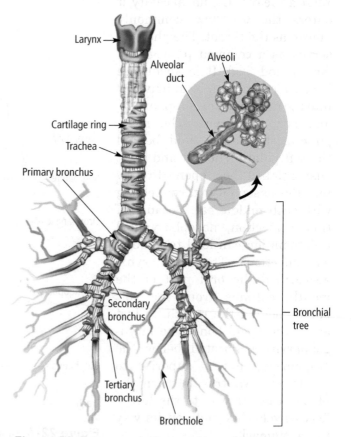

Figure 22–5 Larynx, trachea, and bronchial tree.

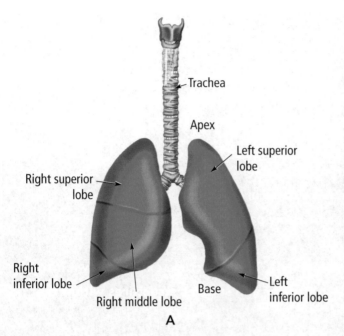

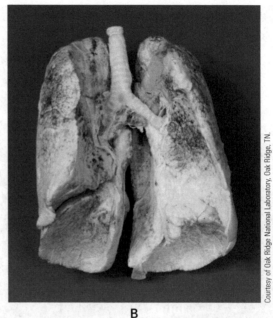

Courtesy of Oak Ridge National Laboratory, Oak Ridge, TN.

Figure 22–6 (A) Structures of the lungs. (B) Human lungs.

cavity (Figure 22–6). They are separated from each other by the mediastinum and the heart. The upper part of the lung, underneath the collarbone, is the apex; the broad, lower part is the base. Each base is concave, allowing it to fit snugly over the convex part of the diaphragm.

Lung tissue is porous and spongy, because of the alveoli and the tremendous amount of air it contains. If you were to place a specimen of a cow lung in a tankful of water, for example, it would float quite easily.

The right lung is larger and broader than the left because the heart inclines to the left side. The right lung is also shorter because of the diaphragm's upward displacement on the right to accommodate the liver. The right lung is divided by fissures (clefts) into three lobes: superior, middle, and inferior.

The left lung is smaller, narrower, and longer than its counterpart. It is subdivided into two lobes: superior and inferior.

The Pleura

The lungs are covered with a thin, moist, slippery membrane of tough endothelial cells, or pleura. There are two pleural membranes. The one covering the lungs and dipping between the lobes is the pulmonary, or visceral, pleura. Lining the

thoracic cavity and the upper surface of the diaphragm is the parietal pleura. Consequently, each lung is enclosed in a double-walled sac. **Pleurisy** is an inflammation of this lining.

The space between the two pleural membranes is the pleural cavity, filled with serous fluid called pleural fluid. This fluid is necessary to prevent friction between the two pleural membranes as they rub against each other during each breath.

The pleural cavity may, on occasion, fill with an enormous quantity of serous fluid. This occurs when there is an inflammation of the pleura. The increased amount of pleural fluid compresses and sometimes causes parts of the lung to collapse. This makes breathing extremely difficult. To alleviate the pressure, a thoracentesis may be performed. This procedure entails the insertion of a hollow, tubelike instrument through the thoracic cavity and into the pleural cavity, to drain the excess fluid.

The Mediastinum

The **mediastinum**, also called the *interpleural space*, is situated between the lungs along the median plane of the thorax. It extends from the sternum to the vertebrae. The mediastinum contains the thoracic viscera: thymus gland,

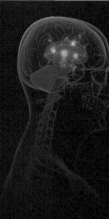

KEY CONCEPT

The primary function of the respiratory system is to exchange oxygen and carbon dioxide in the body. Many structures aid in this process:

- The nasal cavity is where air first enters the body. Here the air is warmed, moistened, and filtered.
- Air next passes into the pharynx (throat).
- The larynx (voice box) is the next structure through which air passes. The vocal cords are housed here, and as air passes these structures it causes vibration, which creates sound.
- Air then enters the trachea (windpipe). This structure extends down into the chest and branches out into smaller and smaller structures within the lungs.
- The bronchi and bronchioles are these smaller structures. The branching of these structures creates more surface area.
- At the end of each bronchiole are alveoli, the structures where the exchange of oxygen and carbon dioxide occurs.
- The lungs are large, cone-shaped organs that hold a tremendous amount of air.
- The pleura is a moist membrane that covers the lungs.
- The mediastinum is the space between the lungs along the median of the thorax.

heart, aorta and its branches, pulmonary arteries and veins, superior and inferior vena cavae, esophagus, trachea, thoracic duct, lymph nodes, and vessels.

RESPIRATION

Respiration is the physical and chemical process by which the body supplies its cells and tissues with the oxygen needed for metabolism, and relieves them of the carbon dioxide formed in energy-producing reactions. Respiration is subdivided into external respiration, which takes place in the lungs; internal respiration, which occurs between the cells of the body and the blood by way of the fluid bathing the cells; and cellular respiration, which occurs within the cells of the body.

External Respiration

External respiration, also known as *breathing* or *ventilation,* is the exchange of oxygen and carbon dioxide between the lungs and the outside environment. The breathing process consists of inspiration (inhalation) and expiration (exhalation). On inspiration, air enters the body, where it is warmed, moistened, and filtered as it passes to the air sacs (alveoli) of the lungs. The concentration of oxygen in the alveoli is greater than in the bloodstream. Oxygen diffuses from the area of greater concentration (the alveoli) to an area of lesser concentration (the bloodstream), then into the red blood cells. At the same time, the concentration of carbon dioxide in the blood is greater than in the alveoli, so it diffuses from the blood to the alveoli. Expiration expels the carbon dioxide from the alveoli of the lungs. Some water vapor is also given off in the process.

Internal Respiration

Internal respiration includes the exchange of carbon dioxide and oxygen between the cells and the lymph surrounding them, plus the oxidative process of energy in the cells. After inspiration, the alveoli are rich with oxygen and transfer it into the blood. The greater concentration of oxygen in the blood diffuses the oxygen into the tissue cells. At the same time, the cells build up a carbon dioxide concentration, which increases to a point that exceeds the level in the blood. This causes carbon dioxide to diffuse out of the cells and into the blood, where it is carried away to be eliminated.

Deoxygenated blood, produced during internal respiration, carries carbon dioxide in the form of bicarbonate ions (HCO_3^-). These ions are transported by both blood plasma and red blood cells. Exhalation expels carbon dioxide from the red blood cells and the plasma; it is released from the body in the following manner:

$$H_2CO_3 \longrightarrow H_2O + CO_2$$

(Bicarbonate ions decompose to form water and carbon dioxide.)

Cellular Respiration

Cellular respiration, or **oxidation**, involves the use of oxygen to release energy stored in nutrient molecules such as glucose. This chemical reaction occurs within the cells. Just as wood, when burned (oxidized), gives off energy in the form of heat and light, so too does food give off energy when it is burned or oxidized in the cells. Much of this energy is released in the form of heat to maintain body temperature. Some, however, is used directly by the cells for such work as contraction of muscle cells. It is also used to carry on other vital processes.

Food, when oxidized, gives off waste products, including carbon dioxide and water. The carbon dioxide is carried away through the process of internal respiration. The water is used by the body or eliminated by the kidneys if in excess. The process of respiration is illustrated in Figure 22–7.

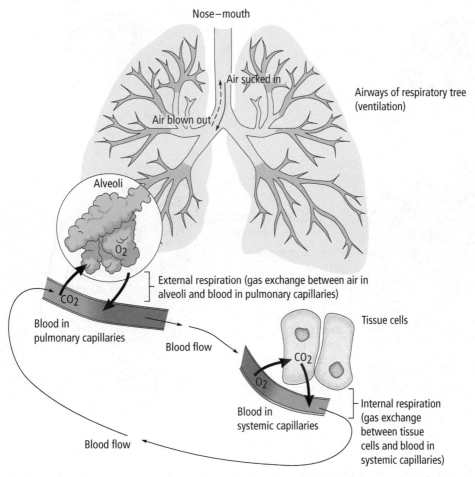

Figure 22-7 Respiration.

MECHANICS OF THE BREATHING

Pulmonary ventilation (breathing) in the lungs is accomplished by changes in pressure within the chest cavity. The normal pressure within the pleural space is always negative; that is, less than atmospheric pressure. The negative pressure helps to keep the lungs expanded. The variation in pressure is brought about by cellular respiration and mechanical breathing movements.

Inhalation/Inspiration

The two groups of intercostal muscles are external intercostals and internal intercostals. Their muscle fibers cross each other at an angle of 90 degrees. During inhalation, or **inspiration**, the external intercostals lift the ribs upward and outward (Figure 22–8). This increases the volume of the thoracic cavity. Simultaneously, the sternum rises along with the ribs, and the dome-shaped diaphragm contracts and becomes flattened, moving downward. As the diaphragm moves downward, pressure is exerted on the abdominal viscera. This causes the anterior muscles to protrude slightly, increasing the space within the chest cavity in a vertical direction. A decrease in pressure results. Because atmospheric pressure is now greater, air rushes in all the way down to the alveoli, resulting in inhalation.

Exhalation/Expiration

In exhalation, or **expiration**, the opposite takes place. Expiration is a passive process; all the contracted intercostal muscles and diaphragm relax. The ribs move down and the diaphragm moves up. In addition, the surface tension of the fluid lining the alveoli reduces the elasticity of the lung tissue and causes the alveoli to collapse. This action, coupled with the relaxation of contracted respiratory muscles, relaxes the lungs; the space within the thoracic cavity decreases, thus increasing the

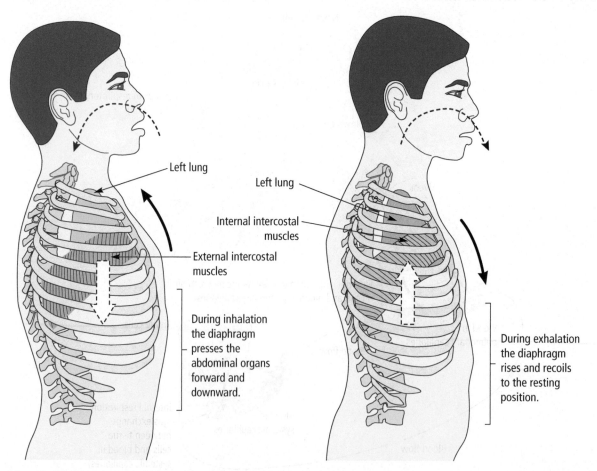

Figure 22–8 Mechanics of breathing—inhalation and exhalation.

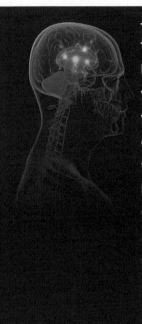

KEY CONCEPT

Respiration is the process by which the body supplies its cells with oxygen and relieves them of carbon dioxide. This takes place through breathing, the process by which air enters and leaves the body. Air enters the thoracic cavity upon inhalation or inspiration. During exhalation or expiration, air leaves the lungs as a result of the decreased volume within the thoracic cavity.

internal pressure. Increased pressure forces air from the lungs, resulting in exhalation.

The lungs are extremely elastic and able to change capacity as the size of the thoracic cavity is altered, an ability known as *compliance*. When lung tissue becomes diseased and fibrotic, the lung's compliance decreases and ventilation decreases.

Respiratory Movements and Frequency of Respiration

The rhythmic movements of the ribcage when air is drawn in or expelled from the lungs constitute the respiratory movements. Inspiration and expiration combined count as one respiratory movement. Thus, the normal rate in quiet breathing for an adult is about 14 to 20 breaths per minute. This rate is variable. The respiratory rate can be increased by muscular activity, increased body temperature, and certain pathological disorders such as hyperthyroidism. It changes with sex: females have a higher rate, at 16 to 20 breaths per minute. The respiratory rate also changes with age. For example, at birth the rate is 40 to 60 breaths per minute; at 5 years, it is 24 to 26 breaths. The body's position also affects the respiration rate. When one is asleep or prone, the rate is 12 to 14 breaths per minute; when in a sitting position, it is 18; when in a standing position, it is

20 to 22 breaths per minute. Emotions play a role in decreasing or increasing the respiratory rate, probably through the hypothalamus and pons. Other situations that can affect the respiratory rate are:

- *Coughing*—a deep breath is taken, followed by a forceful exhalation from the mouth to clear the lower respiratory tract.
- *Hiccoughs (hiccups)*—caused by a spasm of the diaphragm and a spasmodic closure of the glottis; believed to be the result of an irritation to the diaphragm or the phrenic nerve.
- *Sneezing*—occurs like a cough except that air is forced through the nose to clear the upper respiratory tract.
- *Yawning*—a deep, prolonged breath that fills the lungs believed to be caused by the need to increase oxygen within the blood.

CONTROL OF BREATHING

The rate of breathing is controlled by neural (nervous) and chemical factors. Although both have the same goal—that of respiratory control—they function independently.

Chemical control of respiration depends on the level of carbon dioxide in the blood. When blood circulates through active tissue, it receives carbon dioxide and other metabolic waste products of cellular respiration. As blood circulates through the respiratory center, the respiratory center senses the increased carbon dioxide in the blood and increases the respiratory rate. For example, a person performing vigorous exercise or physical labor breathes more deeply and quickly to meet the need for more oxygen and rid the body of the excess carbon dioxide produced.

Other chemical regulators of respiration are the chemoreceptors found in carotid arteries and the aorta. These chemoreceptors are sensitive to blood oxygen levels. As the arterial blood flows around these carotid and aortic bodies, the chemoreceptors sense the amount of oxygen present. If oxygen declines to very low levels, impulses are sent from the carotid and aortic bodies to the respiratory center, which will stimulate an increase in the rate and depth of respiration.

The respiratory center can be affected by drugs such as depressants, barbiturates, and morphine.

LUNG CAPACITY AND VOLUME

A device called a **spirometer** measures the volume and flow of air during inspiration and expiration (lung capacity). Comparing the reading with the norm for a person's age, height, weight, and sex, can determine if any deficiencies exist. Disease processes such as chronic obstructive pulmonary disease (COPD) affect lung capacity (Figure 22–9).

- **Tidal volume** is the amount of air that moves in and out of the lungs with each breath. The normal amount is about 500 milliliters.

- *Inspiratory reserve volume (IRV)* is the amount of air you can force a person to take in over and above the tidal volume. The normal amount is 2,100 to 3,000 milliliters.

- *Expiratory reserve volume (ERV)* is the amount of air you can force a person to exhale over and above the tidal volume. The normal amount is 1,000 milliliters.

- *Vital lung capacity* is the total amount of air involved with tidal volume, inspiratory reserve volume, and expiratory reserve volume. The normal vital capacity is 4,500 milliliters.

- *Residual volume* is the amount of air that cannot be voluntarily expelled from the lungs. It maintains the continuous exchange of gases between breaths. The normal residual volume is 1,500 milliliters.

- *Functional residual capacity* is the sum of the expiratory reserve volume plus the residual volume. The normal amount is 2,500 milliliters.

- *Total lung capacity* includes tidal volume, inspiratory reserve, expiratory reserve, and residual air. The normal amount is 6,000 milliliters.

DISORDERS OF THE RESPIRATORY SYSTEM

Many diseases and disorders can affect the proper operation of the respiratory system. Some of the most common are asthma, bronchitis, emphysema, lung cancer, cystic fibrosis, pulmonary fibrosis, pneumonia, and whooping cough.

Asthma

Asthma, a disease that affects the lungs, has become the most common long-term disease in children. A growing percentage of adults are also afflicted with this disease. Asthma affects a considerable percentage of athletes as well. During an asthma attack, the muscles around the airways tighten, or *spasm*, and the lining inside the airways swells or thickens and gets clogged with thick mucus. This makes it harder to move air in and out of the lungs. The cause of asthma is not well known, but environmental factors may play a key role. Asthma can be controlled by the use of special medications and inhalers.

Exercise-induced asthma is a condition in which vigorous physical activity triggers airway narrowing. This reversible airway obstruction occurs during or after exertion. This type of asthma can occur in otherwise healthy people who do not have chronic asthma. Exercise is the only stimulus for their asthma symptoms. Exercise-induced asthma may occur in people who have chronic asthma and are not aware that their symptoms during exercise are a manifestation of asthma.

SIGNS AND SYMPTOMS The symptoms of exercise-induced asthma include coughing, wheezing, dyspnea (difficulty in breathing), and chest tightness.

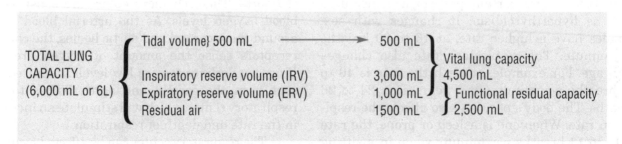

TOTAL LUNG CAPACITY (6,000 mL or 6L) {	Tidal volume} 500 mL	→	500 mL }	Vital lung capacity 4,500 mL
	Inspiratory reserve volume (IRV)		3,000 mL	
	Expiratory reserve volume (ERV)		1,000 mL	} Functional residual capacity
	Residual air		1500 mL	2,500 mL

Figure 22–9 Lung capacity and volume.

TREATMENT Treatment for chronic asthma and exercise-induced asthma differ. It is important that any new patient with asthma symptoms be assessed to determine whether the asthma is chronic or exercise induced.

In athletes, **bronchoconstriction** (narrowing of the bronchials) develops after 6 to 8 minutes of vigorous exercise. The maximal decrease in pulmonary function occurs about 15 minutes after exercise begins. Pulmonary function returns to its original level 30 to 60 minutes after exercise has ended. All athletes who have exercise-induced asthma should carry a quick-acting inhaler with them during exercise to relieve any symptoms that develop. If asthma symptoms are well controlled, exercise-induced asthma should not limit performance.

CHEST (THORAX) INJURIES

Most athletic injuries to the chest are the result of a direct blow. The majority of these injuries are superficial, involving the chest or ribcage. However, athletic injuries may involve the contents of the chest cavity, such as the lungs, heart, and vessels. Injuries to the chest can be life threatening and should be a primary concern when they do occur.

Injuries to the chest that can occur during athletics are described in the following subsections.

Rib Contusions

Rib contusions are caused by a forceful blow to the ribcage that bruises the intercostal muscles. The intercostal muscles lie between the ribs and aid in breathing. Bruising of these muscles will cause pain upon both inhalation and exhalation.

Rib contusions are common in contact sports such as football, rugby, soccer, wrestling, and basketball. A direct blow to the ribcage can also damage the soft tissue surrounding the ribs.

SIGNS AND SYMPTOMS Rib contusions result in point tenderness and pain when the chest is palpated and compressed at or near the site of injury. The athlete may feel sharp pain during breathing.

TREATMENT Immediate care of rib contusions begins with removal from the sport activity. The

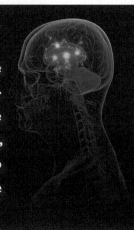

athlete should apply ice to the injured area for 20 minutes every 3 to 4 hours. It is important that the athlete be closely monitored for signs of a more serious injury. These signs may include shock.

REHABILITATION The athlete should be checked by the family physician and receive clearance before returning to play. If football is the sport, the athlete should have the shoulder pads checked to be sure that they fit properly and cover the chest. The athlete should also be fitted with additional padding for protection.

Rib Fractures

A **rib fracture** is a break in the bony structure of the thorax. Rib fractures are fairly common in collision sports such as football, wrestling, and soccer. These injuries are most often the result of a direct blow to the ribcage. Rib fractures can be serious and cause additional damage to the organs that they normally protect. Displaced fractures of three or more consecutive ribs on the same side of the chest can cause a condition known as **flail chest**. A flail chest does not allow normal inhalation and exhalation of the lungs. In fact, the normal movements of breathing will be reversed, or **paradoxical** (Figure 22–10). This condition causes a great deal of pain and requires immediate medical attention. Displaced, fractured ribs can puncture the lungs and the heart and must be considered life threatening.

The mechanism of injury in a rib fracture is similar to that of a rib contusion. The only difference is the degree of force required to cause a fracture. Rib fractures occur only when a violent force is applied directly to a specific area of the ribs. The ribs have a certain amount of movement, which is

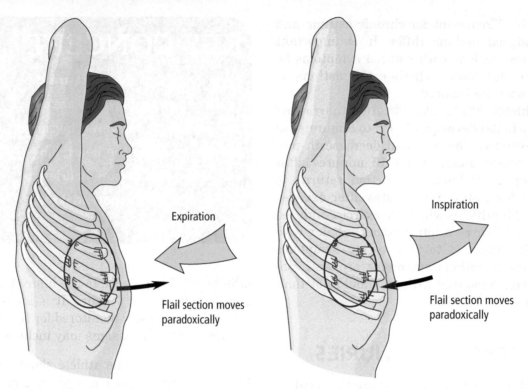

Expiration

Flail section moves
paradoxically

Inspiration

Flail section moves
paradoxically

Figure 22–10 A flail segment impairs breathing because of its paradoxical motion.

required for respiration; thus, the force needed to cause a fracture is much greater than the force that would cause a contusion. Another mechanism of injury is a forceful compression of the ribcage, as in a pile-up in a football game.

SIGNS AND SYMPTOMS The athlete will experience severe pain during breathing and point tenderness to the touch. The athlete may have **crepitus**, a feeling of grating as the ends of the bones rub together. An athlete with a rib fracture will generally refrain from breathing deeply, taking rapid, shallow breaths instead; he or she may also hold the injured side in an attempt to restrict painful movement of the chest. Palpation of the ribs with gentle compression will reveal pain at the fracture site.

TREATMENT Because a fracture may involve more than the ribs, immediate medical treatment must be sought. The athlete should cease to practice or play.

Supporting the fracture site with a pillow will help to manage the pain. The athlete should be treated for shock and be reassured until emergency medical services (EMS) personnel arrive.

REHABILITATION After the athlete has been cleared by the family physician to return to play, he or she should wear additional padding. The athlete should be monitored for several days to be sure no additional symptoms occur.

Chest Contusions

A **chest contusion**, bruising over the central area of the chest, results from a compressive, forceful blow to the body. Chest contusions are the most frequent injuries to the chest wall. The severity depends on the amount of force applied to the tissue. These injuries involve the skin, subcutaneous tissues, muscles, or periosteum of the ribs or sternum.

SIGNS AND SYMPTOMS Contusions of the chest wall will reveal an area of localized tenderness and possible swelling. This type of injury usually does not cause pain during breathing or restrict motion of the ribcage, unless the injured athlete takes very deep respirations.

As with all contusions, they will be tender to the touch, and the tissues involved tend to swell. Contusion of the heart muscle must be considered if the chest contusion is determined to be severe. If this is possible, medical treatment should be sought.

TREATMENT Ice should be applied to the injured area for 15 to 20 minutes every 3 hours and continued until risk of further swelling has passed—typically 24 to 72 hours. Compression using a large, 6-inch, double-length elastic wrap will help to minimize swelling. As with any injury to the chest or abdomen, the athlete should be monitored closely for signs of shock.

REHABILITATION Athletes with chest contusions can normally continue with athletics as long as they have been cleared by the certified athletic trainer or physician. Those with severe chest contusions will need a few days of rest before returning to activity. The athlete should be fitted with additional padding to protect the injured area, if appropriate for the sport activity.

Myocardial Contusion and Aortic Rupture

A contusion to the heart is called a **myocardial contusion**. This injury is relatively rare, but can occur if the force applied to the sternum is great enough to compress the heart against the spine. Blows from baseballs and softballs, or a barbell dropped onto the chest, can cause this injury. Outside of athletics, this injury often results from a car accident in which the driver's chest hits the steering wheel.

SIGNS AND SYMPTOMS Signs and symptoms of this injury are immediate, severe pain in the chest with rapid onset of shock. A myocardial contusion may have the following effects: bleeding into the membrane that surrounds the heart, which can cause **cardiac tamponade** (buildup of fluid in the pericardium, which is the thin membrane around the heart); abnormality in the transmission of the electrical impulses that control the heartbeat; congestive heart failure (a condition in which the heart's decreased pumping ability causes fluid to back up into the lungs); damage to heart valves; death of areas of heart muscle; and rupture of the heart chamber walls and nearby structures; or weakening of the heart muscle. This type of injury may also cause an aortic rupture, which normally results in immediate death.

TREATMENT Management of this injury requires quick, decisive action, beginning with activation of emergency medical services. Monitor the victim and treat for shock until help arrives. Be ready to administer CPR if needed. Document the time of injury.

REHABILITATION A return to normal athletics after a myocardial contusion is doubtful for the remainder of the season and perhaps the rest of the year. The athlete must have a physician's clearance before returning. Addition of padding on the chest should be a requirement for return.

Sudden Death Syndrome in Athletes

This catastrophic condition occurs in people younger than 35 years of age. Cardiac arrest is the leading cause of death in young athletes, resulting in 1 in 50,000 deaths each year. **Sudden death syndrome** is usually caused by some form of heart disease. (For victims under the age of 30, only 20% of the cases were noncardiac in nature.) The most common heart diseases causing sudden death are **hypertrophic cardiomyopathy** (thickening of the cardiac muscle), coronary artery abnormalities, Marfan's syndrome (abnormality of the connective tissue that weakens the structure of the aorta and cardiac valves), and congenital heart disease.

The most common cause of noncardiac sudden death in athletes is use of alcohol, cocaine, or other illegal drugs. Cerebral aneurysm (weakness in an artery or vein in the brain that breaks and results in catastrophic bleeding) and head trauma may also cause sudden death.

SIGNS AND SYMPTOMS Signs of this condition include chest pain, discomfort during exercise, heart palpitations, shortness of breath, profuse sweating, and loss of consciousness caused by inadequate supply of oxygen to the brain. This condition occurs in individuals who are apparently healthy and show no signs of physical impairment prior to its onset.

TREATMENT Provide CPR until EMS arrives.

Pneumothorax

Pneumothorax occurs when air enters the thoracic cavity between the chest wall and the lung. The difference in pressure causes the lung to collapse. A pneumothorax can occur if a foreign object or fractured rib penetrates the skin on the chest and creates an open chest wound. It can also occur if an intense impact tears the lung itself.

Three additional conditions may arise as a result of a chest wound—sucking chest wound, spontaneous pneumothorax, and tension pneumothorax:

- A **sucking chest wound** occurs when the chest cavity has been injured and air moves through the wound but remains in the **pleural space** outside the lung. This creates a pneumothorax. The air passing through the wound makes a sucking sound. Treatment is to seal the wound on three sides with a large, occlusive dressing (Figure 22–11), allowing air to exit as the victim breathes.

- A **spontaneous pneumothorax** is normally caused by rupture of a weakened area on the surface of the lung. This rupture allows air to escape into the pleural space and create a pneumothorax.

- **Tension pneumothorax** occurs when air enters the pleural space but cannot exit. The air leaking into the pleural space accumulates with every breath, compromising the affected lung. As pressure increases, the collapsed lung will begin to press against the unaffected lung and then the heart (Figure 22–12). Death can

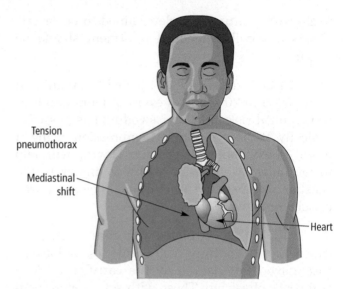

Figure 22–12 Increasing pressure in the lungs pushes the heart and the great vessels to the side of the chest.

result quickly if the athlete does not receive proper medical treatment. As described earlier, sealing a chest wound on three sides only will allow air to escape and help prevent a tension pneumothorax. It is important to note that a tension pneumothorax is not limited to open chest wounds. Activating the EMS system immediately is crucial.

SIGNS AND SYMPTOMS Signs of a pneumothorax are severe chest pain, difficulty breathing, cyanosis (bluish discoloration of the skin), unequal expansion of the right and left sides of the chest upon inhalation, and the absence of breathing sounds on the side of the collapsed lung.

TREATMENT Call EMS immediately. Apply an occlusive dressing over any open chest wound that may allow air to enter the chest. An occlusive dressing will help to keep the pneumothorax from enlarging. Reassure the athlete so that breathing can be kept mode-rate and controlled. Treat for shock and monitor vital signs until EMS personnel arrive.

REHABILITATION After the athlete has recovered, no further management should be necessary. Additional padding may be required to help deflect any blunt trauma that may occur, especially in contact sports.

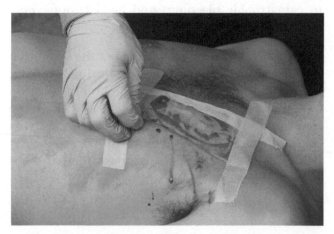

Figure 22–11 A sucking chest wound is covered with an occlusive dressing; three sides are secured and one side is left open as a vent.

Hemopneumothorax

This condition, also known as a hemothorax, can occur with both open and closed chest injuries, and often accompanies a pneumothorax. In a **hemopneumothorax**, blood accumulates in the pleural space between the chest wall and the lung. This compromises the lungs' ability to operate, as does a pneumothorax. With the loss of blood, the certified athletic trainer must be concerned about the onset of shock.

SIGNS AND SYMPTOMS Signs and Symptoms of this injury are similar to those of a pneumothorax.

TREATMENT Activate the EMS system immediately. Treat for shock and monitor vital signs until medical help arrives.

REHABILITATION Physician's orders must be followed as to the type and intensity of future contact permitted in sports. Additional chest protection and padding will be required to limit exposure in contact sports.

Pulmonary Contusions

A *pulmonary contusion* is a bruise on the lung caused by a direct blow from an object or a competitor. This causes bleeding in the lung tissue, which leads to **edema** (swelling), hemorrhaging, and increased lung secretions. A collision or impact by another player, piece of equipment, or the ground could cause a pulmonary contusion.

SIGNS AND SYMPTOMS About 24 to 48 hours after the injury occurred, the athlete may experience shortness of breath, chest pain, coughing, **hemoptysis** (coughing up blood), and **rales** (a crackling sound to the breathing).

TREATMENT If a pulmonary contusion is suspected, the athlete should be transported to a hospital immediately and be closely monitored for shock.

REHABILITATION The athlete can return to participation pursuant to physician's orders. In football, shoulder pads should be checked to be certain the chest area is properly covered. A specially padded "flak jacket" worn under the shoulder pads will provide additional protection for this area of the chest.

Blows to the Solar Plexus

The most common intra-abdominal injury is a blow to the **celiac plexus** (solar plexus). This is commonly known as "having the wind knocked out." This network of nerves lies deep in the upper middle region of the abdomen. A blow to this area can cause transitory paralysis of the diaphragm. A blow to the upper middle region of the abdomen, whether from another athlete or hitting the ground when falling, can cause this condition.

SIGNS AND SYMPTOMS Although the athlete may become very anxious because of perceived inability to breathe, this injury is usually of short duration, and no treatment is necessary. The condition responds to a few moments of rest and reassurance.

TREATMENT Reassure the athlete. Loosen belts and any constricting clothing. This is a transitory condition that resolves quickly. If complete recovery does not occur within minutes, or if pain, tenderness, and signs of shock appear, intra-abdominal injury should be suspected and the athlete taken to the hospital at once.

REHABILITATION The athlete should be cleared to continue participation as soon as breathing has returned to normal and no further injuries are suspected or seen.

FUN FACTS

Physician Henry Heimlich's procedure for saving a choking victim was developed in the mid-1970s and made his name a household word. By applying sudden pressure to the abdomen by various means, a rescuer can force air upward through the windpipe, thereby dislodging the obstruction and reopening the airway. This is the *Heimlich maneuver.*

Hyperventilation

Hyperventilation is usually brought on by anxiety stress, or hysteria. Hyperventilation involves breathing at a rate faster than required for the proper exchange of oxygen and carbon dioxide.

SIGNS AND SYMPTOMS Carbon dioxide is depleted from the blood, causing chest pain, dizziness, and a numbing sensation of the lips, fingers, and toes. If hyperventilation is not controlled, the athlete will eventually lose consciousness. Loss of consciousness is the body's safety mechanism to return the athlete's vital signs to normal.

TREATMENT Talk in a calm, reassuring manner to encourage the athlete to relax and regulate breathing to a slower, controlled pace. Try to get the athlete to talk, as this will also help control the rate of respiration. If the athlete loses consciousness, contact EMS. Normally, the athlete will regain consciousness very quickly.

If the athlete has a history of hyperventilation, the certified athletic trainer should counsel the athlete about ways to prevent future attacks.

REHABILITATION The athlete may return to competition or practice as soon as the condition is resolved.

Side Stitches

Side stitches can occur during vigorous exercise such as running. They seem to occur more commonly in novice exercisers who have not yet established proper pacing, and whose breathing tends to be quick and shallow (Figure 22–13). About 30% of all runners will experience side stitches at some point.

SIGNS AND SYMPTOMS The pain of a side stitch usually occurs just under the ribs, often while the athlete is running. Some causes of side stitches include an unconditioned diaphragm, food allergies, intestinal gas, or having eaten just before running. Running a greater distance than usual, or at a faster pace than usual, may also cause side stitches.

The *diaphragm* is a muscle that separates the chest cavity from the abdomen. It moves down

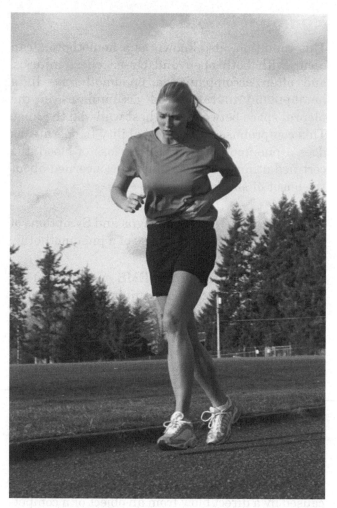

Figure 22–13 Side stitches are painful and usually occur on the right side of the abdomen.

upon inhalation and up upon exhalation. When it is subject to more or faster exercise than it is accustomed to, it can "cramp" and cause pain. Side stitches seem to occur most often on the right side of the body. It is possible that the liver alters the motion of the diaphragm more on that side because of its larger right lobe.

TREATMENT There are many theories as to the best way to alleviate side stitches. Some of these include stretching, relaxing, altering one's breathing patterns, and walking briskly rather than running. What works with one athlete may not work with another.

REHABILITATION The athlete should do a warmup that gradually increases running speed. Taking deep, full breaths while running allows the

KEY CONCEPT

Chest injuries in athletics, which are usually the result of a direct blow to the area, include:

- Rib contusions, which is bruising of the intercostal muscles between the ribs. The area should be iced for 20 minutes every 3 to 4 hours. The athlete must be closely monitored for signs of a more serious injury or shock.

- Rib fracture, which is the breakage of one or more ribs. Breaks in more than one consecutive rib can result in a flail chest. Immediate medical treatment must be sought, as the risk of additional injury is high.

- Chest contusion, which is bruising of the chest wall. The affected area should be iced for 20 minutes every 3 to 4 hours for 24 to 72 hours. The athlete should be monitored for additional injury and shock.

- Myocardial contusion, which is bruising of the heart muscle and results from a direct and forceful blow to the middle chest area. It can also result in aortic rupture if the force is great enough to tear or sever the aorta. EMS must be activated.

- Sudden death syndrome, which is usually the result of an unknown cardiac abnormality. Provide CPR and activate EMS.

- Pneumothorax, an injury in which air enters the pleural cavity between the chest wall and the lung and causes the lung to collapse. If unrecognized, this can progress to a tension pneumothorax, in which pressure is exerted on the heart and the heart and trachea are pushed away from center. EMS must be activated.

- Hemopneumothorax, which is similar to a pneumothorax except that blood rather than air enters the pleural space. As with a pneumothorax, EMS must be activated.

- Pulmonary contusions, which are bruises to the area or structures of the lungs. EMS must be activated.

- Solar plexus injury ("having the wind knocked out"), which occurs when a blow to the middle region of the chest affects the nerves in the solar plexus. This condition usually resolves itself in minutes.

(continued)

(continued)

- **Hyperventilation, meaning breathing too fast for normal respiratory processes. treatment should be aimed at calming and relaxing the athlete and encouraging slower breathing.**
- **Side stitches, which occur during vigorous exercise and result in pain under the ribs. Treatments vary, and not all treatments work with all athletes. Proper training and conditioning can help prevent side stitches from occurring.**

diaphragm to fully lower and reduces the stress on it. If the athlete takes many shallow breaths when exercising or running, the diaphragm remains consistently high and never lowers enough to relax. The diaphragm becomes stressed, and a "stitch" may result. Stretching, proper hydration, and avoiding eating one hour prior to running or exercise may also help to control side stitches.

INJURY PREVENTION FOR THE CHEST

Injury prevention begins with proper equipment and education. Good, well-maintained, equipment that fits properly will reduce the chance of injuries to the chest. Athletes who are at higher risk of chest injuries, because of the nature of their sport or the positions they play, should wear additional protection. An example is the quarterback who may get hit while his arm is elevated. He is at greater risk because of his inability to protect himself in this position. Additional padding can help to prevent injuries.

Education can also help minimize the risk of trauma to the chest. Athletes need to be trained on how to protect themselves while participating in contact sports. Use of proper techniques help the athlete avoid situations that could cause injury.

THE ABDOMINOPELVIC CAVITY

The **abdominopelvic cavity** is actually one large cavity, with no separation between the abdomen and pelvis. To avoid confusion, the areas of this cavity are usually referred to separately as the abdominal cavity and the pelvic cavity. The **abdominal cavity** contains the stomach, liver, gallbladder, pancreas, spleen, small intestine, appendix, and part of the large intestine. The kidneys are close to but behind the abdominal cavity. The urinary bladder, reproductive organs, rectum, remainder of the large intestine, and appendix are in the **pelvic cavity**.

PROTECTION OF THE ABDOMINAL ORGANS

The abdominal area is vulnerable to injury during most athletic activities, especially contact sports. The muscular abdominal wall is the area most commonly involved.

Athletic injuries to the contents of the abdominal cavity occur infrequently. The musculature of the abdominal wall provides the intra-abdominal viscera adequate protection from most injuries. Serious athletic injuries to the intra-abdominal contents do occur, though, and can become life threatening. These injuries, usually associated with contact or collision sports, occur as the result of some type of direct trauma to the abdomen or lower back. The structures most often associated with serious intra-abdominal injuries are the solid organs, such as the kidneys, spleen, and liver—all of which have rich blood supplies.

Intra-abdominal conditions can develop quickly. The certified athletic trainer must be alert to the signs and symptoms, such as shock, that may indicate possible intra-abdominal injury.

ORGANS OF THE ABDOMINOPELVIC CAVITY

Many of the body's organs are housed within the abdominopelvic cavity. Each has at least one specific function.

Stomach

The **stomach** is found in the upper part of the abdominal cavity, just to the left of and below the diaphragm. Its shape and position are determined by several factors: the amount of food contained within the stomach, the stage of digestion, the position of the person's body, and the pressure exerted on the stomach from the intestines below.

The stomach is divided into three portions: the upper part or *fundus;* the middle section, called the *body* or *greater curvature;* and the lower portion, called the *pylorus.* The opening from the esophagus into the stomach is through a circle of muscle, called the **cardiac sphincter**, which controls passage of food into the stomach. It is called the cardiac sphincter because of its proximity to the heart. Toward the other end of the stomach lies the **pyloric sphincter** valve, which regulates entrance of food into the **duodenum** (the first part of the small intestine) (Figure 22–14).

The stomach wall consists of four layers: mucous, submucous, muscular, and serous.

1. The mucous coat, the thick, innermost layer, is made up of small gastric glands embedded in connective tissue. When the stomach is not distended with food, the gastric mucosa is thrown into folds called *rugae.*

2. The submucosa coat is made of loose areolar connective tissue.

3. The muscular coat consists of three layers of smooth muscle: the outer, longitudinal layer; a middle, circular layer; and an inner, oblique layer. These muscles help the stomach perform peristalsis, which pushes food into the small intestine.

4. The serosa is the thick outer layer covering the stomach. It is continuous with the peritoneum. The serosa and peritoneum meet at certain points, surrounding the organs around the stomach and holding them in a kind of sling.

Small Intestine

The small intestine has the same four layers as the stomach: the mucosa, submucosa, muscle layer, and serosa (Figure 22–15).

The final preparation of food to be absorbed occurs in the small intestine. This coiled portion of the alimentary canal can be as long as 20 feet. The small intestine is divided into three sections: the duodenum, the **jejunum**, and the **ileum**. The small intestine is held in place by the mesentery. The small intestine lining secretes digestive juices and is covered with villi that absorb the end products of digestion (Figure 22–16).

The first segment of the small intestine is the duodenum. This 12-inch structure curves around the head of the pancreas. A few inches into the duodenum is the ampulla of Vater, which is the site where the pancreatic duct and the common bile duct of the liver enter. The pancreatic duct empties the digestive juices of the pancreas. The common bile duct empties bile from the liver. The next section of the small intestine is the jejunum, which is about 8 feet long, and the ileum, which is 10 to 12 feet long.

Absorption is possible because the lining of the small intestine is not smooth. It is covered with millions of tiny projections called **villi**. Each microscopic villus contains a network of blood and lymph capillaries (Figure 22–16). The digested portion of food passes through the villi into the bloodstream and on to the body cells. The indigestible portion passes to the large intestine.

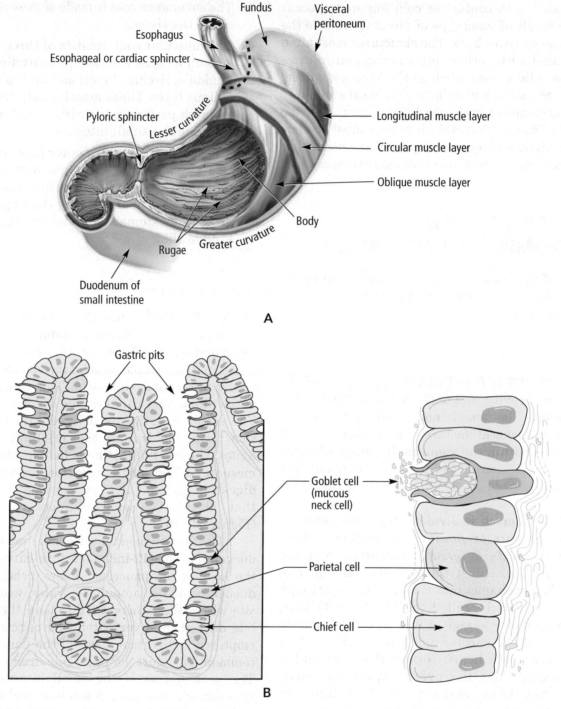

Figure 22–14 (A) Parts of the stomach. (B) The three types of gastric gland cells making up the gastric glands that line the stomach.

Pancreas

The pancreas is a feather-shaped organ located behind the stomach (Figure 22–17). It functions both as an exocrine gland, meaning it has a duct that carries away its secretions, and as an endocrine gland, meaning it is ductless and the secretions are emptied directly into the bloodstream. The digestive juices are carried by the pancreatic duct into the duodenum, at the sphincter of Oddi (Figure 22-17).

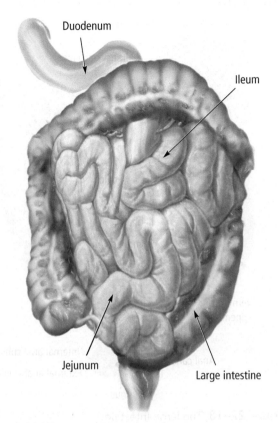

Figure 22–15 The small intestine.

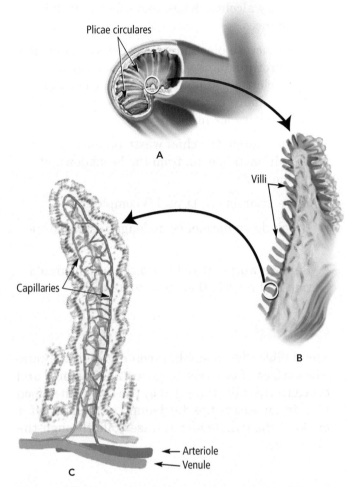

Figure 22–16 Structures of absorption in the small intestine. (A) Plicae circulares. (B) Villi. (C) Capillaries.

Liver

The liver is the largest organ in the body. It is located below the diaphragm, in the upper right quadrant of the abdomen (Figure 22–17). The portal vein carries the products of digestion from the small intestine to the liver. Some of the liver's many functions are as follows:

- Manufacture bile, a yellow to green fluid that is necessary for the digestion of fat. About 800 to 1,000 cc of bile are produced daily. Bile contains bile salts, bile pigments (mainly **bilirubin**, which comes from breakdown of the hemoglobin molecule), cholesterol, phospholipids, and some electrolytes. The **hepatic duct** from the liver joins with the **cystic duct** of the gallbladder to form the **common bile duct**, which carries the bile to the duodenum. If this duct is blocked, bile may enter the bloodstream and cause **jaundice**, which gives the skin and sclera of the eyes a yellowish color.

- Produce and store glucose in the form of **glycogen**.

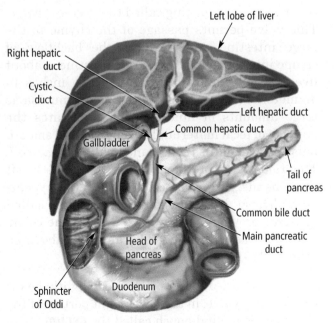

Figure 22–17 Liver, gallbladder, and pancreas.

- Detoxify alcohol, drugs, and other harmful substances.

- Manufacture blood proteins such as fibrinogen and prothrombin, which are necessary for blood clotting; albumin, which is needed for fluid balance in the cells; and globulin, which is necessary for immunity.

- Prepare urea, the chief waste product of protein metabolism, from the breakdown of amino acids.

- Store vitamins A, D, and B complex.

- Break down hormones no longer useful to the body.

- Remove worn-out red blood cells from circulation and recycle their iron content.

Gallbladder

The **gallbladder**, a small, green organ in the inferior surface of the liver (Figure 22–17), stores and concentrates bile unneeded by the body. When food high in fat enters the duodenum, at the sphincter of Oddi, the gallbladder releases bile through the cystic duct.

Large Intestine

The ileum empties its intestinal chyme (semiliquid food) into the side wall of the large intestine through an opening called the *ileocecal valve*. This valve permits passage of the chyme to the large intestine and prevents the backflow of chyme into the ileum. The large intestine is about five feet long and approximately two inches in diameter. The secretion of the colon mucosa is large amounts of mucus, which lubricates the passage of fecal material. The longitudinal smooth muscle layer is in three bands called *tenae coli*. The remainder of the colon is gathered to fit these bands, giving the colon a puckered appearance. These little puckers or pockets, called *haustra*, provide more surface area in the colon. The **colon**, as it is also called, frames the abdomen (Figure 22–18).

CECUM AND APPENDIX Located slightly below the ileocecal valve, in the lower right portion of the abdomen, is a blind pouch called the **cecum**.

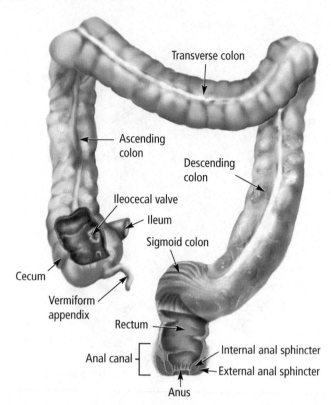

Figure 22–18 The large intestine.

To the lower left of the cecum is the **vermiform appendix**. The appendix is a finger-like projection protruding into the abdominal cavity (see Figure 22–18). It has no digestive function. Appendicitis, is an inflammation of the appendix, is a very painful condition that requires immediate medical care.

ASCENDING, TRANSVERSE, AND DESCENDING COLON The colon continues upward, along the right side of the abdominal cavity, to the underside of the liver (hepatic flexure), forming the **ascending colon**. Then it veers to the left across the abdominal cavity, to a point below the spleen (splenic flexure), forming the **transverse colon**. The **descending colon** travels down from the splenic flexure on the left side of the abdominal cavity. As the descending colon reaches the left iliac region, it enters the pelvis in an S-shaped bend. This section, known as the **sigmoid colon**, extends some seven or eight inches as the **rectum**. The rectum opens into the anus (see Figure 22–18).

Kidneys

The kidneys are bean-shaped organs resting high against the dorsal wall of the abdominal cavity; they lie on either side of the vertebral column, between the peritoneum and the back muscles. Because the kidneys are located behind the peritoneum, they are said to be **retroperitoneal**. They are positioned between the twelfth thoracic and the third lumbar vertebrae. The right kidney is situated slightly lower than the left because of the large area occupied by the liver.

Each kidney and its blood vessels are enclosed within a mass of fat tissue called the *adipose capsule*. In turn, both kidneys and adipose capsules are covered by a tough, fibrous tissue called the **renal fascia**.

There is an indentation along the concave medial border of the kidney called the **hilum**. The hilum is a passageway for the lymph vessels, nerves, renal artery and vein, and the ureter. At the hilum the fibrous capsule continues downward, forming the outer layer of the ureter. Cutting the kidney in half lengthwise reveals its internal structure. The upper end of each ureter flares into a funnel-shaped structure known as the **renal pelvis** (Figure 22–19).

The kidneys have the potential to work harder than they actually do. Under ordinary circumstances, only a portion of the nephron (the functional unit of the kidney) is used. Should one kidney not function, or have to be removed, more nephrons and tubules open up in the second kidney to take over the work of the nonfunctioning or missing kidney.

MEDULLA AND CORTEX The kidney is divided into two layers: an outer, granular layer, the **cortex**, and an inner, striated layer, the **medulla**. The medulla is red and consists of radially striated cones called the *renal pyramids*. The base of each renal pyramid faces the cortex, while its apex (*renal papilla*) empties into cup-like cavities called *calyces*. These, in turn, empty into the renal pelvis.

The cortex is reddish brown and consists of millions of microscopic functional units of the kidney called *nephrons*. Cortical tissue is interspersed between renal pyramids, separating and supporting them. These interpyramidal cortical supports are the *renal columns*. The renal columns

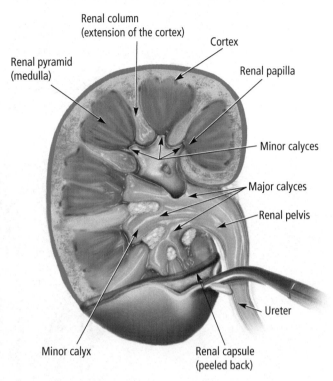

Figure 22–19 Structures of the kidney.

and the renal pyramids alternate with one another (Figure 22–19).

NEPHRON The **nephron** is the basic structural and functional unit of the kidney. The nephron is located mostly within the cortex, with only a small, tubular portion in the medulla. Each kidney has more than 1 million nephrons, which altogether comprise 140 miles of filters and tubes.

A nephron begins with the **afferent arteriole**, which carries blood from the renal artery. The afferent arteriole enters a double-walled, hollow capsule, the **Bowman's capsule** (named for Sir William Bowman [1816–1892], English anatomist). Within the capsule the afferent arteriole finely divides, forming a knotty ball called the **glomerulus**, which contains some 50 separate capillaries. The combination of the Bowman's capsule and the glomerulus is known as the *renal corpuscle*. The Bowman's capsule sends off a highly convoluted (twisted) tubular branch, the **proximal convoluted tubule**.

The proximal convoluted tubule descends into the medulla to form the **loop of Henle**. In Figure 22–20, observe that the loop of Henle has a

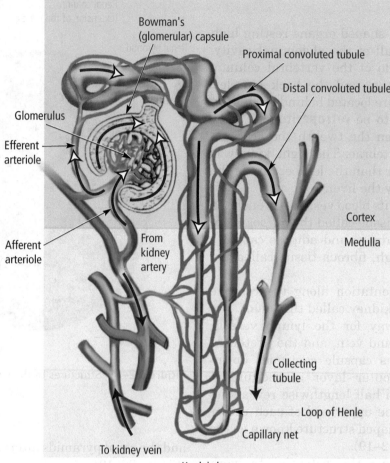

Figure 22–20 Structures of the nephron.

straight, descending limb, a loop, and a straight ascending limb. When the ascending limb of Henle's loop returns to the cortex, it turns into the **distal convoluted tubule**. Eventually this convoluted tubule opens into a larger, straight vessel known as the **collecting tubule**. Several distal convoluted tubules join to form this single straight collecting tubule. The collecting tubule empties into the renal pelvis, then into the ureter.

As Figure 22–20 shows, the walls of the renal tubules are surrounded by capillaries. After the afferent arteriole branches out to form the glomerulus, it leaves the Bowman's capsule as the **efferent arteriole**. The efferent arteriole branches to form the peritubular capillaries surrounding the renal tubules. All of these capillaries eventually join together to form a small branch of the renal vein, which carries blood from the kidney.

FUN FACTS
Each kidney has more than 1 million nephrons, which altogether comprise 140 miles of filters and tubes.

URETERS Urine passes from the kidneys' collecting tubules into the renal pelvis, down the ureter, into the urinary bladder. There are two **ureters** (one from each kidney) carrying urine from the kidneys to the urinary bladder. They are long, narrow tubes, less than 1/4 inch wide and 10 to 12 inches long. Mucous membrane lines both renal pelves and the ureters. Beneath the mucous membrane lining of the ureters are smooth muscle fibers. When these muscles contract, peristalsis is initiated, pushing urine down the ureter into the urinary bladder.

Urinary Bladder

The **urinary bladder**, a hollow, muscular organ made of elastic fibers and involuntary muscle, acts as a reservoir, storing the urine until about 1 pint (500 mL) is accumulated. The bladder then becomes uncomfortable and must be emptied. Emptying the bladder, or voiding, takes place by muscular contractions of the bladder that are involuntary, although they can be controlled to some extent through the nervous system. Contraction of the bladder muscles forces the urine through a narrow canal, the **urethra**, which extends to the outside opening, the **urinary meatus**.

Terms Referring to Regions in the Abdominopelvic Cavity

To locate the abdominal and pelvic organs more easily, anatomists have subdivided the abdominopelvic cavity into nine regions (Figure 22–21), located in the upper, middle, and lower parts of the abdomen:

- The upper or **epigastric region** is located just below the sternum (breastbone), and the right hypochondriac and left hypochondriac regions are located below the ribs.

- The middle or **umbilical area** is located around the navel or umbilicus, and the right lumbar

and left lumbar regions extend from anterior to posterior. (Pain may refer from this area to the back.)

- The lower or **hypogastric region**, also referred to as the *pubic area;* the left iliac and right iliac may also be called the left and right *inguinal areas.*

ABDOMINAL INJURIES

Collision sports such as football and hockey can produce a host of injuries. The usual musculoskeletal injuries are identified quite easily by a certified athletic trainer, but internal injuries are not as obvious. Thus, abdominal injuries, even when mild, must be treated carefully.

Abdominal injuries in athletics are rare. However, when they do happen they can be life threatening. A direct blow to the abdomen can affect any number of organs. Strong abdominal musculature is good protection against blows to the abdomen, but sometimes it is not enough.

Organs in the abdomen are either solid or hollow. The stomach, intestines, and bladder are all hollow organs. They are seldom injured because the hollow organs are usually not full when an athlete is competing, thus lessening the chance of injury because they can "give" a bit if struck.

Figure 22–21 The nine regions of the abdomen.

Right hypochondriac region — Epigastric region — Left hypochondriac region — Umbilical region — Right lumbar region — Left lumbar region — Right iliac region (inguinal) — Hypogastric region (pubic area) — Left iliac region (inguinal)

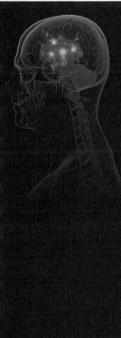

KEY CONCEPT

Abdominal injuries in athletics are rare. However, injuries to the abdomen can affect a number of organs and have the potential to be life threatening if they go unrecognized. Even mild injuries must be monitored and treated carefully. The solid organs found within the abdominal cavity, when damaged, will bleed profusely and may cause life-threatening hemorrhage.

Solid organs are a different story. Organs such as the liver, spleen, and kidneys are particularly susceptible to abdominal blows. Because of their rich blood supplies, injuries to the solid organs can cause severe hemorrhage.

Kidney Contusion

Contusions to the kidney are uncommon in athletics, but they do occur. The certified athletic trainer should suspect a **kidney contusion** when any athlete sustains a violent blow to the upper posterior abdominal wall. This can occur in contact sports such as football and hockey, and occasionally in other sports.

SIGNS AND SYMPTOMS An athlete who has sustained a kidney contusion may have pain located high in the posterior abdomen and radiating into the lower abdominal region. He or she may show signs of shock, nausea, vomiting, rigidity of the back muscles, and **hematuria** (blood in the urine).

TREATMENT An athlete with a suspected kidney contusion must be taken to the hospital immediately for diagnosis and observation.

REHABILITATION The athlete's physician may require a two- to four-week recuperation period before activity can be resumed, depending on the severity of the injury. In some cases the athlete will be restricted for the remainder of the season.

Liver Contusion

The liver, which lies just beneath the ribs on the right, is the largest solid organ in the abdomen. The liver is a large mass of blood vessels and cells packed tightly together. Blood flow to the liver is very high, because blood that is pumped from the abdomen passes through the liver before it returns to the heart. An injury to the liver is a probable life-threatening injury that demands immediate medical attention.

Liver contusions from athletics are not common. However, a hard blow to the right side of the ribcage can tear or contuse the liver.

SIGNS AND SYMPTOMS Liver contusions can cause severe bleeding and shock. This requires immediate surgery for repair. An injury to the liver commonly produces a referred pain just below the right scapula, right shoulder, and substernal area; the pain may also radiate to the left side of the chest.

TREATMENT The EMS system must be activated immediately for a liver contusion, a life-threatening injury. Treat for shock and reassure the athlete until help arrives.

REHABILITATION The athlete must follow physician's instructions as to if and when he or she can return to participation.

Injuries to the Spleen

The **spleen** is a large mass of lymphatic tissue found behind the lower ribs on the left side of the abdomen, slightly behind and to the left of the stomach. It acts as a blood filter and helps launch the body's immune system.

The spleen has the unique ability to splint itself after an injury, only to rupture later with little or no apparent traumatic cause. A ruptured spleen may radiate pain to the left shoulder and arm. This referred pain can complicate the evaluation of an abdominal injury. Spleen injuries are responsible for many deaths each year, so any suspected injury to this area is a medical emergency. A person can live without the spleen, although its removal increases the risk of bloodstream infection.

The spleen is the organ of the abdominal region most commonly injured. Injury to the spleen normally results from a blow to the left upper quadrant, the lower left ribcage, or the left side of the back (Figure 22–22).

SIGNS AND SYMPTOMS Pain will be located in the upper-left quadrant of the body. Referred pain may be felt in the left shoulder, radiating one-third of the way down the left arm. This referred pain is called **Kehr's sign**. The athlete may go into shock and have low blood pressure.

TREATMENT The medical staff must activate the EMS system for immediate transportation to the hospital. The athlete should be treated for shock. Calm and reassure the athlete until help arrives.

REHABILITATION The athlete must follow a physician's instructions as to if and when he or she can return to participation. Thereafter, additional padding to protect the upper and lower quadrants of the body may be helpful.

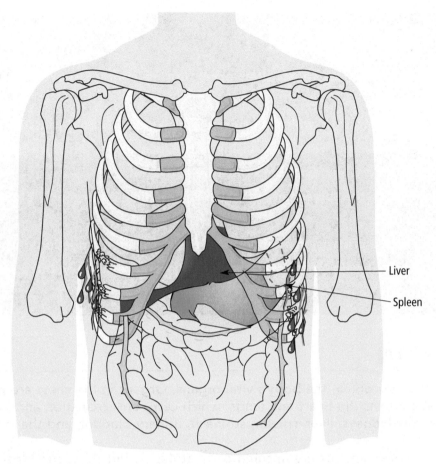

Figure 22–22 Lower rib fractures can result in injury to the liver or spleen.

Hernias

The National Center for Health Statistics estimates that about 5 million people in the United States have abdominal hernias (see the NCHS website at http://www.cdc.gov/nchs/ for many interesting health facts and statistics). A **hernia** is a protrusion of abdominal tissue through a portion of the abdominal wall. Inguinal (groin) hernias, which occur most often in men, and femoral hernias, which most often occur in women, are the prevalent types. Hernias can be congenital or occur as a result of activity, such as athletics.

Hernias can be caused by a chronic cough, straining to lift heavy objects, persistent sneezing, straining during bowel movements or urination, and obesity. Participating in athletics does not increase the risk of developing an abdominal hernia.

SIGNS AND SYMPTOMS A hernia usually first becomes noticeable as a bulge somewhere in the abdomen or pelvic area, or in the scrotum for men.

If the bulge is reducible, it may enlarge when the person is standing and become smaller when he or she lies down. The changes in the size of a hernia are due to the increased gravitational pressure on the abdominal wall when the person is standing. A hernia may cause sharp or dull pain that worsens when having a bowel movement, during urination, or while lifting a heavy object. The pain might worsen as the day progresses, especially after long periods of standing, because of gravitational pressure.

TREATMENT Most hernias eventually require surgery. Hernias normally are not emergency situations, but the athlete should see a physician as soon as possible. If not treated, a hernia can worsen over time, sometimes to the point that emergency medical treatment is required.

REHABILITATION The athlete can return to play only with a physician's consent. Use of a commercial support for a hernia may be considered as a preventative measure to avoid recurrence.

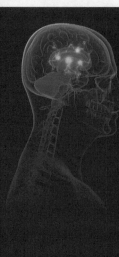

KEY CONCEPT

Abdominal injuries most often occur during contact sports. These injuries include:

- Kidney contusion, which is bruising of the kidneys. **EMS** must be activated.
- Liver contusion, which is bruising of the liver and is uncommon. This can cause severe bleeding. **EMS** must be activated.
- Injuries to the spleen, any of which is a medical emergency. **EMS** must be activated.
- Hernias, a protrusion of abdominal tissue through a portion of the abdominal wall. Most hernias eventually require surgery, but a hernia is not normally an emergency.

CONCLUSION

The chest and abdomen contain the body's vital organs. Organs in the chest are protected by the ribcage. The chest contains the heart and lungs, which carry out circulation and respiration; the abdomen contains the kidneys, liver, spleen, stomach, urinary bladder, and the intestines, among other organs.

Chest and abdominal injuries are uncommon in athletics, but do occur. Most of the internal organs are very vascular and can bleed profusely if injured. Proper recognition and treatment of these injuries are vital to the health and well-being of the athlete.

REVIEW QUESTIONS

1. What are the organs of the thoracic and abdominal cavities?
2. What is the difference between true ribs and false ribs?
3. Explain external and internal respiration.
4. Why is the right lung larger than the left lung?
5. What is the normal rate of respiration for an adult?
6. How is respiration dependent on chemical factors in the blood?
7. What is the significance of thoracic and abdominal injuries?
8. Why would a flail chest be considered life threatening?
9. What is the pleural space?
10. Explain sudden death syndrome in athletics.
11. Explain the difference between a pneumothorax, tension pneumothorax, and hemopneumothorax.
12. How does the treatment for a pneumothorax and a tension pneumothorax differ?
13. Have you ever had a blow to your celiac plexus? If so, what did it feel like? If not, ask someone who has and report his or her description.
14. What is the first aid for hyperventilation?
15. Why do side stitches differ from one athlete to another?

16. What is the difference between the small and large intestine?
17. Explain where the liver and kidneys are located.
18. Explain where the spleen is located.
19. What is Kehr's sign?
20. Explain what a hernia is and how it is treated.

PROJECTS AND ACTIVITIES

1. Where is the EMS location closest to your school? How many miles is it from your school to this location? How long do you think it would take EMS to arrive on the scene of a medical emergency at your school? Ask the school nurse or certified athletic trainer for specific time estimates.
2. Using the Internet, research sudden death syndrome in athletes. Report your findings to the class.
3. Talk with the cross-country or track coach at your school about side stitches. Ask how he or she deals with this condition. Is the coach's method different from the methods explained in this chapter? How do you explain the differences in technique?
4. If an athlete has to have the spleen removed because of an injury, will he or she live a normal life? Research this topic and report your findings.
5. If an athlete has only one kidney genetically or because of injury or disease, can he or she continue to play contact sports? Why?
6. Pick one of the chest or abdominal injuries explained in this chapter. Write a research paper on this topic. This paper should be detailed and reflect a thorough understanding of this condition.
7. Talk with the certified athletic trainer at your school about thoracic and abdominal injuries. Ask if he or she carries or uses any special equipment to help them recognize these injuries.

LEARNING LINKS

- Search for the Internet for further information on various chest and abdominal injuries that result from athletic trauma on the Internet. Learn more about their Signs and Symptoms, and how to manage them.

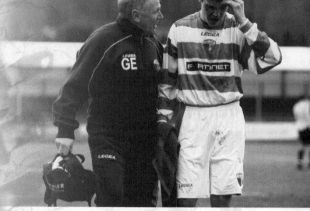
Rosli Othman/Shutterstock.com.

CHAPTER 23

The Head and Face

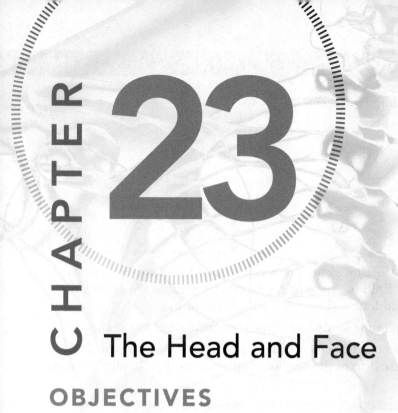

OBJECTIVES

Upon completion of this chapter, the reader should be able to:

- Describe the anatomy of the head and face
- Explain what sports are responsible for the majority of eye injuries
- Discuss common injuries to the head, face, teeth, eyes, nose, ears, and scalp
- Describe how facial injuries can be prevented
- Explain the treatment for epistaxis
- Explain various injuries of the brain that a person might suffer as a result of athletic participation
- Explain the signs and symptoms of a concussion
- Explain how concussions can be prevented
- Demonstrate on-field management and assessment of concussions

KEY TERMS

antegrade amnesia *A loss of memory for events that occur immediately after the injury.*

anterior chamber *The space between the cornea and the iris.*

anvil *The second of the three bones in the middle ear; also known as the incus.*

aphasia *Loss of speech or comprehension.*

aqueous humor *The watery fluid found in the anterior and posterior chambers of the eye.*

arachnoid *The web-like middle protective membrane covering the brain and spinal cord.*

auricle *The visible part of the ear; consists of the pinna; also called the outer ear.*

AVPU *A method of determining level of consciousness.*

KEY TERMS CONTINUED

baseline testing *A test that allows a pre-test to be done prior to participation. This allows for a "baseline" of information to be available in case of a concussion. Comparing the two can help with assessment and diagnosis.*

brainstem *The lowest part of the brain, which merges with the spinal cord.*

cauliflower ear *Deformity of the ear caused by destruction of the underlying cartilage of the outer ear.*

cerebellum *The part of the brain that controls muscular coordination and complex actions.*

cerebral concussion *Injury to the brain from a forceful impact causing temporary dysfunction.*

cerebral contusion *Bruising or laceration of the brain tissues from contact of the skull with underlying tissues.*

cerebrospinal fluid (CSF) *A clear, colorless fluid that contains small quantities of glucose and protein. Cerebrospinal fluid fills the ventricles of the brain and the central canal of the spinal cord.*

cerebrum *The largest and most highly evolved part of the brain.*

choroid coat *The middle layer of the eye.*

ciliary body *The part of the choroid body in the eye from which the ligaments that suspend the lens extend.*

cochlea *Spiral cavity within the inner ear that contains the hearing sensory.*

concussion *A more serious form of closed head injury characterized by one or more of the following: loss of consciousness, amnesia, seizure, or a change in mental state.*

cones *Structures of the eye responsible for color vision.*

conjunctiva *The outermost layer of the eye; covers the sclera.*

conjunctivitis *Infection of the outermost layer of the eye; also known as pink eye.*

contrecoup *Mechanism of injury in which the brain rebounds off the other side of the skull after an initial impact.*

cornea *A circular, clear area in front of the sclerotic coat.*

corneal abrasion *A scratch or small cut of the cornea of the eye.*

cranium *The bony skull.*

dura mater *The outermost membrane covering the brain and spinal cord.*

ear canal *The passageway for sound in the ear.*

eardrum *The tympanic membrane between the ear canal and the cavity of the middle ear.*

epidural hematoma *A collection of blood between the skull and the dura mater.*

epistaxis *Nosebleed.*

eustachian tube *The passageway from the throat to the middle ear; equalizes the pressure in the middle ear.*

extrinsic eye muscles *The muscles responsible for moving the eye within the orbital socket.*

foramen magnum *Large opening at the base of the skull through which the spinal cord passes.*

fovea centralis *The structure of the eye that contains the cones for color vision.*

frontal bone *The strong, anteriormost bone in the skull that constitutes the forehead.*

KEY TERMS CONTINUED

Glasgow Coma Scale (GCS) *A standard guide used to rate various states of consciousness.*

hammer *The first of the three bones in the middle ear; also known as the malleus.*

hard palate *The front portion of the roof of the mouth.*

hyphema *A buildup of blood in the anterior chamber of the eye.*

incus *The second of the three bones in the middle ear; also known as the anvil.*

inner ear *An extremely intricate series of structures contained deep within the bones of the skull; consists of the cochlea, the semicircular canals, and two additional organs involved with balance.*

intracranial hematoma *Pooling of blood because of damage to blood vessels within the brain.*

intrinsic eye muscles *The muscles that help the iris control the amount of light entering the pupil.*

iris *The colored, muscular layer surrounding the pupil in the eye.*

labyrinth *A maze of winding passageways found in the ear.*

lens *A crystal structure in the eye that refracts light rays.*

malleus *The first of the three bones in the middle ear; also known as the hammer.*

mandible *The bone of the lower jaw.*

mastoid sinus *An air-filled space within the mastoid process of the temporal bone behind the ears.*

maxilla *The bone of the upper jaw.*

meatus *An opening; in this instance, the opening to the ear canal.*

meninges *Protective membranes covering the brain and spinal cord.*

middle ear *A small cavity between the eardrum and the inner ear.*

occipital bone *The most posterior bone of the skull.*

optic disc *An area of the eye devoid of visual reception; also known as the blind spot.*

orbit *The deep, bony socket that houses the eye.*

ossicle *Any small bone; here, referring to the three small bones of the ear.*

outer ear *The visible part of the ear; consists of the pinna; also called the auricle.*

parietal bone *The largest of the bones of the skull.*

pia mater *The innermost membrane covering the spinal cord and brain.*

pinna *Part of the outer ear.*

postconcussion syndrome *A condition that may develop following a concussion; exhibited by persistent headache, dizziness, fatigue, irritability, and impaired memory or lack of concentration.*

posterior chamber *The space between the iris and the lens.*

pupil *The opening in the iris of the eye that permits passage of light.*

pupillary dilation *Widening of the pupils due to increased intracranial pressure compressing the third cranial nerve.*

retina *The innermost layer of the eye, containing the rods and cones.*

retrograde amnesia *A loss of memory for events that occurred before the injury.*

KEY TERMS CONTINUED

rods *Cells in the retina that are sensitive to dim light.*

sclera *The tough, white, external coating of the eye.*

secondary impact syndrome (SIS) *Rapid swelling and herniation of the brain after a second head injury that occurs before the first injury has resolved.*

semicircular canal *Structures in the inner ear involved with equilibrium.*

soft palate *The back portion of the roof of the mouth.*

stapes *The third of the three bones found in the middle ear; also known as the stirrup.*

stirrup *The third of the three bones found in the middle ear; also known as the stapes.*

sty *Infection of a gland along the eyelid.*

subdural hematoma *A collection of blood between the surface of the brain and the dura mater.*

suspensory ligaments *The structures that hold the lens of the eye in place.*

sutures *Immovable joints composed of connective tissue in the skull where the cranial bones meet.*

swimmer's ear *An infection of the skin covering the outer ear canal.*

temporal bone *The cranial bone that forms the base of the skull, behind and at the sides of the face.*

temporomandibular joint (TMJ) *The joint that connects the mandible to the skull.*

tympanic membrane *The membrane that separates the external ear from the middle ear; also called the eardrum.*

tympanic rupture *Perforation of the tympanic membrane between the middle ear and the ear canal.*

vestibule *A small cavity at the beginning of a canal.*

vestibulocochlear nerve *The eighth cranial nerve, which sends sound and balance signals to the brain.*

vitreous humor *Transparent, gelatin-like substance that fills the greater part of the eyeball.*

THE HEAD AND FACE

The term *head injury* describes damage to the scalp, skull, or brain. Head injuries can occur in any sport, and in various ways; however, most are caused by the application of some type of sudden force to the head, usually a direct blow. Trauma of this type may be caused by collision with another athlete or an object such as a goalpost, wall, bleacher, or the floor/ground. It may also occur if the athlete is struck by some sort of athletic equipment, such as a baseball bat, golf club, or hockey stick. In addition, the head may be injured by a blow from a projectile such as a baseball, golf ball, discus, or hockey puck.

The head can be divided into two anatomical groups: the face and cranium. The face includes the eyes, ears, nose, jaw, and mouth (Figure 23–1).

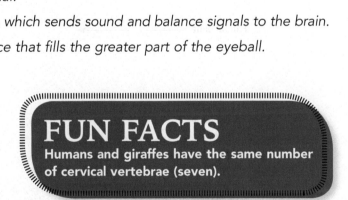

FUN FACTS
Humans and giraffes have the same number of cervical vertebrae (seven).

The cranium (skull) contains the brain and spinal cord attachments (Figure 23–2).

THE EYE

The human eye is a tender sphere about 1 inch (2.5 cm) in diameter. It is protected by the orbital socket of the skull and the eyebrows, eyelids, and eyelashes (Figure 23–3). The eyes are continuously bathed in fluid by tears secreted from lacrimal glands, which are located above the lateral

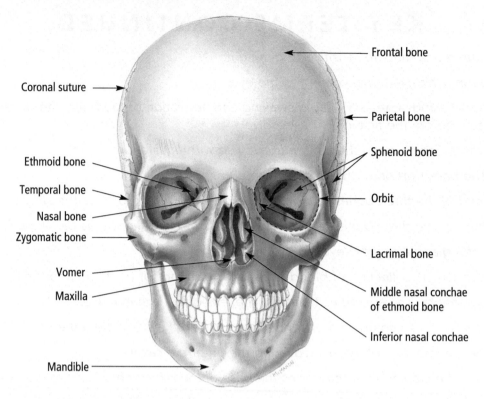

Figure 23–1 The facial bones.

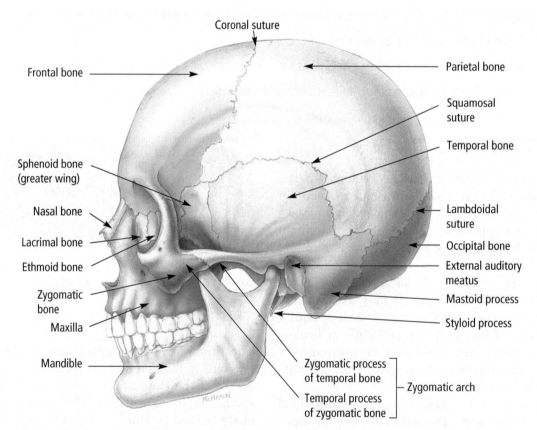

Figure 23–2 The cranial bones.

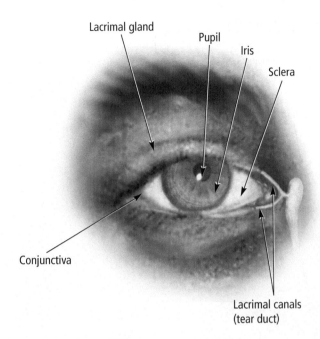

Figure 23–3 External view of the eye.

area of each eye. The tears flow across the eye into the lacrimal duct, which is located in the corner of the eye and empties into the nasal cavity. This explains why, when we cry, we may also need to blow the nose. Lacrimal secretions have some antibiotic properties: Tears cleanse and moisten the eyes on a continuous basis.

Along the border of each eyelid are glands that secrete an oily substance that lubricates the eye. An infection of this gland is called a **sty**.

The **conjunctiva** is the thin membrane that lines the eyelids and covers part of the eye. It secretes mucus that helps to lubricate the eye.

The location of the eyes in front of the head allows superimposition of images from each eye. This enables us to see stereoscopically in three dimensions (length, width, and depth).

The wall of the eye is made up of three concentric layers, or coats, each with its specific function. These three layers are the sclera, choroid, and retina (Figure 23–4).

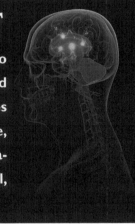

KEY CONCEPT

The head can be divided into two anatomical groups, the face and the cranium. The face includes the structures of the eye, nose, mouth, ears, and jaw. The cranium includes the brain, skull, and spinal cord attachments.

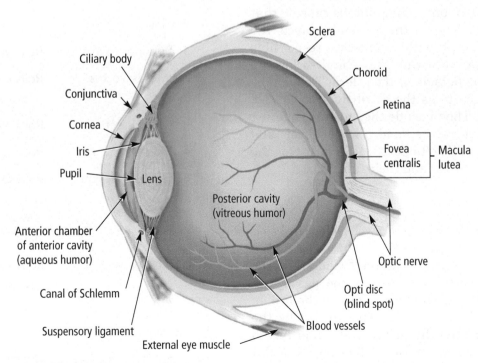

Figure 23–4 Internal view of the eye.

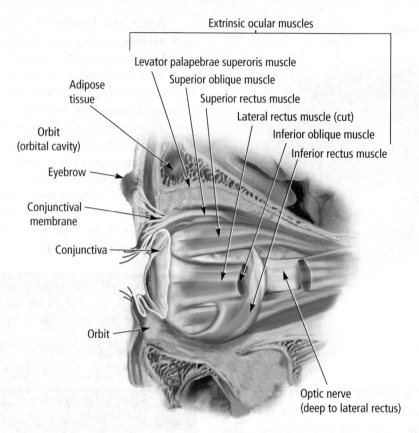

Figure 23–5 Extrinsic eye muscles.

Sclera

The outer layer is called the **sclera**, or white of the eye. It is a tough, unyielding fibrous capsule that maintains the shape of the eye and protects the delicate structures within. Muscles responsible for moving the eye within the orbital socket are attached to the outside of the sclera. These muscles are referred to as the **extrinsic eye muscles** (Figure 23–5). They include the superior, inferior, lateral, medial rectus, and the superior and inferior oblique. See Table 23–1 for a list of the extrinsic eye muscles and their functions.

Cornea

In the very front center of the sclerotic coat lies a circular, clear area called the **cornea**. The cornea is sometimes referred to as the "window" of the eye. It is transparent to permit the passage of light rays. This transparency is due to the lack of blood vessels. Thus, corneal cells are fed by the movement of lymph through interstitial or lymph spaces. The cornea consists of five layers of flat cells arranged much like sheets of plate glass.

Table 23–1 Extrinsic and Intrinsic Eye Muscles	
EYE MUSCLE	FUNCTION
A. Extrinsic	
1. Superior rectus	Rolls eyeball upward
2. Inferior rectus	Rolls eyeball downward
3. Lateral rectus	Rolls eyeball laterally
4. Medial rectus	Rolls eyeball medially
5. Superior oblique	Rolls eyeball on its axis, moves cornea downward and laterally
6. Inferior oblique	Rolls eyeball on its axis, moves cornea upward and laterally
B. Intrinsic	
1. Sphincter pupillae	Constricts pupil

Possessing pain and touch receptors, it is sensitive to any foreign particles that come in contact with its surface. An injury to the cornea may cause scarring and impaired vision.

Choroid Coat and the Iris

The middle layer of the eye is the **choroid coat**. It contains blood vessels to nourish the eye, and a nonreflective pigment that renders it dark and opaque. The pigment provides the choroid coat with a deep, red-purple color; this darkens the eye chamber, preventing light reflection within the eye. In front, the choroid coat has a circular opening called the **pupil**. A colored, muscular layer surrounds the pupil; this is the **iris**, or colored part of the eye. The iris may be blue, green, gray, brown, or black. Eye color is related to the number and size of melanin pigment cells in the iris. If there is little melanin present, the eye is blue, because light is scattered to a greater extent. With increasing quantities of melanin, eye color ranges from green to black. The total absence of melanin results in a pink eye color, characteristic of albinism. Such irises are pink because the blood inside the choroid blood vessels shows through the iris.

Within the iris are two sets of antagonistic smooth muscles, the sphincter and the dilator pupillae. These **intrinsic eye muscles** help the iris to control the amount of light entering the pupil. When the eye is focused on a close object or stimulated by bright light, the sphincter pupillae muscle contracts, rendering the pupil smaller. Conversely, when the eye is focused on a distant object or stimulated by dim light, the dilator pupillae muscle contracts. This causes the pupil to grow larger, permitting as much light as possible to enter the eye.

Lens and Related Structures

The **lens** is a crystalline structure located behind the iris and pupil. It has concentric layers of fibers and crystal-clear proteins in solution. It is an elastic, disc-shaped structure with anterior and posterior convex surfaces, thus forming a biconvex lens. However, the posterior surface is more curved than the anterior. The curvature of each surface alters with age. During infancy, the lens is spherical; in adulthood, it is medium convexed; in the elderly, it is almost flattened. The capsule surrounding the lens

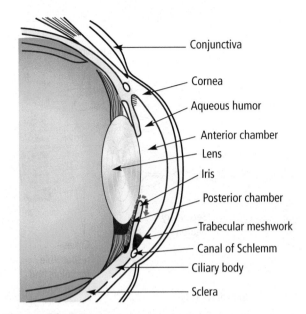

Labels:
- Conjunctiva
- Cornea
- Aqueous humor
- Anterior chamber
- Lens
- Iris
- Posterior chamber
- Trabecular meshwork
- Canal of Schlemm
- Ciliary body
- Sclera

Figure 23–6 Flow of aqueous humor.

also loses its elasticity over time. The lens is held in place behind the pupil by **suspensory ligaments** from the **ciliary body** of the choroid body.

The **anterior chamber** and **posterior chamber** are filled with a watery fluid called **aqueous humor**, and it is constantly replenished by blood vessels behind the iris (Figure 23–6). **Vitreous humor**, a transparent, jellylike substance, fills the space behind the lens. Both substances help to maintain the eyeball's spherical shape, refracting (bending) light rays as they pass through the eye.

Retina

The **retina**, the innermost, third coat of the eye, is located between the vitreous humor and the choroid coat. The retina does not extend around the front portion of the eye. It is upon this light-sensitive layer that light rays from an object form an image. After the image is focused on the retina, it travels via the optic nerve to the visual part of the cerebral cortex (occipital lobe). If light rays do not focus correctly on the retina, the condition may be corrected with contact lenses or eyeglasses, which bend the light rays as required.

The retina contains pigment and specialized cells, known as **rods** and **cones** (Figure 23–7), which are sensitive to light. The rod cells are sensitive to dim light, and the cones are sensitive to bright light. The cones are also responsible for color vision. There are three types of cone cell, each sensitive to a specific color. The part of the retina

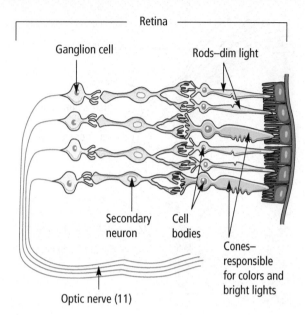

Figure 23–7 Diagram of visual neurons showing rods and cones.

where the nerve fibers enter the optic nerve to go to the brain lacks these specialized cells.

THE OPTIC DISC AND THE FOVEA Viewing the retina through an ophthalmoscope, one can observe a yellow disc called the *macula lutea*. Within this disc is the **fovea centralis**, which contains the cones for color vision (see Figure 23–4). The area around the fovea centralis is the extrafoveal or peripheral region, where the rods for dim and peripheral vision can be found.

Slightly to the side of the fovea centralis lies a pale disc called the **optic disc** or blind spot. Nerve fibers from the retina gather here to form the nerve. The optic disc contains no rods or cones; therefore, it is devoid of visual reception. See Figure 23–8 to help you locate your blind spot.

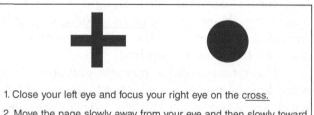

1. Close your left eye and focus your right eye on the <u>cross.</u>
2. Move the page slowly away from your eye and then slowly toward your eye.
3. At a distance of about 6–8 inches the black <u>circle</u> "disappears."

Figure 23–8 Testing for the blind spot.

PATHWAY OF VISION

Images in the light $\longrightarrow$ cornea $\longrightarrow$ pupil $\longrightarrow$ lens $\longrightarrow$ where the light rays are bent or refracted $\longrightarrow$ retina $\longrightarrow$ rods and cones (nerve cells) pick up the stimulus $\longrightarrow$ optic nerve $\longrightarrow$ optic chiasma (where the two optic nerves cross) $\longrightarrow$ optic tracts $\longrightarrow$ occipital lobe of the brain for interpretation.

EYE INJURIES

According to the American Academy of Ophthalmology, about 40,000 people suffer sports-related eye injuries in the United States each year (American Academy of Ophthalmology, 2008). Most injuries occur in younger people: Nearly three-quarters of sports- and recreation-related eye injuries affect people under the age of 25, and about half affect children under the age of 15.

The sports that cause most of these injuries are basketball, baseball, and racquet sports. Any sport involving a projectile is considered hazardous to the eyes. The most common eye injury occurs in basketball, usually due to a finger or elbow penetrating the eye. However, baseball, racquetball, hockey, and other sports also frequently cause eye injuries that range from corneal abrasions and bruises to fractured eye sockets and facial bones, eye hemorrhages and retinal detachments, and even blindness from a direct hit that crushes the eyeball.

More than 90% of sports-related eye injuries can be prevented by use of protective athletic eyewear, which should be considered necessary equipment for *all* sports activities. Eyeglasses and contact lenses do not provide protection and may actually put an athlete at increased risk for eye injury, because plastic and glass lenses often shatter when struck by a projectile such as a ball. Protective athletic eyewear is made with polycarbonate plastics that are highly resistant to impact. Table 23–2 correlates sports and the recommended type of protective eyewear that should be worn.

Injuries to the eye and orbit are not very common in competitive athletics. If an eye injury is not treated properly, the result could be a loss of visual acuity or permanent loss of sight in the affected eye. Proper treatment of eye injuries is paramount.

Table 23–2 Recommended Eye Protection for Sports Activities

SPORT	MINIMAL EYE PROTECTOR*	COMMENT
Baseball/Softball Batter or Baserunner	ASTM+ F910	Face guard attached to helmet
Baseball/Softball Fielder	ASTM+ F803 for baseball	ASTM+ specifies age ranges
Basketball	ASTM+ F803 for basketball	ASTM+ specifies age ranges
Bicycling	Helmet plus streetwear ANSI+ Z80, industrial ANSI+ Z87.1 or sports ASTM F803 eyewear	Use only polycarbonate lenses
Boxing	None available—not permitted in sport	Participation is contraindicated for functionally one-eyed athletes
Fencing	Protector with neck bib	Test requirements of the International Federation of Fencing
Field Hockey, Men's and Women's	Goalie: full face mask-; ASTM+ F803 for women's lacrosse	Protectors that pass for women's lacrosse also pass for field hockey
Football	Polycarbonate eye shield attached to helmetmounted wire face mask-	
Ice Hockey	Goaltenders: ASTM+ F1587; ASTM+ F513 face mask on helmet-	HECC+ or CSA+ certified full face shield
Lacrosse, Men's	NOCSAE+ face mask attached to lacrosse helmet-	
Lacrosse, Women's	ASTM+ F803 for women's lacrosse	Face guard attached to helmet
Martial Arts, Full-Contact	None available—not permitted in sport	Participation is contraindicated for functionally one-eyed athletes
Paintball	ASTM+ F1776 for paintball	
Racquet Sports	ASTM+ F803 for specific sport	Racquet sports include squash, badminton, tennis, paddle tennis, handball, and racquetball
Soccer	ASTM+ F803 for selected sport	No specific standard for soccer; ASTM+ F803 for any specified sport is recommended
Street Hockey	ASTM+ 513 face mask on helmet-	Must be HECC+ or CSA+ certified
Track and Field	Streetwear with polycarbonate lenses/fashion eyewear	Use only polycarbonate lenses

(continued)

Table 23–2	Recommended Eye Protection for Sports Activities *(continued)*	
SPORT	**MINIMAL EYE PROTECTOR***	**COMMENT**
Water Sports	Swim goggles with polycarbonate lenses	Water sports include swimming and water polo
Wrestling	No standard is available	Custom protective eyewear can be made

*Eyewear should be made with highly shatter-resistant 3-mm polycarbonate or Trivex lenses, unless there is a specific reason for another lens material.

⁺ASTM (American Society of Testing and Materials); ANSI (American National Standards Institute); NOCSAE (The National Operating Committee on Standards for Athletic Equipment); HECC (Hockey Equipment Certification Council); CSA (Canadian Standards Association)

⁻For sports in which a face mask or helmet with an eye protector is worn, functionally one-eyed athletes and those who have had previous eye trauma or surgery, and for whom an ophthalmologist has recommended eye protection, must also wear sports protective eyewear that conforms to ASTM F803 requirements.

Eye Specks

It is not uncommon for dirt and other debris to find its way into the eyes. Because the eyes are very sensitive, any foreign object on them will create pain. A scratch or cut caused by dirt or some other foreign object can cause a **corneal abrasion**, a scratch or small cut of the cornea of the eye.

Corneal abrasions can be caused by sand, dust, dirt, wood shavings, or metal filings that get in the eye. The cornea can also be scratched by a fingernail, a tree branch, or a contact lens. Rubbing the eyes very hard can also cause a corneal abrasion. Outdoor sports put participants at greater risk from foreign-object eye injuries. Care and protective eyewear should be used to minimize the risk of this injury.

TREATMENT The examiner should wash hands before assisting an injured athlete. The athlete should be seated in a well-lighted area. Try to locate the object in the eye visually. Examine the eye by gently pulling the lower lid down and instructing the athlete to look upward. Reverse the procedure for the upper lid. Hold the upper lid and examine the eye while the athlete looks downward. If a foreign object is found embedded in the eyeball, cover the athlete's eye with a sterile pad or a clean cloth. Do not try to remove the object.

Objects in the eye should be washed out by splashing clean water into it. It is important to avoid rubbing the eye because of the risk of further injury. If something is on the white part of the eye, a soft tissue or cotton swab can be used to gently lift it out. If the particle cannot be removed, or if there does not seem to be anything in the eye, the athlete should see a physician immediately.

REHABILITATION An athlete can return to competition or practice as soon as the object has been removed from the eye and the athlete no longer complains of discomfort.

Blows (Contusions) to the Eye

The eye is located in a deep socket called the **orbit** (refer to Figure 23–1). This is nature's way of protecting one of the most important organs of the body. A black eye is often a minor injury, but it can also appear when there is significant eye injury or head trauma (Figure 23–9).

Blows to the eye are not uncommon and can occur during almost any sport or activity. Common mechanisms of this injury include contact of the orbit with elbows in basketball, baseballs hit or thrown, and other athletes. Protective eyewear is available for every sport and activity and should be worn.

SIGNS AND SYMPTOMS Injuries to any part of the eye or orbit are painful. Swelling and discoloration may occur quickly. The athlete will guard the injury by placing a hand over the injured eye. This is a safety mechanism to protect the site from further damage. The medical staff will need

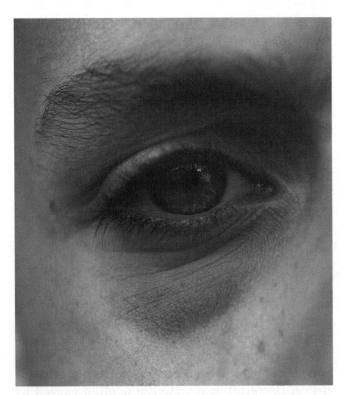

Figure 23–9 A blow to the eye can cause bruising. Courtesy of Photodisc

to assess the injury to determine the course of action to be taken.

TREATMENT The athlete should apply a cold compress immediately for 15 minutes, and each hour as needed, to reduce pain and swelling. Discoloration or blackening of the eye could indicate that internal damage has occurred. If bruising occurs, the athlete should consult a physician immediately.

REHABILITATION The athlete may return to competition or practice if cleared by the medical staff. Protective eyewear should be worn until the eye and its surrounding tissues have completely healed. The athlete should wear protective eyewear as a preventative measure thereafter.

Cuts, Punctures, and Abrasions of the Eye or Eyelid

Wounds that penetrate the eye can cause infection and blindness. These injuries are considered medical emergencies. Penetrating wounds to the eye can occur from any object, including fingers accidentally stuck in the eye. Fortunately, these injuries are rare in athletics.

TREATMENT If initial assessment indicates that an object has penetrated the eye, the athlete should receive emergency medical care and promptly be transported to the nearest medical facility.

To treat cuts or punctures to the eye, bandage the eye without any pressure and seek emergency medical care immediately. Do not attempt to wash the eye or remove any object stuck in the eye. A paper cup held over the injured eye can help protect it until the athlete can receive medical care.

REHABILITATION The athlete can return to play with a physician's approval. Proper protective eyewear should be worn upon return to competition or play.

Orbital Blow-Out Fracture

An orbital blow-out fracture consists of a fracture of the bones of the eye socket. This may involve the orbital floor, walls, or roof. Most cases involve the orbital floor of the eye socket itself.

An orbital blow-out fracture is almost always secondary to a blunt blow from a relatively large object, such as a fist, elbow, or baseball bat. The force of a nonpenetrating object that is larger than the orbital entrance causes the characteristic fracture pattern that gives this injury its name.

SIGNS AND SYMPTOMS Most athletes will have pain and tenderness around the eye, swelling, and double vision. Pain upon attempted eye movement is also common. The athlete may notice bruising around the eye, double vision (*diplopia*), protrusion of the eye (*proptosis*), or numbness in the cheek and upper jaw areas.

TREATMENT Immediate treatment is to bandage both eyes and apply an ice compress for 15 to 20 minutes. The athlete will need to see an ophthalmologist immediately for evaluation and treatment.

REHABILITATION The athlete will not be allowed to return to athletics until cleared by the doctor. Protective eyewear will be required for further athletic participation.

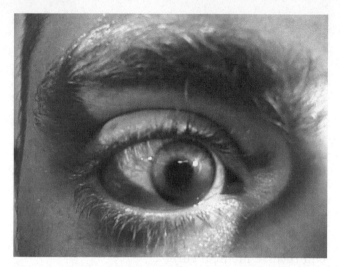

Figure 23–10 Blood in the front of the eye is called a hyphema. Courtesy of Kevin Reilly, MD, Albany Medical Center, NY.

Hyphema

Hyphema, bleeding in the anterior chamber (the space between the cornea and the iris) of the eye (Figure 23–10), occurs when blood vessels in the iris bleed and leak into the clear aqueous fluid.

Bleeding in the anterior chamber is most often caused by blunt trauma to the eye. In athletics, this can occur when a ball or finger strikes the eye. It may also be associated with surgical procedures. Other causes include abnormal vessel growth in the eye and certain ocular tumors.

SIGNS AND SYMPTOMS In the initial stage, the athlete will complain of dramatically decreased vision. As the hyphema sinks to the inferior part of the anterior chamber, vision will return to normal.

TREATMENT Athletes who have sustained an eye injury resulting in hyphema should be seen by an ophthalmologist. The treatment depends on the cause and severity of the hyphema. Frequently, the blood is reabsorbed over a period of days to weeks. During this time, the ophthalmologist will carefully monitor the athlete. The ophthalmologist may recommend yearly follow-ups to detect long-term complications of hyphema such as traumatic glaucoma or retinal detachment.

REHABILITATION Athletes with significant hyphemas must rest and avoid strenuous activity to allow the blood to reabsorb. The timing of return to play is a decision for the ophthalmologist.

Conjunctivitis

Conjunctivitis, commonly known as *pink eye*, is an infection of the conjunctiva (the outermost layer of the eye that covers the sclera). The three most common types of conjunctivitis are viral, allergic, and bacterial. Each requires different treatment. With the exception of the allergic type, conjunctivitis is typically contagious.

Viral conjunctivitis is often associated with an upper respiratory tract infection, cold, or sore throat. The allergic type occurs more frequently among those with allergic conditions. When related to allergies, the symptoms are often seasonal. Allergic conjunctivitis may also be caused by intolerance to substances such as cosmetics, perfume, or drugs. Bacterial conjunctivitis is often caused by bacteria such as staphylococcus and streptococcus. The severity of the infection depends on the type of bacteria involved.

SIGNS AND SYMPTOMS The first symptom of conjunctivitis is discomfort in the eye, followed by redness and inflammation of the conjunctiva, the tissue covering the eye and inner surface of the eyelids. There is some pain associated with conjunctivitis, but the athlete likely will complain of discomfort that is not relieved by rubbing or a sensation of something that feels like sand in the eye.

After a day or so of these symptoms, a white, yellow, or green discharge from the eyes may be present. In bacterial conjunctivitis, the discharge will be somewhat thick. In viral conjunctivitis, the discharge may be thinner, and may even be clear.

TREATMENT Conjunctivitis requires medical attention. The appropriate treatment depends on the cause of the problem. For mild cases of the allergic type, cool compresses and artificial tears sometimes relieve discomfort. In more severe cases, nonsteroidal anti-inflammatory medications and antihistamines may be prescribed. Some patients with persistent allergic conjunctivitis may also require topical steroid drops.

Bacterial conjunctivitis is usually treated with antibiotic eyedrops or ointments that cover a broad range of bacteria. Like the common cold, there is no cure for viral conjunctivitis; however, the symptoms can be relieved with cool compresses and artificial tears (available in most pharmacies). For the worst cases, topical steroid drops may be prescribed to reduce the discomfort from inflammation. Viral conjunctivitis usually resolves within three weeks.

REHABILITATION Because conjunctivitis is contagious, the athlete will need to be cleared by a physician for return to athletics.

THE EAR

The ear is the organ of hearing and balance. It consists of three parts: the **outer ear**, the **middle ear**, and the **inner ear** (Figure 23–11). The outer ear and middle ear are the apparatus for collecting and transmitting sound. The inner ear is responsible for analyzing sound waves and also

KEY CONCEPT

Eye injuries:

- **Dirt and debris can become embedded in the structures of the eye and cause pain or a corneal abrasion. A corneal abrasion is a cut or scratch on the cornea. Attempts can be made to wash objects out by splashing water into the eye.**

- **However, embedded objects should not be removed, and the athlete should be instructed to see a physician.**

- **A blow or contusion to the eye often results in a black eye. Application of a cold compress for 15 minutes immediately after the injury will aid in reducing pain and swelling.**

- **Cuts, punctures, or abrasions to the eye or eyelid can cause infection and blindness. These are medical emergencies, and the athlete should be promptly transported to a medical facility.**

- **An orbital blow-out fracture is a break in the bones that house the eye. Immediate treatment consists of bandaging both eyes and applying an ice compress for 15 to 20 minutes. The athlete should seek immediate treatment from an ophthalmologist.**

- **Hyphema is a buildup of blood in the anterior chamber of the eye. Treatment will depend on the cause, but the athlete should seek the care of an ophthalmologist.**

- **Conjunctivitis is an infection of the outermost layer of the eye. This is usually contagious and requires medical attention.**

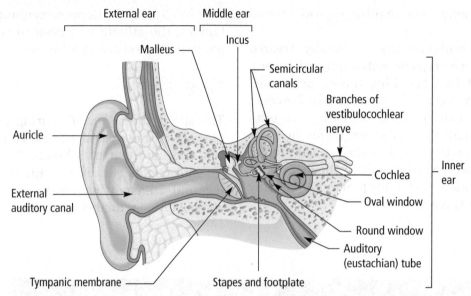

Figure 23–11 The external, middle, and inner ear, and organs of the ear.

contains the mechanism by which the body maintains balance. The outer ear is composed of the **pinna** and **ear canal**; the middle ear contains the **eardrum**, **hammer**, **anvil**, **stirrup**, and **eustachian tube**; and the inner ear consists of the **vestibule**, **semicircular canals**, and **cochlea**. Sensory impulses from the inner ear pass to the brain via the **vestibulocochlear nerve**.

The Outer Ear

The pinna (also called the **auricle**), the visible part of the ear, is composed of folds of skin and cartilage. The pinna leads into the ear canal (also called the **meatus**), which is about 1 inch (or 2.5 cm) long in adults and closed at its inner end by the **tympanic membrane** (eardrum). The part of the canal nearest the outside is made of cartilage. The cartilage is covered with skin that produces wax. The tiny hairs in the canal trap dust, pollen, pollution, and small foreign bodies.

The Middle Ear

The middle ear, a small cavity between the eardrum and the inner ear, conducts sound to the inner ear by means of a chain of three tiny, linked, movable bones called **ossicles**. The ossicles link the eardrum to an oval window in the bony wall on the opposite inner side of the middle-ear cavity.

The bones are named for of their shapes. The **malleus**, or *hammer*, is joined to the inside of the eardrum. The **incus**, or anvil, has one broad joint with the malleus (which lies almost parallel to it) and a delicate joint to the third bone, the **stapes**, or *stirrup*. The base of the stapes fills the oval window that leads to the inner ear.

The middle ear is cut off from the outside by the eardrum, but it is not completely airtight. A ventilation passage, the eustachian tube, runs forward and down into the back of the nose. The eustachian tube is normally closed, but it opens due to muscular contraction when yawning or swallowing.

The middle ear acts as a transformer. It passes on the vibrations of sound from compression and decompression of the outside air. The air is a thin medium that carries the sound into the inner ear; the fluid in the inner ear, a thicker medium, resonates with the sound vibration.

The Inner Ear

The inner ear is an extremely intricate series of structures contained deep within the bones of the skull. It consists of a maze of winding passageways collectively known as the **labyrinth**. The front part, the *cochlea*, is a coiled tube resembling a snail's shell and is related to hearing. The rear part, which consists of three semicircular canals and two other organs, is related to balance. The semicircular canals are set at right angles to each other and are connected to a cavity known as the *vestibule*. These canals contain hair cells bathed in fluid. Some of these cells are sensitive to gravity and acceleration, and others respond to head position and movement (side to side, up and down, or tilted). Posture and directional information is registered by the relevant cells and conveyed by nerve fibers to the brain.

INJURIES TO THE EAR

In athletics, injuries to the ear usually involve the external ear. Even in mandatory-helmet sports, lacerations and abrasions occur. These may be due to an opponent's fingernail or a player bending the ear during placement of a helmet. Common athletic injuries include cauliflower ear (hematology *auras*), swimmer's ear (Otis *extern*), tympanic membrane (eardrum) rupture, and foreign bodies in the ear.

Cauliflower Ear

Cauliflower ear is caused by destruction of the underlying cartilage of the outer ear (pinna). Blood collects between the ear cartilage and the skin. There is a thickening of the entire outer ear, which may be so extensive that the normal shape becomes completely distorted and unrecognizable. The ear is said to look like a piece of cauliflower. This condition is typically seen in wrestlers and boxers who have had repeated trauma to the ear.

SIGNS AND SYMPTOMS When trauma causes a blood clot under the skin of the ear, the clot disrupts the connection of the skin to the ear cartilage. The cartilage has no other blood supply, so if the skin separates from the cartilage, the cartilage is deprived of nutrients and dies, shriveling up to form the classic cauliflower ear.

TREATMENT The physician may drain the hematology (the blood clot) through an incision in the ear and apply a compressive dressing to sandwich the two sides of the skin against the cartilage. When treated promptly and aggressively, the development of cauliflower ear deformity is unlikely. Delay in diagnosis and treatment makes management of this problem more difficult and may result in greater ear deformity.

REHABILITATION Return to athletics requires a physician's approval. Well-fitting headgear will be required for future participation.

Swimmer's Ear

Swimmer's ear is an infection of the skin covering the outer ear canal. Acute swimmer's ear is commonly a bacterial infection caused by the streptococcus, staphylococcus, or pseudonymous types of bacteria.

Swimmer's ear is usually caused by excessive water exposure. When water pools in the ear canal (where it is frequently trapped by wax), the skin will become soggy and serve as a good culture medium for bacteria. This is a common condition in athletes involved with water sports (Figure 23–12).

SIGNS AND SYMPTOMS The first sign of infection is that the ear feels full and may itch. The ear canal will swell, and ear drainage will follow. At this stage the ear will be very painful, especially with movement of the outside portion of the ear. The ear canal may swell shut, and the side of the face can become swollen. The glands of the neck may enlarge, and it can become difficult to open the jaw.

TREATMENT Moisture and irritation will prolong this problem. For this reason, the ear should be kept dry. While showering or swimming, the athlete should wear an earplug that is designed to keep water out.

REHABILITATION The athlete may return to activity after treatment has begun and proper steps have been taken to minimize water exposure of the ear canal.

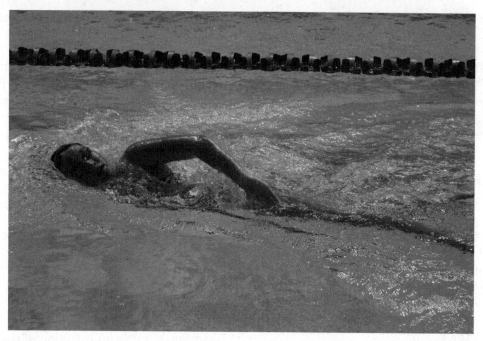

Figure 23–12 Swimmer's ear is a common complaint of athletes involved in water sports.

Foreign Bodies in the Ear

A number of objects can get into the ear canal and be very difficult to remove. Because of the size of the ear canal, objects are very hard to grasp. Insects can also crawl or fly into the ear canal. Insects often do not have enough room to turn around inside of the ear canal and can become stuck.

This condition usually occurs in children under the age of five. Athletes rarely encounter this problem because of athletic participation.

SIGNS AND SYMPTOMS Foreign bodies in the ear may cause the following symptoms: mild to severe ear pain, drainage from the ear, fever, nausea and vomiting, coughing, tearing from the eye, dizziness, and a foul odor from the ear caused by infection.

TREATMENT Treatment will depend on the depth and type of foreign body in the ear. Some foreign bodies will fall out of the ear naturally without having to be removed. Gentle flushing of the ear canal with warm water can remove other objects. Removal of some foreign bodies requires long, specially designed instruments. Live insects are usually immobilized or killed (with a liquid or gel) prior to removal. Surgery is occasionally needed to remove a foreign body or to treat damage to the ear from the foreign body.

REHABILITATION The athlete may return to play immediately.

Tympani (Eardrum) Rupture

The eardrum, also called the *tympanic membrane*, separates the middle ear from the ear canal. The eardrum is delicate and easily perforated (torn). Most often it is ruptured by an infection of the middle ear (Otis *media*), but other types of trauma may also cause tears or ruptures.

Trauma is the most common cause of a **tympanic rupture**. Rupture of the eardrum can also occur when fluid behind the eardrum builds up in the middle ear, causing pressure on the eardrum. The pressure increases until the eardrum breaks, allowing the fluid to drain out of the ear. A very loud noise, such as an explosion, can also cause the membrane to rupture. In athletics, trauma to the head, such as a skull fracture or a blow to the ear, can cause this injury.

SIGNS AND SYMPTOMS The person may have severe ear pain that dimi-nishes or ceases when the eardrum ruptures and relieves the pressure.

A ruptured eardrum usually drains suddenly. The drainage often looks like pus and smells bad.

TREATMENT The athlete should be taken to a physician immediately for evaluation and treatment. After a rupture, the eardrum usually heals on its own in one to two weeks, usually without hearing loss. Antibiotics may be prescribed to manage potential infection.

REHABILITATION The athlete may return to activity with a physician's approval.

THE NOSE

The nose is a triangular composition of bone, cartilage, and skin that projects from the frontal bone of the cranium and the maxillae of the face. Because of its location, it is susceptible to injury during athletic activities.

The human nose serves as an air passage between the nostrils and the throat, and as the organ for the sense of smell. The nose warms, moistens, and filters the air that enters the nostrils and travels down to the lungs. It can detect about 10,000 different smells. Smell accounts for about 90% of what we think of as taste.

INJURIES TO THE NOSE

Injuries to the nose are often caused by impact and blunt trauma, which can easily occur in contact sports. Pain, swelling, and bruising are common with any type of injury to the nose. The nose is highly vascular and often will bleed, sometimes profusely, when injured (Figure 23–13). Other facial and neck injuries may also be present with injuries to the nose.

Epistaxis

Epistaxis is the medical term for nosebleed. Epistaxis usually refers to major nosebleeds that are difficult to stop, or recurrent nosebleeds. Nosebleeds that are easy to stop, and simple, blood-tinged, nasal secretions, rarely come to the attention of the physician. Most of these are caused by nasal dryness or very minor trauma to the nose. Major or recurrent epistaxis may suggest a more serious problem that requires the assistance of a physician.

Epistaxis can be classified as anterior, when it arises in the front of the nasal cavity, or posterior, when it arises in the back of the nasal cavity. Fortunately, anterior epistaxis is more common and much easier to treat. The most

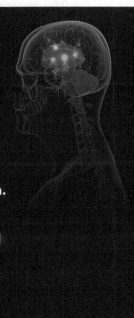

KEY CONCEPT

Ear injuries:

- **Cauliflower ear is a deformity caused by damage to the cartilage in the outer ear. Drainage of the blood buildup will help keep this from occurring, if done early.**

- **Swimmer's ear is an infection of the skin covering the outer ear canal. The ear must be kept dry, as moisture will irritate and prolong the problem.**

- **Foreign bodies may become lodged in the ear. Treatment is removal of the object, but the method of removal will depend on the type of material lodged in the ear and how far in the ear it is lodged.**

- **Tympani rupture is perforation of the tympanic membrane. The athlete should immediately be taken to a physician for treatment.**

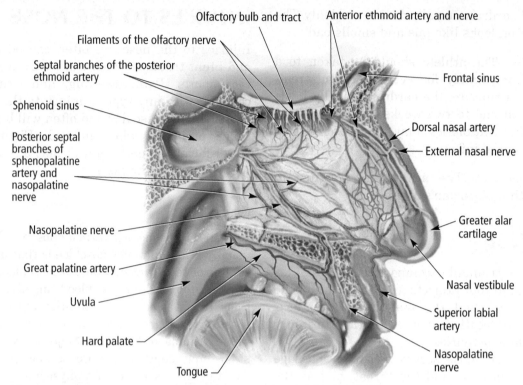

Figure 23–13 The vascular and nervous structures of the nasal cavity.

common cause of anterior epistaxis is nasal dryness. Nosebleeds are most common in the winter months when the humidity is low; certain types of heating may further dry the air indoors.

The second most common cause of anterior epistaxis, and the most common cause of posterior epistaxis, is vascular disease (with or without high blood pressure). As blood vessels become damaged by high blood pressure, high cholesterol, or aging, they become brittle and break more frequently. If blood pressure is high, the epistaxis will be more difficult to stop. Other causes of epistaxis are nasal trauma, nasal tumors, or abnormal blood clotting due to medicines or diseases such as leukemia or liver failure.

In athletics, nosebleeds are common, especially in wrestling. Wrestling requires close physical contact that frequently results in forceful contact with the nose.

SIGNS AND SYMPTOMS The certified athletic trainer will need to determine the severity of the injury. If the bleeding is posterior, little or no blood may be discharged from the nostrils, but the athlete will probably complain of swallowing blood. There is no way for the certified athletic

trainer to stop this type of bleeding. The athlete must rely on the natural clotting mechanism to stop the bleeding. Posterior nosebleeds can be life threatening and should be considered medical emergencies. The certified athletic trainer should activate the EMS system.

Blood flowing from the nostrils is an anterior nosebleed and can normally be managed conservatively.

TREATMENT Management of superficial bleeding during contact sports is of paramount importance to the sports medicine professional. Because of the possibility of cross-contamination by bloodborne pathogens, the sports medicine professional must be equipped to stop a flow of blood, prevent recurrent bleeding, contamination, and infection, and appropriately clean up the situation. In addition, these actions must occur in a timely manner in order to get the athlete back into competition, as an athlete who is actively bleeding will not be allowed to continue.

During a wrestling match, for example, a wrestler who sustains a traumatic, bleeding injury can lose the match on an injury default if the bleeding is not stopped. When bleeding begins, the referee will stop the match regardless of the match score or situation. Wrestling cannot resume until the bleeding is stopped, and both athletes and the mat are cleaned up. The amount of time allowed to stop the bleeding and prevent a recurrence may vary from 5 minutes to an unlimited period, but pressure will be on the sports medicine professional to get the job done in a hurry.

The first step in treating epistaxis is to stop the bleeding. The athlete should sit down and lean slightly forward so that the blood will drain out of the nose instead of down the back of the throat. Keeping the head at a level above the heart will make the nose bleed less. If the athlete leans back, he or she may swallow the blood. This can cause nausea, vomiting, and diarrhea.

Have the athlete use the thumb and index finger to squeeze together the soft portion of the nose. This area is located between the end of the nose and the hard, bony ridge that forms the bridge of the nose. This should be done for 5 minutes. If the nose still bleeds, repeat the squeeze for 10 minutes. The athlete can place a cold compress or an ice pack across the bridge of the nose.

Certain precautions, such as refraining from nose blowing and strenuous activity, will help keep a nosebleed from returning.

REHABILITATION If the athlete can return to competition after a nosebleed, nasal packing with sterile gauze or nasal tampons may be required. Wrestling is an example of a sport in which an athlete may need to continue the match. Normally play can be resumed safely after packing of the nasal cavity.

Nasal Fractures and Septal Deviations

The nasal bone's protruding position, along with its relative lack of support, predisposes it to fracture and deviation. Prompt evaluation and treatment will help prevent functional and cosmetic changes. Because of the central location of the nose and its proximity to other important structures, the certified athletic trainer should carefully search for other facial injuries when there is a nasal fracture.

Nasal fractures in athletes occur as a result of direct blows, especially in contact sports, and as a result of falls. Any force directed to the mid-face, either frontally or laterally, can disrupt the nasal anatomy, causing bony or cartilaginous injury. The nasal bones are the most commonly fractured bony structures of the face.

SIGNS AND SYMPTOMS Signs of nasal fracture include deformity, swelling, skin laceration, ecchymosis, epistaxis, and leakage of **cerebrospinal fluid (CSF)**.

TREATMENT Immediate treatment of nasal fractures and septal deviations is to control bleeding with careful, direct pressure. Ice should be applied, and the athlete should sit down with head tilted slightly forward to avoid posterior bleeding and swallowing of blood. The athlete should be sent to a physician for additional care and treatment.

KEY CONCEPT

Nasal injuries:

- **Expistaxis (nosebleed) is a concern only when the bleeding is difficult to stop or is recurrent. Infection control procedures must be maintained when dealing with a nosebleed. The athlete should sit down, lean forward, and squeeze the soft portion of the nose to try to stop the bleeding.**

- **A nasal fracture is a break in the bone or damage to the cartilaginous structures of the nose. Control bleeding, apply ice, and refer the athlete to a physician for further treatment.**

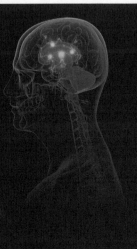

REHABILITATION Athletes with nasal fractures can return to activity after clearance by a physician. Special face masks are available and should be worn to protect the nose from further injury.

THE MOUTH AND JAW

The mouth and jaw are complex structures that are vulnerable to athletic injury. The mouth is composed of a **soft** and **hard palate**, mucous membranes, and the tongue. The mouth consists of 32 teeth, the lips, and the cheeks (Figure 23–14).

The jaw is made up of the **maxilla** and the **mandible**. The maxilla is a fixed bone that does not move. The mandible, in contrast, moves forward, backward, and sideways. This allows the teeth to bite and chew. The mandible and maxilla are attached to the skull at the **temporomandibular joint (TMJ)**.

INJURIES TO THE MOUTH AND JAW

Possible injuries to the jaw and mouth include fractures, TMJ dislocation and dysfunction, and damage to the teeth and soft tissues of the mouth. Generally, these injuries fall into three categories:

- Soft-tissue injuries such as cuts or lacerations to the lips, the tongue, the inside of the mouth, or the face.

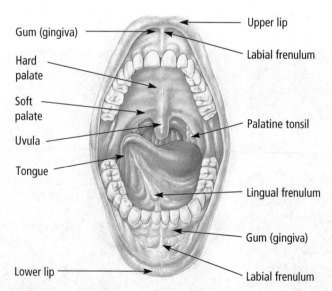

Gum (gingiva)
Hard palate
Soft palate
Uvula
Tongue
Lower lip
Upper lip
Labial frenulum
Palatine tonsil
Lingual frenulum
Gum (gingiva)
Labial frenulum

Figure 23–14 The mouth and its structures.

- Dental injuries to the teeth. Examples include fractured teeth, teeth that are partially or totally knocked out, and injuries to tooth-related structures (such as the braces).

- Jaw-related or bone-related injuries in which some bruising or fracturing of the jaw bones occurs. This includes alveolar fracture, which is a break in the bone that houses the teeth, and upper-jaw or lower-jaw fractures. Bruises or contusions to the bone in the lower jaw may also occur.

The fractures and injuries to bone are probably the most severe of the three and require the most attention.

Jaw Fractures

A broken jaw is a fracture of the mandible (bone of the lower jaw). The mandible is a sturdy bone that is horseshoe-shaped in the middle, but angled at the right and left sides. At either end, the mandible meets the skull's temporal bones to form the right and left temporomandibular joints in front of each ear.

Whenever an impact fractures the mandible, damage may occur in the tooth-bearing middle portion, at the angle, or at the extreme condyles (ends) near the ears. In more than 50% of cases, at least two fractures will be present. One will be the "direct" fracture at the actual site of impact; the second will be an "indirect" fracture somewhere else along the jaw. Most often, this second fracture is located near one of the condyles of the mandible, close to the temporomandibular joint. The second fracture occurs because the force of impact travels upward along the jaw and snaps the relatively thin portion of the mandible just below the ear.

Jaw fractures are the third most common type of facial fractures, after fractures of the nose and cheek. Fractures of the mandible are normally a result of a direct blow to the jaw.

SIGNS AND SYMPTOMS Symptoms may include severe pain at the fracture site, swelling, blood at the base of the teeth near the fracture site, deformity, tenderness, and sometimes numbness. If an athlete receives a blow to the jaw, fracture should be suspected if there is obvious deformity, if the teeth do not meet as they did before, or if sharp bits of bone can be felt in the mouth. Fractures of the lower jaw may be confined to the temporomandibular joint, in which case they will produce pain on biting; there may or may not be a change in the bite. Nerves may be damaged by the fracture, leading to numbness of the upper or lower lip.

TREATMENT Treatment includes immobilization of the athlete, application of ice, and treatment for shock. The athlete should be transported to a physician immediately.

REHABILITATION In most cases, the prognosis is very good, especially when the fracture is treated promptly and properly. The athlete must be cleared by the physician before continuing with athletics. Special protective helmets, shields, or mouthpieces may be required for future participation.

Temporomandibular Joint Injury

The temporomandibular joint (TMJ) allows the mouth to open and close. The TMJ is affected by the resulting action of the joint on the other side of the jaw, the muscles of the jaw and tongue, and the relationship of the teeth as they meet (Figure 23–15). As these all work together, a change in one part will cause a change in the function of the other parts.

SIGNS AND SYMPTOMS TMJ pain can be the result of direct trauma to the jaw or face, malocclusion (teeth not coming together), muscle imbalance, postural imbalance, or all of these.

A TMJ dislocation will result in inability to close the mouth, severe pain, deformity, and swelling. TMJ sprains are less severe than dislocations and are caused by overstretching one or more ligaments in the temporomandibular joint. Sprains involving two or more ligaments cause considerably more disability than single-ligament sprains. When the ligament is overstretched, it becomes tense and gives way at its weakest point, either where it attaches to bone or within the liga-ment itself. If the ligament pulls loose a fragment of bone, it is called a *sprain fracture*. The athlete will experience severe pain at the time of the injury. A popping feeling, along with difficulty opening and closing the mouth, is also a sign of injury. There may be tenderness, swelling, and bruising at the injury site.

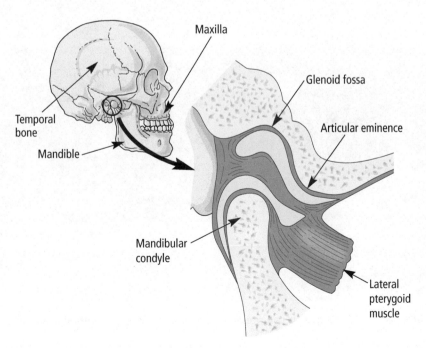

Figure 23–15 Temporomandibular joint.

TREATMENT Treatment includes application of ice and referral to a physician.

REHABILITATION Athletes may have to wear a dental appliance to support the TMJ. A mouthpiece may be required gear for future participation. A physician's clearance is required prior to return to athletics.

Injuries to the Teeth

According to the American Dental Association, more than 200,000 oral injuries are prevented annually in the United States by sports mouthguards (Figure 23–16). According to Massachusetts Dental Society, athletes are 60 times more likely to suffer damage to the mouth when not wearing a protective mouthguard. These oral traumas happen to athletes from the elementary grades to college level. Dental injuries are the most common type of orofacial injury sustained during participation in sports.

The benefits of sports mouthguard protection have been well documented. In 1995, Dr. Raymond Flanders' study on the high incidence of oral injuries showed that in football, where mouthguards are mandatory, only .07% of all injuries involved teeth and the oral cavity.

Conversely, in basketball, where mouthguards are not worn, 34% of all injuries to players involved teeth or the oral cavity (Flanders & Bhat, 1995). Whatever the sport, injuries to the teeth and oral cavity will be the result of direct trauma or impact on or around the head.

SIGNS AND SYMPTOMS Athletes will complain of loose, chipped, or missing teeth. There will be pain in the teeth involved, and in the gums anchoring the teeth.

TREATMENT If a tooth is knocked out or is hanging from the socket, place it back into the socket and have the athlete maintain pressure on the tooth to keep it in place. Transport the athlete to a dentist immediately. If it is not possible to reinsert the tooth, wrap it in sterile, moist gauze and have the athlete take the tooth to the dentist. The longer it is out of the mouth, the less likely it is that the tooth can be saved.

Chipped teeth usually do not require immediate care. Remove any tooth chips from the mouth so that they do not impede the airway. The athlete should be instructed to consult a dentist.

REHABILITATION An athlete who has had a tooth knocked out needs to obtain clearance to return to

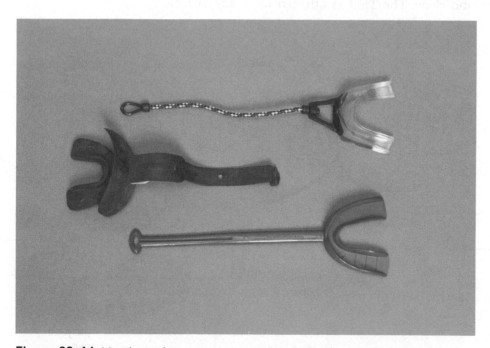

Figure 23–16 Mouthguards can prevent many injuries to the mouth and teeth.

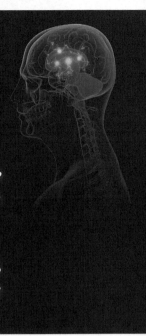

KEY CONCEPT

Injuries to the mouth and jaw:

- **A jaw fracture is a break in the lower jawbone. The athlete should be immobilized, ice should be applied, and the athlete should be monitored for shock. Treatment by a physician is necessary.**
- **Dislocation of the temporomandibular joint can cause severe pain, swelling, and deformity. Apply ice and refer the athlete to a physician for treatment.**
- **Injuries to the teeth can result in loose, chipped, or missing teeth. If a tooth is knocked out or hanging from the socket, place the tooth back in the socket, maintaining pressure to keep it in place. If that is not possible, wrap the tooth in moist gauze so the athlete can take it to the dentist for possible reimplantation.**

participation from a dentist. As stated earlier, mouthguards will prevent most dental injuries. The athlete should be required to use a mouthguard for all future athletic endeavors.

THE HEAD

As stated earlier, the skull consists of multiple facial bones and several bones that make up the cranium (see Figures 23–1 and 23–2).

The **cranium is an** oblong, egg-shaped collection of bones designed to protect the important anatomic structure underlying it, the brain. The anterior bone that makes up the forehead, the **frontal bone**, is very strong. The **temporal bone**, which makes up the sides of the skull, along the temples, is weaker and more easily fractured by a direct blow. Located in the temporal bone, behind the ears, within the *mastoid process,* are the **mastoid sinuses**. (A sinus is a cavity within a bone.)

The most posterior bone in the cranium is the **occipital bone**. The spinal cord passes through the occipital bone through a large opening called the **foramen magnum**, which translated means "big hole."

The largest bone of the skull, the **parietal bone**, by virtue of its size and lateral position protects a large part of the brain.

All the cranial bones are joined at immovable joints called **sutures**.

The Brain

The seat of all higher intellect, the human brain—thought to distinguish us from all other creatures—is in many ways very similar to those of other mammals. The human brain consists of a brainstem, cerebellum, and cerebrum. These areas of the brain have further subdivisions, each of which has its own unique functions. Figure 23–17 shows these subdivisions.

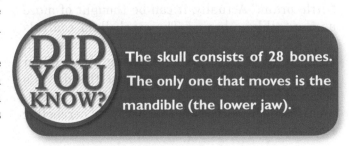

DID YOU KNOW? The skull consists of 28 bones. The only one that moves is the mandible (the lower jaw).

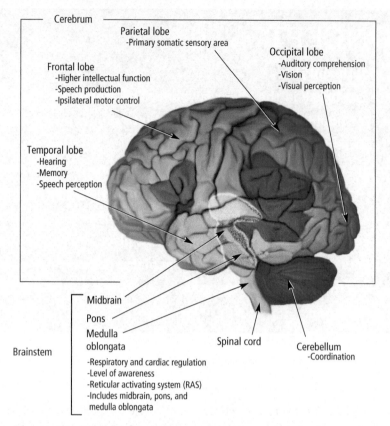

Cerebrum

Parietal lobe
-Primary somatic sensory area

Frontal lobe
-Higher intellectual function
-Speech production
-Ipsilateral motor control

Occipital lobe
-Auditory comprehension
-Vision
-Visual perception

Temporal lobe
-Hearing
-Memory
-Speech perception

Brainstem

Midbrain

Pons

Medulla oblongata

-Respiratory and cardiac regulation
-Level of awareness
-Reticular activating system (RAS)
-Includes midbrain, pons, and medulla oblongata

Spinal cord

Cerebellum
-Coordination

Figure 23–17 The brain and its subdivisions.

THE BRAINSTEM The most basic part of the human brain is the **brainstem**, which acts like a junction box for the complex wiring system of the central nervous system. The upper regions of the brain send all signals to the brainstem to be passed to the spinal cord for distribution to the body. The brainstem consists of the midbrain, pons, and medulla oblongata. All mammals have a brainstem that is involved in the control of life-sustaining functions such as breathing and heartbeat.

THE CEREBELLUM The word **cerebellum** means "little brain." Actually, it can be thought of more as the "athletic brain." The cerebellum controls muscular coordination and complex actions, such as shooting a basketball or driving a car. When police officers stop a car and test the driver's sense of balance as part of a drunk-driver assessment, they are testing the person's cerebellar functions.

THE CEREBRUM The seat of all higher thinking is the **cerebrum**. The cerebrum is the largest area of the brain and occupies the majority of the cranial vault. It is divided into a right and a left hemisphere and can be further divided into different lobes, each of which has specific duties and functions.

THE MENINGES The brain is protected by a hard, bony shell. Inside the shell there are membranes, called **meninges**, that surround the brain and continue along the spinal cord. These meninges pad the brain from impact. The innermost layer, the **pia mater**, clings to every surface of the brain. The next layer of the meninges is the **arachnoid**. The arachnoid spreads, web-like, over the entire brain. The outermost layer is called the **dura mater**, which literally means "tough mother" because it was once thought to give rise to every membrane of the body. Together, the pia mater, the arachnoid, and the dura mater act together to "pad" the brain from injury.

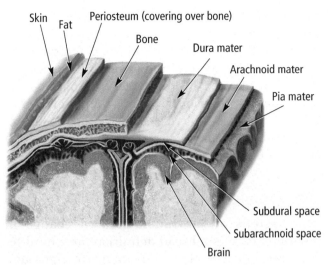

Skin Fat Periosteum (covering over bone) Bone Dura mater Arachnoid mater Pia mater Subdural space Subarachnoid space Brain

Figure 23–18 The meninges consist of the pia mater, arachnoid, and dura mater.

There is a great deal of cerebrospinal fluid (CSF) within the skull that further absorbs impact. The CSF also carries nutrients to and removes some wastes from the brain cells.

The combination of the bony skull, the protective meninges, and the shock-absorbing CSF protects the brain itself from impact and injury. These protective layers are illustrated in Figure 23–18.

HEAD INJURIES

Approximately half of the trauma-related deaths in the United States are due to head injuries. The mortality rate after a severe head injury is approximately 35%. More than half of those who do survive are left with serious disability as a result of injury to the brain.

Scalp Injuries

Injuries to the scalp may or may not involve the skull or brain. An athlete may incur a severe brain injury without any observable trauma to the scalp. Conversely, an athlete may have a dramatic-looking scalp injury but suffer little or no brain damage.

Common athletic injuries to the scalp are contusions and lacerations. These injuries are fairly common in sports, such as soccer, that do not require protective helmets.

SIGNS AND SYMPTOMS The scalp is highly vascularized and may bleed profusely if cut. Scalp wounds often appear worse than they actually are. Contusions about the scalp are marked by local tenderness and swelling. Bleeding between the skin and underlying tissue may result in a hematoma, which is commonly referred to as a "goose egg."

TREATMENT The source of bleeding should be located, and the bleeding controlled by direct pressure, before evaluation of the head is continued. If a fracture is suspected at the site of the bleeding, additional care should be taken not to depress the fracture site with added pressure.

REHABILITATION The athlete's physician or neurologist will determine when it is safe for the athlete to return to activity. Wearing of a protective helmet may become mandatory.

Skull Fractures

Skull fractures are uncommon in athletics but may occur if an athlete who lacks head protection receives a severe blow. Fractures of the skull may range from a simple linear fracture to a severe compound depressed fracture, in which bone fragments lacerate brain tissue. This type of trauma is more common in sports that require the use of a bat or club, but also occur in soccer because headgear is not required.

SIGNS AND SYMPTOMS Bleeding or cerebrospinal fluid draining from the ear or nose may be the only indication of a skull fracture. With any significant scalp injury, the certified athletic trainer should check for signs of a skull fracture.

TREATMENT If a skull fracture is suspected, the athlete should be immobilized and treated for shock while EMS is called. This should be treated as a significant head injury. If bleeding is present, light pressure with several layers of sterile gauze should control the bleeding.

REHABILITATION As with all head injuries, the athlete's physician or neurologist will determine when it is safe for the athlete to return to activity. Wearing of a protective helmet may become mandatory.

BRAIN INJURIES

Injuries to the brain constitute by far the most serious threat to an athlete. These injuries usually result from movement of the brain within the skull. The semisolid brain, surrounded by cerebrospinal fluid, has limited freedom to move about within the skull. The brain is vulnerable to accelerative forces in a variety of contact and collision sports. Whenever a sudden force or impact is applied to the head, there can be an abrupt movement of the brain within the skull.

A sudden, forceful impact to the head can cause agitation of the brain, resulting in transient dysfunction (**cerebral concussion**). The brain may also be injured by direct transmission of force from the skull to the underlying tissue. This can result in the brain being contused (**cerebral contusion**) or lacerated as it collides with the skull. The brain can be injured when it rebounds against the opposite side of the skull. This mechanism,

called a **contrecoup** injury, is possible because the brain can move within the skull. The extent of the injury to the brain depends on the magnitude and direction of impact and the structural features of the brain affected by the force. Any blow to the head may be injurious to the brain. However, a brain injury is not necessarily the result of a single blow; it may be the cumulative effect of a series of blows.

Concussions

Concussions or "a trauma-induced change in mental status" is a broad definition for a hard-to-diagnose injury with a wide range of signs and symptoms; as defined by the Cantu Concussion Center, Emerson Hospital, Concord, Massachusetts. Robert Cantu, one of the world's leading experts on concussions and their effects on the human body, states that the signs and symptoms of concussions are:

PHYSICAL	EMOTIONAL	COGNITIVE	SLEEP DISTURBANCE
Headaches	Depression	Difficulty concentrating	Sleeping more or less than usual
Nausea	Nervousness	Troubles with memory	Trouble falling asleep
Vomiting	Irritability	Feeling mentally slow or as in a fog that will not lift	
Balance and/or visual problems	Panic attacks		
Dizzy Spells			
Sensitivity to light and/or noise			
Fatigue and/or low energy			

A traumatic brain injuries (TBI) occur commonly during sports. They range in severity from momentary disorientation to a blow resulting in loss of consciousness. Coaches, as well as trainers, therapists, and physicians covering athletic contests, need to understand concussions and the immediate treatment for

athletes who suffer these injuries. Inappropriate care may have serious and sometimes lifelong consequences.

In the United States, between 1.6 and 3.8 million sports- and recreation-related concussions occur annually; as reported by the Center for Disease Control and Prevention (CDC).

This is double the numbers reported only a decade ago. The likelihood of suffering a concussion while playing a contact sport has been estimated as high as 10% per year of play. More than 300,000 concussions are sustained each year in high school contact sports. For football in particular, college athletes experience an estimated 6.3 concussions per 1,000 athletic exposures, a number that includes all practices and games. High school rates were at 11.2 concussions per 1,000 athletic exposures. Concussions often cause significant, sustained neuropsychological impairments in information processing speed, problem solving, planning, and memory. These impairments worsen with multiple concussions.

BASELINE TESTING Prior to participation in any collision sport, it is important to have a **Baseline Test** completed. Baseline Testing should be done by a medical health professional trained to administer these tests. As defined by the Sports Concussion Institute, "A Baseline Concussion Test is an important piece to concussion management. Each concussion is unique, so it is important to treat individuals on a case-by-case basis. Comparing post-injury test scores of an individual to their own baseline test scores from before the concussion is considered best practice. Without a baseline test to use for comparison, an individual's post-injury test scores can only be compared to the general population. Whenever possible, we want to compare apples to apples, and Baseline Concussion Tests allow us to do just that."

The Baseline Test should be repeated annually to establish a valid test result for comparison. If using a computerized or written test, these tests should be repeated every two years. If an athlete has sustained a concussion, these tests should be administered as needed.

In February 2018 the United States Food and Drug Administration (FDA) approved the first ever blood test for mild traumatic brain injury (mTBI). Availability of a blood test for a suspected concussion will help health care professionals determine the need for a CT scan in patients suspected of having mTBI and help prevent un-necessary neuroimaging and associated radiation exposure to patients. The blood test will aid in concussion evaluation.

The blood test Indicator works by measuring levels of proteins, known as UCH-L1 and GFAP, that are released from the brain into blood and measured within 12 hours of a head injury. Levels of these blood proteins after a concussion can help predict which patients may have intracranial bleeding visible by CT scan and which won't. Being able to predict if patients have a low probability of intracranial bleeding can help health care professionals in their management of patients and the decision to perform a CT scan. Test results can be available within 3 to 4 hours.

TREATMENT Management of concussion includes a review of the history of the athlete's injury, inspection, palpation, and neurological screening. The history includes the mechanism or cause of injury, symptoms associated with the injury, and the level of consciousness. The inspection and palpation include the cervical vertebrae and musculature. Neurological screening includes sensory and motor testing.

Several different scales exist for grading concussions. The **Glasgow Coma Scale (GCS)** is an effective method often used to describe various states of consciousness. The advantage of the GCS is that it is a standard guide for rating various conditions that allows for easy identification of a change in an athlete's level of consciousness. This saves time because observations are rated numerically. The aims in developing the scale were that it should be widely acceptable and should complement, not replace assessments of other neurological functions. The GCS evaluates three different responses:

1. Eye opening
2. Motor responses
3. Verbal responses

Each is evaluated independent of the others, and each is assigned a numerical value. Higher scores are awarded to athletes who are more responsive. The total score reflects the level of brain functioning, with the highest score being 15 and the lowest score a 3. Table 23–3 outlines the GCS.

The American College of Surgeons Committee on Trauma has adopted the **alert/verbal/painful/unresponsive (AVPU)** method of determining levels of consciousness. This method investigates whether the individual is alert, responsive to verbal stimuli, responsive to painful stimuli, or unresponsive. Within seconds, the certified athletic trainer can assess an athlete's pupil size, reaction, and best motor response. The examiner also notes whether the athlete responds appropriately to commands, responds only to painful stimuli, or exhibits no movement at all. This method can be used in conjunction with the Glasgow Coma Scale. Table 23–4 outlines the AVPU scale.

Table 23–3	Glasgow Coma Scale		
EYE OPENING			
CRITERION	**OBSERVED**	**RATING**	**SCORE**
Open before stimulus	✓	Spontaneous	4
After spoken or shouted request	✓	To sound	3
After finger tip stimulus	✓	To pressure	2
No opening at any time, no interfering factor	✓	None	1
Closed by local factor	✓	Non testable	NT
VERBAL RESPONSE			
CRITERION	**OBSERVED**	**RATING**	**SCORE**
Correctly gives name, place and date	✓	Orientated	5
Not orientated but communication coherently	✓	Confused	4
Intelligible single words	✓	Words	3
Only moans / groans	✓	Sounds	2
No audible response, no interfering factor	✓	None	1
Factor interferring with communication	✓	Non testable	NT
BEST MOTOR RESPONSE			
CRITERION	**OBSERVED**	**RATING**	**SCORE**
Obey 2-part request	✓	Obeys commands	6
Brings hand above clavicle to stimulus on head neck	✓	Localising	5
Bends arm at elbow rapidly but features not predominantly abnormal	✓	Normal flexion	4
Bends arm at elbow, features clearly predominantly abnormal	✓	Abnormal flexion	3
Extends arm at elbow	✓	Extension	2
No movement in arms / legs, no interfering factor	✓	None	1
Paralysed or other limiting factor	✓	Non testable	NT

Table 23–4 AVPU

ALERT	YES/NO
Verbal—response to verbal command	Yes/No
Pain—response to painful stimulus	Yes/No
Unresponsive	Yes/No

Careful evaluation of pupil size and response to light is essential at the initial assessment and during further observation. Raised intracranial pressure and temporal lobe herniation will cause compression of the third cranial nerve (oculomotor). The result is **pupillary dilation**, which nearly always occurs initially on the side where the pressure is raised. The pupil will at first remain reactive to light, but subsequently becomes sluggish and then fails to respond to light at all. As the intracranial pressure increases, pupil response on the other side may also be affected.

CLASSIFICATION OF CONCUSSIONS Over the past few decades there has been numerous concussion grading systems and return to play protocols. All have been helpful and used by many health professionals. The major thing lacking was a consensus of all the best practices that are known to date.

The International Conference on Concussion in Sport is held each year in a different city worldwide. The goal of this group was to come to consensus on a single protocol that everyone could adopt and utilize. They meet each year to share newest scientific studies and best practices. Each year the protocol may be modified depending on new research. Tables 23-5 and 23-6 show return to play protocol developed in the 2017 conference.

PREVENTION As part of the history of injury, information regarding protective equipment used at the time of the injury should be sought.

Table 23–5 Graduated return to sport strategy

CONCUSSION GRADE	CANTU GRADING SYSTEM (2001 REVISION)	1991 COLORADO MEDICAL SOCIETY GUIDELINES	1997 AMERICAN ACADEMY OF NEUROLOGY GUIDELINES
Grade 1 (mild)	• No LOC • Either PTA or postconcussion signs and symptoms that clear in less than 30 minutes	• Transient mental confusion • No PTA • No LOC	• No LOC • Transient confusion • Symptoms or abnormalities clear in less than 15 minutes
Grade 2 (moderate)	• LOC lasting less than 1 minute and PTA or • Postconcussion signs or symptoms lasting longer than 30 minutes but less than 24 hours	• No LOC • Confusion with PTA	• No LOC • Symptoms or abnormalities last more than 15 minutes
Grade 3 (severe)	• LOC lasting more than 1 minute or • PTA lasting longer than 24 hours or • Postconcussion signs or symptoms lasting longer than 7 days	• Any LOC, however brief	• Any LOC, either brief (seconds) or prolonged (minutes)

Table 23–6 Postconcussion Symptoms Scale

	NONE			MODERATE			SEVERE
				RATING			
Headache	0	1	2	3	4	5	6
Nausea	0	1	2	3	4	5	6
Vomiting	0	1	2	3	4	5	6
Drowsiness	0	1	2	3	4	5	6
Numbness or tingling	0	1	2	3	4	5	6
Dizziness	0	1	2	3	4	5	6
Balance problems	0	1	2	3	4	5	6
Sleeping more than usual	0	1	2	3	4	5	6
Sensitivity to light	0	1	2	3	4	5	6
Sensitivity to noise	0	1	2	3	4	5	6
Feeling slowed down	0	1	2	3	4	5	6
Feeling as if "in a fog"	0	1	2	3	4	5	6
Difficulty concentrating	0	1	2	3	4	5	6
Difficulty remembering	0	1	2	3	4	5	6
Trouble falling asleep	0	1	2	3	4	5	6
More emotional than usual	0	1	2	3	4	5	6
Irritability	0	1	2	3	4	5	6
Sadness	0	1	2	3	4	5	6
Nervousness	0	1	2	3	4	5	6
Other	0	1	2	3	4	5	6

Such information can guide modification and optimization of the protective equipment. However, research shows that there are relatively few methods by which concussive brain injury can be minimized in sport (McCrory 2001; McIntosh & McCrory 2000). The brain is not an organ that can be conditioned to withstand injury. Thus, extrinsic mechanisms of injury prevention (i.e., protective equipment and rule changes to limit contact with the head) must be sought.

Helmets help to protect the head and reduce the risk of brain injury. In sports where there may be high-speed collisions, or that have the potential for missile injuries (e.g., baseball) or falls onto hard surfaces (e.g., football, ice hockey), published evidence proves that sport-specific helmets help reduce the number and severity of head injuries (McIntosh & McCrory, 2000).

The National Operating Committee on Standards for Athletic Equipment (NOCSAE) is a non-profit organization operating in the United States; whose mission is to reduce athletic injuries and death through standards and certification for athletic equipment. Schools and universities look to NOCSAE certification of equipment, particularly helmets, to protect players and reduce liability. NOCSAE data indicate a significant reduction in athlete fatalities and brain injuries when using NOCSAE-certified equipment. This, along with rule changes and better coaching

KEY CONCEPT

Signs of a concussion include:

- Unaware of surroundings, dates, time, or place
- Loss of consciousness
- Confusion
- Amnesia
- Headache
- Dizziness
- Nausea
- Unsteadiness/loss of balance
- Ringing in ears

- Double vision or seeing flashes of light
- Sleepiness
- Sleep disturbance
- Convulsions
- Exhibition of inappropriate emotions
- Vacant stare
- Slurred speech

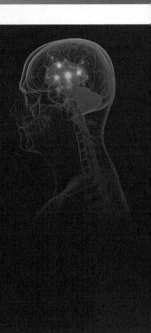

techniques, will help to further protect all athletes from catastrophic injury.

The use of correctly fit mouth guards can reduce the rate of dental orofacial and mandibular injuries (Park et al., 1993; Lanze, 2003), but evidence that they reduce cerebral injuries is largely theoretical, and clinical evidence of a beneficial effect in reducing concussion rates has not yet been demonstrated scientifically (McCrory, 2001).

Rule enforcement is a critical aspect in reducing and preventing concussions. Referees play a key role in enforcing new rules that are intended to reduce injuries to the brain and body as a whole.

Athletes and health care providers alike must be educated regarding the detection of concussion, its clinical features, assessment techniques, and principles of safe return to play. Many valuable methods of improving education, including Internet resources, educational videos, outreach programs, concussion working groups, and various sport groups, are available today.

AMNESIA Amnesia may take the form of **retrograde amnesia**, in which there is a loss of memory for events that occurred before the injury; or **antegrade amnesia**, in which there is a loss of memory for events occurring immediately after

awakening from a loss of consciousness. Dizziness, tinnitus (ringing in the ears), unsteadiness, blurred vision, double vision, nausea, and headaches are also common and may be experienced in varying combinations.

Normally, an athlete who has suffered a concussion will improve rapidly to an alert state of consciousness. The greatest concern of anyone who is responsible for caring for an athlete with a head injury is the possible development of an expanding intracranial or intracerebral bleed. The signs and symptoms of a concussion normally are reversible; that is, they will appear to be worst on the initial evaluation and then improve. If the signs and symptoms become progressively worse, the deterioration suggests that there may be problems within the cranium.

POSTCONCUSSION SYNDROME **Postconcussion syndrome** is a poorly understood condition that occurs following a concussion. It consists of a persistent headache, dizziness, fatigue, irritability, anxiety, insomnia, ringing in the ears, blurry vision, sensitivity to light and noise, and impaired memory or lack of concentration. The symptoms may persist for days, weeks, or perhaps a year or more. These symptoms must be monitored periodically, and the athlete withheld from activity for as long as they persist.

Brain Contusions

Contusions, or bruising of the brain, result when the brain collides against the skull or is raked over bony irregularities, especially on the floor of the skull. Contusions to the hemispheres of the brain may result in a lack of nerve function of the bruised portion of the brain, but usually do not result in a loss of consciousness. The difference between a brain contusion and a concussion is the fact that a concussion involves a widespread trauma due to a blow to the head.

SIGNS AND SYMPTOMS Signs suggesting that an athlete may have a cerebral contusion are numbness, weakness, loss of memory, **aphasia** (loss of speech or comprehension), or general misbehavior when the athlete is alert. An athlete with a cerebral contusion remains stable or begins improving. Any deterioration suggests additional intracranial involvement and problems.

Hemorrhage (Bleeding)

Intracranial hemorrhaging is a potentially life-threatening consequence of a head injury. Hemorrhaging can lead to a rapid deterioration of the athlete's condition and must be recognized if death or disability is to be averted. The same sudden forces that may result in a concussion or contusion (to any area) of the brain may also damage blood vessels, causing a hemorrhage. Hemorrhaging forms a hematoma, which may continue to enlarge after the injury. Hematomas are classified by their locations within the skull:

- A **subdural hematoma** develops when bridging cerebral vessels that travel from the brain to the overlying dura are torn. This condition is the most frequent cause of death from trauma in athletics. Rupturing of the cerebral vessels can occur as a result of a twisting motion of the cerebral hemispheres, or from stretching of the vessels on the side opposite the point of impact. Hemorrhaging can result in low-pressure venous bleeding or rapid arterial bleeding into the subdural space of the cerebrum (Figure 23–19). The hematoma may progress rapidly, or not become evident for hours, or even days, after the injury.

- An **epidural hematoma** develops when a dural artery is ruptured. Usually this hematoma is

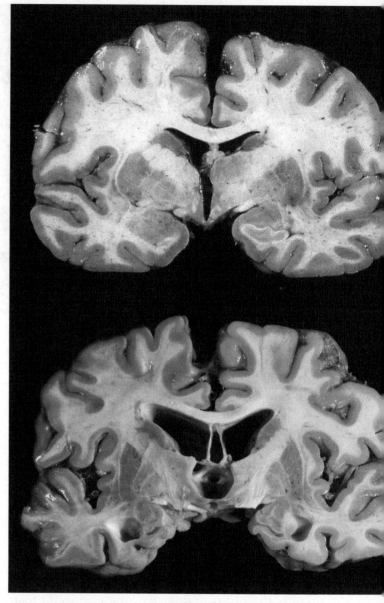

Figure 23–19 A subdural hematoma usually results from the tearing of small veins under the dura mater. Courtesy of Ann McKee and Boston University

associated with a skull fracture and is commonly caused by a tear of the meningeal artery. The bleeding occurs between the dura mater and the skull (Figure 23–20). The clot formation is usually rapid, and signs and symptoms may occur in a matter of minutes to hours.

- An **intracranial hematoma** develops when blood vessels within the brain are damaged. This may occur when a cerebral contusion is accompanied by significant bleeding.

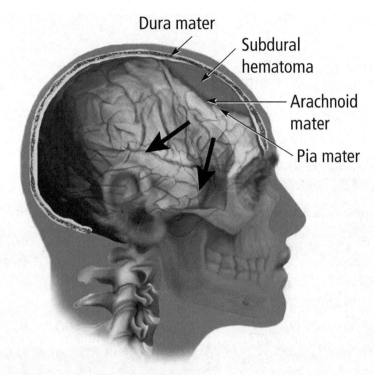

Figure 23–20 An epidural hematoma is often associated with a skull fracture and an arterial injury.

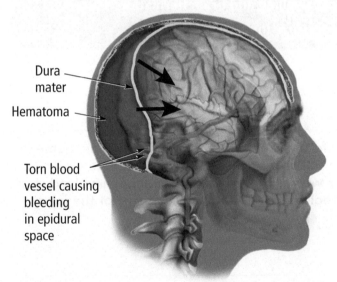

Figure 23–21 An epidural hematoma is often associated with a skull fracture and an arterial injury.

Each type of hematoma can cause an increase in intracranial pressure and shifting of the hemispheres away from the hematoma. This accounts for the deteriorating neurologic signs and symptoms such as decreasing levels of consciousness, loss of movements, slowing of pupil reactions, or dilating pupils. The importance of continuing evaluation cannot be overemphasized. A certified athletic trainer *must* continue to evaluate an athlete who has suffered a head injury for neurological signs that may indicate hemorrhaging and an expanding lesion within the cranium. Failure to do so can result in disability or death for the athlete.

Secondary Impact Syndrome

Secondary impact syndrome (SIS) involves rapid swelling and herniation of the brain after a second head injury that occurs before the symptoms of a previous injury have been resolved. Although rare, SIS is dangerous and can be deadly. The second impact may be relatively minor; in some cases, SIS may occur even without an impact to the head. A blow to the chest or back may create enough force to move the athlete's head suddenly and send acceleration/deceleration forces to an already compromised brain.

Prevention is the only sure cure. It is essential that an athlete who is symptomatic from a head injury not be allowed to participate in contact or collision activities until all cerebral symptoms have subsided.

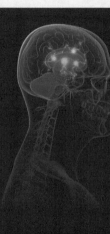

KEY CONCEPT

Head injuries:

- Scalp injuries can involve the skull and the brain. A severe brain injury can exist without serious visible trauma to the scalp. Bleeding should be controlled, and then a further evaluation of the head done.

- Skull fractures are breaks in any of the bones of the skull. Bleeding or leakage of cerebrospinal fluid from the nose or ears may be the only indication of a skull fracture. Immobilize the athlete, treat for shock, and call **EMS**.

Brain injuries:

- Concussions range in severity and can result in significant neurological impairment. Treatment should begin with the athlete's injury history, inspection, palpation, and neurological screening.

- Contusions are bruising of the brain, and may result in lack of nerve function in the bruised area.

- Hemorrhage is bleeding within the spaces in the brain. This is a serious condition and **EMS** must be activated.

- Secondary impact syndrome is rapid swelling and brain herniation following a second injury that occurs before the first injury has healed.

CONCLUSION

Injuries to the head and neck can be serious and life threatening. Proper care and management of these injuries can mean the difference between full or partial recovery. A complete understanding of the anatomy of the head and brain, as well as the mechanism of injury involved in an accident, will give medical personnel the proper tools for an accurate assessment of the injury, proper treatment, and an eventual return to sport.

REVIEW QUESTIONS

1. What sports are responsible for the majority of facial injuries? Why?
2. How can facial injuries be prevented?
3. Write a brief explanation of the different types of injuries to which the eyes are susceptible in athletics.
4. What is cauliflower ear, and how can it be prevented and treated?
5. What is the cause of swimmer's ear?
6. Describe the treatment for epistaxis.
7. Explain temporomandibular joint injuries.
8. You are responsible for the medical coverage of a softball game. One of the girls is hit in the mouth with the softball. The impact knocks out one of her teeth. What do you do?

9. How does a mouthguard help prevent injuries to the teeth and mouth?
10. Why do scalp injuries bleed so profusely?
11. Explain the difference between a cerebral concussion and a cerebral contusion.
12. What is a contrecoup injury?
13. Explain the different methods used for assessing various states of consciousness.
14. What are the return-to-play criteria for an athlete suffering a concussion?
15. What are the signs and symptoms of a concussion?
16. What is the difference between retrograde and antegrade amnesia?
17. Describe the three different types of hematomas that can occur within the skull.
18. Why is secondary impact syndrome a concern with head injuries?
19. How can concussions be prevented?

PROJECTS AND ACTIVITIES

1. Draw a picture of the ear. Label all of the parts listed in the Key Terms section.
2. Explore sites on the Internet that offer TMJ advice and support. Write down your findings.
3. Ask your family dentist what is done for someone who has lost a tooth to injury. Write a report on what you found out.
4. Write a report on catastrophic head injuries in athletics.
5. Ask the football coach at your school how he fits helmets for his athletes. Ask him to fit you with one. How does the helmet feel? Do you believe you are protected against a head injury?

LEARNING LINKS

- Search http://www.physsportsmed.com and for articles on the types of head and facial injuries discussed in this chapter.
- Search the Internet for information on various types of prevention techniques and protective equipment available to prevent the occurrence of head and facial injuries.

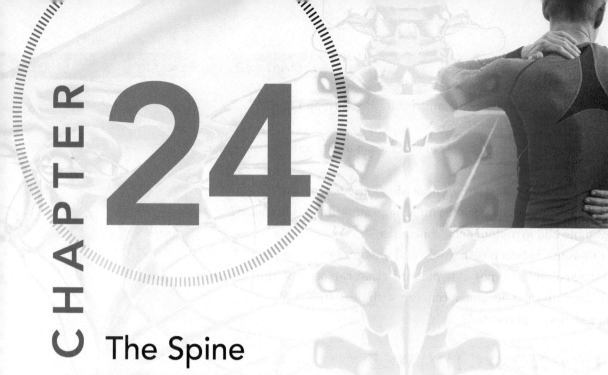
Albina Glisic/Shutterstock.com.

CHAPTER 24

The Spine

OBJECTIVES

Upon completion of this chapter, the reader should be able to:

- Describe how the nervous system works
- Describe the peripheral and autonomic nervous systems
- Describe the function of the sympathetic system
- Explain common injuries to the spine
- Explain how one would give aid to an athlete with a neck injury
- Describe the management protocols for an athlete with a back injury
- Explain the symptoms of intervertebral disc herniation

KEY TERMS

afferent nerve *A nerve that carries nerve impulses from the periphery to the central nervous system; also known as a sensory nerve.*

annulus fibrosus *Rings of collagen fibers that surround the intervertebral disk.*

articular facet *The small, articulating surface of the vertebrae.*

atlas *The first cervical vertebra; articulates with the axis and occipital skull bone.*

autonomic nervous system *A division of the peripheral nervous system; consists of a collection of nerves, ganglia, and plexuses through which visceral organs, heart, blood vessels, glands, and smooth muscles receive their innervation.*

axial loading *Compression of the spinal cord from a blow to the top of the head when the neck is slightly flexed.*

axis *The second cervical vertebra.*

bilateral *On both sides.*

central nervous system *The body system that consists of the brain and the spinal cord.*

KEY TERMS CONTINUED

cervical nerve syndrome *An injury to the neck resulting from a forced lateral flexion that causes the nerves to be stretched or impinged.*

cervical vertebrae *The first seven bones of the spinal column.*

coccyx *The last bone of the spinal column; tailbone.*

cranial nerves *Twelve pairs of nerves that begin in the brain and transmit messages to and from various parts of the face and head to stimulate various functions, and receive sensory information.*

effector *The organ that responds to a stimulus.*

efferent nerve *A nerve that carries messages from the brain and spinal cord to muscles and glands; also known as a motor nerve.*

gray matter *The inner part of the spinal cord.*

intervertebral disc herniation *Dislocation of a disc, resulting in pressure against the spinal cord.*

lumbar vertebrae *The five vertebrae located in the lower lumbar region of the back.*

meninges *Any of the three linings that enclose the brain and spinal cord.*

mixed nerve *A nerve composed of both afferent and efferent fibers.*

motor nerve *A nerve that carries messages from the brain and spinal cord to muscles and glands; also known as an efferent nerve.*

neuropraxia *The cessation of function of a nerve without degenerative changes.*

nucleus pulposus *A gelatin-like substance in the center of the vertebral disc.*

parasympathetic nervous system *Division of the autonomic nervous system that inhibits or opposes the effects of the sympathetic system.*

paresthesia *Sensation of tingling, crawling, or burning of the skin.*

pars interarticularis *The area between the superior and inferior articulations of the vertebrae; a common site of fractures due to spondylolysis.*

peripheral nervous system *A division of the central nervous system, made up of 12 pairs of cranial nerves and 31 pairs of spinal nerves.*

plexus *A network of spinal nerves.*

quadriparesis *Partial paralysis in all four extremities.*

quadriplegia *Paralysis in all four extremities.*

receptor *A sensory nerve that receives a stimulus and transmits it to the central nervous system.*

reflex *Any involuntary action.*

sacroiliac joint *The area between the sacrum and the ilium.*

sacrum *The wedge-shaped bone below the lumbar vertebrae at the end of the spinal column.*

sciatic nerve *The largest nerve in the body; originates in the sacral plexus and runs through the pelvis and down the leg.*

sensory nerve *A nerve that carries nerve impulses from the periphery to the central nervous system; also known as an afferent nerve.*

KEY TERMS CONTINUED

spinal cord *Part of the central nervous system within the spinal column; begins at the foramen magnum of the occipital bone and continues to the second lumbar vertebra.*

spinal nerves *Thirty-one pairs of nerves originating in the spinal cord.*

spondylolisthesis *The slippage of one vertebra on the vertebra directly below it.*

spondylolysis *The breakdown of the structure of the vertebrae.*

stenosis *Narrowing of a duct or canal.*

stimulus *Any action that excites or produces a temporary reaction in the whole organism or in any of its parts.*

subcutaneous spinous process *Area just under the skin over each protrusion of the vertebrae.*

subluxation *An incomplete or partial dislocation of a joint.*

sympathetic nervous system *The division of the autonomic nervous system that prepares the body for action.*

thoracic vertebrae *The 12 segments of the vertebral column that articulate with ribs to form part of the thoracic cage.*

unilateral *On one side only.*

white matter *The outer part of the spinal cord.*

THE NERVOUS SYSTEM

The nervous system is the body's information gatherer, storage center, and control system. Its overall function is to collect information about external conditions in relation to the body's internal state, analyze this information, and initiate appropriate responses to satisfy certain needs. The most powerful need is survival. The nerves do not form one single system, but rather several that are interrelated. Some of these are physically separate; others differ in function only.

The brain and spinal cord make up the **central nervous system**. The nervous system's other division is the **peripheral nervous system**. The nervous system uses electrical impulses, which travel along the length of the cells at up to 250 miles per hour. The cells process information

from the sensory nerves and initiate an action within milliseconds.

THE PERIPHERAL AND AUTONOMIC NERVOUS SYSTEMS

Peripheral Nervous System

The peripheral nervous system includes all the nerves and ganglia (groups of cell bodies) of the body outside the brain and spinal cord (Figure 24–1). It connects the central nervous system to the various body structures. The **autonomic nervous system**, a specialized part of the peripheral system, controls the involuntary, or automatic, activities of the vital internal organs.

The three functions of the peripheral nervous system are:

1. To connect the body to the central nervous system.
2. To control the automatic or involuntary activities of the body.
3. To act as the reflex center of the body.

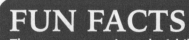

FUN FACTS
There are approximately 1 billion neurons in a human spinal cord.

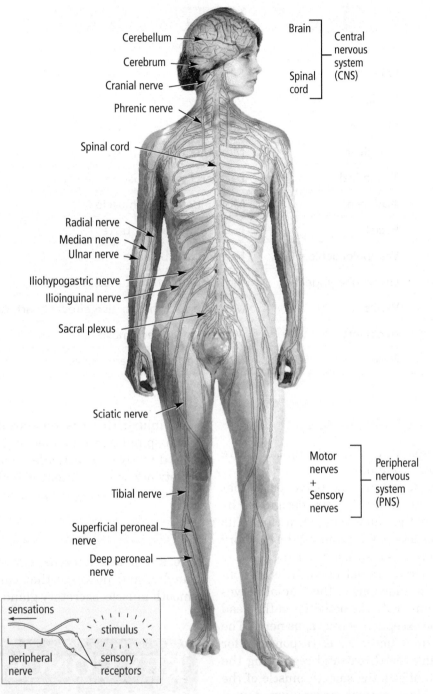

Cerebellum
Cerebrum
Cranial nerve
Phrenic nerve
Spinal cord
Radial nerve
Median nerve
Ulnar nerve
Iliohypogastric nerve
Ilioinguinal nerve
Sacral plexus
Sciatic nerve
Tibial nerve
Superficial peroneal nerve
Deep peroneal nerve

Brain
Spinal cord
Central nervous system (CNS)

Motor nerves + Sensory nerves
Peripheral nervous system (PNS)

sensations
stimulus
peripheral nerve
sensory receptors

Figure 24–1 The peripheral nervous system connects the central nervous system to structures of the body.

Nerves

A *nerve* consists of bundles of nerve fibers enclosed by connective tissue. If the nerve's fibers carry impulses from the sense organs to the brain or spinal cord, it is called a **sensory**, or **afferent nerve**; if its fibers carry impulses from the brain or spinal cord to muscles or glands, it is known as a **motor**, or **efferent nerve**; if it contains both sensory and motor fibers, it is called a **mixed nerve**.

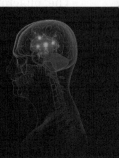

KEY CONCEPT

The nervous system uses electrical impulses, which travel along the length of the cells, to initiate an action.

Table 24–1 Cranial Nerves

NUMBER	NAME	FUNCTION
I	Olfactory	Smell
II	Optic	Vision, eyesight
III	Oculomotor	Movement of eye muscle
IV	Trochlear	Movement of eye muscle
V	Trigeminal	Face and teeth muscles, chewing
VI	Abducens	Movement of eye muscle
VII	Facial	Facial expressions, taste
VIII	Vestibulocochlear	Hearing and balance
IX	Glossopharyngeal	Movement of throat muscle, taste
X	Vagus	Movement of throat; also affects heart, digestive system
XI	Accessory	Movement of neck muscles
XII	Hypoglossal	Movement of tongue muscles

Cranial and Spinal Nerves

The cranial and spinal nerves make up the entire peripheral nervous system.

The **cranial nerves** are 12 nerve pairs that begin in areas of the brain. They are designated by number and name; the name may give a clue to its function (see Table 24–1). For example, the olfactory nerve, cranial nerve I, is responsible for the sense of smell. The optic nerve, cranial nerve II, is responsible for vision. The functions of the cranial nerves are concerned mainly with the activities of the head and neck, with the exception of the vagus nerve. The vagus nerve, cranial nerve X, is responsible for activities involving the throat and regulating the heart rate; it also affects the smooth muscle of the digestive tract. Most cranial nerves are mixed nerves: They carry both sensory and motor fibers. The olfactory, optic, and vestibulocochlear nerves, however, consist only of sensory fibers, meaning they pick up only the stimuli.

The **spinal nerves** originate at the spinal cord and go through openings in the vertebrae. There are 31 pairs of spinal nerves, and all are mixed nerves. The spinal nerves are named in relation to their location on the spinal cord. They carry messages to and from the spinal cord and brain, and to all parts of the body. Therefore, after a spinal cord injury, there is no sensation or movement. Each spinal nerve divides and branches; either it goes directly to a particular body segment or forms a network with adjacent spinal nerves and veins, called a **plexus** (Figure 24–2 and Table 24–2).

Autonomic Nervous System

The autonomic nervous system includes nerves, ganglia, and plexuses that carry impulses to all smooth muscle, secretory glands, and heart muscle

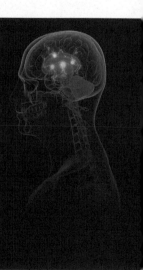

KEY CONCEPT

The peripheral nervous system connects the central nervous system to various body structures. The autonomic nervous system is a specialized portion of the peripheral nervous system that controls the involuntary activities of the vital organs.

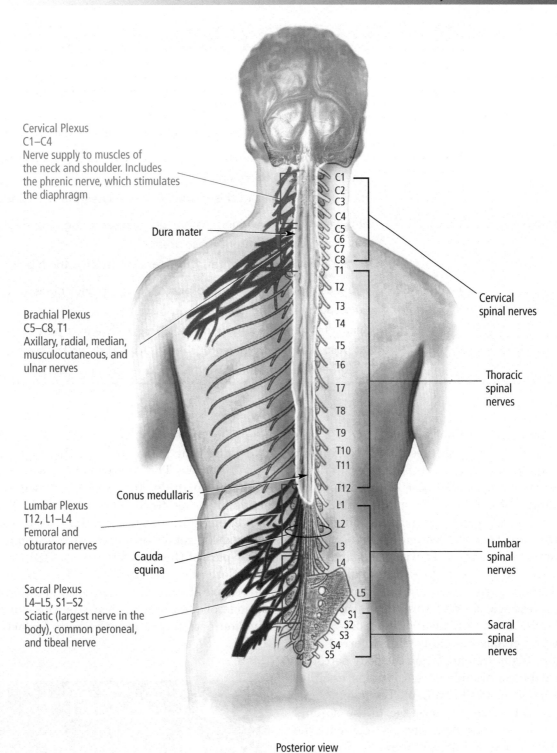

Cervical Plexus
C1–C4
Nerve supply to muscles of
the neck and shoulder. Includes
the phrenic nerve, which stimulates
the diaphragm

Dura mater

C1
C2
C3
C4
C5
C6
C7
C8

Cervical
spinal nerves

T1
T2
T3
T4
T5
T6
T7
T8
T9
T10
T11
T12

Thoracic
spinal
nerves

Brachial Plexus
C5–C8, T1
Axillary, radial, median,
musculocutaneous, and
ulnar nerves

Conus medullaris

Lumbar Plexus
T12, L1–L4
Femoral and
obturator nerves

Cauda
equina

Sacral Plexus
L4–L5, S1–S2
Sciatic (largest nerve in the
body), common peroneal,
and tibeal nerve

L1
L2
L3
L4
L5

Lumbar
spinal
nerves

S1
S2
S3
S4
S5

Sacral
spinal
nerves

Posterior view

Figure 24–2 Spinal nerve plexus and important nerves.

(Figure 24–3). It regulates the activities of the visceral organs (heart and blood vessels, respiratory organs, alimentary canal, kidneys, urinary bladder, and reproductive organs). The activities of these organs are usually automatic—not subject to conscious control.

The autonomic system has two divisions, sympathetic and parasympathetic. These two divisions may be antagonistic in their action. The sympathetic system may accelerate the heartbeat in response to fear, whereas the parasympathetic slows it down. Normally the two divisions are in

Table 24–2 Spinal Nerve Plexus

NUMBER	NAME	FUNCTION
Cervical plexus	C1–C4	Supplies motor movement to muscles of neck and shoulders and receives messages from these areas. Phrenic nerve is part of this group and stimulates the diaphragm.
Brachial plexus	C5–C8, T1	Supplies motor movement to shoulder, wrist, and hand and receives messages from these areas. Radial nerve is part of this group and stimulates the wrist and hand.
Lumbar plexus	T12, L1–L4	Supplies motor movement to buttocks, anterior leg, and thighs and receives messages from these areas. Femoral nerve is part of this group and stimulates the hip and leg.
Sacral plexus	L4–L5, S1–S2	Supplies motor movement to posterior of leg and thighs and receives messages from these areas. Sciatic nerve is the largest nerve in the body and is part of this group. It passes through the gluteus maximus and down the back of the thigh and leg. It extends the hip and flexes the knee.

balance; the activity of one or the other becomes dominant as dictated by the needs of the organism.

The **sympathetic system** consists primarily of two cords, beginning at the base of the brain, proceeding down both sides of the spinal column, and consisting of nerve fibers and ganglia of nerve cell bodies. The cord between the ganglia is a cable of nerve fibers closely associated with the spinal cord. Sympathetic nerves extend to all the vital internal organs, including the liver and pancreas, heart, stomach, intestines, blood vessels, the iris of the eye, sweat glands, and the bladder (Figure 24–3). The sympathetic nervous system is often referred to as the "fight-or-flight system." When the body perceives that it is in danger or under stress, it prepares either to run away or to stand and fight. The sympathetic nervous system sends the message to the adrenal medulla, which secretes its hormones to prepare the body for this action. Think about how you feel when you are facing a major test or are waiting in the doctor's office for test results. You can feel your heart beating faster and your mouth going dry—results of the automatic response to danger. When the danger passes, the parasympathetic nervous system helps restore balance to the body system. If the system gets excessive stress hormones, health problems may result. Learning to live with stress is the key to a healthier body.

The **parasympathetic nervous system** has two important active nerves: the vagus and the pelvic nerves. The vagus nerve, which extends from the medulla and proceeds down the neck, sends branches to the chest and neck. The pelvic nerve, emerging from the spinal cord around the hip region, sends branches to the organs in the lower part of the body (Figure 24–3B).

Both the sympathetic and parasympathetic nerves are strongly influenced by emotion. During periods of fear, anger, or stress, the sympathetic division acts to prepare the body for action. The

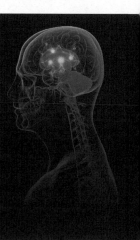

KEY CONCEPT

The sympathetic system consists of nerves that extend to all internal vital organs. This system prepares the body to respond to an external stimulus that it perceives as dangerous; this is the fight-or-flight response.

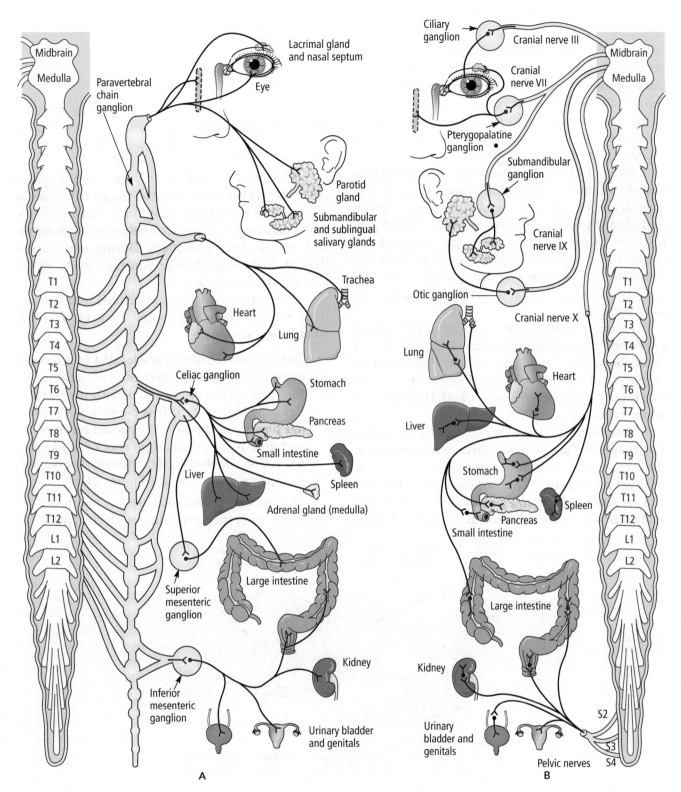

Figure 24–3 (A) The sympathetic division of the autonomic nervous system. (B) The parasympathetic division of the autonomic nervous system.

effects of the parasympathetic division are generally to counteract the effects of the sympathetic. For example, the sympathetic nervous system increases the rate of heart muscle contraction, and the parasympathetic decreases the rate. The two systems operate as a pair, striking a nearly perfect balance when the body is functioning properly.

Reflex Act

The simplest type of nervous response is the **reflex act**, which is unconscious and involuntary. The blink of the eye when a particle of dust touches it, the removal of a finger from a hot object, the secretion of saliva at the sight or smell of food, and the functions of the heart, stomach, and intestines are all examples of reflex actions.

Every reflex act is preceded by a change in the environment, called a **stimulus**. Examples of stimuli are sound waves, light waves, heat energy, and odors. Special structures called **receptors** pick up these stimuli. For example, the retina of the eye is the receptor for light; special cells in the inner ear are receptors for sound waves; and special structures in the skin are the receptors for heat and cold.

A simple reflex is one in which only a sensory nerve and a motor nerve are involved. The classic example is the knee-jerk reflex. The knee is tapped, and the leg extends (Figure 24–4). This test is used by physicians to test both the muscular and nervous systems.

Reaction to a stimulus is called the *response*. The response may be in the form of movement; in that case, the muscles are the **effectors**, or responding organs. If the response is in the form of a secretion, the glands are the effectors. Reflex actions, or autonomic reflexes, involving the skeletal muscles are controlled by the spinal cord. They also may be called *somatic reflexes*.

THE SPINE

The spine, or vertebral column, is strong and flexible. It supports the head and provides for the attachment of the ribs. The spine also encloses the spinal cord of the nervous system.

The spine consists of small bones called *vertebrae*, which are separated from each other by pads of cartilage tissue called *intervertebral disks*. These disks serve as cushions between the vertebrae and act as shock absorbers. During our lifetime these disks become thinner, which accounts for the loss of height as we age.

The vertebral column is divided into five sections named according to the area of the body where they are located:

1. **Cervical vertebrae** (7) are located in the neck area. The **atlas** is the first cervical vertebra that articulates, or is jointed, with the occipital bone of the skull. This permits us to nod our heads. On the **axis**, the second cervical vertebra, is the *odontoid process*, which forms a pivot on which the atlas rotates; this permits us to turn our heads (see Figure 24–5).
2. **Thoracic vertebrae** (12) are located in the chest area; they articulate with the ribs.

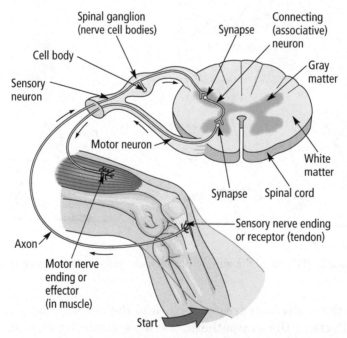

Figure 24–4 In this example, tapping the knee (patellar tendon) results in extension of the leg, producing the knee-jerk reflex.

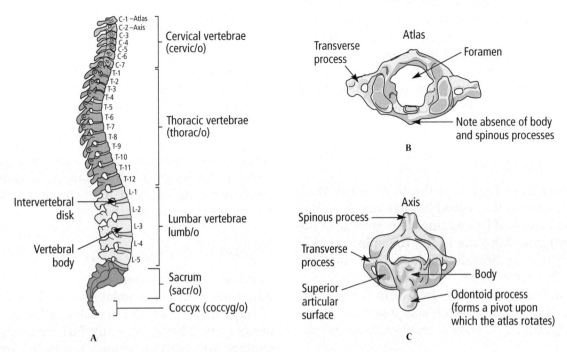

Figure 24–5 (A) Lateral view of the spine. (B) View of the atlas. (C) View of the axis.

3. **Lumbar vertebrae** (5) are associated with the lower back. They have large bodies that bear most of the body's weight.
4. **Sacrum**, a wedge-shaped unit formed by five fused bones, forms the posterior pelvic girdle and serves as an articulation point for the hips.
5. **Coccyx**, also known as the *tailbone,* is formed by four fused bones.

The spinal nerves enter and exit the spinal cord through the openings (foramen) between the vertebrae. When you study a model of the human skeleton, note that the spine is curved instead of straight. A curved spine has more strength than a straight one would. Before birth, the thoracic and sacral regions are convex curves. As the infant learns to hold up its head, the cervical region becomes concave. When the child learns to stand, the lumbar region also becomes concave. This completes the four curves of a normal, adult human spine.

A typical vertebra, as seen in Figure 24–6, contains three basic parts: body, foramen, and

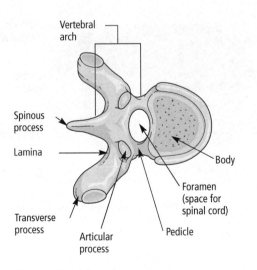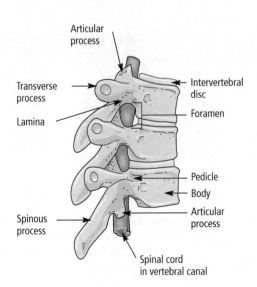

Figure 24–6 A typical vertebrae.

(several) processes. The large, solid part of the vertebra is known as the *body;* the central opening for the spinal cord is called the *foramen.* Above the foramen protrude two wing-like, bony structures called *transverse processes.* The roof of the foramen contains the spinous process (spine) and the articular processes.

Spinal Cord

The **spinal cord** begins at the base of the skull and continues to the second lumbar vertebra. It is white and soft and lies within the vertebrae of the spinal column. Like the brain, the spinal cord is submerged in cerebrospinal fluid and is surrounded by the three **meninges** (membranes). The **gray matter** in the spinal cord is located in the internal section; the **white matter** composes the outer part. Figure 24–7 shows cross-sections of the spinal cord.

In the gray matter of the cord, connections made between incoming and outgoing nerve fibers provide the basis for reflex action. The spinal cord functions as a reflex center and a conduction pathway to and from the brain.

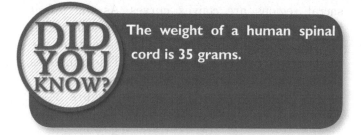

DID YOU KNOW? The weight of a human spinal cord is 35 grams.

INJURIES TO THE SPINE

The human spine is a remarkable structure. During activity (particularly athletic activity), the spine is able to withstand tremendous stresses and forces, while at the same time remaining flexible and mobile. The spine, or vertebral column, encases and provides protection for the spinal cord. Trauma to the spine can produce devastating injuries, which can be fatal or cause irreversible spinal-cord damage that results in permanent paralysis.

Cervical Spine Injuries

Cervical spine injuries range in severity from minor neck pain to complete paralysis or death. It is imperative that the certified athletic trainer protect the athlete from any further injury when damage to the cervical spine is suspected. Improper handling and transportation may cause irreparable spinal-cord damage in an athlete who has suffered a cervical spine fracture or dislocation.

Mechanism of injury to the cervical spine can involve vertebrae, facet joints, intervertebral discs, ligaments, muscles, nerve roots, or the spinal cord. These structures can be injured in many ways. The most common mechanism of injury to the neck is forced movement of the head on the cervical spine or excessive motion of the neck. This can occur when the athlete receives a blow that forces the head beyond its normal limits of motion, resulting in hyperextension, flexion, lateral flexion, rotation, or a combination of these.

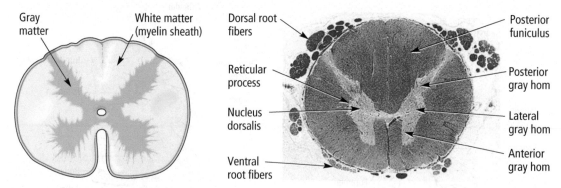

Figure 24–7 Cross-sections of the spinal cord. (Image on right is from Bergman, Afifi, and Heidger, *Atlas of Microscopic Anatomy: A Functional Approach: Companion to Histology and Neuroanatomy,* 2e, 1999. Reprinted with permission. http://www.vh.org/Providers/Textbooks/MicroscopicAnatomy /MicroscopicAnatomy.html.)

The most serious injuries to the cervical spine usually occur as a result of **axial loading** or cervical compression. This may occur when an athlete receives a blow straight to the top or crown of the head, especially when the neck is slightly flexed. This mechanism may cause a fracture of the vertebra or force the **articular facets** to slide away from each other. The neck can also be injured by a direct blow. This mechanism usually results in contusions or bruising on the neck. It can also result in a serious spinal injury, depending on the force of the blow, the object involved, and the position of the cervical spine at the time and in relation to the force.

SIGNS AND SYMPTOMS Do not move the athlete except from immediate danger or for basic trauma management. It is estimated that 50% of neurologic injuries are created after the initial traumatic event. It is also difficult to determine immediately if a neck injury is stable or unstable.

If the athlete has fallen on the field and a neck or spine injury is suspected, keep the athlete still until an initial evaluation has been completed. A neck injury must be assumed if the athlete is unconscious, has numbness and paralysis, and has neck pain or pain with neck movement.

If the athlete is alert, the history of the injury can be as important as the physical exam. How the athlete responds to questions can help in further assessing the level of consciousness. Important questions to ask are:

- How did the injury happen?
- Are you having any weakness, numbness, or tingling?
- Are you feeling any pain?
- Have you had a prior neck injury?

Most experts agree that severe neck injuries are usually accompanied by pain and sometimes neurologic symptoms. An athlete without pain and neurologic symptoms has a very low probability of having a severe neck injury, and therefore can be helped off the field for further evaluation.

TREATMENT When a neck injury is suspected, airway management is of primary importance. If the athlete is not breathing, the jaw-thrust technique has been shown to be the safest method for opening the airway. In this technique, the caregiver places the fingers behind the angle of both sides of the patient's jaw and lifts up, bringing the mandible forward (Figure 24–8). If this technique is inadequate, the modified jaw-thrust/head-tilt maneuver, in which the jaw is pulled upward and the head tilted back as little as possible, can be used.

If a football player has a suspected neck injury, do not remove the helmet. Jostling the head and neck can cause severe neurologic complications if the patient has an unstable fracture. If airway access is necessary, the face mask may be cut using a device designed for this purpose (a technique covered later in this chapter.)

In assessing circulation, first check for a carotid pulse. If it is absent, begin chest compressions in accordance with basic life-support guidelines.

The two classes of spinal cord injury are complete and incomplete. Complete injury renders the athlete without movement or sensation below the level of injury. Incomplete injury leaves the patient with some preserved motor or sensory function. An athlete with neck pain should have the cervical spine immobilized, and emergency medical services should be activated immediately. Immobilization of the cervical spine includes reassuring the athlete and supporting the head and neck in a way that eliminates any movement. Manually immobilizing the head is the best way to keep the athlete's head and neck aligned. Kneel in front of the athlete's head and, using both hands, hold it in place until EMS personnel arrive and take over care of the athlete.

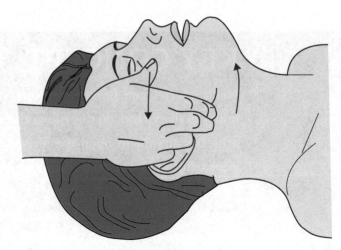

Figure 24–8 The jaw-thrust maneuver.

The best way to handle cervical spine injuries is to be prepared for them. It is important to have an emergency plan, with all equipment inspected and readily accessible and all personnel involved trained to use it. Communication among all members of the emergency medical team should be established before the competition. Transportation to an emergency medical facility should be immediately available.

REHABILITATION All injuries of the spine must be evaluated by a physician, who will make the decisions about return to play. The physician may place limits on future participation in certain sports.

Cervical Sprains and Strains

Some of the more common injuries to the neck are cervical sprains and strains. These injuries vary in severity. Slight trauma may result in only mild injury of little consequence.

SIGNS AND SYMPTOMS In mild cases, the athlete will express no feelings of weakness or instability. Although there may be tenderness and pain at the injury site, the athlete can easily demonstrate a normal range of motion in the neck. With a moderate sprain and strain, the athlete may have limited motion of the cervical spine, but without radiation of pain or **paresthesia** (abnormality of sensation). With a more severe injury, the athlete will usually resist moving the neck through a full range of motion. More severe

injuries may cause localized pain and muscle spasm, and the athlete may complain of an insecure feeling about the neck.

TREATMENT Any athlete with less than a full, pain-free range of cervical motion, or who has persistent paresthesia or weakness, should be protected and excluded from further athletic activity. He or she should be referred to a physician for further radiographic and neurologic evaluations.

Cervical Nerve Syndrome

Another common athletic injury to the neck is **cervical nerve syndrome**. This injury results from forced lateral flexion, which causes the nerve roots to be either stretched or impinged. Known as a *pinched nerve, burner, or stinger*, it is characterized by sharp, burning, radiating pain.

SIGNS AND SYMPTOMS The athlete may complain of pain shooting into the posterior scalp, behind the ear, around the neck, or down the top of the shoulder. If the brachial plexus (see Chapter 21) is involved, the athlete may complain of radiating pain, numbness, and loss of function in the arm and possibly the hand. Symptoms of cervical nerve syndrome usually subside in minutes, but such injuries may leave residual soreness and paresthetic (numbness, tingling) areas.

REHABILITATION Athletes may return to athletic activity if all paresthesia has completely

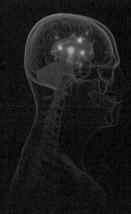

KEY CONCEPT

Neck injuries can be very serious, so proper management is critical. If a neck injury is suspected, do not move the athlete. It is very important to maintain the athlete's airway. To open the airway, use the jaw-thrust technique. If the athlete is wearing a helmet, do not remove it; a face mask can be cut away to allow access to the airway. Once the airway has been opened and is being managed, check for a pulse. The spine should be manually immobilized. EMS should be activated and will replace the manual immobilization with a neck collar.

subsided; they can demonstrate full muscle strength in the muscles of the upper extremity; and they exhibit full, pain-free range of cervical motion. Subsequent occurrences must be referred to the doctor for further analysis.

Cervical Fractures and Subluxations

Serious injuries of the cervical spine, such as fractures or dislocations, are not common in athletics, but the potential for this type of an injury is inherent in almost any sport. Football players are at greatest risk for serious cervical spine injuries because the head is often used in blocking and tackling. Diving and gymnastics also provide mechanisms for devastating neck injuries. Most fatal or paralyzing injuries occur when an athlete's neck is in flexion and he or she receives a blow to the crown of the head. An example is when the head is down and the top of the head makes contact with an opponent. This type of force can cause either a fracture or a **subluxation** (incomplete or partial dislocation) of the vertebrae, which may produce injuries to the spinal cord. The spinal cord may be completely or partially transected, contused, or concussed.

SIGNS AND SYMPTOMS A spinal cord contusion can cause swelling within the cord, resulting in various degrees of temporary or permanent damage. A spinal cord concussion may cause transitory paralysis and symptoms, but usually there is complete recovery.

The major signs and symptoms that may indicate a serious neck injury include unremitting neck pain, muscle spasms, and evidence of spinal-cord involvement. Spinal-cord involvement may manifest as numbness, loss of sensation, weakness, paresthesia, and partial or complete paralysis of the limbs.

Athletes may experience transient **quadriparesis** or **quadriplegia** from a cervical spine injury—also called **neuropraxia**—means the cessation of function of a nerve in the absence of degenerative changes. Symptoms include burning pain, numbness, tingling, loss of sensation, weakness, or complete paralysis. Recovery of complete motor and sensory function usually occurs within a few minutes, but may take 36 to 48 hours. Athletes exhibiting neuropraxia or transient quadriparesis should be referred for further medical evaluation. Possible causes other than a cervical fracture or dislocation may be a spinal **stenosis** (narrowing), congenital abnormality, cervical instability, or intervertebral disk herniation.

Because most mechanisms of cervical spine injury involve forces to the head, injuries to the head and neck must be considered together. Whenever there is a possibility of neck injury, treat the athlete as if he or she has a serious cervical spine injury until proven otherwise.

HELMET MANAGEMENT IN SUSPECTED SPINAL INJURIES The first rule of management for an athlete who is on the field with a neck injury is to *stabilize the neck*. It is important to keep the helmet on if possible. For football and ice hockey players in the supine position, shoulder pads elevate the trunk. If the helmet is removed, the head drops and the neck hyperextends. Leaving the helmet in place keeps the neck from hyperextending. Helmets fit snugly and cradle the head, minimizing head and neck motion.

If an injured athlete is breathing and does not require airway management, the helmet should be left on to help support the head and neck. The face mask should be removed, however, because EMS protocols require removal of the mask before transport. When an athlete requires airway intervention, the face mask must be removed immediately for access to the airway, while the helmet stays on. Ideally, the helmet is left in place until the cervical spine can be imaged with radiography. In most situations, the only reasons to remove the helmet are inability to establish an airway or failure of the helmet to stabilize the head adequately. At this point, a neck collar will replace the football helmet.

A special tool is used to snip the plastic clips that hold the face mask onto the helmet (Figure 24–9). Care should be taken not to disturb the helmet when removing the face mask.

Thoracic Spine Injuries

Common athletic injuries to the thoracic spine include contusions, sprains, and strains. Contusions caused by a blow to the thoracic area commonly

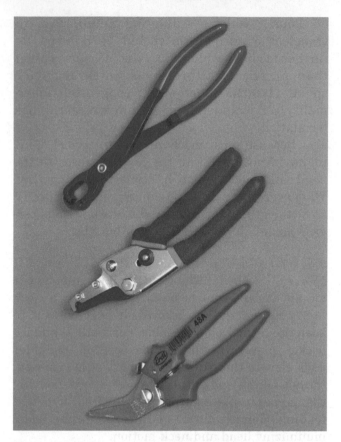

Figure 24–9 There are different tools designed for removal of face masks. The certified athletic trainer should practice removing face masks each season to be prepared in case this skill is needed.

involve the *paraspinal muscles* (the muscles lateral to the spinous processes). Sprains and strains may be caused by overstretching the soft tissue surrounding the thoracic vertebrae or by violent muscular contraction against resistance. Serious injuries to the thoracic spine are extremely rare in athletic activities. Fractures or dislocations are unusual because of the spine's stable anatomy in the region. The most common serious injury is a compression fracture to the body of one of the thoracic vertebrae. The mechanism of injury is usually forced forward flexion of the thoracic spine, which compresses the anterior portion of the adjacent vertebral bodies. Typically, the athlete will give a history of sharp forward flexion, resulting in a jackknifing effect. This can occur as an athlete falls violently on the buttocks or is forced into extreme flexion of the thoracic spine.

SIGNS AND SYMPTOMS On examination, it may be difficult to distinguish between a sprain and a strain. With either injury there may be tenderness, spasms, and increased pain with active contraction or stretching. An athlete with a moderate or severe injury may exhibit a very stiff back, and may resist any motion or movement of the thoracic spine.

An athlete with a compression fracture will usually have no neurological complaints and will be able to move around, even walk. However, he or she will complain of constant localized pain, which may increase with any movement of this area of the spine.

TREATMENT The athlete should be referred to a physician for further evaluation.

Lumbar Spine Injuries

The lumbar spine, or lower back, area is subjected to many types of stresses and forces during both athletic and nonathletic activity. The lower back is very susceptible to injury. Occasionally, low back pain is caused by structural defects in the vertebrae or intervertebral discs. All conditions affecting the lumbar spine can be aggravated by various contributing factors such as inadequate or inappropriate conditioning, inflexibility, congenital anomalies, and poor postural habits.

Common athletic injuries to the lower back are contusions, sprains, and strains. Contusions are more common in the paraspinal muscles, but may also occur over the **subcutaneous spinous processes** (see Figure 24–6). The athlete often has an injury history of a direct blow to the lumbar area, with localized tenderness and pain on movement. Sprains and strains in the multiplicity of muscles and ligaments in the lower back are common. These injuries can be caused by the same types of mechanisms and can occur simultaneously. Violent muscle contractions against resistance, overuse, and overstretching are common mechanisms resulting in sprains or strains in the soft tissues along the spine. It is difficult to differentiate between a sprain and a strain in this area.

Severe injuries to the lumbar spine such as fractures and dislocations are extremely rare in athletic activity. Neurological damage as a result of such an injury is not as likely as in the cervical spine, because the spinal cord ends at about the first lumbar vertebrae. Compression fractures, as previously described with regard to the thoracic spine, can occur to the bodies of the lumbar vertebrae. However, the most common fractures in the lower back involve the spinous or transverse processes and usually occur as a result of a direct blow or violent muscle contraction. Without radiographs, fractures of this type are sometimes indistinguishable from severe strains or contusions.

Spondylolysis

The most common structural defect of the lumbar spine in an athlete is a condition called **spondylolysis**, which is a defect in the **pars interarticularis** of the vertebrae (Figure 24–10).

If this defect is **bilateral** (on both sides), it may allow the vertebra to slip forward on the

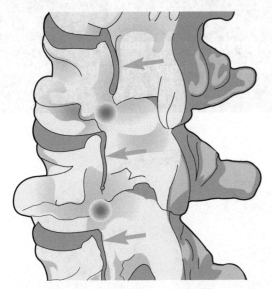

Figure 24–10 The arrows show the facet joints, and the dots show the pars interarticularis.

vertebra or sacrum below—a condition called **spondylolisthesis**. Spondylolisthesis may develop in athletes who undertake strenuous exercise or competition. Many medical experts consider this condition to be a stress fracture, the result of repeated trauma and stress, rather than an acute fracture. It is also believed that spondylolysis and spondylolisthesis can be congenital.

SIGNS AND SYMPTOMS The athlete with spondylolisthesis will usually complain of low back pain associated with increased activity. With rest or inactivity the pain diminishes, only to return when activity is resumed. In addition to pain in the lower back, the athlete may complain of pain radiating into the buttocks and upper thighs. The appearance of radiating pain, as well as recurrent episodes of low back pain with activity, are signals to refer the athlete to a physician for diagnosis.

Intervertebral Disc Herniation

Another structural defect that may occur in the lumbar spine of an athlete is **intervertebral disc herniation**. In this condition, the **nucleus pulposus** herniates through the **annulus fibrosus** and presses against the spinal cord or the spinal nerve roots (Figure 24–11). This condition is more common in people in their 30s and 40s, although it can occur in younger athletes as well.

SIGNS AND SYMPTOMS The athlete with a ruptured or herniated disc normally has extreme pain and stiffness in the lower back, pain in the buttocks, and a unique type of radiating leg pain if the compression is severe. This leg pain is usually **unilateral** (one-sided) and follows the route of the

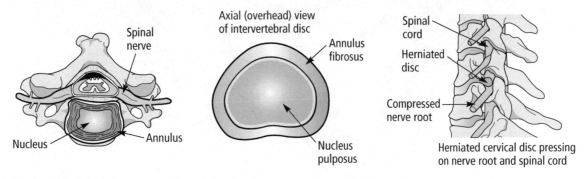

Figure 24–11 The anatomy of a spinal disc.

sciatic nerve, which is formed by the fourth and fifth lumbar nerves and the first, second, and third sacral nerves. Pain may radiate down into the thigh, calf, and foot, depending on the nerve roots involved. Sitting for prolonged periods of time, standing with both legs straight, and bending over will be especially uncomfortable for the athlete. Additional signs that may indicate a herniated disc include unilateral muscle weakness, sensory loss, or reflex loss in the leg.

TREATMENT Athletes with signs and symptoms of this type must be referred to a physician for further evaluation.

Sacroiliac Injuries

Sacroiliac injuries are usually sprains that occur as a result of acute or chronic trauma. They may result from a single maneuver, twist, or awkward movement, or from overuse associated with poor

KEY CONCEPT

A ruptured or herniated disk is usually characterized by:

- **Severe pain**
- **Stiffness in the lower back**
- **Pain in the buttocks**
- **Unilateral radiating leg pain if the compression of the spinal cord is severe**

Associated signs may include muscle weakness, sensory loss, or loss of reflexes in the leg.

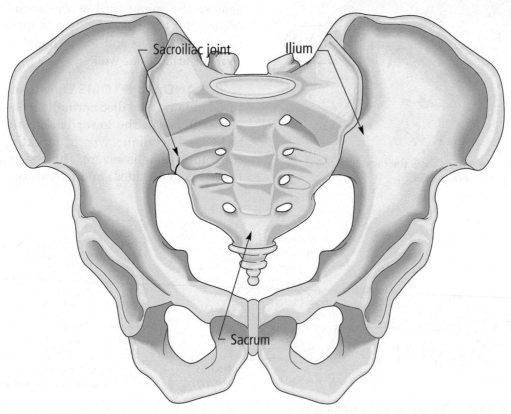

Figure 24–12 Sacroiliac joint.

posture, bad lifting techniques, or strenuous maneuvers repeated many times.

SIGNS AND SYMPTOMS Symptoms of a sacroiliac sprain include stiffness or a consistent soreness of the **sacroiliac joint** area (see figure 24–12) that is better in the morning but gets worse as the day goes on. There are no neurologic signs, but there may be referred pain in the back of the thigh, groin, or hamstrings. Heat generated during activity may diminish the discomfort, but the pain returns as soon as the athlete cools down.

KEY CONCEPT

Athletic competition produces tremendous forces and stresses on the spine, which can cause injury. Common injuries to the spine include:

- Cervical spine injuries, which range in severity from neck pain to paralysis. Very serious cervical spine injuries can result in death. These are emergency situations; special care must be taken when managing and treating an athlete with a cervical spine injury so as not to make the injury worse.
- Cervical sprains and strains—the most common neck injuries—vary in severity. Injuries of this nature should be checked by a physician.
- Cervical fracture and subluxation, which are breakage or dislocation of the structures of the spine. These injuries are not common.
- Thoracic spine injuries, such as contusions, sprains, and strains, should be treated by a physician.
- Lumbar spine injuries, usually consisting of contusions, sprains, and strains, should be treated by a physician.
- Spondylolysis, the breakdown of the structures of the spine. This is often attributed to overuse.
- Intervertebral herniated disk, which is displacement of the material inside the disk so that it presses against the spinal cord. This condition should be treated by a physician.
- Sacroiliac injuries, which are usually sprains resulting from acute or chronic trauma.

CONCLUSION

The spine is the central support structure of the body. It can withstand tremendous stresses and forces while remaining flexible and mobile. The spine, or vertebral column, encases and provides protection for the spinal cord. Trauma to the spine can produce spinal-cord damage and result in devastating injuries to the athlete.

Injuries to the cervical, thoracic, lumbar, or sacral areas must be handled correctly by sports medicine personnel. All members of the sports medicine team should be equipped with the proper knowledge and tools to handle these emergencies. A team approach ensures the best possible care for the injured athlete.

REVIEW QUESTIONS

1. How does the nervous system work?
2. Explain the difference between the peripheral and autonomic nervous systems.
3. Describe the function of the sympathetic system.
4. What are the differences between the motor nerve, efferent nerve, and a mixed nerve?
5. What is a plexus? Name the different plexuses in the body.
6. Describe the reflex act.
7. List and explain common injuries to the spine.
8. Describe the management protocols for an athlete with a back injury.
9. What are the symptoms of intervertebral disc herniation?
10. As an athletic training student aide, what would you do if an athlete complains of neck pain after a collision?

PROJECTS AND ACTIVITIES

1. If the nervous system sends electrical impulses at 250 miles per hour, how long would it take for an impulse to reach the foot of an athlete who is six feet tall?
2. What are some disorders of the autonomic nervous system? The peripheral nervous system? Use the Internet as a resource for this project.
3. Draw a sketch of the spinal column. Label each vertebra.

LEARNING LINKS

Learn more about spinal injuries and treatment of spinal injuries at https://www.mayoclinic.org/diseases-conditions/spinal-cord-injury/symptoms-causes/syc-20377890.
• View the animations of spinal anatomy and spinal injuries at http://www.spine-health.com.

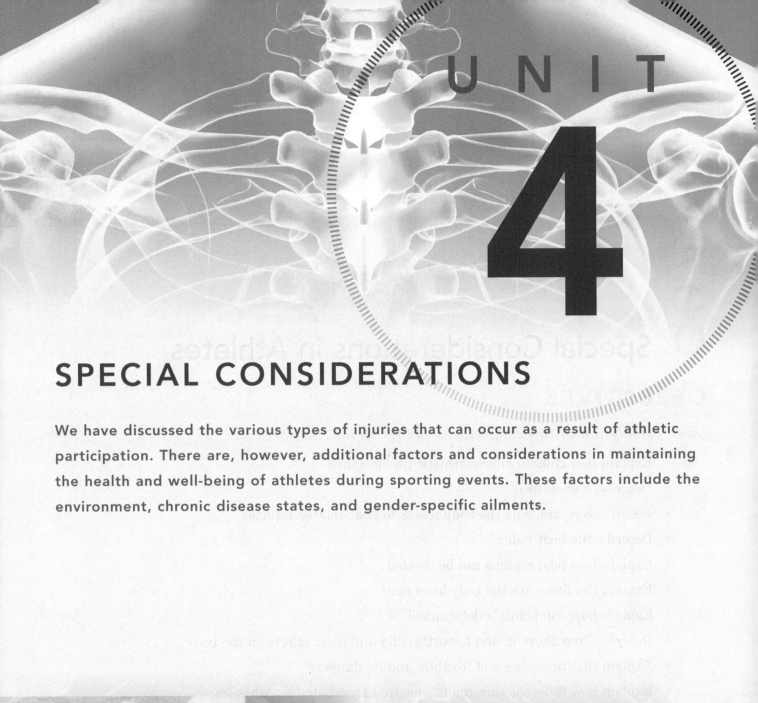

4

SPECIAL CONSIDERATIONS

We have discussed the various types of injuries that can occur as a result of athletic participation. There are, however, additional factors and considerations in maintaining the health and well-being of athletes during sporting events. These factors include the environment, chronic disease states, and gender-specific ailments.

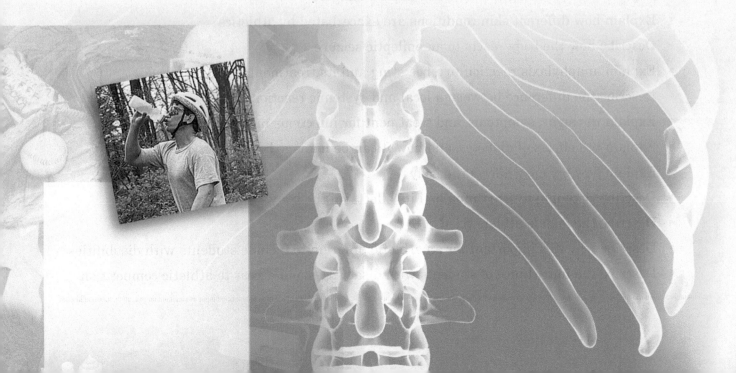

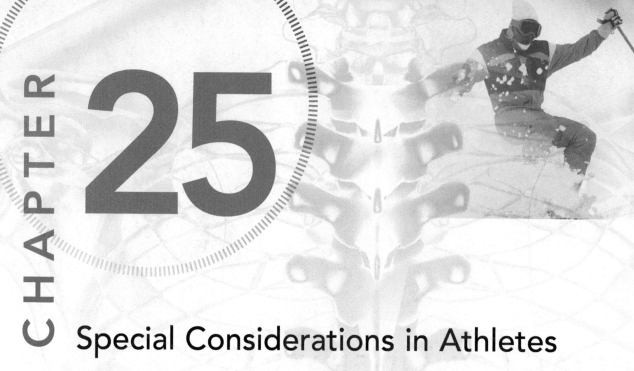

CHAPTER 25

Special Considerations in Athletes

OBJECTIVES

Upon completion of this chapter, the reader should be able to:

- Explain how climate affects athletic performance
- Describe homeostasis
- Describe how and why the body reacts to heat-related injuries
- Describe the heat index
- Explain how heat cramps can be treated
- Explain the five ways the body loses heat
- Explain how wind chill is determined
- Describe hypothermia and hyperthermia and their effects on the body
- Explain the three stages of frostbite and its dangers
- Explain how different skin conditions are exacerbated by athletics
- Describe how the body reacts to an epileptic seizure.
- Explain anaphylaxis reaction to a bee sting and its treatment
- Describe the difference between a local and systemic reaction
- Explain the signs, symptoms, and treatment for infectious mononucleosis
- Explain the effects of diabetes, and how it can be managed
- Explain how epilepsy affects the body
- Describe circadian dysrhythmia and its effects on the body
- Describe the female athlete triad
- Describe why it is important for an athletic program to include students with disabilities
- Describe the importance of students with disabilities and access to athletic competition

KEY TERMS

acne mechanica *A form of acne that results from heat, pressure, occlusion, and friction.*

amenorrhea *Lack of a menstrual flow.*

beta cells *The cells responsible for making insulin.*

Circadian dysrhythmia *Circadian rhythm disorders are disruptions in a person's circadian rhythm. The circadian rhythm, or "internal body clock" regulates the 24-hour cycle of biological processes.*

conduction *The loss of heat through transfer to a cooler object.*

convection *Heat loss through air currents passing by a warm surface.*

core body temperature *The temperature of the human body necessary to maintain homeostasis (about 98.6°F).*

diabetes *A disease in which the body does not produce insulin or does not produce enough insulin for the body to properly absorb glucose.*

diabetic coma *A condition in which there is too much sugar and too little insulin in the blood, resulting in body cells receiving inadequate nourishment.*

epilepsy *A condition in which seizures occur regularly throughout the affected person's life.*

epinephrine *A medication that dilates the airway and constricts the blood vessels.*

EpiPen *An auto-injecting device used to administer epinephrine to those with severe allergic reactions.*

evaporation *The loss of heat through perspiration.*

female athlete triad *A disorder that affects female athletes; characterized by disordered eating, amenorrhea, and osteoporosis.*

frostbite *Damage to skin tissue and blood vessels due to prolonged exposure to temperatures below 32°F.*

generalized tonic-clonic seizure *A type of seizure characterized by a sudden cry and fall, rigidity, jerking of muscles, shallow breathing, and loss of bladder and bowel control. This usually lasts for a couple of minutes.*

heat cramps *Painful, involuntary muscle spasms caused by exposure to heat and dehydration.*

heat exhaustion *The mildest form of generalized heat-related illness, characterized by multiple symptoms and often by dehydration.*

heat index *A reference point indicating the risk associated with outdoor exercise; based on a combination of air temperature and relative humidity.*

heat stress *The inability of the body to maintain homeostasis because of high temperatures.*

heat syncope *Fainting that occurs when the body attempts to cool itself by dilating the blood vessels.*

heatstroke *A life-threatening form of heat illness that involves a rise in body temperature and altered mental status.*

herpes gladiatorum *A type of herpes infection commonly seen in wrestlers.*

homeostasis *A state of balance within the body.*

hyperthermia *A condition in which body temperature rises above normal.*

hypothalamus *A part of the diencephalon; the temperature-regulating center of the brain.*

KEY TERMS CONTINUED

hypothermia *A condition in which body temperature drops below normal.*

insulin *A hormone produced by the pancreas; necessary for glucose absorption.*

insulin reaction *The body's response to excess insulin; the level of sugar in the blood decreases, causing brain cells to suffer.*

jogger's nipples *A condition caused by chafing between a runner's nipples and shirt.*

local reaction *Pain, swelling, redness, itching, and formation of a weal at the site of an insect bite or sting.*

MRSA *Methicillin-resistant staphylococcus aureus (MRSA) is a bacterium that causes infections in different parts of the body. It is tougher to treat than most strains of staph infection because of its resistance to commonly used antibiotics.*

osteoporosis *Bone loss.*

pancreas *An organ, located near the stomach, that produces insulin.*

plantar warts *Small, hard growths on the bottom of the foot.*

radiation *The loss of heat through the transfer of infrared rays into the cooler environment.*

seizure *A sudden attack or convulsion due to involuntary electrical activity in the brain.*

simple partial seizure *A type of seizure in which a jerking motion begins in one part of the body; the victim remains awake and aware.*

sunburn *Injury to the skin from the sun's rays (ultraviolet light).*

systemic reaction *A generalized reaction to an insect sting or bite, characterized by flushing of the skin and an itchy rash; more serious symptoms such as wheezing, nausea, vomiting, palpations, and faintness can also occur.*

thermoregulation *The process by which body temperature is maintained.*

tinea cruris *A fungal infection found in the groin area; often referred to as "jock itch."*

tinea pedis *A fungal infection that thrives in warmth and dampness; often referred to as "athlete's foot" or ringworm.*

wind chill *The rate of heat loss from the human body resulting from the combined effect of cold temperature and wind.*

SPECIAL CONSIDERATIONS IN ATHLETICS

Depending on the size of the school or program, there may be hundreds of athletes involved in sports throughout the year. Each athlete brings unique conditions or concerns that are important for the athletic staff to know. These conditions range from previous injuries, to potentially life-threatening allergies, to bee stings. The training staff needs to be aware of an athlete's medical condition, so they can be prepared if an emergency should arise.

ENVIRONMENTAL CONDITIONS AND ATHLETIC PARTICIPATION

Environmental conditions can have a negative effect on athletic performance. The certified athletic trainer, as well as the coach and athlete, must prepare for difficult environmental conditions that can also have an adverse impact on the athlete's health.

Stress

Heat stress occurs when the human body cannot maintain **homeostasis** (internal equilibrium);

body temperature begins to rise, and heat-related illnesses and disorders may develop. **Hyperthermia** is the general name given to a variety of heat-related illnesses.

The temperature-regulating center of the brain, the **hypothalamus**, is responsible for controlling the amount of heat lost from the body. Approximately 80% of total heat loss is through the skin via evaporation and perspiration. The hypothalamus regulates this heat loss by changing the dilation of blood vessels in the skin. This, as well as perspiration, helps to keep the body from overheating. The process by which body temperature is maintained is referred to as **thermoregulation**.

Assessing the Risk

Athletes need to be well hydrated, rested, and in good physical condition if the body's heat-regulating mechanisms are to work properly. When an athlete is not conditioned properly, the body will work harder, therefore placing more strain on its heat-regulating system.

Air temperature alone is not adequate to assess whether conditions are safe for intense exercise. Relative humidity (the percent of mois-

ture in the air) also plays an important role. These two criteria are combined in the **heat index**, which provides a reference point for estimating the various levels of risk associated with exercise in heat and humidity. Tables 25–1 and 25–2 illustrate guidelines for training in heat and the heat index.

It is important to note that the heat index is calculated for conditions in the shade. Exercise in direct sunlight poses an even greater risk when temperature and humidity rise. The greater the heat-index temperature, or apparent temperature, the more moisture is in the air. In this situation, the body progressively loses its ability to adequately evaporate moisture. This can cause a potentially dangerous increase in body core temperature. There are degrees of heat illness, but even the milder ones can become life threatening if not properly treated.

GENERAL CARE OF HEAT ILLNESS The most effective methods of reducing body temperature include moving the victim to a cool location, removing unnecessary clothing, and pouring cool water over the extremities. This should be followed by fanning the victim to increase air circulation and evaporation. Another method of reducing body

Table 25–1 Temperature and Humidity Training Guidelines		
TEMPERATURE	HUMIDITY	PROCEDURES
80–90°F	<70%	Carefully observe athletes with special weight considerations.
80–90°F	>70%	Athletes should rest and drink water frequently (10 minutes every hour).
90–100°F	<70%	Athletes should rest and drink fluid frequently (10 minutes every hour). Clothing should be changed when it becomes wet, because dampness acts as an insulator under these conditions. All athletes should be carefully observed for signs of heat-related illness.
90–100°F over 100°F	>70%	Discontinue or shorten practice, or move the practice to a climate-controlled location such as a gym. Have the athletes change into cooler clothing if possible. Athletes should rest and drink water frequently (10 minutes every hour). Clothing should be changed when it becomes wet to avoid insulating effects. All athletes should be carefully observed for signs of heat-related illness.

Table 25–2 Heat Index

AIR TEMPERATURE (°F)	RELATIVE HUMIDITY (%)												
	40	45	50	55	60	65	70	75	80	85	90	95	100
110	136												
108	130	137											
106	124	130	137										
104	119	124	131	137									
102	114	119	124	130	137								
100	109	114	118	124	129	136							
98	105	109	113	117	123	128	134						
96	101	104	108	112	116	121	126	132					
94	97	100	103	106	110	114	119	124	129	136			
92	94	96	99	101	105	108	112	116	121	126	131		
90	91	93	95	97	100	103	106	109	113	117	122	127	132
88	88	89	91	93	95	98	100	103	106	110	113	117	121
86	85	87	88	89	91	93	95	97	100	102	105	108	112
84	83	84	85	86	88	89	90	92	94	96	98	100	103
82	81	82	83	84	84	85	86	88	89	90	91	93	95
80	80	80	81	81	82	82	83	84	84	85	86	86	87

With Prolonged Exposure or Physical Activity

Caution
Fatigue Possible

Extreme Caution
Heatstroke, Muscle Cramps, or Heat Exhaustion Possible

Danger
Heatstroke, Muscle Cramps, or Heat Exhaustion Likely

Extreme Danger
Heatstroke Highly Likely

Source: National Weather Service. http://weather.noaa.gov/weather/hwave.html. December 2000.

temperature is to immerse the victim in cool (not cold) water. The victim's extremities should then be vigorously massaged to promote circulation of cooled blood in the extremities back to the heart. Once body temperature has dropped to 102°F, cooling should be stopped to avoid hypothermia and shivering.

The keys to avoiding heat-related illness are prevention, addressing the environment, acclimatization, and proper hydration. Athletes should be weighed before and after exercise to determine fluid loss. The certified athletic trainer must monitor the environment and modify practices accordingly. At-risk athletes (e.g., those who are coming back from an injury, are overweight, or have other medical conditions) should be carefully monitored. Unlimited water access and timely water breaks are essential.

Dehydration

On average, a person will lose between three and six liters of water each day. Perspiration is responsible for one to two liters on an average day, but that amount can climb to one to two liters per hour during periods of vigorous exercise. It is estimated that one hour of exercise can demand approximately a 50% increase in the amount of water the body uses.

SIGNS AND SYMPTOMS Signs of dehydration are at first subtle. The athlete's urine turns a light yellow. He or she gets a mild headache and becomes fatigued. When an athlete is further dehydrated (after one hour of practice or competition), endurance may be reduced by 22%, and the maximum oxygen uptake (a measure of heart and lung efficiency) can be 10% lower. This is when the athlete begins to feel thirsty. After two hours of strenuous exercise (three to four liters of water lost), the athlete's endurance decreases 50%, and oxygen uptake is reduced by almost 25%. The urine is now dark yellow. Signs of serious dehydration include disorientation, irritability, rapid pulse, and complete exhaustion.

There are three levels of dehydration:

- *Mild:* the mucous membranes dry out; pulse is normal; urine is noticeably yellow; the athlete feels mild thirst.

- *Moderate:* the mucous membranes are extremely dry; pulse is weak and rapid; urine is very dark; the athlete feels very thirsty.

- *Severe:* the mucous membranes are completely dry; the athlete is disoriented and drowsy; there is no urine output; the eyes are unable to make tears; beginning stages of shock appear (rapid, weak pulse, rapid breathing, and pale skin).

TREATMENT Proper hydration and fluid replacement begin prior to exercise or competition, and do not end until well after the athlete has finished. Recommendations include:

- Before exercise, athletes should weigh themselves to establish a starting point, and begin hydrating 2 to 3 hours before exercising.

- Another 7 to 10 ounces should be consumed after the warmup (10 to 15 minutes before activity).

FUN FACTS
The thermoregulatory responses to exercise in the heat differ between child athletes and adult athletes. Children sweat less, create more heat per body mass, and acclimatize slower to warm environments. As a result, child athletes may be more at risk of heat-related injuries in hot, humid conditions.

- During exercise, drink enough fluids to prevent excessive dehydration. Depending upon the athlete's condition level and heat index, each athlete will be different.

- Each athlete should develop a hydration plan based on fluid needs, monitoring of fluid intake, and the constraints of the sport.

- After exercise, athletes should replace lost fluids (sweat and urine). It is important that athletes weigh themselves to determine how much fluid was lost. Significant weight loss (two to three pounds) may require 24 to 48 hours for complete recovery (Figure 25–1). Athletes must replenish lost fluid before the next exercise period.

SPORTS DRINKS The advantages of sports drinks as compared to plain water have been debated for some time. The primary purpose of using sports drinks containing carbohydrates is to maintain a sufficient concentration of blood

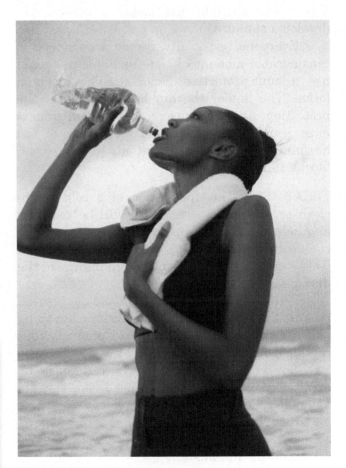

Figure 25–1 Athletes need to drink plenty of water before, during, and after exercise. Courtesy of Photodisc.

glucose and to sustain a high rate of energy production from blood glucose and glycogen stored in muscles. This becomes important with athletes who exercise more than 60 minutes. Less than this, water is sufficient. Sports drinks also taste good, thereby encouraging athletes to drink more fluids.

Another advantage for the athlete is electrolyte replacement. When you sweat excessively, you begin to lose electrolytes such as sodium, potassium, phosphate, calcium, magnesium and chlorine. Low electrolyte levels can cause muscle cramps, dizziness, confusion and nausea.

Sunburn

Athletes who spend a considerable amount of time practicing and competing outdoors are at risk of overexposure to ultraviolet (UV) light, which can lead to skin cancer and premature aging. In addition to athletes who are outdoors during the intense midday sun, skiers and hikers need to be especially cautious. Research shows that the higher the altitude, the faster a person will develop a **sunburn**.

Everyone, especially people who spend a considerable amount of time in the sun, should use a sun protective factor (SPF) sunscreen lotion. The higher the number, the greater the protection. An SPF sunscreen of 30 will protect most people adequately and block 97% of the harmful, ultraviolet B radiation. No sunscreen blocks 100%.

TREATMENT The application of a cold washcloth or a soak in a cool bath will be soothing and help the athlete cope with the pain and discomfort of sunburn. Use of an over-the-counter (OTC) pain reliever may also help minimize the discomfort.

Petroleum-based products should not be used because they prevent heat and sweat from escaping and can worsen a burn. First-aid products that contain benzocaine should also be avoided, because they can cause irritation or allergic reactions. The application of a moisturizing lotion or aloe vera gel will help relieve itching.

Blistering of the skin is a signal of a serious sunburn. The athlete should seek medical advice for sunburns that blister.

PREVENTION To protect against skin cancer, the American Academy of Dermatology recommends that everyone wear a broad-spectrum sunscreen with an SPF of 15 or higher. Even on cloudy days, wear protective clothing and avoid the sun from 10 A.M. to 4 P.M. when its rays are the strongest.

Heat Cramps

Heat cramps are common, but should not be overlooked, as they may signal the first stage of heat illness.

SIGNS AND SYMPTOMS Heat cramps occur most commonly in the calf muscles, but may also affect the quadriceps, hamstrings, or abdominal muscles. These cramps are caused by rapid water and electrolyte loss through perspiration.

TREATMENT Care of heat cramps includes slow, passive stretching of the involved muscle in combination with the application of ice. Immediate fluid and electrolyte replacement are vital to prevent further progression. Cool water cools the body better and is more rapidly absorbed by the stomach than warm water.

REHABILITATION Athletes may return to competition after all symptoms have subsided, but should be allowed to drink plenty of liquids and rest before returning.

Heat Syncope

Heat syncope, or fainting, occurs when the body attempts to cool itself by dilating the blood vessels in the skin to speed up evaporation.

SIGNS AND SYMPTOMS Because the blood supply to the brain is reduced, the athlete may suffer lightheadedness, dizziness, headache, nausea, and vomiting, as well as fainting.

TREATMENT Heat syncope is also associated with dehydration, so it can be treated by drinking fluids. To avoid heat syncope, all activity should be stopped when symptoms occur.

REHABILITATION Exercise should not be resumed until the symptoms have completely subsided.

Heat Exhaustion

Heat exhaustion is the condition of near-total body collapse. An athlete suffering from heat exhaustion may have trouble dissipating heat, but the body's heat control mechanism will remain intact.

SIGNS AND SYMPTOMS The skin will be cool, moist, and pale. The athlete may suffer from generalized weakness, dizziness, and nausea. Breathing is often rapid but shallow, and the pulse rapid and weak. This condition may progress to heatstroke if not treated.

TREATMENT Treatment for heat exhaustion should be initiated immediately. The athlete should be moved to the shade. Fluid replacement is vitally important. It is also imperative that the body be cooled, using ice towels if necessary. Table 25–3 summarizes heat-related illnesses and their care.

REHABILITATION The athlete suffering from heat exhaustion should not return to practice or play that day. Excessive weight loss (through perspiration) should be monitored, and the individual should not return to activity until the water lost has been replaced. Each episode of heat exhaustion predisposes the athlete to additional, more serious episodes of heat exhaustion that can progress to heatstroke.

Heatstroke

The most severe heat-related condition, **heatstroke**, involves a breakdown of the body's heat-regulation mechanism.

SIGNS AND SYMPTOMS Heatstroke is caused by your body overheating; usually as a result of prolonged exposure to or physical exertion in high temperatures and/or high humidity. The certified athletic trainer should monitor the heat index closely on days where excessive heat/humidity is present. Heatstroke can occur if your body temperature rises to 103°F (40°C) or higher. Symptoms include hot, dry skin, mental confusion, nausea and vomiting, flushed (red) skin, rapid breathing and heat rate, as well as possible headache.

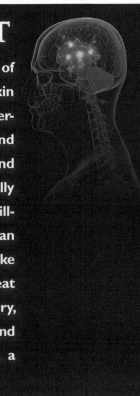

KEY CONCEPT

Heat exhaustion is a mild form of heat illness characterized by skin that is cool, moist, and pale; generalized weakness; dizziness; and nausea. Fluid replacement and cooling of the body are vitally important at this stage of heat illness. If not treated, heat illness can progress to heatstroke. Heatstroke is a life-threatening form of heat illness characterized by hot, dry, red skin, mental confusion, and unconsciousness. Heatstroke is a medical emergency.

The chief symptoms of heatstroke are hot, dry, red skin. There is commonly a strong and rapid pulse, with possible mental confusion and unconsciousness.

TREATMENT Heatstroke requires immediate emergency treatment.

It is imperative that the athlete be moved to the shade and cooled immediately. Excessive clothing should be removed. Icing should be initiated with ice towels. Ice packs may be placed in the axilla and groin areas. Misting the skin with cool water, followed by fanning the skin, will help lower body temperature. This is a *true medical emergency!*

Untreated heatstroke can quickly cause damage to your brain, heart, kidneys, as well as muscles. The damage worsens the longer treatment is delayed, increasing the risk of serious complications or death. Individuals suffering from heatstroke must be immediately transported to an emergency room by EMS. Table 25–3 summarizes heat-related illnesses and their care.

Table 25–3 Care and Treatment of Heat-Related Illnesses

HEAT DISORDER	CAUSES	SYMPTOMS	FIRST AID
Sunburn	Prolonged exposure to the sun.	Redness and pain. In severe cases, swelling of skin, blisters, fever, headaches.	Ointment for mild cases if blisters appear. If blisters break, apply dry, sterile dressing. Serious, extensive cases should be seen by a physician.
Heat cramps	Dehydration, fatigue.	Painful spasms, usually in muscles of legs, although abdomen is possible. Heavy sweating.	Stretch cramping muscles; give gentle massage to relieve spasm. Give sips of water. If nausea occurs, discontinue use.
Heat exhaustion	Dehydration, fatigue.	Heavy sweating; weakness; skin cold, pale, and clammy. Pulse weak and rapid. Normal or subnormal temperature possible. Possible fainting and vomiting.	Get victim out of sun. Have victim lie down and loosen clothing. Apply cool, wet cloths. Fan or move victim to air-conditioned room. Give sips of water to replace lost fluids; if nausea occurs, discontinue. If vomiting continues, seek immediate medical attention.
Heatstroke (sunstroke)	Failure of the thermoregulatory system. Work or exercise in hot environment. Lack of acclimation to warm environment.	High body temperature (106°F or higher). Hot, dry skin. Rapid, strong pulse. Possible unconsciousness.	Heat stroke is a severe medical emergency. Summon medical assistance or get the victim to a hospital immediately. Delay can be fatal. Move the victim to a cooler environment. Reduce body temperature with cold bath or sponging. Apply ice packs/cold compresses to armpits, groin, neck, and extremities. Cool victim immediately by whatever means available. Use extreme caution. Remove clothing; use fans and air conditioners. Do not give fluids.

Cold Stress

The body loses heat in five ways: respiration, evaporation, conduction, radiation, and convection.

Loss of heat through respiration occurs when heat escapes during exhalation. This can be reduced by covering the mouth and nose.

Evaporation occurs when perspiration evaporates from the skin and moisture is exhaled from the lungs (Figure 25–2), contributing to heat loss. The athlete should control the amount of evaporation by wearing clothing that can be ventilated or removed. Clothing should be made

Evaporation of sweat into environment

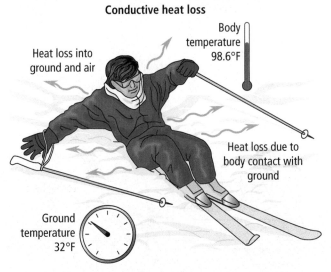

Losing heat

Body temperature 101°F

Figure 25–2 Evaporation is one method used to disperse excess heat from the body.

of fabric that will not absorb water, but allow it to pass through, thereby not trapping moisture next to the skin.

When there is a temperature difference between the body and an outside surface, the warmer of the two will transfer heat to the other. This is **conduction** (Figure 25–3). An example is sitting on cold ground; the warmth of the body will warm the surface of the ground. The body will lose heat, and the ground will gain heat, until equilibrium is reached. Other examples of heat conduction are touching cold equipment, swimming in cold water, or being wet when the moisture is cooler than the body, thus reducing body heat.

Radiation is heat transfer by infrared rays. If the body is hotter than the environment, it will lose heat to the environment by radiation (Figure 25–4). In direct sunlight, the body absorbs radiant heat from the sun. Radiation causes the largest heat loss from uncovered skin, particularly the head, neck, and hands. It is important to cover these areas to keep warm and prevent further heat loss.

The primary function of clothing is to keep a layer of warm air next to the skin, while allowing

Conductive heat loss

Heat loss into ground and air

Body temperature 98.6°F

Heat loss due to body contact with ground

Ground temperature 32°F

Figure 25–3 Heat loss by conduction transfers heat from a warm object to a cooler object.

water vapor (perspiration) to pass outward. The body continually warms this layer of air close to the body. This is **convection** (Figure 25–5). A wet-suit works on the same theory, but when a person wearing wetsuit gets into the water, he or she is

Radiation heat loss

Body temperature 101°F

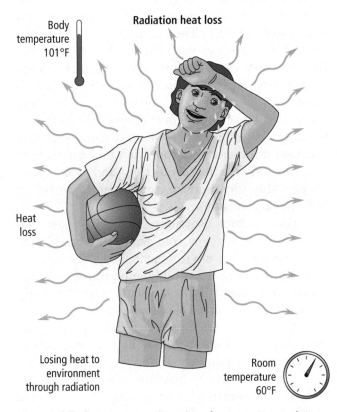

Heat loss

Losing heat to environment through radiation

Room temperature 60°F

Figure 25–4 Radiation is heat loss from a warmer object into the cooler environment.

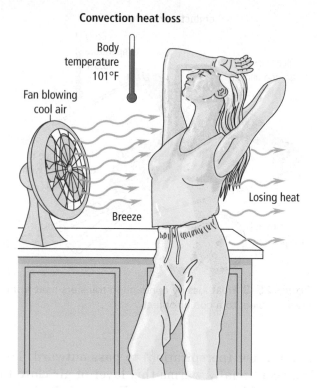

Convection heat loss

Body temperature 101°F

Fan blowing cool air

Breeze

Losing heat

Figure 25–5 Convection is heat loss through air currents.

KEY CONCEPT

The body loses heat in five ways:

- **Respiration**—heat escapes during exhalation
- **Conduction**—heat escapes to a cooler surface
- **Evaporation**—heat escapes through the skin via perspiration
- **Radiation**—heat escapes to the cooler environment
- **Convection**—heat escapes to circulated air currents

chilled for a few moments before the water next to the skin is warmed by the body. A drysuit has less initial shock because water does not get inside to start with. The clothing worn under the drysuit retains the warmth in the trapped air. Heat is lost rapidly with the slightest breeze unless a windproof (nylon or Gore-Tex) shell is worn over clothing to prevent warm air from being lost. The cooling effect of wind chill is equal to that of much lower actual temperatures because of increased evaporation and convection. Clothing with wind protection and good insulating value (dead-air space) is needed to retain body heat at a safe level.

Four factors contribute to cold stress: cold temperatures, high or cold wind, dampness, and cold water. A cold environment forces the body to work harder to maintain its temperature. Cold air, water, and snow all draw heat from the body. Anyone working in a cold environment may be at risk of cold stress. Older people may be at more risk than younger adults, because they are not able to generate heat as quickly.

Also, certain medications may prevent the body from generating heat normally. These include antidepressants, sedatives, tranquilizers, and some heart medications.

Wind Chill

Wind chill is the term used to describe the rate of heat loss from the human body resulting from the combined effect of low temperature and wind. As winds increase, heat is carried away from the body faster, driving down both skin temperature and eventually internal body temperature. Exposure to low wind chills can be life threatening to humans and animals alike.

Wind-chill temperature is a measure of relative discomfort due to combined cold and wind. Originally developed in 1941, it was revised in November 2001 (NOAA/NCAR, 2001). The current index makes use of the advances in science, technology, and computer modeling to provide a more accurate, understandable, and useful formula for calculating wind chill.

The wind-chill chart (Table 25–4) is based on physiological studies of the rate of heat loss for various combinations of ambient temperature and wind speed. The effects of wind chill depend strongly on the amount of clothing and other protection worn, as well as on age, health, and body characteristics. Wind-chill temperatures near or below 0°F create a risk of frostbite or other injury to exposed flesh. The risk of hypothermia because of inadequate clothing also depends on the wind-chill.

Table 25–4 Wind-Chill Chart

WIND SPEED (MPH)	AIR TEMPERATURE (°F)														
	40	35	30	25	20	15	10	5	0	–5	–10	–15	–20	–25	–30
5	36	31	25	19	13	7	1	–5	–11	–16	–22	–28	–34	–40	–46
10	34	27	21	15	9	3	–4	–10	–16	–22	–28	–35	–41	–47	–53
15	32	25	19	13	6	0	–7	–13	–19	–26	–32	–39	–45	–51	–58
20	30	24	17	11	4	–2	–9	–15	–22	–29	–35	–42	–48	–55	–61
25	29	23	16	9	3	–4	–11	–17	–24	–31	–37	–44	–51	–58	–64
30	28	22	15	8	1	–5	–12	–19	–26	–33	–39	–46	–53	–60	–67
35	28	21	14	7	0	–7	–14	–21	–27	–34	–41	–48	–55	–62	–69
40	27	20	13	6	–1	–8	–15	–22	–29	–36	–43	–50	–57	–64	–71
45	26	19	12	5	–2	–9	–16	–23	–30	–37	–44	–51	–58	–65	–72
50	26	19	12	4	–3	–10	–17	–24	–31	–38	–45	52	–60	–67	–74

Exposed flesh freezes in 30 minutes.
Exposed flesh freezes in 10 minutes.
Exposed flesh freezes in 5 minutes.

Source: NOAA, 2001.

Hypothermia

When a person is in a cold environment, most of the body's energy is used to maintain its internal temperature. Over time, the body will begin to shift blood flow from the extremities (hands, feet, arms, and legs) and outer skin to the core (chest and abdomen). This allows exposed skin and the extremities to cool rapidly and increases the risk of frostbite and hypothermia.

Hypothermia, meaning "low heat," is a potentially serious health condition. Hypothermia occurs when body heat is lost (from being in a cold environment) faster than it can be replaced.

SIGNS AND SYMPTOMS When body temperature drops below the normal 98.6°F to around 95°F, normally the onset of symptoms begins. The victim begins to shiver and stomp the feet to generate heat. As body temperature falls, slurred speech, lack of coordination, and memory loss develop, and the person will stop shivering. Once body temperature falls to around 85°F, the person may become unconscious; at 78°F, death may occur.

People who have experienced trauma often go into shock and shiver, a warning sign of hypothermia. Physical or mental trauma limits the body's capability to regulate its own temperature.

At the onset of hypothermia, the individual realizes that she or he is cold. Shivering may occur, but is controlled when the person becomes active. As hypothermia progresses, the feet feel stiff, the muscles become tense, and the victim has a feeling of fatigue and weakness. Coordination begins to decrease. The skin takes on a waxy pallor, and numbness occurs. Curiously, many victims of hypothermia deny that they have any symptoms. Denial is the main reason so many cases of hypothermia are fatal.

As moderate hypothermia takes over the body, the temperature ranges between 93 and 95°F. Shivering becomes less intense, and normal activity becomes uncomfortable because blood vessels are severely constricted. At this stage, the victim has poor coordination and trouble staying balanced. Speech may become slurred, and the victim may appear to be intoxicated. The hypothermic individual can no longer make responsible decisions and experiences feelings of apathy and confusion. The individual's breathing becomes shallow, and he or she experiences an overwhelming urge to sleep.

As **core body temperature** decreases, severe hypothermia sets in. An individual with severe hypothermia is extremely weak; the skin turns blue and the pupils become dilated. At this stage, the victim may still deny that a problem exists and may become violent. However, unconsciousness gradually ensues. Breathing becomes so shallow that the victim appears to be dead. When hypothermia reaches this level, the individual's only option is to be taken to a medical facility where the body can be warmed properly.

Individuals with diabetes often experience poor circulation, making them more prone to hypothermia because it is difficult for them to recognize numbness in their feet, arms, and legs. Persons with diabetes must be especially careful when outside in frigid temperatures.

Alcohol can be a contributing factor in the onset of hypothermia; it numbs the senses and thins the blood, making it difficult for anyone under the influence of alcohol to recognize the warning signs of hypothermia.

Hypothermia causes dehydration, which depletes the body of important nutrients. In some cases this may cause an erratic heartbeat.

TREATMENT Never attempt to bring a hypothermia victim's body back to normal temperature by placing him in hot water, giving him alcohol, or wrapping him in an electric or hot blanket. If body temperature rises too fast, it could induce cardiac arrest.

Move an individual suspected of suffering from hypothermia inside, out of the elements. Remove wet or cold clothing and replace with clothes that are warm and dry. The victim should avoid all physical activity and lie prone until medical help arrives.

IMPENDING HYPOTHERMIA:
- Seek or build a shelter to get the person out of the cold, windy, wet environment.

- Get a stove going or start a fire or to provide warmth. Provide the individual with a warm drink.

- Halt further heat loss by insulating the person with extra clothes, blankets, and the like. The victim should recover from the condition quickly.

MILD HYPOTHERMIA:
- Remove or insulate the individual from the cold environment, keeping the head and neck covered. This prevents further heat loss and rewarms the body.

- Provide the person with a warm, sweetened drink (no alcohol), and some high-energy food. Limited exercise may help to generate some internal heat, but it depletes energy reserves.

MODERATE HYPOTHERMIA:
- Activate EMS.

- Remove or insulate the person from the cold environment, keeping the head and neck covered.

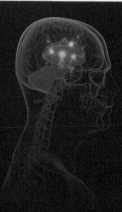

KEY CONCEPT

Hyperthermia is a condition in which body temperature increases above normal. The key to managing hyperthermia is to cool the body by moving the athlete to a shaded area, removing any unnecessary clothing, applying cool water to the extremities, fanning the athlete, and giving the athlete cool water to drink.

Hypothermia is a condition in which body temperature decreases below normal. The key to managing hypothermia is to warm the body by removing the athlete from the cold climate, removing wet or cold clothes, applying warm clothes or a blanket, and providing warm liquids to drink.

Apply mild heat (comfortable to your elbow) to the head, neck, chest, armpits, and groin of the victim.

- Use hot-water bottles, wrapped Thermo-Pads, or warm, moist towels.

- This treatment may have to continue for some time. Offer sips of warm, sweetened liquids (no alcohol) if the individual is fully conscious, is beginning to rewarm, and is able to swallow. Victims of hypothermia should be seen by a physician.

SEVERE HYPOTHERMIA:

- Activate EMS.

- Place the individual in a prewarmed sleeping bag with one or two other people. Skin-to-skin contact in the areas of the chest (ribs) and neck is effective. Exhale warm air near the person's nose and mouth or introduce steam into the area.

- Try to keep the individual awake; ignore pleas of "Leave me alone, I'm okay." This person is in serious trouble. Keep a close, continuous watch over the victim.

- Apply mild heat, with the aim of stopping the body temperature drop, not rewarming.

- If the victim loses consciousness, be very gentle, because at this point the heart is extremely sensitive. Always assume that the individual is revivable; do not give up.

- Check for pulse at the carotid artery. If after two minutes you do not find a pulse, check on the other side of the neck for two minutes.

- If there is any breathing or pulse, no matter how faint, do not give CPR, but keep very close watch for changes in vital signs.

- If no pulse is found, begin CPR immediately, stopping only when the heart begins to beat or the person applying CPR cannot carry on any longer without personal danger.

- Medical help is imperative, and hospitalization is needed.

Frostbite

Frostbite occurs when skin tissue and blood vessels are damaged from exposure to temperatures below 32°F. Frostbite most commonly affects the toes, fingers, earlobes, chin, cheeks, and nose—the body parts that are often left uncovered in cold temperatures. Frostbite can occur gradually or rapidly. The speed with which frostbite progresses will depend on how cold or windy it is and the duration of exposure to those conditions.

SIGNS AND SYMPTOMS Frostbite has three stages of progression.

In the first stage, the individual experiences a pins-and-needles sensation, and the skin turns very white and soft. This is called *frostnip*. No blistering occurs. This stage produces no permanent damage and may be reversed by soaking the affected body part in warm water or breathing warm air on the affected area.

In the second stage, blistering may occur. The skin feels numb, waxy, and frozen, indicating superficial frostbite (Figure 25–6). Ice crystals form in the skin cells, but the rest of the skin remains flexible.

The third stage, deep frostbite, is the most serious. In this stage, blood vessels, muscles, tendons, nerves, and bone may be frozen (Figure 25–7). Deep frostbite can lead to permanent damage, blood clots, and gangrene in severe cases. No feeling is experienced in the affected area, and there is usually no blistering. Serious infection and loss of limbs frequently occur after frostbite reaches this stage. However, even with deep frostbite, some frozen limbs may be saved if medical attention is quickly obtained.

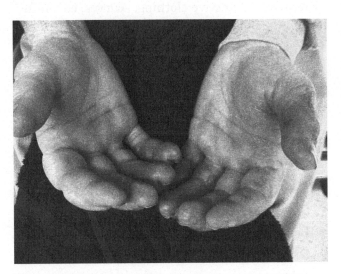

Figure 25–6 Superficial frostbite can be quite painful. Courtesy of Kevin Reilly, M.D., Albany Medical Center, Albany, NY.

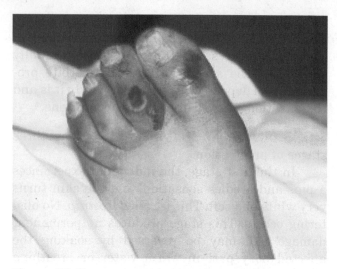

Figure 25–7 Deep frostbite results in permanent damage to tissue. Courtesy of Dr. Deborah Funk, Albany Medical Center, Albany, NY.

TREATMENT Frostbite risk can be reduced by the following:

- Wear several layers of clothing when in extremely cold conditions; the air pockets between the layers will help to retain warmth.
- Limit use of alcohol and tobacco. Alcohol causes the blood to cool quickly, and tobacco inhibits circulation to the extremities.
- Avoid going outdoors during extremely cold weather.
- When outside, shield the face and other body parts from cold wind and temperatures by wearing protective clothing, scarves, earmuffs, gloves, and so on.
- Wear waterproof skin moisturizer on exposed areas.
- Do not spend extended periods in extreme temperatures when exhausted, intoxicated, wet, or under the influence of certain drugs.

Seek emergency care if, after being in extremely cold conditions, any of the following are experienced:

- Skin swelling
- Loss of limb function and absence of pain
- Drastic skin color changes
- Blisters
- Slurred speech
- Memory loss

If the person cannot be transported to a hospital immediately, the following rewarming techniques may help until arrival at an emergency facility:

- Bring the individual indoors as soon as possible.
- Apply warm towels or immerse the affected area in circulating lukewarm water for 20 minutes. Hot water should not be used, and the area should not be rubbed in any way. If blisters are present, leave them intact.
- Do not hold the affected area near fire; the area may be burned because of the reduced feeling in the area.
- Offer the individual warm fluids, if alert, but never alcohol.
- Keep the affected area raised.

After rewarming, a superficial frostbite will redden and become painful as circulation resumes in the area. Blisters are likely to form within 24 hours.

A deep frostbite injury will remain hard and cool to the touch, and may turn blue or black. Blisters may form. Skin surrounding the affected

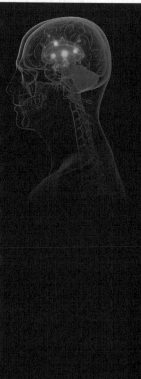

KEY CONCEPT

Environmental conditions can greatly affect the health and well-being of athletes. During summer sports, pay close attention to the heat index; during winter sports, pay attention to the wind chill. These are both good gauges for determining the risk posed by environmental exposure. At all times, athletes should remain adequately hydrated. This will help protect them from the possible risks of environmental exposure.

area may become swollen and remain swollen for more than a month. If gangrene develops, amputation may be necessary.

While a frostbite injury is healing:

- Avoid infection by leaving blisters intact.
- Watch for signs of infection, such as redness, swelling, fever, oozing pus, and red streaks on the skin.
- Take all prescribed medications.
- Do not expose the affected area to cold temperatures until cleared to do so by a physician.

SKIN CONDITIONS IN ATHLETES

Among the most serious conditions that afflict athletes are the various infections caused by bacteria, fungi, and viruses transmitted by skin-to-skin contact with other athletes or athletic equipment. Athletes are susceptible to skin infections because sweating softens and impairs the skin; the body's main barrier. Athletic equipment covers the skin, thereby creating a warm, moist environment in which microorganisms can grow. Athletes also often suffer from skin traumas, such as cuts or scrapes, which facilitate the entry of microorganisms.

Athletes can reduce their risk of becoming affected by bacterial, viral, and fungal infections by practicing basic hygiene and making sure their equipment and shoes fit properly.

Acne Mechanica

Acne mechanica is a form of acne, often seen in athletes, that results from heat, pressure, occlusion, and friction. It usually occurs in areas that are covered by protective gear, such as the shoulders, back, and head. Tight clothing (especially that made of synthetic materials) and equipment such as helmets and shoulder pads are primary culprits of acne mechanica.

TREATMENT Methods for preventing and treating acne mechanica include wearing clean clothing, made of cotton or a material that wicks away moisture, against the skin or underneath a uniform. Application of an OTC acne medication may also be effective. Washing the affected areas immediately following athletic activity will help minimize any outbreak.

Plantar Warts

Plantar warts are small, hard growths that occur on the bottom of the foot. The warts are pressed into the foot when walking and can be painful. Plantar warts are more common in children than in adults.

Because plantar warts are under pressure, they grow inward, causing pain. They can be differentiated from simple calluses by characteristic dark specks in the center. If shaved, these marks will show pinpoint bleeding. Plantar warts are caused by human papillomavirus and are contagious.

TREATMENT Warts may vanish spontaneously in time with no treatment. The treatment of warts involves cutting, burning, or freezing (with liquid nitrogen). The use of chemicals may also be effective. These treatments all depend on the body having enough immunity to prevent the wart from regrowing.

Not walking barefooted in locker rooms will help keep plantar warts from spreading to others. A dermatologist can develop a proper treatment.

Herpes Gladiatorum

Herpes simplex infection in wrestlers, **herpes gladiatorum**, is a well-known, frequently reported condition. Rapid identification and treatment of this condition is essential to prevent epidemics that may otherwise sweep through entire wrestling teams, and to avert missed practices and competitions for an individual athlete.

Herpes gladiatorum is transmitted through skin-to-skin contact. Abrasions and cuts ease the transmission of fungal organisms, and moisture and occlusive clothing provide an optimal environment for organism growth.

A similar contagion is impetigo, a superficial infection of the skin caused by *staphylococcus* (staph) and *streptococcus* (strep) bacteria. Impetigo is more common in children 2- to 5-year-olds than in adults. It is most likely to occur in warm, humid environments and is most commonly spread by close contact.

TREATMENT Therapy may include both topical and oral antifungal medications. In addition to treatment with antifungals, measures should be taken to ensure that the infection is not transmitted to other wrestlers. Wrestlers are typically excluded from participation until they complete 10 days of topical therapy or 15 days of oral treatment. Unfortunately, it is not known how long a patient requires treatment before he or she is considered noninfectious.

Close observation by coaches and certified athletic trainers is important in keeping all wrestlers eligible to compete. Any suspicious skin lesion should be evaluated by a physician as soon as possible. Upon diagnosis of herpes gladiatorum, appropriate therapy should be instituted without delay.

Fungal Infections

Typically referred to as "jock itch," ringworm, or "athlete's foot," **tinea pedis** is a fungal infection that thrives in warmth and dampness. Tinea pedis lives off the dead skin cells and calluses of the feet, especially between the toes. Fungal infections can also be found in the groin area, in which case they are called **tinea cruris**.

SIGNS AND SYMPTOMS Symptoms include inflammation, burning, itching, scaling, and blistering. Athlete's foot and jock itch are prevalent in gyms and locker rooms because the fungus thrives in warm and moist conditions. Tinea cruris is promoted by tight clothing that does not allow air to circulate.

TREATMENT Perspiration is a crucial factor in the development of fungal infections. Fungal medications will alleviate, control, and eliminate such infections. Fungal infections are more of a problem for men because they tend to perspire more heavily than women.

Prevention includes the following measures:

- At home, take shoes off and expose feet to the air.
- Change socks and underwear every day, especially in warm weather.
- Dry the feet carefully (especially between the toes) after using a locker room or public shower.
- Avoid walking barefoot in public areas. Instead, wear flip-flops, sandals, or water shoes.
- Do not wear thick clothing for long periods of time in warm weather. It will increase the amount of sweating.
- Throw away worn-out exercise shoes. Never borrow other people's shoes.
- Do not share towels or headgear.

MRSA

Athletic trainers and coaches must be on alert for infections that don't respond to conventional treatment. Methicillin-resistant staphylococcus aureus, **MRSA,** is a bacterium that causes infections in different parts of the body. It is tougher to treat than most strains of staph infection because it is resistant to commonly used antibiotics.

MRSA is spread by contact. Athletes can contract MRSA by touching another person who has it on the skin, or by touching objects that have the bacteria on them. MRSA is carried by about 2% of the population (or 2 in 100 people), although most of them are not infected.

SIGNS AND SYMPTOMS The symptoms of MRSA depend on where one is infected. Most often, it causes mild infections on the skin, like sores or boils. But it can also cause more serious skin infections or infect surgical wounds, the bloodstream, lungs, or the urinary tract. Though most MRSA infections aren't serious, some can be life threatening. Many public health experts are alarmed by the spread of tough strains of MRSA.

TREATMENT Suspected MRSA must be treated by a doctor. It is important to take precautions to keep the lesion from making contact with anyone else. Cover well, and have the athlete seek immediate care. MRSA is constantly adapting to antibiotics on the market and is becoming more dangerous. Because it is hard to treat, MRSA is sometimes called a "superbug."

Infectious Mononucleosis

Infectious mononucleosis is a contagious disease commonly known as "mono." It is typically the result of the Epstein-Barr virus (EBV). However, other viruses also cause this disease. Infectious mononucleosis is common among teenagers and young adults, especially college students. It is estimated that at least one out of four teenagers and young adults who get infected with EBV will develop infectious mononucleosis.

Typically, these viruses spread most commonly through bodily fluids, especially saliva, and can also be spread through blood and semen during sexual contact.

SIGNS AND SYMPTOMS Symptoms usually appear four to six weeks after being infected. Many symptoms will appear slowly, but not always at the same time. Symptoms include extreme fatigue, head and body aches, fever, rash, sore throat, and swollen lymph nodes in the neck and armpits, as well as a swollen liver and or spleen.

TREATMENT There is no vaccine to protect against infectious mononucleosis. Prevention includes protecting yourself by not kissing or sharing drinks, food, or personal items, like toothbrushes, with people who have infectious mononucleosis.

Symptoms can be lessened by drinking plenty of fluids, lots of rest, and taking OTC medications to lessen pain and lower fever. Because the spleen may become enlarged as a result of infectious mononucleosis, those infected should avoid contact sports until fully recovered. Participating in contact sports may cause the spleen to rupture.

Blisters

Playing sports involves a considerable amount of movement. Athletic equipment and poorly fitting shoes can cause friction to the skin. This friction, along with heat and moisture that may develop as a result, increases the risk of blistering.

Blisters appear when a tear occurs within the upper layers of the skin, forming a space between the layers but leaving the surface intact. Fluid then seeps into this space, causing the skin to bubble. The soles of the feet and palms of the hands are most commonly affected, because the hands and feet often rub against shoes, skates, racquets, and other athletic equipment.

TREATMENT If an athlete gets a blister, the goals will be to relieve the pain, keep the blister from enlarging, and avoid infection. To relieve the pain, the athlete will need to correct the situation that caused the blister in the first place. Special padding and blister foams will help to dissipate friction and allow the blister to heal.

The best protection against infection is a blister's own skin. Care should be taken to not break the skin or pop a blister. This creates a direct route for entry of infectious microorganisms. If the blister does pop and drain, clean the area with an antibacterial soap and an application of an antibiotic ointment such as bacitracin with polymyxin B (double-antibiotic ointment) or bacitracin alone. Avoid ointments that contain neomycin, because they are more likely to cause an allergic reaction. The blister should then be covered with a bandage. The bandage should be changed daily, or more frequently if it gets wet.

Larger or painful blisters that are intact may have to be drained by a physician because of the risk of infection.

To prevent blisters, athletes should keep the skin well lubricated to reduce friction and decrease moisture. Properly fitting shoes are critical in preventing blisters, as are acrylic or other synthetic-material socks that are designed to decrease friction and wick away moisture. Athletes may also find that wearing two pairs of socks and applying talcum powder before practice reduces the occurrence of blisters.

Abrasions

Sports participation puts the unprotected skin of athletes at risk of injury. Abrasions, a common complaint, are normally caused by poorly fitting equipment or rubbing of the skin against another athlete or surface.

The epidermis is the superficial, outermost layer of skin; the dermis is the deeper layer that imparts firmness and flexibility to the skin. *Abrasion* typically refers to an injury that removes these layers of skin.

TREATMENT Treatment of abrasions includes cleaning the wound with mild soap and water, applying an antibiotic cream, and bandaging. Bandages should be replaced daily. Abrasions should be checked periodically for signs of infection.

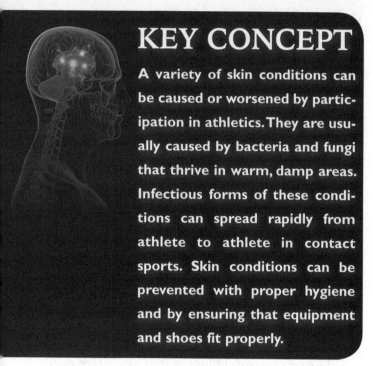

KEY CONCEPT

A variety of skin conditions can be caused or worsened by participation in athletics. They are usually caused by bacteria and fungi that thrive in warm, damp areas. Infectious forms of these conditions can spread rapidly from athlete to athlete in contact sports. Skin conditions can be prevented with proper hygiene and by ensuring that equipment and shoes fit properly.

Athletes should use special wraps or padding to protect an abrasion until it has healed.

Jogger's Nipples

Another condition caused by friction that affects runners is known as **jogger's nipples**. Constant chafing between a runner's nipples and shirt, particularly during long runs, can cause painful, crusted lesions that often bleed and show through the shirt.

To prevent jogger's nipples, dermatologists recommend applying petroleum jelly, patches, or a bandage over the nipples prior to long runs. Semisynthetic or other soft-fiber sports bras and shirts can also help prevent jogger's nipples.

DIABETES

Diabetes is a disease in which the body does not produce or properly use **insulin**. Insulin is a hormone needed to make cells absorb sugar from the blood, where it is converted into the energy used in daily life. The causes of diabetes continue to be a mystery, although both genetics and environmental factors (such as obesity and lack of exercise) appear to play roles.

According to the American Diabetes Association (2015), approximately 30.3 million people in the United States, or 9.4% of the population, have diabetes. Although an estimated 23.1 million have been diagnosed, 7.2 million people (or one-third) are unaware that they have the disease. The two major types are Type 1 and Type 2 diabetes.

Type 1 Diabetes

Type 1 diabetes results from the body's failure to produce insulin. An estimated 1.2 to 2.4 million people, or 5 to 10% of the population, have Type 1 diabetes. Type 1 diabetes is usually diagnosed in children and young adults and was previously known as *juvenile diabetes*.

In Type 1 diabetes, the body does not produce insulin, a hormone that is necessary for the body to be able to use sugar. Sugar is the basic fuel for the cells in the body. Insulin takes sugar from the blood and delivers it by "unlocking" the cells of the body, allowing glucose to enter and fuel them. When sugar builds up in the blood instead of going into cells, it can cause two problems: Cells may be starved for energy, and, over time, high blood sugar levels may damage eyes, kidneys, nerves, or the heart.

The **pancreas**, an organ near the stomach, produces insulin in special **beta cells**. Sometimes, beta cells die and cannot produce insulin. Many things can kill beta cells, but in most people with Type 1 diabetes the immune system makes a mistake. Cells that normally protect the body from germs attack and kill beta cells instead. Without beta cells, insulin cannot be made. Sugar therefore builds up in the blood, resulting in diabetes.

Many people who have Type 1 diabetes live long, healthy lives. The key is keeping blood sugar levels within the target range. This can be done with meal planning, exercise, and insulin. People with Type 1 diabetes need to check their blood sugar levels regularly.

Type 2 Diabetes

Type 2 diabetes, also called *adult onset diabetes*, occurs when the body still makes insulin, but either does so in insufficient amounts or produces insulin that does not function properly. Type 2 is by far the most common form of the condition, affecting 90 to 95% of all diagnosed cases in adults. Persons with Type 2 diabetes usually do not require insulin injections because control is achievable through careful diet and exercise.

Diabetic Emergencies

Persons with diabetes are subject to two very different types of emergencies: insulin reaction (or insulin shock) and diabetic coma.

Insulin reaction occurs when there is too much insulin in the body. This condition rapidly reduces the level of sugar in the blood, causing brain cells to suffer. Insulin reaction can be caused by taking too much medication, failing to eat, heavy exercise, or emotional factors.

Diabetic coma occurs when there is too much sugar and too little insulin in the blood; in this state, the body cells do not get enough nourishment. Diabetic coma can be caused by eating too much sugar, not taking prescribed medications, stress, or infection.

SIGNS AND SYMPTOMS Signs and symptoms of insulin reaction include fast breathing, fast pulse, dizziness, weakness, change in the level of consciousness, vision difficulties, sweating, headache, numb hands or feet, and hunger.

Signs and symptoms of a diabetic coma develop more slowly than those of insulin shock, sometimes over a period of days. Signs and symptoms include drowsiness, confusion, deep and fast breathing, thirst, dehydration, fever, a change in the level of consciousness, and peculiar, sweet or fruity-smelling breath.

TREATMENT OF INSULIN REACTION AND DIABETIC COMA Knowing and examining for the signs and symptoms of diabetic emergencies will help in giving proper aid. In addition, if the patient is conscious, two very important questions need to be asked to determine the nature of the problem:

- Ask, "Have you eaten today?" Someone who has eaten but not taken prescribed medication may be in a diabetic coma.

- Ask, "Have you taken your medication today?" Someone who has not eaten but did take the medication may be having an insulin reaction.

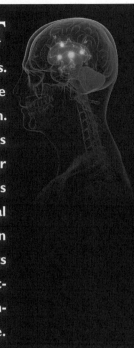

KEY CONCEPT
There are two forms of diabetes. Type I diabetes results from the body's failure to produce insulin. Individuals with Type I diabetes need to maintain blood-sugar levels within a target range. This is often accomplished through meal planning, exercise, and insulin injections. Type 2 diabetes results from insufficient bodily production of insulin and can be controlled through diet and exercise.

Distinguishing between the two types of diabetic emergencies can be difficult. Always check for a medical bracelet that will reveal a person's condition.

Of the two conditions, insulin shock is a true emergency that requires prompt action. A person in insulin shock needs sugar. If she is conscious, give her sugar in any form: candy, fruit juice, or a soft drink. Sugar can save the life of a person who is in insulin shock. If the person is suffering from diabetic coma, sugar is not required, but will not cause her further harm. Monitor the victim carefully and seek professional help.

SEIZURE DISORDERS

Seizures are disruptions of normal brain activity. The brain is a complex organ that functions by creating and sending messages in the form of electrical signals to control, for example, the muscles. Signals can also go from the body to the brain, sending sensory information such as sight, sound, touch, taste, temperature, and balance. Most of the brain's electrical messages, however, are sent from one part of the brain to another. These internal messages account for our ability to think, to perceive sensations, and to be conscious, self-motivated individuals.

To function normally, the brain's messages must be sent from place to place in an orderly manner. Congress has special rules of order dictating who can speak when, and about what; similarly, the brain has special rules to maintain order. If all members of Congress were to speak at once, there would be mayhem, and Congress would be unable to function. A seizure is, in effect, many parts of the brain speaking at once. Order is disrupted, and the brain cannot carry out its normal functions.

Seizures are a fairly common experience. About 5 to 7% of the U.S. population will suffer a seizure during their lifetime, but simply having an isolated seizure does not constitute epilepsy. **Epilepsy** is a condition in which seizures recur regularly throughout the affected person's lifetime. About 1% of the population will develop epilepsy; for about half of these people, a cause can be established. For the remainder, the cause of their epilepsy is unknown.

Many processes disrupt normal brain functions and induce either a single seizure or a few seizures over a relatively short period. These processes include infections, high fever, brain tumors, drugs, strokes, bleeding in the brain, trauma to the brain, and low blood glucose, sodium, or calcium. Seizures caused by these processes usually cease when the underlying problem is solved and therefore are not classified as epilepsy. Only when the underlying cause cannot be found or treated, and the seizures recur indefinitely, is epilepsy diagnosed.

Physical injury to the brain can cause epilepsy. For example, many people, after suffering a stroke, develop epilepsy originating in the part of the brain that was injured by the stroke. Penetrating injuries to the brain can cause epilepsy. Such injuries might occur following a skull fracture if bone fragments are forced into the brain.

Epilepsy can also be caused by events that are far more subtle than physical insult to the brain. For example, alterations in brain chemistry, brought about by some street drugs, or workplace exposure to certain toxic chemicals, can cause seizures. Unfortunately, the common thread that ties all these different causes together—the ultimate cause of epilepsy—is not known.

There are different types and severities of seizures. A **simple partial seizure** is when jerking begins in one area of the body, such as an arm, leg, or the face. It cannot be stopped, but the person stays awake and aware. Jerking may proceed from one area of the body to another, and sometimes spreads to become a convulsive seizure. Partial sensory seizures may not be obvious to an onlooker, but the person experiences a distorted environment. Victims may see or hear things that are not there, or they may feel unexplained fear, sadness, anger, or joy. A person having a seizure may become nauseated, experience odd smells, and have a generally "funny" feeling in the stomach.

No first aid is required for a simple partial seizure unless the seizure becomes convulsive.

Generalized tonic-clonic seizures, also called *grand mal seizures,* are characterized by a sudden cry, falling, and rigidity, followed by muscle jerks, shallow breathing or temporarily suspended breathing, bluish skin, and possible loss of bladder or bowel control. The seizure usually lasts a couple of minutes, after which normal breathing resumes. There may be some confusion or fatigue, followed by return to full consciousness.

First aid for a grand mal seizure includes looking for medical identification and protecting the victim from nearby hazards. Loosen ties or shirt collars and protect the victim's head from injury. Turn the victim on the side to keep the airway clear, unless an injury exists. Reassure the victim as consciousness returns. If a single seizure lasts less than five minutes, ask the victim

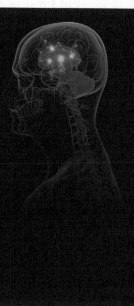

KEY CONCEPT

Epilepsy is a chronic condition with a variety of causes. However, the ultimate cause of epilepsy is unknown. Seizures resulting from epilepsy can be either partial, affecting only one area of the body, or generalized, affecting the entire body and causing a temporary decrease in the level of consciousness.

if he or she desires hospital evaluation. If there are multiple seizures, or if one seizure lasts longer than five minutes, call an ambulance. If the person is pregnant, injured, or diabetic, call for aid at once.

INSECT BITES AND STINGS

The two greatest risks from most insect stings and bites are allergic reactions and infections.

A bee sting is always potentially serious. The severity and duration of a reaction will vary from one person to another. In addition, a given individual's reaction to bee stings may differ between occurrences. Most persons experience a local, nonserious allergic reaction to bee venom; however, the reaction will depend on the location and number of stings received. The ever-present possibility of a severe allergic reaction to bee venom makes a sting a potentially life-threatening occurrence.

SIGNS AND SYMPTOMS Two kinds of reactions are usually associated with insect stings—local and systemic i.e., allergic or life threatening).

A **local reaction** is generally characterized by pain, swelling, redness, itching, and a weal surrounding the wound made by the stinger. This is the reaction of the vast majority of persons, and those suffering it are considered to be at little risk of death.

Systemic reactions are generalized reactions occurring within a few minutes of a sting. Mildest symptoms are flushing of the skin, followed by an itchy nettle rash. More serious symptoms include chest wheezing, nausea, vomiting, abdominal pains, palpitations, and faintness. The speed of the onset of a reaction is an indication of its seriousness. Anaphylaxis occurs within seconds or minutes of a sting. Common initial symptoms are chest wheezing, nausea, vomiting, and confusion, followed by falling blood pressure leading to death.

Epinephrine by injection is the only effective immediate treatment. The use of an **EpiPen**, an automatic injector, can save the life of someone suffering anaphylaxis. EpiPens are designed to inject a premeasured, single dose of epinephrine. If the victim is unable to administer the dose personally, a bystander can assist. EpiPens are designed to be administered in the front part of the leg, through

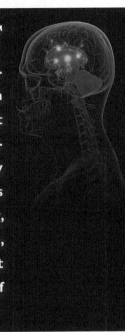

KEY CONCEPT

A systemic reaction is a generalized reaction occurring within just a few minutes of an insect sting or bite. The mildest symptoms are flushed skin and an itchy rash. More serious symptoms include difficulty in breathing, nausea, vomiting, palpitations, and fainting. The time of onset indicates the degree of severity of the reaction.

clothing. This is done by thrusting the EpiPen into the leg and holding it there for 10 seconds.

Remove the EpiPen and massage the site of the injection for several seconds. When the EpiPen is removed, the needle should be visibly protruding from the unit; this indicates that the medication was delivered. The effects of the epinephrine injection will last 15 to 20 minutes. Activate EMS. It is important that the victim be taken to the emergency room immediately for observation.

TREATMENT First aid for bee stings includes:

- Notifying a companion in case assistance becomes necessary
- Immediately removing the sting apparatus by scraping it out of the skin
- Applying ice, which helps reduce swelling and pain
- Seeking medical assistance if you suspect a serious reaction

PREVENTION Chemicals in certain hair sprays, deodorants, and perfumes or colognes can attract bees. Athletes must take care not to wear anything that might do so while outdoors. Any person who is allergic to bee stings should have on them at all times a medical identification bracelet or card, and also carry an anaphylaxis kit.

THE FEMALE ATHLETE TRIAD

Some physically active women are at risk for a group of symptoms called the **female athlete triad**. Each part of the triad can impair health and sport performance. This often unrecognized disorder is a combination of three conditions:

- Disordered eating
- Amenorrhea (lack of menstrual periods)
- Osteoporosis

The competitive nature and strong discipline that help shape a good athlete may also be part of the equation leading to this disorder. Competitive athletes may be at higher risk than more casual athletes, because of their more rigorous training schedules and the "play-to-win" nature of their sports. Athletes who participate in endurance sports (such as cross-country running), aesthetic sports (such as gymnastics or ballet), and sports that require form-fitting uniforms (such as swimming) tend to be at greater risk. The emphasis on appearance and the perception that carrying less weight will universally improve performance increase this risk.

An underfueled athlete is a slowed and weakened athlete. No matter the sport, if muscles lack sufficient and proper fuel, performance will decline. A first sign of disordered eating might simply be early fatigue. As the fuel deficit worsens, actual loss of strength and muscle size can occur, as the body uses skeletal muscle to fuel essential body functions like heart function and breathing. Lack of fuel can also impair concentration. The athlete with strength loss and poor concentration is more easily injured, and injuries in a poorly fueled body are slow to heal.

Loss of menstrual periods (**amenorrhea**) may signal a change in the body's intricate and complicated hormone system. Hormonal imbalance from underfueling the body can result in lowered estrogen production (although there are other causes of lowered estrogen levels). Diminished estrogen level can have many effects; the most immediately apparent one is bone loss. Bone loss that occurs as a result of amenorrhea can begin after just a few months with no periods.

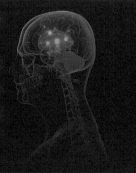

KEY CONCEPT
Competitive athletes may be at higher risk than casual athletes due to a more rigorous training schedule and the "play-to-win" nature of their sports.

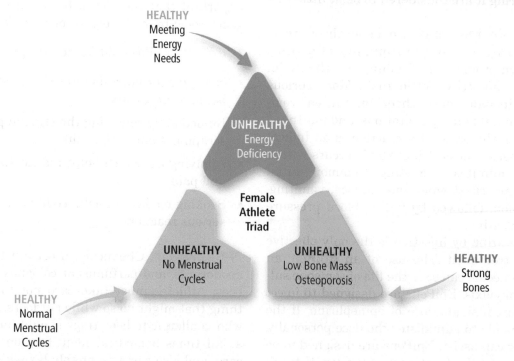

Figure 25–8 Female Athlete Triad Model

Loss of bone, or **osteoporosis**, especially in an athlete, can be an unfortunate setup for injury. Stress fractures can sideline the athlete from sports activity and will be slow to heal if the body is underfueled. Repeated stress fractures and unexplained injuries should be a red flag for further evaluation of the athlete's eating and exercise patterns. Bone loss that occurs because of amenorrhea can be permanent.

Warning Signs

The warning signs of the female athlete triad include:

- Frequent or unexplained injuries, especially stress fractures

- Excessive or compulsive exercise (not being psychologically able to skip a day of exercise or reduce the time spent exercising)

- Change in performance (loss of endurance, speed, or strength)

- Impaired concentration

- Absent or irregular menstrual periods

- Restrictive eating masked as a "performance-enhancing" meal plan

- Use of weight-loss products or supplements

Prevention

Prevention of the female athlete triad includes:

- Choosing an activity that complements the individual's natural body strengths.

- Realizing that health is more important than competitive success.

- Avoiding frequent weigh-ins, weight comments, and punitive consequences for weight gain.

- Appreciating a healthy, active body. Do not make comparisons to others, especially those portrayed in the media. Optimal weight for health and performance differs for everyone.

- Realizing that the thinnest athletes are not necessarily the fastest or the strongest.

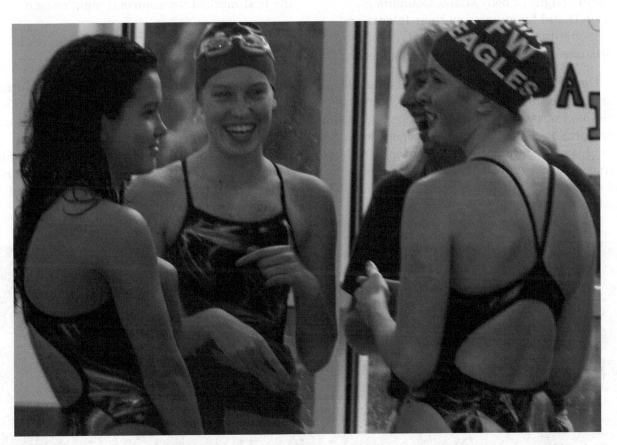

Figure 25–9 A good coach-athlete relationship is important in identifying and working through an athlete's health concerns.

- Thinking of fuel as the ultimate performance enhancer.

- Not starving the bones. The fuel mix should include several servings of calcium sources such as milk, yogurt, cheese, calcium-fortified juices, and soy products. A lactose-intolerant athlete can try lactose-free dairy products. Green, leafy vegetables, almonds, and beans also contain calcium.

- Being a role model with words and actions. Speak up when negative comments are made about weight or body shape. Compliment friends and teammates on their talents and personality, not their looks. Take a positive attitude about fueling and enjoying foods.

Disordered eating, whether manifested as restrictive eating behaviors, binging, purging, or excessive exercise, can lead to changes in normal body hormone levels. Normal estrogen levels are needed to maintain calcium content in bone. Estrogen levels may be lowered by amenorrhea and cause loss of calcium content in the bone. The result is osteoporosis, or porous bones.

Circadian Dysrhythmia Disorder

Circadian dysrhythmia is a disruption in a person's circadian rhythm. The circadian rhythm, or "internal body clock," regulates the 24-hour cycle of biological processes. Linked to this 24-hour cycle are metabolic functions such as hormone production, cell regeneration, and other biological activities. Patterns of brainwave activity are also linked to the circadian rhythm.

The circadian rhythm is important in determining sleeping patterns, such as when we sleep and when we wake, every 24 hours. Normally the circadian clock is set by the light-dark cycle over 24 hours. Causes of this disorder are routine change (such as staying up too late at night) shift work, time zone changes, jet lag, pregnancy, medications, and certain medical disorders.

Treatment depends on the type of disorder the person is experiencing. For example, someone suffering from this disorder because of staying up too late at night would need to regulate his or her sleep cycle and go to bed at approximately the same time nightly. A consistent pattern of sleep is the best method for a normal night's sleep.

Students with Disabilities and Participation in Athletic Programs

According to the National Center for Education Statistics (2015), public schools have a significant number of students with disabilities; often up to 13% of the total enrollment. It is paramount that certified athletic trainers understand the unique needs of these students, and work with parents and coaches to create a medically safe and fostering environment.

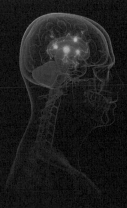

KEY CONCEPT

The female athlete triad is characterized by disordered eating, amenorrhea, and osteoporosis. Competitive athletes are at higher risk for the disorder than are more casual athletes. The triad also occurs more often in athletes who participate in sports in which body image is important. Disordered eating can lead to a loss of strength, poor concentration, and additional injuries. Amenorrhea contributes to bone loss and may lead to osteoporosis. Osteoporosis places the athlete at great risk of fractures.

Federal Laws such as the 2004 Individuals with Disabilities Education Act (IDEA), the Rehabilitation Act of 1973 (Section 504), the Americans with Disabilities Act of 1990 (ADA), as well as state and local codes have included regulations and provisions for the participation of individuals with disabilities.

The benefits and opportunities afforded by an educationally based athletic program that includes our disabled students cannot be overstated.

CONCLUSION

Many health and safety factors must be considered when participating in athletics. Factors such as the environment can turn a positive practice or game situation into a dangerous one. Understanding the causes of environmental-related illnesses helps the athlete plan ahead and stay within safe limits.

Other concerns are specific medical conditions that may limit or curtail athletic competition. The athlete must be made aware of the different illnesses and conditions that affect performance and health. Quick recognition and treatment will ensure good health and optimal performance.

It is important to recognize that all athletes must be given equal access to athletic participation and competition. Coaches and parents, working in conjunction with local school personnel, can develop and implement an athletic program beneficial to everyone.

REVIEW QUESTIONS

1. What is homeostasis?
2. Explain first aid for heat cramps.
3. What is the difference between heat exhaustion and heatstroke? Does the immediate care differ? How?
4. Explain each of the five ways in which the body loses heat.
5. Explain the heat index.
6. How is wind chill determined?
7. Describe hyperthermia and the effects on the body.
8. Explain the steps that should be taken to aid a person with moderate hypothermia.
9. Explain the three stages of frostbite.
10. Can a person lose fingers and toes to frostbite? How?
11. What SPF lotion would protect the majority of people?
12. What types of skin infections are common for athletes?
13. What are the signs, symptoms, and treatment for infectious mononucleosis?
14. What are the two diabetic emergencies? How are they treated?
15. Explain how epilepsy affects the body.
16. What is an anaphylactic reaction to a bee sting?
17. What is the difference between a local and a systemic reaction?
18. List and explain the three parts of the female athlete triad.
19. How can the female athlete triad be prevented?
20. What is circadian dysrhythmia, and how does it affect the body?
21. Why is it important to include students with disabilities in an athletic program?
22. Should athletes with disabilities compete with athletes without disabilities? Explain your answer, including pros and cons.

PROJECTS AND ACTIVITIES

1. What is the mathematical formula for wind chill? If the wind speed is 20 miles per hour and the air temperature is 35°F, what is the wind-chill temperature?

2. Take two plastic, one-gallon milk jugs and fill them with 70°F water. "Dress" one of them with wool and the other with cotton. Set them outside for two hours. Check the temperature of each jug. Is there any difference? Explain your findings. What type of heat loss is this? (This experiment can only be done during the late fall or winter months when the outside temperature is below 40°F.)

3. An athlete should not lose more than 3% of his or her body weight during any practice session. Create a chart indicating weight loss of 3%. The vertical axis of your chart should represent current body weight, and the horizontal axis should represent weight after a 3% loss.

4. On the Internet, find an article about someone who has suffered severe hypothermia and lived. Write a review of what you read.

5. Talk with the wrestling coach at your school about skin diseases and wrestlers. What does he or she do to prevent skin diseases among the wrestlers?

6. What products on the market today cure tinea pedis?

7. Ask your school nurse or certified athletic trainer about the percentage of athletes who are allergic to bee stings. What is this number? What is done if one of these individuals is stung?

8. Set up an interview with the gymnastics, girls' swimming, or girls' cross-country coach. Talk about the female athlete triad. What did you learn?

LEARNING LINKS

- Visit the website https://www.ncbi.nlm.nih.gov/pmc/articles/PMC3435916/ to research more about the female athlete triad.

- Visit the website of the American Diabetes Association, at http://www.diabetes.org, to learn more about the maintenance of diabetes.

- Visit the National Federation of State High School Associations (NFHS) and read their position statement on inclusion of students with disabilities into the sports program. http://nfsh.org

GLOSSARY

abdominal cavity The area of the body that contains the stomach, liver, gallbladder, pancreas, spleen, small intestine, appendix, and part of the large intestine.

abdominopelvic cavity The area from below the diaphragm to the pubic floor; there is no separation between the abdomen and pelvis.

abduction Movement of the limbs away from the midline of the body.

abrasion An injury that occurs when several layers of skin are torn loose or totally removed.

absorption The passage of a substance into body fluids and tissues.

acetylcholine The chemical released when a nerve impulse is transmitted.

Achilles tendon A tendon in the back of the ankle and foot that attaches the gastrocnemius and soleus muscles to the calcaneus.

acne mechanica A form of acne that results from heat, pressure, occlusion, and friction.

acromioclavicular joint The joint formed by the acromion of the scapula and the clavicle; commonly known as the AC joint.

acromioclavicular separation A traumatic sprain to the acromioclavicular (AC) joint, usually caused by a direct blow to the shoulder.

acromion process The lateral triangular projection of the spine of the scapula that forms the point of the shoulder and articulates with the clavicle.

action potential The electric change occurring across the membrane of a nerve or muscle cell during transmission of a nerve impulse.

active motion Movement through a range of motion done by the athlete during examination to assess injury.

adaptation The systematic application of exercise stress sufficient to stimulate muscle fatigue, but not so severe that breakdown and injury occur.

adduction Movement of the limbs toward the midline of the body.

adductor muscles A muscle group that aids in adduction of the hip; consists of the adductor longus, adductor brevis, and adductor magnus muscles.

automated electronic defibrillator (AED) Device used to shock the heart back to normal rhythm.

afferent arteriole Structure that takes blood from the renal artery to the Bowman's capsule.

afferent nerve A nerve that carries nerve impulses from the periphery to the central nervous system; also known as a sensory nerve.

afferent neuron A neuron that carries nerve impulses from the periphery to the central nervous system; also known as a sensory neuron.

allied health profession Any area of health care that contributes to or assists the professions of physical medicine, dentistry, optometry, pharmacy, and podiatry.

alveolar sacs (alveoli) Air sacs found in the lung.

amenorrhea Lack of a menstrual flow.

American Council on Exercise (ACE) Fitness certifying organization founded in 1985. Provides certification for Personal Trainer, Group Fitness Instructor and Lifestyle and Weight Management Consultant.

amphiarthroses (singular: amphiarthrosis) Slightly movable joints connected by fibrocartilage.

anabolic-androgenic steroids Manmade substances related to male sex hormones

491

that are used to build muscle and enhance masculine characteristics.

anabolic steroids Substances that are used to enhance metabolism and thus act to build up body tissues.

anatomical snuffbox A depression on the side/back of the hand, just beneath the thumb, that is formed by two tendons (the extensor pollicis brevis and the extensor pollicis longus).

androstenedione A steroid produced naturally in both men and women that can change or enhance the growth and development of masculine or feminine traits.

angiogenesis The formation of new blood vessels.

annulus fibrosus Rings of collagen fibers that surround the intervertebral disk.

anorexia nervosa A psychophysiological disorder characterized by an abnormal fear of becoming obese, a distorted self-image, persistent unwillingness to eat, and severe weight loss.

antagonist A muscle whose action opposes the action of another muscle.

antegrade amnesia A loss of memory for events that occur immediately after the injury.

anterior chamber The space between the cornea and the iris.

anterior compartment Contains the tibialis anterior, extensor digitorum longus, peroneus tertius, and extensor hallucis muscles.

anterior cruciate ligament (ACL) A ligament in the knee that attaches to the anterior aspect of the tibial plateau, restricting anterior movement of the tibia on the femur.

anterior shoulder dislocation Dislocation of the humerus that occurs in the anterior inferior direction.

anthropomorphic data Statistics on size, weight, body structure, gender, strength, and maturity level of particular individuals.

anvil The second of the three bones in the middle ear; also known as the incus.

aorta The heart's main artery, which carries nutrient-rich blood away from the heart to the body's cells.

aphasia Loss of speech or comprehension.

appendicular skeleton Bones of the pelvis and shoulder girdles, and limbs.

aqueous humor The watery fluid found in the anterior and posterior chambers of the eye.

arachnoid The web-like middle protective membrane covering the brain and spinal cord.

arteries Blood vessels that carry blood from the heart to all organs and cells in the body.

arterioles The smallest of the arteries.

arthritis An inflammation of an entire joint.

arthrology The study of joints.

articular cartilage Thin layer of connective tissue covering the ends of long bones.

articular facet The small articulating surface of the vertebrae.

ascending colon The portion of the colon that travels up the right side of the abdominal cavity.

assessment Orderly collection of objective and subjective data on an athlete's health status.

asthma Airway obstruction caused by an inflammatory reaction to a stimulus.

Athlete's Bill of Rights Policies and standards for fair treatment of athletes.

Athlete's Circle of Care All individuals involved in care of the athlete; may include coaches, parents, certified athletic trainer, family doctor, school nurse, massage therapist, sports psychologist, physical therapist, nutritionist, personal trainers, and chiropractor.

athletic code of ethics A tool to clarify and distinguish proper practices from those that can be detrimental and harmful.

athletic training The rendering of specialized care (prevention, recognition, evaluation, and care of injuries) to individuals involved in exercise and athletics.

athletic training student aide (ATSA) A student interested in a career in sports medicine and athletic training who begins studying the field as an assistant to the athletic director in a high school or college sports medicine program.

atlas The first cervical vertebra; articulates with the axis and occipital skull bone.

atria (singular: atrium) The upper chambers of the heart.

atrophy Weakness and wasting away of muscle tissue.

auricle The visible part of the ear; consists of the pinna; also called the outer ear.

autonomic nervous system A division of the peripheral motor nervous system; consists of a collection of nerves, ganglia, and plexuses through which visceral organs, heart, blood vessels, glands, and smooth muscles receive their innervation.

AVPU A method of determining level of consciousness (alert/verbal/painful/unresponsive).

avulsion An injury in which layers of the skin are torn off completely or only a flap of skin remains.

axial loading Compression of the spinal cord from a blow to the top of the head when the neck is slightly flexed.

axial plane A horizontal flat surface dividing the body into upper and lower parts; also known as the transverse plane.

axial skeleton The bones of the head and trunk (skull, spine, sternum, and ribs).

axis The second cervical vertebra.

ball-and-socket joints Freely movable joints in which a rounded end of one bone fits into an indented end of another bone; allows the widest range of motion.

ballistic stretching A rhythmical, bouncing action that stretches the muscles a little further each time; this technique has fallen out of favor.

baseball (mallet) finger An injury to the finger resulting from tearing of the finger tendon and damage to the cartilage.

baseline testing A test that includes a pretest prior to participation. This allows for a "baseline" of information to be available in case of a concussion. Comparison of the two can help with assessment and diagnosis.

belly The central part of a muscle.

beta cells The cells responsible for making insulin.

biceps tendon The tissue that connects the biceps muscle to the shoulder girdle.

biceps tendonitis Inflammation of the tendon that connects biceps to the shoulder girdle.

bigorexia Obsessive preoccupation with a delusional belief that one's own body is too small, too skinny, or insufficiently muscular. This is a mental disorder normally found in men.

bilateral On both sides.

bilirubin One of two pigments that determines the color of bile; reddish in color.

blind spot An area of the eye devoid of visual reception; also known as the optic disc.

body mass index (BMI) A medical standard used to define obesity.

boutonnière deformity A tear of the extensor tendon of the PIP joint, at the middle of the finger, and the DIP joint that controls the fingertip.

Bowman's capsule The double-walled capsule around the glomerulus of a nephron.

boxer's fracture A break in the fifth metacarpal leading to the little finger.

brachial plexus A group of peripheral nerves that leave the spinal cord and extend from the vertebrae into the shoulder.

brainstem The lowest part of the brain, which merges with the spinal cord.

bronchiole One of the small subdivisions of a bronchus.

bronchoconstriction Narrowing of the bronchioles.

bronchus One of the primary branches of the trachea.

bulimia An eating disorder characterized by episodic binge eating, followed by feelings of guilt, depression, and self-condemnation.

burnout Mental and physical exhaustion that causes an athlete to drop out of a sport or quit an activity that was once enjoyable.

bursitis Inflammation of the bursa (a padded cavity around a joint that decreases the friction between two surfaces) caused by excessive stress or tension.

CAB An acronym standing for circulation, airway, and breathing.

caffeine An alkaloid present in coffee, many soft drinks, and chocolate that acts as a stimulant and is believed to enhance endurance and improve reaction times.

calorie The energy needed to raise the temperature of one gram of water from 14.5° to 15.5°C.

capillaries Tiny, microscopic blood vessels that connect arteries to veins.

carbohydrate An essential nutrient that provides the primary source of fuel for the body; sugars and starches.

cardiac conduction system The heart's electrical system, consisting of specialized cells within heart muscle that carry an electrical signal, which regulates the pumping of the heart.

cardiac muscle The type of muscle that makes up the heart.

cardiac sphincter Circular muscle fibers around the cardiac end of the esophagus.

cardiac tamponade A buildup of fluid in the pericardium.

cardiorespiratory conditioning An activity that puts increased demand on the lungs, heart, and other body systems; also known as aerobic or endurance training.

cardiorespiratory system The body system that includes the functions of the heart, blood vessels, circulation, and exchange of gases between the blood and the atmosphere.

carpals The eight bones that make up the wrist.

carpal tunnel A passageway that runs from the forearm through the wrist.

carpal tunnel syndrome An inflammatory disorder caused by irritation of the tissues and nerves around the median nerve.

cauliflower ear Deformity of the ear caused by destruction of the underlying cartilage of the outer ear.

cecum A pouch at the proximal end of the large intestine.

celiac plexus A cluster of nerves located in the upper middle region of the abdomen; also known as the solar plexus.

cellular dedifferentiation A form of wound healing in which mature cells produce new cells with the same function.

cellular respiration (or oxidation) The use of oxygen to release energy from the cell.

centralis The structure of the eye that contains the cones for color vision.

central nervous system The body system that consists of the brain and the spinal cord.

central training room A multipurpose facility designed to accommodate a variety of athletic training needs.

cerebellum The part of the brain that controls muscular coordination and complex actions.

cerebral concussion Injury to the brain from a forceful impact causing temporary dysfunction.

cerebral contusion Bruising or laceration of the brain tissues from contact of the skull with underlying tissues.

cerebrospinal fluid (CSF) A clear, colorless fluid that contains small quantities of glucose and protein. Cerebrospinal fluid fills the ventricles of the brain and the central canal of the spinal cord.

cerebrum The largest and most highly evolved part of the brain.

certified athletic trainer (ATC) A professional who has attained a standard level of competence in athletic training. The ATC is involved in the prevention, recognition, and evaluation of injuries, and works closely with others in rehabilitation from injuries.

Certified Strength and Conditioning Specialist (CSCS) A specialist who designs and implements safe, effective strength and conditioning programs.

cervical nerve syndrome An injury to the neck resulting from a forced lateral flexion that causes the nerves to be stretched or impinged.

cervical vertebrae The first seven bones of the spinal column.

chest contusion Bruising over the central area of the chest as a result of a compressive blow to the chest.

chiropractor A health care specialist who provides conservative management of neuromusculoskeletal disorders and functional clinical conditions.

chondroitin A naturally occurring substance found in human and animal cartilage; often used as a supplement to treat osteoarthritis.

choroid coat The middle layer of the eye.

cilia Tiny, lash-like processes of protoplasm.

ciliary body The part of the choroid body in the eye from which the ligaments that suspend the lens extend.

Circadian dysrhythmia Circadian rhythm disorders are disruptions in a person's circadian rhythm. The circadian rhythm or "internal body clock" regulates the 24-hour cycle of biological processes.

circuit training The use of 6 to 10 strength exercises completed one right after another; each exercise is done by performing a specific number of repetitions or for a specific period of time before moving to the next exercise.

circumduction Circular movement of the limbs around an axis.

circumferential Around an extremity or body part.

clearance Permission granted by a physician, based on an athlete's physical examination, to participate in a sporting event.

closed kinematic chain A sequence of action in which the body part farthest from the trunk is fixed during movement.

coccyx The last bone of the spinal column; the tailbone.

cochlea Spiral cavity within the inner ear containing the hearing sensory receptors.

collagen fibers A protein substance found in bone and cartilage.

collecting tubule The structure in the nephron that collects urine from the distal convoluted tubule.

Colles's fracture An injury to the lower arm bone, just above the wrist.

colon The large intestine.

comminuted fracture A break in the bone in which the bone is shattered in many pieces.

common bile duct The passage that brings bile to the duodenum.

compartment syndrome A serious condition that may develop when swelling exists in one or more of the four compartments of the leg or arm.

compound fracture A complete break in the bone where the bone ends separate and break through the skin; also known as an open fracture.

concave A half-circle-shaped indentation to a surface.

concentric contraction A contraction resulting in the shortening of the muscle.

concussion A more serious form of closed head injury characterized by one or more of the following: loss of consciousness, amnesia, seizure, or a change in mental state.

conduction The loss of heat through transfer to a cooler object.

condyle The rounded prominence found at the point of articulation with another bone.

condyloid (ellipsoidal) joints Freely movable joints that allow bones to move in many different directions, but not to rotate.

cones Structures of the eye responsible for color vision.

conjunctiva The outermost layer of the eye; covers the sclera.

conjunctivitis Infection of the outermost layer of the eye; also known as pink eye.

connective tissue Cells whose secretions support and connect organs and tissues in the body.

contractibility The ability to shorten or reduce the distance between the parts.

contrecoup Mechanism of injury in which the brain rebounds off the other side of the skull after an initial impact.

contusion An injury resulting from a direct blow or force that does not interrupt the skin; typically bruising is seen at the injury site.

convection Heat loss through air currents passing by a warm surface.

convex A half-circle-shaped protrusion on a surface.

core body temperature The temperature of the human body necessary to maintain homeostasis (about 98.6°F).

cornea A circular, clear area in front of the sclerotic coat of the eye.

corneal abrasion A scratch or small cut of the cornea of the eye.

coronal plane A vertical flat surface running from side to side of the body; also known as the frontal plane.

coronary arteries The heart's own system of blood vessels.

cortex The outer portion of an organ.

coupling agent A cream or gel, applied to an area before ultrasound treatment, that provides a medium for sonic waves to penetrate the skin.

cramp A sudden, involuntary contraction of a muscle.

cranial nerves Twelve pairs of nerves that begin in the brain and transmit messages to and from various parts of the face and head to stimulate various functions, and receive sensory information.

cranium The bony skull.

creatine monohydrate An amino acid, found naturally in skeletal muscle, that is stored for quick energy and used as a supplement to increase skeletal muscle.

crepitus A grinding noise or sensation within a joint.

cryotherapy The therapeutic use of cooling agents.

cubital tunnel syndrome Irritation, compression, and entrapment of the ulnar nerve.

cystic duct The duct from the gallbladder to the common bile duct.

Daily Value (DV) The percentage per serving of each nutritional item listed on a modern-day food label, based on a daily intake of 2,000 kcal.

deep posterior compartment Contains the popliteus, flexor digitorum longus, flexor hallucis longus, and tibialis posterior muscles.

defined medical emergency A medical illness or traumatic injury that has the potential to be life threatening or progress to a life-threatening event in the absence of treatment.

delayed onset muscle soreness (DOMS) The presence of soreness in the muscles a day or two after overuse of the muscles or a traumatic injury.

depression Movement of a body part downward in a frontal plane.

deQuervain's tenosynovitis Tendonitis originating in the base of the thumb.

descending colon The portion of the colon that travels down the left side of the abdominopelvic cavity.

diabetes A disease in which the body does not produce insulin or does not produce enough insulin for the body cells to properly absorb glucose.

diabetic coma A condition in which there is too much sugar and too little insulin in the blood, resulting in body cells not receiving enough nourishment.

diagnosis Using information from assessment and evaluation findings to establish the cause and nature of an athlete's injury or disease; made only by a physician or other licensed health care provider.

diaphysis The shaft of a long bone.

diarthroses (singular: diarthrosis) Freely movable joints; also known as synovial joints.

diastolic The lowest pressure in the heart; relates to ventricular relaxation.

dietary fat A nutrient that is a source of energy, insulates body tissues, and transports fat-soluble vitamins.

dietary fiber The indigestible component of plants that are consumed by humans.

dietary supplement A product, other than tobacco, intended to enhance the diet that bears or contains one or more of the following dietary ingredients: vitamins, minerals, amino acids, herbs, or other botanicals.

disaccharide A form of carbohydrate consisting of double sugars, such as sucrose, maltose, and lactose. These forms of sugars must be reduced to monosaccharides before they can be absorbed by the body.

dislocation The displacement of any bone from its normal position.

distal convoluted tubule The tubular structure that ascends to the cortex from the loop of Henle.

doping The unnatural use of any substance or means to gain an unfair edge over the competition.

dorsiflexion Movement that flexes the foot.

duodenum The first part of the small intestine.

dura mater The outermost membrane covering the brain and spinal cord.

dynamic (isotonic) exercise An activity that causes the muscle to contract and shorten.

dynamic stability Mobility with steadiness of a joint.

ear canal The passageway for sound in the ear.

eardrum The tympanic membrane between the ear canal and the cavity of the middle ear.

eccentric contraction A contraction of muscle that results in the lengthening of the opposing muscle.

ecchymosis Bruising.

edema Swelling.

effector The organ that responds to a stimulus.

efferent arteriole The structure that carries blood from the glomerulus.

efferent nerve A neuron that carries messages from the brain and spinal cord to muscles and glands; also known as a motor nerve.

efferent neuron A nerve that carries messages from the brain and spinal cord to muscles and glands; also known as a motor neuron.

effusion Swelling within the joint cavity.

elasticity The ability to return to original form after being compressed or stretched.

electrical modality A therapeutic treatment technique that involves the use of electrical stimulation; for example, ultrasound, TENS, and e-stim.

electrical stimulation (e-stim) Use of electrical impulses to produce muscle contractions by stimulating the motor nerves.

elevation Movement of a body part upward in a frontal plane.

emergency action plan (EAP) A formal document outlining the steps to be should be taken in the event of a medical crisis or disaster.

emergency medical service (EMS) system The response system in a particular area that is called upon in the event of a medical crisis or traumatic injury. This usually consists of personnel trained in basic or advanced life support, and an ambulance or equipped emergency vehicle to transport them and the injured victim to a hospital emergency room.

energy The power used to do work or to produce heat or light.

emergency preparedness Being properly equipped and trained for any medical crisis or disaster.

energy The power used to do work or to produce heat or light.

ephedra A substance derived from a shrub-like plant; used as a stimulant to boost energy and weight loss.

epicondylitis A chronic strain of the medial or lateral epicondyle in the elbow.

epidural hematoma A collection of blood between the skull and the dura mater.

epigastric region The upper region of the abdomen.

epiglottis Elastic cartilage that prevents food from entering the trachea.

epilepsy A condition in which seizures occur regularly throughout the affected person's life.

epinephrine A medication that dilates the airway and constricts the blood vessels.

EpiPen An auto-injecting device used to administer epinephrine to those with severe allergic reactions.

epiphyseal plate The growth plate on the end of a bone.

epiphyseal plate fracture A break in the bone at the growth plate (typically at the wrist or ankle).

epiphysis The end of a long bone.

epistaxis Nosebleed.

ergogenic aid Any agent that enhances energy utilization, including energy production and efficiency.

eustachian tube The passageway from the throat to the middle ear; equalizes the pressure in the middle ear.

evaporation Loss of heat through perspiration.

eversion Movement of the sole of the foot outward.

examination Screening of the athlete by a specialist who is responsible for specific aspects of the screening, such as the medical history; height, weight, and vital signs; physical examination; and medical clearance.

excitability The ability to respond to stimuli; also known as irritability.

exercise-induced asthma Airway narrowing as a result of increased physical activity.

expiration Exhalation; the process of breathing air out.

extensibility The ability to lengthen and increase the distance between two parts.

extension Movement that increases the angle between two bones.

external fixation The use of a cast to maintain proper alignment of bones for the purpose of reduction.

external respiration Breathing; the act of inspiration and expiration.

extracellular matrix (ECM) Noncellular material that separates connective tissue cells.

extrinsic eye muscles The muscles responsible for moving the eye within the orbital socket.

extrinsic muscle Muscle that is outside a body part, organ, or bone.

false ribs The five pairs of lower ribs that connect to the seventh rib rather than to the sternum, or make no anterior connection.

family doctor The primary physician in the care of the athlete; works in cooperation with the team doctor.

fast-twitch fiber Fiber in a motor unit that produces quick and forceful contractions; these fibers are easily fatigued.

fat-soluble vitamin A vitamin that can be dissolved in fat.

fatty acid A metabolic byproduct of the breakdown of fat.

female athlete triad A collection of symptoms seen in female athletes, consisting of disordered eating, amenorrhea, and osteoporosis (bone loss).

FERPA The Federal Education Rights and Privacy Act (FERPA) was enacted to protect the privacy rights of student records. Generally, schools must have written permission from the parent or eligible student (age 18 or older) in order to release any information from a student's education record.

fibrocartilage Specialized connective tissue with thick collagen fibers.

flail chest A fracture of three or more consecutive ribs on the same side of the chest.

flexibility The ability of a joint to move freely through its full range of motion.

flexion Movement that decreases the angle between two bones.

Food Guide Pyramid An outline for making food selections based on the government's dietary guidelines.

foramen magnum Large opening at the base of the skull through which the spinal cord passes.

fovea centralis The structure of the eye that contains the cones for color vision.

force couple Two forces acting in opposite directions to rotate a part around an axis.

frontal bone The strong, anterior-most bone in the skull that constitutes the forehead.

frostbite Damage to skin tissue and blood vessels due to prolonged exposure to temperatures below 32°F.

functional activity The level of movement at which the athlete can comfortably work and participate.

gallbladder A small, pear-shaped organ that stores and concentrates bile.

gamekeeper's thumb Injury to the thumb that results in tearing or stretching of the MP joint or rupture of the ulnar collateral ligament.

ganglion A small, hard lump above a tendon or in the capsule that encloses a joint.

gauze dressing A woven, flexible, absorbent cloth applied to a wound.

generalized tonic-clonic seizure A type of seizure characterized by a sudden cry and fall, rigidity, jerking of muscles, shallow breathing, and loss of bladder and bowel control. This usually lasts for a couple of minutes.

Glasgow Coma Scale (GCS) A standard guide used to rate various states of consciousness.

glenohumeral joint The synovial ball-and-socket joint of the shoulder.

glenoid fossa A slightly concave projection of the scapula.

glenoid labrum A ring of cartilage attached to the margin of the glenoid cavity of the scapula.

gliding joint A freely movable joint that allows bones to make a sliding motion.

glomerulus Capillaries inside the Bowman's capsule.

glottis The space within the vocal cords of the larynx.

glucosamine A substance produced naturally in the body; often used as a supplement to maintain joint cartilage.

glycogen A polysaccharide formed and stored in the liver.

goal setting Identifying clearly defined, specific objectives that are measurable.

gomphoses (singular: gomphosis) An immovable joint in which a conical process fits into a socket held in place by ligaments.

gout An accumulation of uric acid crystals in the joint at the base of the large toe and other joints of the feet.

gray matter The inner part of the spinal cord.

greater sciatic notch A space in the pelvis through which the sciatic nerve travels to the legs.

greenstick fracture An incomplete break in the shaft of the bone; occurs in children.

ground fault interrupter (GFI) A small circuit breaker that will stop the flow of electricity in the event of a short or contact with water.

growth hormone An ergogenic aid; a supplement of a substance produced naturally by the pituitary gland that works to increase conversion of amino acids into protein.

hammer The first of the three bones in the middle ear; also known as the malleus.

hamstring muscles A muscle group that aids in hip movement; consists of the biceps femoris, semitendinosus, and semimembranosus muscles.

hard palate The front portion of the roof of the mouth.

head of the humerus The upper portion of the humerus bone, where the bone attaches to the scapula.

heat cramps Painful, involuntary muscle spasms caused by exposure to heat and dehydration.

heat exhaustion The mildest form of generalized heat-related illness; characterized by multiple symptoms and often by dehydration.

heat index A reference point indicating the risk associated with outdoor exercise; based on a combination of air temperature and relative humidity.

heat stress The inability of the body to maintain homeostasis because of high temperatures.

heatstroke A life-threatening form of heat illness that involves a rise in body temperature and altered mental status.

heat syncope Fainting that occurs when the body attempts to cool itself by dilating the blood vessels.

hematoma The formation caused by pooling of blood and fluid within a tissue space.

hematuria Blood in the urine.

hemopneumothorax An accumulation of blood in the pleural space.

hemoptysis Coughing up blood.

hepatic duct The structure that carries bile from the liver to the common bile duct.

hernia A protrusion of abdominal tissue through a portion of the abdominal wall.

herpes gladiatorum A type of herpes infection commonly seen in wrestlers.

Hill-Sachs lesion Indentation of the posterior humeral head (visible on x-ray), resulting from the humerus hitting the glenoid during dislocation.

hilum The indentation along the medial border of the kidney.

hinge joint A freely movable joint that allows flexion and extension.

hip flexors A muscle group that aids in flexion of the hip; consists of the iliopsoas, sartorius, pectineus, and rectus femoris muscles.

HIPAA The Health Insurance Portability and Accountability Act (HIPAA) of 1996 was enacted to protect patients' privacy and provide privacy standards to protect patients' medical records and other health information provided to health plans, doctors, hospitals, and other health care providers.

Hippocratic Oath Declaration made to Hippocrates, the "father of Western Medicine," by his students; it has become a fundamental part of the practice of medicine.

homeostasis A state of balance within the body.

H.O.P.S. An acronym for the approach to the secondary injury survey: history, observation, palpation, and special tests.

humerus The bone of the upper arm.

hydrocollator A stainless-steel container filled with hot water that is used to heat moist packs for superficial heat therapy.

hydrotherapy A form of superficial heating that uses agitated, heated water in a specially designed piece of equipment.

hyperextension Movement beyond the natural range of motion.

hypermobility The ability of a body part to move beyond the normal range of motion.

hyperthermia A condition in which the body temperature rises above normal.

hypertrophic cardiomyopathy Thickening of the cardiac muscle.

hypertrophy An increase in the size of muscle tissue.

hyperventilation Breathing faster than required for proper exchange of oxygen and carbon dioxide.

hyphema A buildup of blood in the anterior chamber of the eye.

hypoallergenic Reduced potential for causing an allergic reaction.

hypogastric region The lower region of the abdomen.

hypothalamus A part of the diencephalon; the temperature-regulating center of the brain.

hypothermia A condition in which the body temperature drops below normal.

ice massage The technique of rubbing ice over the injured area.

ileum The lower part of the small intestine, extending from the jejunum to the large intestine.

iliac crest The upper ridge of the ilium.

iliac crest contusion A painful injury caused by a direct blow to the hip, resulting in ecchymosis, tenderness, and swelling; also known as a hip pointer.

iliac fossa The broad, slightly concave inner surface of the ilium.

ilium A broad, flared bone that makes up the upper and lateral sections of the pelvis.

imagery The process of reviewing and training in the mind only, using visualization.

impetigo Bacterial skin infection causing red sores that can break open, ooze fluid, and develop a yellow-brown crust.

impingement syndrome A condition that occurs when the space between the humeral head below and the acromion above becomes narrowed.

incus The second of the three bones in the middle ear; also known as the anvil.

Infectious mononucleosis A contagious disease commonly known as "mono," mononucleosis is typically the result of the Epstein-Barr virus.

inflammation Process that occurs when tissues are subjected to chemical or physical trauma; pain, heat, redness, and swelling occur.

inner ear An extremely intricate series of structures contained deep within the bones of the skull; consists of the cochlea, the semicircular canals, and two additional organs concerned with balance.

insertion The part of the skeletal muscle that is attached to the movable part of a bone.

inspiration Inhalation; the process of breathing air in.

insulin A hormone produced in the pancreas, necessary for glucose metabolism; lowers the level of glucose in the blood by stimulating cells to absorb glucose.

insulin reaction The body's response to excess insulin; the level of sugar in the blood decreases, causing brain cells to suffer.

intercranial hematoma Pooling of blood because of damage to blood vessels within the brain.

internal fixation Surgical alignment of bones for the purpose of reduction.

internal respiration The exchange of carbon dioxide and oxygen between the cells and the lymph surrounding them; the oxidative process of energy in the cells.

interneuron A nerve that carries messages from a sensory neuron to a motor neuron; also known as an associative neuron.

intervertebral disc herniation Dislocation of a disc resulting in pressure against the spinal cord.

intrinsic eye muscles The muscles that help the iris control the amount of light entering the pupil.

intrinsic muscle Muscle that relates to a specific body part or bone.

inversion Movement of the sole of the foot inward.

iris The colored muscular layer surrounding the pupil in the eye.

ischemia Decreased blood supply to an organ or tissue resulting from pressure, swelling, trauma, or a fracture.

ischium The portion of the pelvis that attaches to the pubis in front and the ilium laterally in the back; bears the weight of the body when sitting.

isokinetic exercise A type of exercise in which a machine is used to control the speed of contraction within the range of motion.

isometric exercise An activity that causes tension in the muscle to increase but does not cause the muscle to shorten.

jaundice A buildup of bilirubin and bile in the bloodstream, which tints skin and eyes a yellowish color.

jejunum The section of small intestine between the duodenum and the ileum.

jersey finger An injury to the finger resulting in tearing of the flexor tendon in the fingertip.

jogger's nipples A condition caused by chafing between a runner's nipples and the shirt.

joint articulation The connecting point of two bones.

Kehr's sign Pain that radiates to the left shoulder and down the left arm; results from a spleen injury or rupture.

kidney contusion Bruising of the kidney.

kinesiology The multidisciplinary study of physical activity or movement; encompasses anatomy, biomechanics, physiology, psychomotor behavior, and social and cultural factors.

labyrinth A maze of winding passageways found in the ear.

laceration An injury that results from a tear in the skin; also known as a cut.

larynx The voice box.

lateral collateral ligament (LCL) A ligament that attaches to the femur and the fibula; maintains stability of the lateral aspect of the knee joint.

lateral epicondyle The bony end of the humerus that lies to the outside of the elbow joint.

lateral longitudinal arch One of the three arches of the foot; composed of the calcaneus, talus, cuboid, and the fourth and fifth metatarsals; lower and flatter than the medial longitudinal arch.

lateral meniscus Cartilage in the knee between the lateral femoral condyle and the lateral tibial plateau.

lens A crystal structure in the eye that refracts light rays.

leukocytes White blood cells.

ligamentous laxity Degree of looseness in the ligaments of a joint.

local reaction Pain, swelling, redness, itching, and formation of a weal at the site of an insect bite or sting.

loop of Henle The proximal convoluted tubule that descends into the medulla.

lumbar vertebrae The five vertebrae located in the lower lumbar region of the back.

lymphocyte A group of white blood cells of crucial importance to the body's immune system.

malleoli Large, bony prominences located on either side of the ankle.

malleus The first of the three bones in the middle ear; also known as the hammer.

mandible The bone of the lower jaw.

manorexia Eating disorders in men.

manual resistance training A form of dynamic exercise accomplished utilizing a training partner.

mastoid sinus Air-filled spaces within the mastoid process of the temporal bone behind the ears.

maxilla The bone of the upper jaw.

meatus An opening; in this instance, the opening to the ear canal.

mechanical modality A therapeutic treatment technique that involves manipulation of the muscles in the body—for example, massage, vibration, and mobilization.

mechanism of force All energies involved at the time of an impact, including the direction, intensity, duration, activity, and position of the body or body part.

medial collateral ligament (MCL) A flat longitudinal band found on the medial side of the knee joint.

medial epicondyle The bony end of the humerus that forms with the elbow joint.

medial longitudinal arch The highest of the three arches of the foot; composed of the calcaneus, talus, navicular, cuneiforms, and the first three metatarsals.

medial meniscus Cartilage in the knee between the femoral condyle and the medial tibial plateau.

medial tibial stress (shin splints) Pain that occurs below the knee, on either the front outside portion or the inside of the leg.

median nerve Nerve within the brachial plexus that crosses the anterior elbow, passes between the heads of the pronator teres, and runs distal to the joint.

mediastinum The intrapleural space separating the sternum in front and the vertebral column behind.

medical kit A portable storage container for medical supplies such as bandages, gauze, antiseptics, ice packs, gloves, and so on. There are many different varieties: softsided bags, fanny packs, and hard-shell boxes.

medicinal herbs Plant matter, used in the form of powders, extracts, teas, or tablets, believed to have therapeutic benefits.

medulla The inner portion of an organ.

medullary canal The center of the shaft of the long bone.

membrane excitability The ability of nerves to carry impulses by creating electrical charges.

meninges Protective membranes covering the brain and spinal cord.

metacarpals The bones that form the structure of the hand.

middle ear A small cavity between the eardrum and the inner ear.

mineral An inorganic substance that participates in many biochemical and physiological processes required for the growth, maintenance, repair, and health of tissues and bones.

mixed nerve A nerve composed of both afferent and efferent fibers.

modalities Treatment of injuries, including heating, cooling, and mechanical/electrical methods.

monocytes Large, circulating white blood cells.

mononuclear phagocytes White blood cells that engulf and destroy waste material and foreign bodies in the bloodstream.

monosaccharide The simplest form of carbohydrate, consisting of sugars that cannot be further reduced by the body, such as glucose, fructose, and galactose.

monounsaturated fatty acid Fats that do not contain high levels of hydrogen in combination with carbon atoms; these types of fats are found mainly in vegetable, olive, and peanut oils.

motivation An internal state or condition (need or desire) that serves to activate or energize behavior and give it direction.

motor nerve A nerve that carries messages from the brain and spinal cord to muscles and glands; also known as an efferent nerve.

motor unit A motor nerve plus all the muscle fibers it stimulates.

MRSA Methicillin-resistant staphylococcus aureus (MRSA) is a bacterium that causes infections in different parts of the body. It is tougher to treat than most strains of staph infection because of its resistance to commonly used antibiotics.

muscle fatigue The result of accumulation of lactic acid in the muscle.

muscle tone The state of partial contraction in which muscles are maintained.

myelin sheath The layers of cell membrane that wrap around nerve fibers; provides electrical insulation and increases the velocity of impulse transmission.

myocardial contusion Bruising of the heart muscle.

myositis ossificans A calcification that forms within the muscle; results from an improperly managed contusion.

nasal septum The partition between the two nasal cavities.

National Academy of Sports Medicine (NASM) Provides education and credentials for fitness, sports performance, and sports medicine professionals.

National Strength and Conditioning Association Certified Personal Trainer (NSCA-CPT) A specialist who designs and implements safe, effective strength and conditioning programs with individual clients.

nephron The functional unit of the kidney.

neuroma A ball-like growth of nerve fibers that creates a nerve scar.

neuromuscular junction The point between the motor nerve axon and the muscle cell membrane.

neuropraxia The cessation of function of a nerve without degenerative changes.

neutrophils White blood cells that engulf and kill bacteria.

nonemergency Any medical illness or injury that does not pose a serious threat to life or limb.

nucleus pulposus A gelatin-like substance in the center of the vertebral disc.

nutrition The process by which a living organism assimilates food and uses it for growth and replacement of tissues; the science or study that deals with food and nourishment.

obturator foramina The large openings in the ischium through which blood vessels and nerves pass to the legs.

occipital bone The most posterior bone of the skull.

occlusive dressing A petroleum-based dressing with a thin plastic film, designed to keep air and moisture from entering or escaping a wound.

Occupational Safety and Health Administration (OSHA) A federal agency that develops regulations for employees whose jobs may put them at risk of bloodborne pathogens.

office-based pre-participation physical examination A complete health screening done by the athlete's family physician.

olecranon bursitis Inflammation of the bursa located over the olecranon process of the elbow.

olfactory nerves Nerves that supply the nasal mucosa and provides a sense of smell.

open kinematic chain A sequence of action in which the body part farthest from the trunk is free during movement.

opposition Movement of the thumb to touch each finger.

optic disc An area of the eye devoid of visual reception; also known as the blind spot.

orbit A deep, bony socket that houses the eye.

origin The part of the skeletal muscle that is attached to the fixed part of a bone.

ossicle Any small bone; here, refers to the any of the three small bones of the ear.

ossification The process of bone formation.

osteoarthritis A degenerative joint disease.

osteoblast Type of bone cell involved in the formation of bony tissue.

osteoclast Type of bone cell involved in the resorption of bony tissue.

osteocyte A bone cell.

osteoporosis Bone loss.

outer ear The visible part of the ear; consists of the pinna; also called the auricle.

overload Progressive overwork of muscles, at a controlled, increased rate, to achieve consistent gains in strength.

oxidation The use of oxygen to release energy from the cell.

palpation Touching during examination to determine extent of injury.

pancreas An organ, located near the stomach, that produces insulin.

paradoxical The opposite of what is expected.

parasympathetic nervous system Division of the autonomic nervous system that inhibits or opposes the effects of the sympathetic system.

paresthesia Sensation of tingling, crawling, or burning of the skin.

parietal bone The largest of the bones of the skull.

pars interarticularis The area between the superior and inferior articulations of the vertebrae; common site of fractures due to spondylolysis.

passive motion Movement through a range of motion performed by the examiner while the athlete relaxes all muscles.

patella The kneecap.

patellar tendon The tendon that encompasses the patella and extends distally across the front of the knee.

patellofemoral joint The point where the kneecap and femur are connected in the trochlear groove.

pelvic cavity The area of the body containing the urinary bladder, reproductive organs, rectum, and the remainder of the large intestine.

peripheral nervous system A division of the nervous system, made up of 12 pairs of cranial nerves and 31 pairs of spinal nerves.

periosteum The fibrous tissue that covers the bone.

peroneal compartment Contains the peroneus longus and peroneus brevis muscles.

pes ansurine The area where the sartorius, gracillus, and semitendinosus muscles attach to the anteriomedial tibia.

phalanges The finger bones.

pharynx The throat.

physical therapist (PT) A health care specialist who is responsible for performing treatments that require special training in therapeutic exercises, hydrotherapy, and electrotherapy; and for performing procedures dealing with individual muscles and muscular movement.

physical therapy assistant (PTA) A health care specialist who works with physical therapists to assist in developing treatment plans for the rehabilitation of injury.

physician assistant (PA) A midlevel health care practitioner who works under the supervision of physicians to provide diagnostic and therapeutic care.

pia mater The innermost membrane covering the spinal cord and brain.

pinna Part of the outer ear.

pivot joint A freely movable joint in which a bone moves around a central axis, creating rotational movement.

plantar fascia Wide, nonelastic, ligamentous tissue that extends from the anterior portion of the calcaneus to the heads of the metatarsals.

plantar flexion Movement that extends the foot.

plantar warts Small, hard growths on the bottom of the foot.

plasma The yellowish, liquid part of blood.

platelets Tiny cell fragments in blood that aid in clotting.

pleura Serous membrane protecting the lungs and lining the internal surface of the thoracic cavity.

pleural space The space between the lung and the chest wall.

pleurisy Inflammation of the lining of the lungs.

plexus A network of spinal nerves.

pneumothorax Condition in which air enters the pleural space between the chest wall and lung.

polysaccharide A form of complex carbohydrate containing combinations of monosaccharides, such as starch, cellulose, and glycogen.

polyunsaturated fatty acid Fats that contain only limited amounts of hydrogen attached to carbon atoms; found mainly in some forms of vegetable oils and seafood.

postconcussion syndrome A condition that may develop following a concussion; exhibited by persistent headache, dizziness, fatigue, irritability, and impaired memory or lack of concentration.

posterior chamber The space between the iris and the lens.

posterior cruciate ligament (PCL) A ligament in the knee that attaches to the posterior aspect of the tibial plateau, restricting posterior movement of the tibia on the femur.

prehabilitation Trying to prevent injuries before they occur, through a preventative management program.

preparticipation physical examination (PPE) A comprehensive assessment of an athlete's overall health and ability to perform a sport at the highest level; emphasizes the areas of greatest concern in sports participation and identifies problem areas in the athlete's history.

preseason conditioning A program, beginning six to eight weeks prior to sports participation, that allows the body to gradually adapt to the demands to be placed on it.

PRICE Acronym for treatment regimen of protection, rest, ice, compression, and elevation.

primary fibrositis An inflammation of the fibrous connective tissue in a joint.

primary injury survey Assessment of life-threatening emergencies and management of airway, breathing, and circulation. EMS should be activated when threats to life are suspected.

prime mover Muscle that provides movement in a single direction.

progressive resistance exercise A type of training in which muscles are worked until they reach their capacity. Once the athlete is able to maintain that capacity, the workload on the muscle is increased to further build strength and endurance.

pronation Movement of the radius and ulna posterior or inferior.

pronator teres syndrome Entrapment or compression of the median nerve.

prophylactic Any agent or method that prevents or guards against injury.

proprioceptive neuromuscular facilitation (PNF) A combined relaxing and contracting of the muscles; an initial isometric contraction against maximum resistance is held at the end of the range of motion, followed by relaxation and passive stretching.

protein An essential nutrient that contains nitrogen and helps the body grow, build, and repair tissue.

protraction Movement of a body part forward in a transverse plane.

proximal convoluted tubule The twisted tubular branch off the Bowman's capsule.

pubis The bone in the pelvis to the front and below the bladder.

pulmonary artery The artery that connects the heart to the lungs.

pulse The rhythmical beating of the heart.

pulse pressure The difference between the diastolic and systolic pressures in the heart.

puncture wound An injury caused by a sharp object that penetrates the skin.

pupil The opening in the iris of the eye that permits passage of light.

pupillary dilation Widening of the pupils due to increased intracranial pressure compressing the third cranial nerve.

pyloric sphincter A valve that regulates the movement of food from the stomach to the duodenum.

quadricep A large group of four muscles in the front of the thigh.

quadriparesis Partial paralysis in all four extremities.

quadriplegia Paralysis in all four extremities.

radial nerve Nerve within the brachial plexus that passes anteriorly to the lateral epicondyle and lies in a tunnel of several muscles and tendons.

radial tunnel syndrome Entrapment of the radial nerve.

radiation The loss of heat through the transfer of infrared rays into the cooler environment.

radius The bone on the thumb side of the forearm.

rales A crackling sound heard when breathing.

receptor A sensory nerve that receives a stimulus and transmits it to the central nervous system.

rectum The portion of the colon that opens into the anus.

reduction The process of putting broken bones back into proper alignment.

referred pain Pain that is felt in one area (such as the shoulder), but that actually originates elsewhere in the body.

reflex Any involuntary action.

regeneration The act of wound healing (tissue rebuilding).

rehabilitation The process of restoring function through programmed exercise, to enable a return to competition.

remodeling The process of absorbing and replacing bone in the skeletal system.

renal fascia The tough, fibrous tissue covering the kidney.

renal pelvis The funnel-shaped structure at the beginning of the ureter.

respiration The physical and chemical process by which the body supplies the cells and tissues with oxygen and rids them of carbon dioxide.

retina The innermost layer of the eye, containing the rods and cones.

retraction Movement of a body part backward in a transverse plane.

retrograde amnesia A loss of memory for events that occurred before the injury.

retropatellar surface The back side of the patella that is covered with a thick layer of articular cartilage.

retroperitoneal Located behind the peritoneum.

reversibility Process of muscle atrophy due to disuse, immobilization, or starvation; leads to decreased strength and muscle mass.

rheumatic fever A bacterial infection that can be carried in the blood to the joints.

rheumatoid arthritis A connective tissue disorder resulting in severe inflammation of small joints.

rib contusion Bruising of the intercostal muscles by a direct blow to the ribs.

rib fracture A break in the bony structure of the thorax.

RICE Acronym for treatment regimen of rest, ice, compression, and elevation.

rods Cells in the retina that are sensitive to dim light.

rotation Movement of a bone on an axis, toward or away from the body.

rotator cuff A collective set of four deep muscles of the glenohumeral joint.

sacroiliac joint The area between the sacrum and the ilium.

sacrum The portion of the vertebral column between the lumbar vertebrae and the coccyx; composed of five fused vertebrae.

saddle joint A freely movable joint between two bones with complementary shapes; allows a wide range of motion.

sagittal plane A vertical flat surface running from front to back of the body.

sarcolemma The muscle cell membrane.

sarcoplasm The material within the muscle cell, excluding the nucleus.

saturated fatty acid Fats that contain the maximum number of hydrogen atoms attached to carbon atoms; found mainly in animal sources.

scaphoidscaphoid fracture A break in the scaphoid bone in the thumb.

scapulothoracic joint The area that provides movement of the scapula over the back side of the ribcage.

scar tissue Fibrous connective tissue that binds damaged tissue.

sciatic nerve The largest nerve in the body; originates in the sacral plexus and runs through the pelvis and down the leg.

sclera The tough, white, external coating of the eye.

secondary impact syndrome (SIS) Rapid swelling and herniation of the brain after a second head injury that occurs before the first injury has resolved.

secondary injury survey A thorough, methodical evaluation of an athlete's overall health to reveal additional injuries beyond the initial injury.

seizure A sudden attack or convulsion due to involuntary electrical activity in the brain.

semicircular canal Structures in the inner ear involved with equilibrium.

sensory nerve A nerve that carries nerve impulses from the periphery to the central nervous system; also known as an afferent nerve.

septum The wall separating the left and right sides of the heart.

sesamoid A small bone formed in a tendon where it passes over a joint.

sharps equipment Instruments such as scalpels, blades, razors, and uncapped needles that can penetrate the skin and cause exposure to bloodborne pathogens.

shin splints Pain that occurs below the knee either on the front outside portion of the leg or on the inside of the leg; also known as medial tibial stress syndrome.

shock A potentially fatal physiological reaction usually characterized by significant drop in blood pressure, reduced blood circulation, and inadequate blood flow to the tissues; may occur in response to several conditions, including illness, injury, hemorrhage, and dehydration.

side stitches Pain that occurs just under the ribcage during vigorous exercise.

sigmoid colon The S-shaped portion of the colon.

simple fracture A break in the bone that may be complete or incomplete, but does not break through the skin; also known as a closed fracture.

simple partial seizure A type of seizure in which a jerking motion begins in one part of the body; the victim remains awake and aware.

simulation The process of making physical training circumstances as close as possible to real competition.

sinuses Recessed cavities of hollow space, filled with air, around the nasal cavity.

skeletal muscle The type of muscle, attached to a bone or bones of the skeleton, that aids in body movements; also known as voluntary or striated muscle.

slow-twitch fiber Fiber in a motor unit that requires a long period of time to generate force; these fibers are resistant to fatigue.

smooth muscle The type of muscle that is not attached to bone and is nonstriated and involuntary; also known as visceral.

soft palate The back portion of the roof of the mouth.

specificity The ability of particular muscle groups to respond to targeted training, so that increased strength is gained in that muscle group only.

sphincter muscle A type of circular muscle.

spinal cord Part of the central nervous system within the spinal column; begins at the foramen magnum of the occipital bone and continues to the second lumbar vertebra.

spinal nerves Thirty-one pairs of nerves originating in the spinal cord.

spirometer A device that measures the volume and flow of air during inspiration and expiration.

spleen Large lymphatic organ that filters blood and helps activate the immune system.

spondylolisthesis The slippage of one vertebra on the vertebra directly below it.

spondylolysis The breakdown of the structure of the vertebrae.

spongy bone Bone permeated by large, marrow-filled spaces.

spontaneous pneumothorax The rupture of a weakened area of the lung, which allows air to escape into the pleural space.

sports medicine The study and application of scientific and medical knowledge to aspects of exercise and injury prevention.

sports nutritionist A health care specialist who designs special diets with the goal of enhancing athletic performance.

sports psychologist A specialist who works with athletes to recover from serious injury through emotional support. They also assist in goal setting and motivation.

sports psychology The study of sport and exercise and the mental (psychological) factors influencing performance.

sport-specific activity Particular types of movement and action that are needed in or related to a particular sport.

sprain An injury resulting from a fall, sudden twist, or blow to the body that forces a joint out of its normal position.

spray adherent An aerosolized liquid that creates a sticky surface to help underwrap and tape stay in place.

standard precautions Infection-control guidelines designed to protect workers from exposure to disease spread by contact with blood or other bodily fluids.

stapes The third of the three bones found in the middle ear; also known as the stirrup.

static stretching A gradual, slow stretching of the muscle through the entire range of motion, then holding the position for 20 to 30 seconds.

station-based pre-participation examination Screening of the athlete by several different specialists who are responsible for specific aspects of the exam, such as the medical history; height, weight, and vital signs; physical examination; and medical clearance.

stenosis Narrowing of a duct or canal.

sternoclavicular joint The area where the clavicle and the sternum connect; also called the SC joint.

stimulus Any action that excites or produces a temporary reaction in the whole organism or in any of its parts.

stinger (burner) An injury caused by stretching or compressing the brachial plexus.

stirrup The third of the three bones found in the middle ear; also known as the stapes.

stomach A major organ of digestion located in the upper left quadrant of the abdominal cavity.

strain A muscle injury caused by the twisting or pulling of a muscle or tendon.

stress Some factor that causes awareness, anxiety, focus, or fear. Stress can be either good or bad; both have positive and negative effects.

stress fracture A small, incomplete break in the bone that results from overuse, weakness, or biomechanical problems.

sty Infection of a gland along the eyelid.

stretching Moving the joints beyond the normal range of motion.

subcutaneous spinous process Area just under the skin over each protrusion of the vertebrae.

subdural hematoma A collection of blood between the surface of the brain and the dura mater.

subluxation (1) An incomplete or partial dislocation of a joint. (2) The abnormal movement of one of the bones that constitute a joint.

subtalar joint A joint in the ankle found between the talus and calcaneus.

sudden cardiac death (SCD) Occurs when an athlete suddenly collapses and dies. This is the result of a previously undiagnosed cardiopulmonary disease.

sucking chest wound An open wound in the chest that allows air to enter and become trapped in the pleural space.

sudden death syndrome The rapid collapse and death of an otherwise healthy person; usually the result of an unknown congenital disorder.

sunburn Injury to the skin from the sun's rays (ultraviolet light).

Sun protective factor (SPF) The value assigned to a spray or ointment used to prevent sunburn. SPF 30 would give a 97% protection factor against harmful, ultraviolet B radiation.

superficial posterior compartment Contains the gastrocnemius, soleus, and plantaris muscles.

supination Movement of the radius and ulna anterior or superior.

suspensory ligaments The structures that hold the lens of the eye in place.

sutures Immovable joints, composed of dense, fibrous connective tissue; found only in the skull, where the cranial bones meet.

swimmer's ear An infection of the skin covering the outer ear canal.

sympathetic nervous system A division of the autonomic nervous system that prepares the body for action.

symphysis The center of the pubis where the two sides of the pubis are fused together.

synapse The space between adjacent neurons through which an impulse is transmitted.

synarthroses (singular: synarthrosis) Immovable joints that lack a synovial cavity and are held together by fibrous connective tissue.

syndesmoses Slightly movable joints where bones are connected by ligaments.

syndrome Pain that occurs below the knee either on the front outside portion of the leg or on the inside of the leg; also known as shin splints.

synergistically Acting together; a group of muscles acts together to enhance the movement of a joint or limb.

synergists Muscles that help steady a joint.

synovial fluid Lubricating substance produced by the synovial membrane; found in joints.

synovial joint Freely movable joint; also known as a diarthrosis.

synovial membrane Layer of tissue that lines joint cavities and produces synovial fluid.

systemic reaction A generalized reaction to an insect sting or bite, characterized by flushing of the skin and an itchy rash; more serious symptoms, such as wheezing, nausea, vomiting, palpations, and faintness can also occur.

systolic The highest pressure in the heart; correlates to ventricular contraction.

talocrural joint A joint in the ankle found between the tibia, fibula, and talus.

target heart rate The percentage of the maximum heart rate that is safe to reach during exercise.

team doctor A physician who specializes in sports medicine and helps the athlete maximize function and minimize time away from sports, work, or school; works in cooperation with the family doctor.

temporal bone The cranial bone that forms the base of the skull, behind and at the sides of the face.

temporomandibular joint (TMJ) The joint that connects the mandible to the skull.

tendonitis Inflammation of the tendons caused by overuse or repetitive motion.

tennis elbow A chronic strain of the lateral epicondyle in the elbow; another name for epicondylitis.

tension pneumothorax Condition in which air entrapped in the pleural space puts pressure on the lung and heart.

tidal volume The amount of air that moves in and out of the lungs with each breath.

thermal modality A therapeutic treatment technique that involves the use of heat or cold—for example, use of the hydrocollator or ice packs.

thermoregulation The process by which body temperature is maintained.

thoracic cavity The upper central area of the body that is subdivided into two cavities: the left pleural cavity (containing the left lung) and the right pleural cavity (containing the right lung).

thoracic vertebrae The 12 segments of the vertebral column that articulate with ribs to form part of the thoracic cage.

tibial plateau The top, flat portion of the tibia.

tibiofemoral joint The point where the tibia meets with the femur.

tinea cruris A fungal infection found in the groin area; often referred to as jock itch.

tinea pedis A fungal infection that thrives in warmth and dampness; often referred to as athlete's foot or ringworm.

Title IX Federal legislation that prohibits discrimination on the basis of sex as to participation in athletics in schools receiving federal funds.

trachea The windpipe.

transcutaneous electrical nerve stimulation (TENS) Use of electrical impulses to reduce pain by stimulating the sensory and pain-signaling nerves.

transdifferentiation A form of wound healing in which mature cells dedifferentiate and produce new cells that are then able to mature into cell types with a completely different function from the originating cells.

trans fatty acid A type of fat that is produced through the process of hydrogenation; found mainly in processed foods such as margarine and snack foods.

transverse arch One of the three arches of the foot; composed of the cuneiforms, the cuboid, and the fifth metatarsal bones.

transverse colon The portion of the colon that veers left across the abdomen to the spleen.

true ribs The first seven pairs of ribs, which connect directly to the sternum.

tympanic membrane The membrane that separates the external ear from the middle ear; also called the eardrum.

tympanic rupture Perforation of the tympanic membrane between the middle ear and the ear canal.

ulna The bone of the inner forearm.

ulnar nerve Nerve within the brachial plexus that passes through the cubital tunnel in the posterior aspect of the medial epicondyle.

ultrasound (US) Therapeutic deep heating that uses high-frequency sound waves; also called ultrasonic diathermy.

umbilical area Area located around the navel.

underwrap A lightweight foam material used as a base for application of tape; helps to reduce irritation caused by tape.

unilateral On one side only.

ureters The long, narrow tubes that convey urine from the kidney to the bladder.

urethra The tube that takes urine from the bladder to the outside of the body.

urinary bladder A muscular, membrane-lined sac that holds urine.

urinary meatus The outside opening of the urethra.

valgus Outward bending or twisting force.

varus Inward bending or twisting force.

veins Blood vessels that carry blood back to the heart.

ventricles The lower chambers of the heart.

venules The smallest of the veins.

vermiform appendix A finger-like projection, of unknown function, that protrudes into the abdominal cavity to the lower left of the cecum.

vestibule A small cavity at the beginning of a canal.

vestibulocochlear nerve The eighth cranial nerve.

villi Hairlike projections within the small intestine.

vitamin A complex organic substance that the body needs in small amounts.

vitreous humor Transparent, gelatin-like substance that fills the greater part of the eyeball.

Volkmann's contracture Condition in which the muscles in the palm side of the forearm shorten, causing the fingers to form a fist and the wrist to bend.

water-soluble vitamin A vitamin that can be dissolved in water.

whirlpool A stainless steel or fiberglass tub with an attached turbine.

white matter The outer part of the spinal cord.

wind chill The rate of heat loss from the human body resulting from the combined effect of cold temperature and wind.

REFERENCES

American Academy of Ophthalmology. (2003). *Hindsight doesn't work if you lose your sight*. San Francisco, CA: Author.

American Academy of Orthopaedic Surgeons. (2000, March). *The shoulder*. Rosemont, IL: Author.

American Academy of Orthopaedic Surgeons. (1999, June). *Report of consensus meeting*. Rosemont, IL: Author.

American Dental Association, Council on Dental Materials. (1984). Mouth protectors and sports team dentists. *Journal of the American Dental Association, 109*, 84–87.

Canadian Academy of Sports Medicine Concussion Committee. (2000). Guidelines for assessment and management of sport-related concussion. *Clinical Journal of Sports Medicine, 10*(3), 209–211.

Cantu, R. C. (1986). Guidelines for return to contact sports after a cerebral concussion. *Physician Sportsmedicine, 14*(10), 75–83.

Cantu, R. C. (2001). Posttraumatic retrograde and anterograde amnesia: Pathophysiology and implications in grading and safe return to play. *Journal of Athletic Training, 36*(3), 244–248.

Concussion in Sport Group. (2001). Guidelines for treatment of concussion: For Salt Lake and beyond; Summary and agreement statement of the First International Conference on Concussion in *Sport*, November 2 and 3, 2001, Vienna, Austria.

European Federation of Sport Psychology. (1998). *Gender and sports participation*.

Experts urge adults to take precautions, prevent burnout of young athletes. (2000, November). *Georgia Tech Sports Medicine & Performance Newsletter*.

Fahey, T. D. (1998, March 7). *Adaptation to exercise: Progressive resistance exercise*. Retrieved August 2003 from http://sportsci.org (Internet Society for Sports Medicine).

Flanders, R. A., & Bhat, M. (1995, April). The incidence of orofacial injuries in sports: A pilot study in Illinois. *JADA, 126*, 491–496.

Frey, C. C. (1998). *The 10 points of proper shoe fit*. Rosemont, IL: American Academy of Orthopaedic Surgeons.

Herring, S. A., & Nilson, K. L. (1987). Introduction to overuse injuries. *Clinical Sports Medicine, 6*(2), 225–232.

Johnston, K. M., McCrory, P., & Mohtadi, N. G. (2001). Evidence-based review of sport-related concussion: Clinical science. *Clinical Journal of Sports Medicine, 11*(3), 150–159.

Kleinginna, P. R., & Kleinginna, A. M. (1981). A categorized list of emotion definitions with suggestions for a consensual definition. *Motivation and Emotion, 5*, 345–379.

Krowchuk, D. P. (1997, January). The preparticipation athletic examination *Pediatric Annals, 26*(1), 37–49.

Lanze, G (2003). Jaw and dental injuries. *ESPN Special Section: Training Room*. http://espn.go.com/trainingroom/s/2000/0105/271531.html.

Louzon, M. (1998, November 9). *Advance for physical therapists and physical therapy assistants*. King of Prussia, PA: Advance Newsmagazines.

Lyznicki, J. M., Nielson, N H., & Schneider, J. F. (2000, August 15). Cardiovascular screening of student athletes. *American Family Physician, 62*, 765–781.

Matheson, G. O. (1998). Participation screening of athletes. *Journal of the American Medical Association, 279*(22), 1829–1830.

McCrory, P. (2001). Do mouth guards prevent concussion? *British Journal of Sports Medicine, 35*(2), 81–82.

McIntosh, A. S., & McCrory, P. (2000). Impact energy attenuation performance of football headgear. *British Journal of Sports Medicine, 34*(5), 337–341.

McKeag, D. B., & Sallis, R. E. (2000). Factors at play in the athletic pre-participation examination. *American Family Physician, 61,* 2683–2690, 2696–2698.

Minnesota State High School League, Sports Medicine Advisory Committee. (2003). *Qualifying physical examination form.*

National Athletic Trainers' Association. (2000). Position statement: Fluid replacement for athletes. *Journal of Athletic Training, 35*(2), 212–224.

National Athletic Trainers' Association. (2009). *Code of ethics.* Dallas, TX: Author.

National Athletic Trainers' Association. (2000). *Primary job markets for athletic trainers.* Dallas, TX: Author.

National Federation of State High School Associations. (2003). *Salary survey.* Indianapolis, IN: Author.

Neer, C. (1972). Anterior acromioplasty for chronic impingement syndrome in the shoulder. *Journal of Bone and Joint Surgery, 54A,* 41–50.

NOAA, Office of Climate, Water, and Weather Services. (2001, November 11). *Wind chill chart.* Silver Spring, MD: National Oceanic and Atmospheric Administration.

Ohio State Athletic Trainers Association. (2003). *Mission statement.* Ohio, OH: Author.

Omey, M. L., & Micheli, L. J. (1999, July 31). Foot and ankle problems in the young athlete. *Medical Science Sports Exercise,* S470–486.

Park, et al. (1993, August). *Methods of improved mouth guards.* Paper presented at the First International Symposium on Biomaterials, Taejon, Korea.

Prevent Blindness America. Retrieved from http://www.preventblindness.org. Last accessed August 2003.

Report of the Quality Standards Subcommittee. (1997). Practice parameter: The management of concussion in sports (summary statement). *Neurology, 48,* 581–585.

Sherman, I., & Sherman, V. (1979). *Biology: A human approach.* New York: New Oxford University Press.

Steindler, A. (1955). *Kinesiology of the human body: Under normal and pathological conditions.* Springfield, MA: Charles V. Thomas.

Sports Medicine Committee. (1990; revised 1991, May). Report: *Guidelines for the management of concussion in sports.* Denver, CO: Colorado Medical Society.

Taber's cyclopedic medical dictionary (20th ed.). (2005). Philadelphia, PA: F.A. Davis.

Throop, R. K., & Castellucci, M. B. (1999). *Reaching your potential: Personal and professional development* (2d ed.). Clifton Park, NY: Delmar Learning.

United States Department of Labor, Bureau of Labor Statistics. (2000). Retrieved June 17, 2003, from http://www.usdol.gov.

RESOURCES

American Academy of Dermatology. (2002). Common skin problems from sports can sideline athletes if left untreated. AAD, Schaumburg, IL.

American Academy of Orthopaedic Surgeons, Des Plaines, IL.

American Academy of Pediatrics, Committee on Sports Medicine and Fitness. (2001). Medical conditions affecting sports participation. *Pediatrics, 107*(5), 1205–1209.

American Academy of Pediatrics, Committee on Sports Medicine and Fitness. (1991). *Head and neck injuries; sports medicine: Health care for young athletes* (2d ed.). Elk Grove Village, IL.

American Heart Association, Dallas, TX.

American Heart Association. (2000). *Guidelines 2000 for cardiopulmonary resuscitation and emergency cardiovascular care.* Chicago, IL.

American Orthopaedic Foot and Ankle Society, 2517 Eastlake Avenue E., Seattle, WA 98102.

American Red Cross, Washington, DC.

Anderson, C. (1993). Neck injuries: Backboard, bench, or return to play? *The Physician and Sportsmedicine, 21*(8), 23–34.

Austin, K., Gwynn-Brett, K., & Marshall, S. (1999). *Illustrated guide to taping techniques.* St. Louis, MO: Mosby.

Bailes, J. E., Hadley, M. N., & Quigley, M. R. (et al.). (1991). Management of athletic injuries of the cervical spine and spinal cord. *Neurosurgery 29*(4), 491–497.

Barone, J. J., & Roberts, H. R. (1996). Caffeine consumption. *Food Chemistry and Toxicology, 34,* 119–129.

Baxter, R. (1998). *Pocket guide to musculoskeletal assessment.* Philadelphia, PA: W. B. Saunders.

Beck, M. F. (1994). *Milady's theory and practice of therapeutic massage* (2d ed.). Chapter 1. Delmar Learning, Clifton Park, NY.

Beck, K. C. (1999). Control of airway function during and after exercise in asthmatics. *Medical Science and Sports Exercise, 31*(supp. 1), S4–S11.

Beebe, R., & Funk, D. (2001). *Fundamentals of emergency care.* Clifton Park, NY: Delmar Learning.

Behrens, S. L., & Michlovitz, S. (1996). *Physical agents: Theory and practice.* Philadelphia, PA: F. A. Davis.

Below, P. R., et al. (1995). *Medicine and Science in Sports and Exercise, 27,* 200–210.

Berne, R., & Levy, M. (2001). *Cardiovascular physiology* (8th ed.). St. Louis, MO: Mosby.

Booher & Thibodeau. (1994). *Athletic injury assessment* (3d ed.). St. Louis, MO: Mosby.

Boston College Eating Awareness Team. Boston College, Boston, MA.

Butler, S. J., & Freeman, J. E. (1996). *Conquering carpal tunnel syndrome and other repetitive strain injuries.* New Harbinger Publications.

Centers for Disease Control and Prevention, 1600 Clifton Road, Atlanta, GA 30333.

Cohen, M. S., & Hasting, H. I. Acute elbow dislocation: Evaluation and management. *Journal of the American Academy of Orthopaedic Surgeons, 6*(1), 15–23.

Cooper, K. (1985). *The aerobics program for total well-being: Exercise, diet, emotional balance.* New York: Bantam/Doubleday Dell.

Coyle, E. E., Coggan, A. R., Hemmert, M. K., & Ivy, J. L. (1986). Muscle glycogen utilization during prolonged strenuous exercise when fed carbohydrates. *Journal of Applied Physiology, 61,* 165–172.

Cummins, R. O. (1994). *Textbook of advanced cardiac life support*. Dallas, TX: American Heart Association.

Disabella, V. (1998). Exercise for asthma patients: Little risk, big rewards. *The Physician and Sportmedicine 26*(6), 75–85.

Donatelli, R. A. (1997). *Physical therapy of the shoulder* (3d ed.). London: Churchill Livingstone.

Engle, A. (2003). *Myology* (3d ed.). New York: McGraw-Hill.

Faigenbaum, A. D., & Michell, L. J. (2000, November). *Preseason conditioning for the young athlete*. American College of Sports Medicine.

Fixelle, S. (n.d.). *The female athlete*. Cardio-vascular and Wellness Nutritionists, A Practice Group of the American Dietetic Association.

Fourré, M. (1991). On-site management of cervical spine injuries. *The Physician and Sportsmedicine, 19*(4), 53–56.

Fulkerson, J. (1996). *Disorders of the patellofemoral joint* (3d ed.). Baltimore, MD: Lippincott, Williams & Wilkins.

Gurley, B. J., Gardiner, S. F., & Hubbard, M. A. (2000). Content versus label claims in ephedra-containing dietary supplements. *American Journal Health System Pharmacy*, 57963–57969.

Goldberger, M. (2001, November 15). JMU School of Kinesiology and Recreational Studies.

Grelsamer & McConnell. (1998). *The patella*. New York: Aspen.

Haller, C. A. & Benowitz, N. L. (2000). Adverse cardiovascular and central nervous system events associated with dietary supplements containing ephedra akaloids. *New England Journal of Medicine, Publication No. 343*, 1833–38.

Haycock, C. E. (1986). How I manage abdominal injuries. *The Physician and Sportsmedicine 14*(6), 86.

Hayes, A. (2000, November 26) *Orthopedics and sports medicine—A developing field for biomedical engineers.*

Hockberger, R., Kirshenbaum, K., & Doris, P. (1992). *Spinal trauma—Emergency medicine: Concepts and clinical practice* (3d ed.). St. Louis, MO: Mosby.

Iannotti, J. P., & Williams, G R. (1999). *Disorders of the shoulder: Diagnosis and management*. Baltimore, MD: Lippincott Williams & Wilkins.

International Olympic Committee, Château de Vidy, Switzerland.

Irwin, Roy. (1983). *Sports medicine*. Upper Saddle River, NJ: Prentice Hall.

Jarjour, N. N (1994). Management of exercise-induced asthma. In J. DeLee, D. Drez, & C. L. Stanitski (Eds.), *Orthopaedic sports medicine* (pp. 320–331). Philadelphia, PA: W. B. Saunders.

Johnston, L. D., O'Malley, P. M., & Bachman, J. G (2001). *Monitoring the future: National survey results on drug use, 1975–2000. Volume I: Secondary school students* (NIH Publication No. 01–4924). Bethesda, MD: National Institute on Drug Abuse.

Johnson, B. (2001, September). *Altru Health System, 4*(1).

Johnson, D. R. (2002). *Introductory anatomy: Respiratory system*. UK: Center for Human Biology.

Kendall, F., & McCreary, E. (1993). *Muscles: Testing and function* (4th ed.). Baltimore, MD: Lippincott Williams and Wilkins.

Kessler, R., & Hertling, D. (1983). *Management of common musculoskeletal disorders*. New York: Harper & Row.

Kibler, W. B. & Herring. (1996). *Functional rehabilitation of sports and musculoskeletal injuries*. New York: Aspen Publishers.

Kiernan, J. A. (1998). *Barr's the human nervous system: An anatomical viewpoint* (7th ed.). Baltimore, MD: Lippincott Williams and Wilkins.

Kinesiology: The field of study. (1997, November). *Report to the American Academy of Kinesiology and Physical Education*.

Lacroix, V. J. (1999, November 12). Exercise-induced asthma. *The Physician and Sportsmedicine 27*(12).

Liang, M. T. C., McKeigue, M. E., & Walker, C. (1988). Nutrition for athletes and physically active adults. *Journal of Osteopathic Sports Medicine, 2*(2), 15.

Louck, S., & Horvath, S. M. (1985). Athletic amenorrhea: A review. *Medical Science Sports Exercise, 17*, 56–72.

Mangine, Robert E. (1995). *Physical therapy of the knee (Clinics in physical therapy)* (2d ed.). London: Churchill Livingstone.

Mind Tools Ltd., London, UK. [1995–2002 editions]

Mosby's Medical, Nursing, & Allied Health Dictionary (5th ed.). St. Louis, MO: Mosby.

National Association of Intercollegiate Athletics, Olathe, KS.

National Collegiate Athletic Association, Indianapolis, IN.

National Diabetes Information Clearinghouse (NDIC), Bethesda, MD.

National Federation of High School Associations, Indianapolis, IN.

National Institute of Health, Bethesda, MD.

National Safety Council, Itasca, IL.

NCAA Injury Surveillance System, NCAA, Indianapolis, IN.

Neumann, D., & Rowan, E. (2002). *Kinesiology of the musculoskeletal system: Foundations for physical rehabilitation.* St. Louis, MO: Mosby.

Occupational Safety & Health Administration, 200 Constitution Avenue, NW, Washington, DC 20210.

O'Connor, P. L., & Schaller, T. M. (2001). *Footworks II.*

Padilla, R. (1995, May 12). *Sport dentistry and prevention of oral injuries.* CDA Sessions, Anaheim, CA.

Painter, J., Rah, J., & Lee, Y. (2002, April). Comparison of international food guide pictorial representations. *Journal of the American Dietetic Association, 102*(4), 483–489.

Physician Assistant Program, Duke University Medical Center, Durham, NC.

Pope, H. G., & Katz, D. L. (1988). Affective and psychotic symptoms associated with anabolic steroid use. *American Journal of Psychiatry, 145*(4), 487–490.

Rizzo, D. C. (2001). *Fundamentals of anatomy and physiology.* Clifton Park, NY: Delmar Learning.

Roberts, W. O. (1998, July). *The Physician and Sportsmedicine, 26*(7).

Rockwood, C. A., & Matsen, F. A. (1998). *The shoulder* (2d ed.). Philadelphia, PA: W. B. Saunders.

Roth, R., & Townsend, C. (2003). *Nutrition and diet therapy* (8th ed.). Clifton Park, NY: Delmar Learning.

Rothman Institute, Philadelphia, PA.

Scott, A., & Fong, E. (2001). *Body structures and functions* (10th ed.). Clifton Park, NY: Delmar Learning.

Smith, L. K., Weiss, E. L., & Lehmkuhl, L. D. (1996). *Brunnstrom's clinical kinesiology* (5th ed.). Philadelphia, PA: F. A. Davis.

Stapleton, T. R. (2002). Hughston health alert. Hughston Sports Medicine Foundation.

"Suggested safety items parents should look for in a high school athletic program," Scott Byrd, ATC/L—Fort Sanders Sports Medicine. http://www.covenanthealth .com.

Sweeney, T. A., & Marx, J. A. (1993). Blunt neck injury. *Emergency Clinics of North America, 11*(1), 71–79.

Tall, R. L., & DeVault, W. (1993). Spinal injury in sport: Epidemiologic considerations. *Clinical Sports Medicine, 12*(3), 441–448.

The Franklin Institute Science Museum, Philadelphia, PA.

The Cleveland Clinic, Department of Patient Education and Health Information, 9500 Euclid Avenue, NA31, Cleveland, OH 44221. http://www.clevelandclinic .org.

Torg, J. S., Vegso, J. J., & O'Neill, M. J. (1990). The epidemiologic, pathologic, biomechanical, and cinematographic analysis of football-induced cervical spine trauma. *American Journal of Sports Medicine, 18*(1), 50–57.

United States Census Bureau. (2000). Census. 4700 Silver Hill Road, Suitland, MD 20746.

United States Department of Health and Human Services, National Institute of Health. (2000, December 14). *Monitoring the future study: Moderating trend among teen drug use continues.*

United States Food and Drug Administration, Rockville, MD.

University of Washington School of Medicine. (2003). *Learning C. P. R.* Seattle, WA. Author.

Wake Forest University Emergency Action Plan, http://www.wfu.edu.

Waldman, S. D. (2002). *Atlas of common pain syndromes*. Philadelphia, PA: W. B. Saunders.

Walker, P., & Wood, E. (2003). *The skeletal and muscular system*. San Diego, CA: Lucent Books.

Wardlaw, G. M., & Insel, P. M. *Perspectives in nutrition*. St. Louis, MO: Mosby.

Watkins, J. (1998, December). *Structure and function of the musculoskeletal system*. Champaign, IL: Human Kinetics Publishers.

Zatsiorsky, V. M. (1998). *Kinematics of human motion*. Champaign, IL: Human Kinetics Publishers.

INDEX